Fifth Edition

Language and Communication Disorders in Children

Deena K. Bernstein
Lehman College
City University of New York

Ellenmorris Tiegerman-Farber
Adelphi University

Allyn and Bacon
Boston • London • Toronto • Sydney • Tokyo • Singapore

BS

Executive Editor and Publisher: Stephen D. Dragin
Editorial Assistant: Barbara Strickland
Marketing Manager: Kathleen Morgan
Editorial-Production Service: Omegatype Typography, Inc.
Composition and Prepress Buyer: Linda Cox
Manufacturing Buyer: Chris Marson
Cover Administrator: Linda Knowles
Photo Research: Elizabeth Wood and Katharine S. Cook
Electronic Composition: Omegatype Typography, Inc.

Between the time Website information is gathered and then published, it is not unusual for some sites to have closed. Also, the transcription of URLs can result in unintended typographical errors. The publisher would appreciate notification where these occur so that they may be corrected in subsequent editions. Thank you.

Library of Congress Cataloging-in-Publication Data

Bernstein, Deena K. (Deena Kahan)
    Language and communication disorders in children / Deena K. Bernstein, Ellenmorris Tiegerman-Farber.—5th ed.
      p. cm.
    Includes bibliographical references and index.
    ISBN 0-205-33635-3
    1. Language disorders in children. 2. Communicative disorders in children. I. Tiegerman-Farber, Ellenmorris. II. Title.
RJ496.L35 B47 2000
618.92'855—dc21

                             2001035528

Printed in the United States of America
10 9 8 7 6 5 4 3 2 1   06 05 04 03 02 01

Photo Credits: pp. 2, 126: Robert Harbison; p. 27: Will Faller; pp. 96, 181: Brian Smith; pp. 256, 315, 354, 388, 436, 510, 565: Will Hart.

3/2/03

Contents

PART II   LANGUAGE ASSESSMENT AND INTERVENTION   95

3   Interactive Teaming: The Changing Role of the Speech-Language Pathologist   96

Ellenmorris Tiegerman-Farber

4   Early Communication Assessment and Intervention: A Dynamic Process   126

Nancy B. Robinson
Michael P. Robb

5

Assessing Children with Language Learning Disabilities   181

Elaine R. Silliman
Sylvia F. Diehl

6

Planning Language Intervention for Young Children   256

Amy L. Weiss

7 Language Intervention in School Settings   315

Nickola Wolf Nelson

8 Language Development and Disorders in Culturally and Linguistically Diverse Children   354

Dolores E. Battle

12   Considerations and Implications for Habilitation of Hearing-Impaired Children   **565**

Christine Radziewicz
Susan Antonellis

Preface

Language and Communication Disorders in Children has proceeded through five editions in the past fifteen years. The changes in this edition reflect the legislative, educational, and clinical changes that have occurred within the professions of speech-language pathology and special education. In this edition, greater emphasis is given to early intervention, the role of the family in assessment and management, multicultural issues, dynamic and curriculum-based assessment and intervention, and educational and clinical accountability.

This volume is divided into three parts. Part I presents the fundamentals of language and communication development; Part II describes the general principles of assessment and best practices for intervention; and Part III focuses on four language disorders populations—children with learning disabilities, mental retardation, autism, and hearing impairment. Included in both Parts II and III are examples and case studies that illustrate how to apply clinical constructs to the actual evaluation and remediation of language difficulties for children with communication disorders.

A number of improvements highlight this edition. In Part I a new chapter (Chapter 2), written by Deena Bernstein and Sandra Levey, presents an overview of language development in children, with increased emphasis on the development of literacy skills.

Part II (Chapters 3–8) addresses assessment and intervention. Three new chapters are included in this section. Chapter 3, written by Ellenmorris Tiegerman-Farber, discusses the role of the family in assessment and educational management; Chapter 5, by Elaine Silliman and Sandra Diehl, provides updated information on language assessment of school-age children; and Chapter 7, by Nickola Wolf Nelson, focuses on service delivery in the schools.

The study of language and communication disorders touches the heart of human experience—the ways children learn language and ways to help children who do not. This book will challenge you to apply theories of child and language development to the rewarding experience of providing language intervention to children with language and communication disorders. We sincerely hope it will motivate you to keep abreast of new research in clinical and educational practice.

Deena K. Bernstein

Ellenmorris Tiegerman-Farber

FROM DEENA K. BERNSTEIN

Acknowledging those who make a text a reality is a risky venture, because a person deserving thanks may be inadvertently omitted.

Thanks to Steve Dragin and Barbara Strickland at Allyn & Bacon, who helped this edition see the light of day; thanks also to the team at Omegatype Typography, Inc. for their assistance with the production of the book.

Our reviewers, Stephen N. Calculator, University of New Hampshire; Charlotte Hubbard, Eastern Kentucky University; and Margery M. Whites, St. Cloud State University, offered suggestions and comments that substantially improved this edition.

Additionally, all the contributors to this text deserve special thanks for their flexibility during the reworking of the manuscript. New contributors Sandra Levey and Sylvia Diehl deserve special thanks for working under the constraints of tight deadlines.

Last, I am grateful to my husband and best friend Josh, for his invaluable support over the years, and to my children Ariella, Chaim Zanvil, and Yakov, who have taught me the lessons of patience and perseverence.

This book is dedicated . . .

To the memory of my parents,
Pearl (Chaya Peryl) and Julius (Yuda) Kahan,
for whom the love and understanding of children
were overriding values.
And
In honor of their great-grandchildren
Chaya Peryl, Yuda, and Moshe D. Bernstein
and
Bracha and Benjamin Z. Isaac Losice.

FROM ELLENMORRIS TIEGERMAN-FARBER

As always, I dedicate this textbook to my family . . .

To my husband Joseph Farber—
You are my soulmate and I thank God for you every morning. I could not have reached for the "stars" without you.

To my parents, Morris and Rita Jacobs—
SLCD could not have started without your house. It has taken fifteen years for me to pay back a debt of gratitude—a house for a house.

To my children, Leslie, Dana, Douglas, Jeremy, Andrew, and Jonathan—
You have taught me to be your mother and I love it.

To my grandchildren, Lindsey, Brandon, and Gabriel—
How wonderful that you are here and that there will be, I am sure, another nine to make an even dozen!

And . . .

To the parents of SLCD—
Never forget the silence, and always cherish your children's words.

To Dr. Christine Radziewicz, Dr. Helene Mermelstein, Dr. Steve Cavallo, Maureen Shapiro, and Karen Katzman—
I could not have done this without your loyalty and support. I will always be committed to all of you wherever life takes me.

To Senator Dean Skelos, Deputy Majority Leader of the New York Senate—
You are the Champion of SLCD and the staunchest supporter of children with special needs in New York State. This School would have never survived without you.

PART I

The Nature of Language and Language Development

CHAPTER 1

Deena K. Bernstein
*Lehman College
City University
of New York*

The Nature of Language and Its Disorders

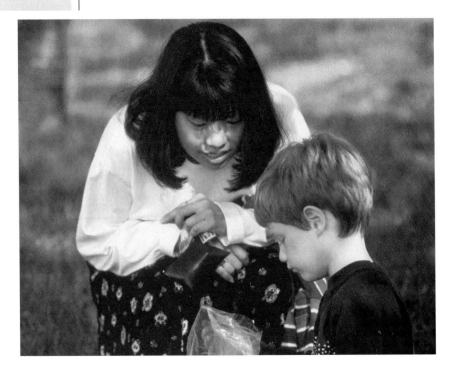

Most children acquire language naturally and, for the most part, without any formal instruction. Some children, however, experience serious difficulties in their acquisition of language. These children are language disordered. To overcome their disorders, such children require the assistance of various professionals, including speech-language pathologists, psychologists, and, in the school setting, special educators and resource room teachers.

The multidisciplinary nature of the study of language disorders is one reason for the complexity of the discipline. Speech-language pathology, special education, sociolinguistics, linguistics, psycholinguistics, and psychology, the disciplines that study language, have their own respective inventories of terms and methods. Diversity of terms, constructs, and even attitudes and biases pervades the study of language and its disorders. A cursory perusal of the writings in this field is enough to convince the student of this diversity.

A second reason for the complexity in studying language disorders relates to the complexity of language itself. Although in the first decade of this century we program computers to process information so that they can control a factory, cook a meal, and even fly a plane, we have not yet succeeded in programming a computer to simulate the generative nature of human language. This may happen someday, but, for the present, language remains too complex for reduction to a simpler format by programming. Comprehending language, theoretically, is a formidable task. Applying theories pragmatically to assess and to provide remediation to individuals who are language disordered is even more complex.

The centrality of language in the human experience is a third factor that complicates the study of language disorders. Language is crucial to all social and educational functioning. Parents are most concerned that their children acquire language because they recognize that a language deficiency may have a serious effect on future educational, social, and vocational opportunities. "Language," it has been said, "may be the most distinctive attribute of human beings; its acquisition is an integral part of human development. It is not surprising that how language is learned and taught are major issues in education and other human service fields" (McCormick & Schiefelbusch, 1984, p. 2).

This first chapter consists of fundamental information on three interrelated subjects relevant to language: the components or elements of language, perspectives on language acquisition, and approaches to language disorders in children. These areas were chosen because speech-language pathologists and special educators must possess a clear understanding of the nature of language and how it is acquired if they are to provide appropriate interventions for children with language and communication disorders.

We will begin, however, by exploring the differences between three seemingly similar but in reality different terms—*communication, speech,* and *language.* We will then further explain the notion of *language* by providing an explanation of its components.

COMMUNICATION, SPEECH, AND LANGUAGE

To the average person, the terms *communication, speech,* and *language* are synonymous. Professionals in the field of speech-language, who spend years studying and treating language-disordered children, often must go into lengthy descriptions of their chosen field of specialization to explain why their area of interest does not include correcting stuttering or improving diction. Confusion about the focus of speech-language specialists probably results from confusion of these terms. To the specialist these terms are very different and denote different aspects of development.

Communication

Communication is the process by which individuals exchange information and convey ideas (Owens, 1990). It is an active process requiring a sender who encodes, or formulates, a message. It also requires a receiver who decodes, or comprehends, the message. Each partner must be alert to the needs of the other to ensure that messages are effectively conveyed and understood.

Although we may primarily use speech and language to communicate, other aspects of communication may enhance or distort the linguistic code. Paralinguistic cues, which include intonation patterns, stress, and speech rate, can signal the attitude and emotions of the speaker and alter the linguistic information. Consider the difference that stress makes in the meaning a speaker wishes to convey when uttering the following:

She grabbed the money from him.

She grabbed the *money* from him.

She grabbed the money from *him*.

Or consider the effect a rising intonation would have on the following sentence:

John kissed her on the lips.

In addition to paralinguistic cues, nonlinguistic cues also contribute to the communication process. Nonlinguistic cues include gestures, body movements, eye contact, and facial expression, which can add to or detract from the linguistic message. All of us are familiar with the individual who looks at us as we talk and may intermittently nod his head, indicating to us that he is actively involved in the communication process. Conversely, the individual who does not make eye contact often communicates a lack of interest or involvement in the communicative interaction, and we in turn may diminish our communication with him.

Speech

Speech is one of the modes that may be used for communication. It is the oral verbal mode of transmitting messages and involves the precise coordination of oral neuromuscular movements in order to produce sounds and linguistic units.

Although we use speech primarily for the purpose of communication, it is not the only means available to us. Writing, drawing, and manual signing are other modes of communication. Individuals select a mode depending on the context, their needs, the needs of the decoder, and the message they wish to transmit.

For some children with disabilities, acquiring speech is not a realistic goal. The limited physical control these children have over the speech mechanism makes it unlikely that they can learn to produce recognizable speech. However, many of these children can acquire the ability to communicate if they are given alternative means. In recent years, a number of alternative and/or augmentative communication systems have been designed for them. These systems allow the child to transmit messages without using speech. Beukelman and Mirenda (1992) and Glennon and DeCoste (1997) describe a number of these systems (Blissymbolics, American Sign Language, computer-operated systems, etc.). In addition, Owens (Chapter 10), Tiegerman-Farber (Chapter 11), and Radziewicz and Antonellis (Chapter 12) also discuss the use of nonspeech modes in the intervention programs for mentally retarded, autistic, and hearing-impaired children.

Language

Language is a socially shared code, or conventional system, that represents ideas through the use of arbitrary symbols and rules that govern combinations of these symbols. There are hundreds of languages, each with its own particular symbols and rules. Language exists because language users have agreed on the symbols and rules to be used. Because these symbols are shared, language users can employ them to exchange information and ideas. The linguistic code allows language users to represent an object, an event, or a relationship with a symbol or a combination of symbols.

Language encompasses complex rules that govern sounds, words, sentences, meaning, and use. These rules underlie an individual's ability to understand language (language comprehension) and his or her ability to formulate language (language production). An individual's implicit knowledge about the rules of his or her language is called linguistic competence. A person who possesses linguistic competence has the knowledge needed to be a language user. He or she knows the rules about sounds and their combination; he or she knows what makes sense and what doesn't. He or she can understand and create an infinite number of sentences and can use language in a variety of social settings. Even though he or she cannot state the rules explicitly, the language user behaves in a way that demonstrates that he or she knows them. Although children give evidence of knowing the rules of language at quite an early age, how this rule learning occurs is still being investigated.

In sum, native speakers/listeners of a language learn a linguistic rule system. This rule system can be divided into three major components: form, content, and use. These components are described more thoroughly in the next section.

THE COMPONENTS OF LANGUAGE

Language is a complex combination of several component rule systems. Bloom and Lahey (1978) have divided language into three major components: form, content, and use.

Form

Form includes the linguistic elements that connect sounds and symbols with meaning. Included in linguistic form are rules that govern sounds and their combination (phonology), rules that govern the internal organization of words (morphology), and rules that specify how words should be ordered to produce a variety of sentence types (syntax).

Phonology

Phonology is the system of rules that govern sounds and their combination. Each language has specific sounds, or phonemes, that are characteristic of that language. Phonemes are combined in specific ways to form linguistic units known as words.

A **phoneme** is the smallest linguistic unit of speech that signals a difference in meaning. The words *bat* and *pat* differ from each other in only one way—their initial sound. Because this initial sound difference produces two different words, the difference is a meaningful one. Therefore, /b/ and /p/ are, by definition, two different phonemes.

Phonemes are classified by their acoustic properties (the pattern of their sound waves), their articulatory properties (where in the oral cavity they are produced, or place of articulation), and their production properties (manner of articulation).

The use of phonemes is governed by two sets of rules. One set describes how sounds can be used in various word positions. These are called distributional rules. In English, for example, the *ng* sound, as in the word *long*, is a single phoneme that never appears at the beginning of a word. The second set of rules determines which sounds may be combined. They are called sequencing rules. In English, for example, the sound sequence *rs* may not appear in the same syllable. In sum, phonological rules govern sounds and their distribution and sequencing within a language.

Morphology

The second component of language—**morphology**—governs word formation. Morphological rules are concerned with the internal structure of words and how they are constructed from morphemes. **Morphemes** are the smallest linguistic unit with meaning (and cannot be broken into any smaller parts that have meaning). Words consist of one or more morphemes. Each of the words *ball, toy,* and *play* consists of one morpheme that can stand alone. Morphemes that can stand alone are called free morphemes. Bound morphemes cannot stand alone and are always found attached to free morphemes. They are affixed to free morphemes as prefixes (*un*happy) or suffixes (tall*est*). Bound morphemes that modify tense, person, or number are called *inflectional morphemes*. Examples of inflectional morphemes include the plural *s* (cat*s*), the past tense *ed* (play*ed*), and the possessive *'s* (Joan*'s*).

Bound morphemes can also be used to change one word into another word that may be a different part of speech. For example, *ness* changes the adjective *sad* into the noun *sadness*. In this case, bound morphemes are called *derivational morphemes*, because they are used to derive new words.

One task for the student of language development and disorders is to determine whether children have knowledge of morphology and to what extent it resembles the rule system of adults.

Syntax

Syntax is the rule system that governs the structure of sentences. It specifies the order words must take and the organization of different sentence types. It allows the individual to combine words into phrases and sentences and to transform sentences into other sentences.

A competent language user can take a basic sentence such as "The boy hit the ball" and transform it into a number of different sentence types.

Did the boy hit the ball? *(interrogative)*

The ball was hit by the boy. *(passive)*

Knowledge of the syntactic system allows a speaker to generate an almost infinite number of sentences (from a finite group of words) and to recognize which sentences are grammatical ("The boy hit the ball") and which sentences are not ("Ball the boy the hit").

Syntactic rules have two additional functions: They describe parts of speech (noun—*house*; verb—*hit*; adjective—*red*) and sentence constituents (noun phrases, verb phrases).

Lightning *hit* (verb) the *red* (adjective) *house* (noun).

The boy (noun phrase) *hit the ball* (verb phrase).

As children produce longer sentences, they begin to build sentences according to syntactic rules. They learn how to construct negative sentences, questions, and imperatives. Later, they add complex structures such as compound sentences and embedded forms. The development of syntax begins at about 18 months and continues for many years. Chapter 2 discusses syntactic growth during the preschool and school years.

Content

The content component of language involves meaning. It maps knowledge about objects, events, and people, and the relationship among them. Included are the rules governing **semantics,** that subsystem of language that deals with words, their meanings, and the links that bind them. It encompasses meanings conveyed by individual words and the speaker's or listener's mental dictionary (called a *lexicon*).

Words are used differently by young children than they are by adults. A very young child may use a word that occurs in the adult linguistic system, but that word may not mean the same thing to him as to the adult. A 2-year-old may say the word *doggie*, but his word may refer to sheep, cows, and horses as well as to a dog. Alternatively, a 2-year-old may use the word *doggie* to refer to a particular dog without knowing it refers to a whole class of animals. Studying children's semantic system involves, in part, examining their understanding and use of words. Lexical acquisition is discussed more fully in Chapter 2.

The content component of language maps an individual's knowledge not only of objects ("big car") but also the relationship that exists between objects, events, and people. Note the use of the following semantic relations in the utterances of three 18-month-old toddlers, Benjy, Eli, and Yuda:

Context	*Utterance*	*Semantic Relation*
Mother and child sitting on the floor.		
Child pushes car and says:	"Push car"	Action–object
Mother and child are sitting in the kitchen. Mother is eating a cookie.		
Child says:	"Mommy eat"	Agent–action
Mother and child are in the kitchen. The child has just finished the milk in her cup. She points to the milk container on the table and says:	"More milk"	Recurrence

A more complete account of the meanings (semantic relations) children convey in their early utterances is given in Chapter 2.

Although most meaning is literal, it can sometimes be nonliteral. For example, if we talk about the "dance of life," we do not mean *dance* in the literal sense. Our meaning is figurative; that is, we are speaking of life in terms of patterns, grace, movement, and change.

Similarly, if I said, "I had a ball," you might infer that I had a good time. The word *ball* is used here in its nonliteral sense. However, note that a literal meaning is also possible (e.g., "I possessed a volleyball," or a baseball, basketball, etc.). Which meaning is appropriate will depend on the context and what has already been said.

In sum, meaning in language is conveyed through the use of words and their combinations. Content maps an individual's knowledge about objects, relationships, and concepts. This knowledge is derived from experiences and is a result of one's cognitive development. Lastly, it is important to remember that meaning can be both literal and nonliteral and is dependent on linguistic and nonlinguistic contexts.

Use

The **use** component of language encompasses rules that govern the use of language in social contexts. These rules are also called **pragmatics** and include rules that govern the reason(s) for communicating (called *communicative functions* or *intentions*) as well as rules that govern the choice of codes to be used when communicating (Bloom & Lahey, 1978).

The functions of language relate to the speaker's intention or goal. Greeting, asking questions, answering questions, requesting information, giving information, and requesting clarification are examples of language functions.

In addition to coding communicative intentions, speakers must use information regarding the listener and the nonlinguistic context to achieve their communicative intention. They must choose from alternative forms of a message the one that will best serve their communicative intention. Speakers must take into account what the listener already knows and does not know about a topic, as well as information about the context. The selection of the words and sentences to use to formulate a message depends on this information. For example, knowing the age and occupation of various listeners influences the choice of words with which to greet them. It is appropriate to say "Hi ya" to a 3-year-old and "How do you do?" to a school principal. The form of the message is also influenced by whether the topics of the message are present in the situation in which the utterance is used. For example, whether a speaker says "The doll is on the floor" or "It's over there" depends on whether the doll and the floor are in the immediate vicinity.

Lastly, pragmatics encompasses rules of conversation or discourse. Speakers must learn to organize their conversations to make them coherent. They must learn how to enter, initiate, and maintain conversations. They must learn how to take turns, how to respond appropriately, and how to tell a cohesive narrative. An individual who is armed with these skills is said to be an effective communicator.

CORRESPONDENCE AND INTEGRATION OF THE COMPONENTS OF LANGUAGE

We began this introductory chapter by defining language and by discussing the components that constitute it. The components of language and their subsystems are depicted in Table 1.1. Although the components of language appear as distinct entities, Bloom and Lahey (1978) have pointed out that they are indeed interrelated (see Figure 1.1).

How a child integrates linguistic components is best exemplified by the 2½-year-old child who looks through a window into the yard while her mother sits in the same

TABLE 1.1	**Language Is**	
	Components	Linguistic Subsystems
	Form	*Phonology*
		Rules that govern speech sounds and their combination
		Morphology
		Rules that govern the organization of words
		Syntax
		Rules that govern word order, sentence structure, and organization of different sentence types
	Content	*Semantics*
		Rules that govern meaning (words and their combinations)
	Use	*Pragmatics*
		Rules relating to the use of language in social contexts

FIGURE 1.1

Bloom and Lahey's Model of Language

Reprinted with the permission of Macmillan Publishing Company from *Language Development and Language Disorders* by Bloom, L. and Lahey, M. Copyright © 1978 by Macmillan Publishing Company.

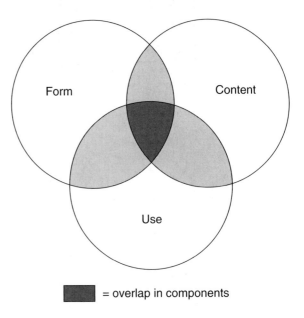

= overlap in components

room reading a book. As the child sees a kitten in the yard, she says to her mother, "Look, baby cat." The child has accomplished three things with this statement. First, she has linguistically coded two communicative intentions (getting attention and describing) by saying "look" and by describing what she sees. Next, she has linguistically coded knowledge about the animal she sees. Finally, she has expressed an utterance containing an acceptable word order. In sum, the child has communicated successfully by integrating pragmatic, syntactic, and semantic rules.

By taking the example a step further to a 3-year-old, we are able to demonstrate the child's integration of phonology and morphology with pragmatic, syntactic, and semantic rules. Both mother and her 3-year-old child are gazing through a window as two puppies are playing in the yard.

Mother: What do you see?

Child: Two puppies.

As in the previous case, the utterance codes knowledge about the animals and contains appropriate word order. In addition, the latter utterance contains the morphological ending that codes plurality. Using phonological rules, the child "knows" that the *s* in *puppies* is pronounced as a *z* because it follows a vowel, in contrast to the *s* in *cats*, which is pronounced as *s*.

Whereas the integration of form, content, and use is observed in the language of nondisabled children, a disruption of the components is often found in the language of children with disabilities. For example, many hearing-impaired youngsters produce language that possesses content but may be deficient in linguistic form. Their vocabulary and their communicative ability may be age appropriate, but their phonological, morphological, and syntactic skills often lag behind. Note the errors (indicated by bracketing) in the sample of David, a 5-year-old who is hearing impaired.

Ye[s]terday I give it to . . . to . . . What[’s] hi[s] name? Oh, Bob? Right. He[’s] not in my cla[ss]. He’s on my bu[s]. Why he can’t come with me?

Or consider the following utterances produced by Sean, an 11-year-old child with autism. Note the inappropriateness of his utterances and the lack of meaning in his sample. Also note the lack of errors in linguistic form.

Clinician: Sean, how are you today?

Sean: Fine, oh so fine, so very very fine and on my mind.

Clinician: Your class went on a trip yesterday. Tell me about it.

Sean: A trip, a trip. Yesterday, today, tomorrow. Hot dogs dogs—all kinds of dogs—bow-wow. It’s October and Halloween. Pepsi the choice of a new generation; Coca-Cola red, white, and blue . . . and soup is good food, too.

The terms and concepts outlined thus far are basic to the study of language and its disorders. Because an understanding of typical language development is crucial to the student who will undertake intervention with language-disordered children, the following section outlines four theoretical perspectives on language acquisition. As this review is merely introductory, the beginning student is strongly urged to supplement it with references noted in the text.

PERSPECTIVES ON LANGUAGE ACQUISITION

Four multidisciplinary approaches to the study of language acquisition have predominated the literature in the past two decades: the behavioral, the psycholinguistic/syntactic, the semantic/cognitive, and the pragmatic. Each approach is summarized in terms of essential elements, emphasizing background, limitations, and contributions. Owens (2001), Nelson (1998), Bohannon and Bonvillian (2001), Berko Gleason (2001), James (1990), and McCormick and Schiefelbusch (1990) provide a more detailed description of these approaches for interested readers.

Behavioral Approach

Background

The behavioral approach to language development was first presented by B. F. Skinner (1957) in *Verbal Behavior*. Language learning, according to this approach, depends on environmental variables, which are mastered by imitation, practice, and selective reinforcement. The result is the acquisition of language through the gradual accumulation of vocal symbols and sequences of symbols. Within the process, parents and significant others are crucial because they model the appropriate utterances that children imitate and practice. By rewarding children’s correct productions, parents shape children’s utterances until they are grammatical and acceptable. In short, children learn language because their verbal behavior is selectively rewarded by others in the environment (Skinner, 1957). Variations on this theme are provided by Osgood (1963), Mowrer (1954), and Staats (1963).

Limitations

Chomsky (1959) faulted Skinner on four counts, the first being that Skinner attempted to explain the process of language acquisition while ignoring the content being learned. Chomsky said, "There is little point in speculating about the process of acquisition without a much better understanding of *what* is acquired" (p. 55).

Second, Chomsky pointed out that children seem to acquire a verbal repertoire far too quickly to depend on environmental conditioning mechanisms alone. Third, Chomsky argued that children produce utterances they never heard adults use—utterances such as "I goed," and "mouses."

Contributions

Although in the early 1960s criticism was leveled at the behavioral school for overemphasizing parental input, recent researchers have revised their thinking to acknowledge its importance in language development. Studies by Snow (1972), Newport (1976), and others have clearly shown the positive effects of parental linguistic input to children's language development. Another contribution made by the behaviorists to the field of speech-language pathology has been to delineate "systematic training designs and their applications to nonspeaking individuals" (McCormick & Schiefelbusch, 1984; Schiefelbusch & Bricker, 1981). Structured behavioral techniques are commonly used in speech-language therapy and provide a basis for many intervention programs used with language-disordered children.

Psycholinguistic/Syntactic Approach

Background

In the late 1950s and early 1960s, linguists, particularly Noam Chomsky, hypothesized that the human brain contains a mental plan to understand and generate sentences (Chomsky, 1957, 1965). This mental plan incorporates the necessary "electronic circuitry" for children to internalize the knowledge necessary for deriving sentences.

Proponents of the psycholinguistic/syntactic approach hold that children have an innate predisposition to apply linguistic rules and that the human infant is "prewired" for language acquisition. According to Chomsky, a baby is born with an innate linguistic mechanism (called the *language acquisition device*, [LAD]) that is activated by exposure to linguistic input. The LAD contains two parts: a set of rules or general principles for forming sentences, and procedures for discovering how these principles are to be applied to the child's particular language.

The child's LAD processes information from the linguistic environment and generates hypotheses about the rules of his language. Using the concept of the preprogrammed LAD, Chomsky was able to explain the seemingly miraculous ability of very young children to acquire language easily and rapidly and to produce an infinite number of novel yet grammatical utterances.

More recently, Chomsky (1981, 1999) revised his ideas of grammar and syntax to account more for language rules and well-formedness as well as for language learnability. The result is called government-language binding theory (GB theory). Chomsky's goal was to present a theory that could account for the constraints on the kinds of hypotheses a child can form about the structure of his or her language no matter what language the child is learning. Government-binding theory attempts to account for the diversity of human languages and to explain the development of grammar by children on the basis of limited input. Chomsky (1999) called the resultant principles *universal grammar*. (For a more complete account of GB theory, see Bohannon & Bonvillian, 2001; Cairns, 1996; Leonard & Loebb, 1988; Nelson, 1998; Owens, 2001).

Limitations

Child development specialists (Schlesinger, 1977; Sinclair-deZwart, 1973) argue that Chomsky treats language learning as if it occurred independently of cognitive development. Citing Piaget's work, Sinclair-deZwart (1973) said that language development is dependent on cognitive development. Schlesinger (1977) pointed out that it is very difficult to ascertain from Chomsky's model precisely what children are born "knowing," as opposed to what they "come to know," and how this knowledge eventually gets linked to words and phrases.

Semanticists (Fillmore, 1968) fault Chomsky by arguing that language depends more on underlying semantic representation than on syntactic rules. Sociolinguists challenge Chomsky's assertion that linguistic input is too fragmented, confused, and unsystematic to facilitate children's acquisition of language. Their data (Nelson, 1973b; Newport, 1976; Phillips, 1973; Snow, 1972) show that parental input enhances language learning. Chapter 2 details the nature of parental input and its facilitating effect on language development.

Contributions

Although the psycholinguistic/syntactic approach is currently viewed as being inadequate to explain language development, Chomsky's work provided the impetus for much in-depth research on the language acquisition process. Investigators began to search for developmental patterns that crossed cultural boundaries. More important, they began to realize the value of naturalistic observations (McCormick & Schiefelbusch, 1984). A host of studies on both normal and disordered language were published in the 1960s (Braine, 1963; Brown & Bellugi, 1964; Brown & Fraser, 1964; Menyuk, 1964), and studies comparing normal and language disordered children's acquisition of morphology and syntax continue to be published (Hansson & Nettelbladt, 1995; Johnston & Shery, 1976; Leonard, 1992). Last, an alternative view of language learning evolved in contrast to the behaviorists' view, with the result that we currently view the child as being active and creative, rather than passive, in the language acquisition process (McLean & Snyder McLean, 1999).

Semantic/Cognitive Approach

Background

With the publication of Bloom's *Language Development: Form and Function of Emerging Grammars* (1970), there appeared a new focus in the study of language development: the meanings conveyed by children's utterances rather than their syntax.

In her seminal study of children's language at the early multiword stage, Bloom (1970) found that one of her subjects used "Mommy sock" on two different occasions. She used it once while she was picking up her mother's sock and once while her mother was putting a sock on her (the child's) foot. Although the form of the child's utterance was the same in both contexts, the *meanings* the child conveyed were clearly different. On the first occasion, she conveyed possession. The sock she was holding belonged to her mother. On the second occasion, the child's utterance conveyed a meaning found between an actor (Mommy) who was doing an action and an object (sock). Bloom concluded that children's language maps meanings. The meaning categories that children use to code relationships among entities found in the world were termed *semantic relations* by Bloom.

Bloom further postulated that children express meanings long before they know anything about syntax and that the meanings they convey are based on their cognitive knowledge.

Following Bloom, the cognitive prerequisites for language acquisition became the subject matter of much research. The works of Piaget (1952, 1954, 1964) were re-explored, and the search began for linkages between the concepts attained in early cognitive development and early linguistic constructions (Sinclair-deZwart, 1973).

The evidence (Nelson, 1973a) tends to show that children begin to use language expressively to talk about what they know and that this knowledge is related to their sensorimotor experiences. A fuller account of the cognitive prerequisite for language acquisition is found in Chapter 2. Rees (1980) best captured the essence of the semantic/cognitive approach when she said that "children say only what they know how to mean" (p. 21).

Limitations

The semantic/cognitive approach to language development highlights the importance of meaning and cognition. However, it does not explain why some children, in spite of age-appropriate cognitive abilities, lag in their linguistic development (Cromer, 1974). It seems that conceptual abilities are not the only abilities important for language learning, but that these other abilities are not accounted for in the semantic/cognitive approach.

Three other criticisms of the semantic/cognitive view have been offered. Bowerman (1978) pointed out that the semantic/cognitive approach does not answer the question of *how* children acquire language, nor does it explain the relationship between later developing cognitive abilities and corresponding linguistic attainments. Schlesinger (1977) observed that the semantic/cognitive approach ignores the role of linguistic input to the language acquisition process. How could language be learned if the child is not exposed to it? Last, McLean and Snyder-McLean (1999) argued that an adequate description of language acquisition must include formulations about the nature and purposes of children's social communicative interactions. They maintained that the social environment of the child is crucial to language development.

Contributions

The semantic/cognitive approach to language development is set against a background of overall development; hence, it gave impetus to multifaceted research on (1) the cognitive prerequisites of language (Bowerman, 1974; Sinclair-deZwart, 1973), (2) the universality of children's cognitive experiences resulting in a universality in their coding of meaning, and (3) the relationship between language and thought (Cromer,

1974; Miller, 1981; Rice, 1983). The role of imitation and play was reexamined (Bates, Benigni, Bretherton, Camaioni, & Volterra, 1979; Sinclair-deZwart, 1973; Westby, 1980) because scholars believed it was rooted in children's symbolic functioning. Last, the importance of contextual support (that is, the nonlinguistic context) was highlighted as being important to understanding the meanings children convey.

The Pragmatic Approach

Background

Because communicative intentions are expressed in social contexts, the pragmatic approach views language development within the framework of social development. According to Bruner (1974/1975), children learn language in order to socialize and to direct the behavior of others. Social interaction and relationships are deemed crucial because they provide the child with the framework for understanding and formulating linguistic content and form.

Within the pragmatic model, caretaker–child interactions are considered to be the originating force for language learning (Rees, 1978). As caretakers respond to infants' early reflexive behaviors and their gestures, the infant learns to communicate intentions. Infants refine these communication skills through repeated communicative interactions with caretakers.

McLean and Snyder-McLean (1978, 1999) summarized the pragmatic model in four major statements:

1. Language is acquired if and only if the child has a reason to talk. Herein it is assumed that the child has learned that he can influence his environment through communication.
2. Language is acquired as a means of acknowledging already existing communication functions.
3. Language is learned in dynamic social interactions involving the child and the mature language user in his environment. The mature language user facilitates this process.
4. The child is an active participant in this transactional process and must contribute to it by behaving in a way which allows him to benefit from the adult's facilitating behavior.

The pragmatic model spawned a range of new research efforts. Expanding on the work of Searle (1965), Dore (1975), Halliday (1975), and Bates (1976) formulated a classification system for categorizing children's communicative intentions, and Bruner (1974/1975), Bates (1976), and others examined the role of parents and caretakers in the language acquisition process.

Limitations

The explanation of language acquisition by the pragmatic approach leaves two major questions unanswered:

1. How do communicative intentions become linked to linguistic structures?
2. How do children acquire symbols for referents?

Two further limitations relate to the newness of the pragmatic view. One, present researchers cannot agree on a common system for classifying communicative intentions; and two, a system for assigning a specific intention to children's utterances has not yet emerged.

Contributions

The pragmatic view highlights the social aspect of language and places language use in center stage. It specifies the contribution of environmental linguistic input and the role of caregiver modeling and feedback. In addition, it has stimulated research on the conditions and contexts in which communication develops (Bates, 1976; Bruner, 1974/1975), and has identified the social prerequisites of language acquisition (see Chapter 2). All of these contributions are aspects of a general communication background, established well before children learn to use language expressively.

Approaches to Language Acquisition Revisited

The four approaches to language acquisition—behavioral, psycholinguistic/syntactic, semantic/cognitive, and pragmatic—contribute to our understanding of language development and enable us to appreciate the complexity of language in the absence of a full-blown model. The need for a complete model of language acquisition, however, remains. Future research may indeed provide it, pending the successful integration of constructs developed in the four approaches reviewed here. This need for integration is best summarized by McLean and Snyder-McLean (1978):

> By nature of its content, language carries within it the products of the cognitive developmental domain; by nature of its function, language carries within it the products of social development; by nature of its form, language carries within it the complex products of all the inputs identified . . . plus the effect of the nature and functions of human physiological and neurological systems. (p. 43)

For the present, without a full model of language, we may view each approach as best describing one or more of the phases in development. As the normal child passes through these phases, different aspects of language acquisition may be emphasized. In the earliest stage of development (infancy), emphasis may be on pragmatic development. In the early preschool years, emphasis may be on syntactic development. Understanding the process of normal language acquisition provides the reader with a firm basis for understanding language disorders.

APPROACHES TO LANGUAGE DISORDERS

There are two major approaches to the study of language disorders in children: the etiological-categorical and the descriptive-developmental. In this section, we define each approach and identify the respective strengths and limitations of each. In conclusion, we present a working definition of language disorders as proposed by the American Speech-Language-Hearing Association (ASHA, 1980).

Etiological-Categorical Approach

The traditional approach to child language disorders involves the classification of disorders by their causes, or etiology. Each etiological category summarizes a cluster of behaviors that differentiates language-disordered children from their normally developing peers.

The use of etiological typologies grew out of the early work of McGinnis (1963) and Myklebust (1954). The etiological categories used by Myklebust (1954) included: (1) mental retardation, (2) deafness and hearing impairment, (3) emotional disturbance and autism, and (4) childhood aphasia and neurologically based disorders. A fifth category, culturally and socially deprived, was later added, reflecting the political-social climate of the 1960s (Kamhi, 1990).

McCormick and Schiefelbusch (1984) classified language disorders into five etiological categories:

1. Language and communication disorders associated with motor disorders. Included in this category are children who possess motor deficits, as well as language disorders due to brain pathology (e.g., cerebral palsy) or damage to the nervous system (e.g., spina bifida). Children in this category possess motor difficulties and may be mentally retarded, visually and hearing impaired, and have seizure disorders. Because of the simultaneous multiple disabilities of these children and the space constraints of this text, we will not discuss this category. Instead, the reader is referred to Cruickshank (1976), McDonald and Chance (1964), and Mysack (1971) for a fuller account of this group.

2. Language and communication disorders associated with sensory deficits. Included in this category are children who have hearing and visual impairments. Because data on the language deficits of the blind are very scanty (Bernstein, 1978), we will discuss only hearing impairments as they relate to language disorders (see Chapter 12).

3. Language and communication disorders associated with central nervous system damage. Damage may be either mild or severe. Children are generally classified as learning disabled when the damage to the central nervous system is mild. When the damage to the central nervous system is severe, however, they are classified as developmental aphasics. Differentiating aphasics from other severely language-disordered children is both difficult and complex (McCormick & Schiefelbusch 1984). Hence, we limit our discussion to the language disorders associated with learning disabilities (see Chapter 9).

4. Language and communication disorders associated with severe emotional-social dysfunctions. Included in this category are children who are classified as psychotic, schizophrenic, and/or autistic. These children experience a profound disruption in the development of their verbal and nonverbal interaction skills. Considerable research on this disruption has been carried out in the area of autism and is reported in Chapter 11.

5. Language and communication problems associated with cognitive disorders. Included in this category are children who are classified as mentally retarded. The

cognitive disabilities of children in this group vary according to the level of retardation. Chapter 10 discusses mental retardation and the language deficits associated with it.

Strengths of the Etiological-Categorical Approach

Etiology is a convenient way of comparing and distinguishing autistic, learning disabled, mentally retarded, and hearing-impaired children. Each classification is like a label that summarizes how a child is similar to, or different from, other children both within and across the disability categories.

A second and practical advantage of the etiological-categorical classification is that often a diagnostic label is needed for a child to receive appropriate services in schools. In many states today, children are placed in special education programs for speech, language, and resource services based on their diagnostic label. Furthermore, special education programs often are tailored to the etiology of a language disorder. Thus, one finds programs for autistic, hearing impaired, or mentally retarded children. In this context, it is understandable that a child must be so labeled in order to be admitted to the appropriate program.

Some advocacy groups have argued vociferously for the continuance of a categorical classification because they believe that it is better to be labeled and to receive attention and services than to be ignored. This has been especially true of advocacy groups for the severely developmentally delayed: the autistic and the mentally retarded.

A third advantage of the etiological-categorical approach is that it provides speech-language pathologists with clues as to what type of remediation might be indicated and the modalities to be used during intervention. For example, knowing that a child possesses cognitive deficits, as in mental retardation, suggests remediation that focuses on teaching the concepts that language codes and on providing the child with redundant and repetitive cues to support the language being taught. Knowing that a child is hearing impaired may lead the speech-language pathologist to search for alternative or augmentative systems to teach language. This may involve teaching some form of manual communication (e.g., sign language) or combining manual and spoken language (e.g., total communication).

Because much of the research concerned with language and communication disorders has focused on groups of children within etiological categories, four chapters—9, 10, 11, and 12—are devoted to explaining these findings. This information should be helpful to speech-language pathologists working in educational or clinical settings in which diagnostic labels are used.

Caution, however, is called for on two accounts: (1) There exists considerable overlap among categories and (2) not all children within a diagnostic category possess similar abilities.

Limitations of the Etiological-Categorical Approach

Drawbacks of the etiological-categorical approach were highlighted by Bloom and Lahey (1978), who pointed out that a particular diagnostic label does not tell the speech-language pathologist what the child really knows about *language* and what he or she needs to learn. Moreover, it is rare to find a child who fits neatly into one diagnostic category. For example, it is not uncommon to find a child who is both mentally retarded and hearing impaired, or a child who is mentally retarded and also has autistic characteristics. In a similar vein, a categorical label implies that there is only *one* cause of the language disorder. This is rarely the case. Although a single factor may appear to be in large part responsible for a language disorder, there are almost always several contributing factors.

A second critique of the etiological-categorical approach has been made by Naremore (1980, 1995), who argued that assessment and intervention are not helped by categorizing. She stated that it would be difficult to find a procedure to assess a group of children defined as either mentally retarded or hearing impaired. Within the group, assessment must be "customized" to each child, with the aim of maximizing the resulting information and the understanding of that child's linguistic system and performance. The goal is to describe the child's linguistic behavior and to prescribe the specific methods and materials for improving his or her linguistic skills.

A third critique of the etiological-categorical model has been made by Kamhi (1990). He noted that an unfortunate outcome of this approach is that it serves "to divide treatment domains" (p. 73). Mentally retarded, autistic, and emotionally disturbed children are considered the province of the psychologist or special educator, whereas hearing-impaired children are the domain of educators of the deaf. This leaves developmentally aphasic and culturally deprived children to be served by speech-language pathologists. Kamhi (1990) pointed out that, in most instances, "speech-language pathologists are the most qualified professionals to treat language disorders regardless of etiological type" (p. 73).

The Descriptive-Developmental Approach

The descriptive-developmental approach *describes* rather than classifies language disorders in children. It involves comparing the language-disordered child's ability to comprehend and formulate language with that of nondisabled children. It assumes that a child with a language disorder needs to learn what the nondisabled child needs to learn at some point in development (Naremore, 1980). McCormick and Schiefelbusch (1984) summarized this point of view:

> There is every reason to think that children with deficient language: (a) need language learning experiences as rich as those provided normal language users, (b) will attend to, understand and talk about many of the same objects, events and relations as typical learners, and (c) want and need to experience the same control over their environment as their more competent peers at the same stage of development. (p. 36)

According to the descriptive-developmental approach, a language disorder is "any disruption in the learning or use of the conventional system of arbitrary signals used by persons in the environment as a code for representing ideas about the world for communication" (Bloom & Lahey, 1978, p. 290). Disruptions occur in either form, content, or use, or in the interactions among them. Based on this construct, Bloom and Lahey (1978) differentiated five types of language disorders in children:

1. Children who exhibit difficulties in learning linguistic form. Included are children whose primary difficulty is in understanding and using phonological, morphological, and syntactic rules.

2. Children who exhibit difficulty in conceptualization and formulation of ideas about objects, events, and relations. Their primary difficulty is related to the semantic component—language content.
3. Children who exhibit difficulties in language use. Included are children who cannot adjust their language to meet listeners' needs, who do not use language to convey a range of communicative functions, and who have difficulties in understanding and speaking in certain contexts. Their primary deficit is in the area of pragmatics.
4. Children who exhibit difficulties in integrating form, content, and use. Bloom and Lahey (1978) termed this group of children as having association problems.
5. Children who exhibit language and communication skills that are similar in all ways to those of younger, typically developing children. Delayed language development is their primary disability.

Strengths of the Descriptive-Developmental Approach

The descriptive-developmental approach focuses on identifying the strengths and weaknesses of children with language deficits. It allows the speech-language pathologist to describe children's language behaviors and to target those areas needing remediation.

Rather than labeling a child, this noncategorical approach is instructionally relevant. It zeroes in on those areas of language that pose difficulty for the child and gives the speech-language pathologist a teaching plan and sequence.

Limitations of the Descriptive-Developmental Approach

Although the descriptive-developmental approach overcomes some of the limitations of the etiological-categorical approach, three problems still prevail:

1. It does not present the clinician with clear-cut procedures as to how to teach those areas needing remediation. Although form, content, and use are useful constructs for understanding language and its disorders, the therapeutic contexts and procedures in which form, content, and use should be taught are not delineated.

2. It assumes that the administration of therapy to a language-disordered child is based on his linguistic disability and is irrelevant to his age or total environment. The descriptive-developmental approach has been criticized by Brown, Nietupski, and HamreNietupski (1976), who have questioned whether it is useful to teach a 16-year-old mentally disabled adolescent who has the developmental skills of a 2-year-old the same vocabulary as one might teach a nondisabled 2-year-old. A strict adherence to the developmental approach without regard to the domestic, educational, and vocational settings in which the child must ultimately function is to Brown and his colleagues not educationally sound.

Brown et al. (1976) advocated an ecological perspective to intervention. The clinician is asked to search the relevant environments in which the child must function for clues as to what to teach. This might be considered the epitome of "customized therapy."

3. The descriptive-developmental approach ignores the practical problems faced by educators in states where a disability label is mandatory for special class placement and/or the receipt of related services (Hobbs, 1978).

LANGUAGE DISORDERS: A DEFINITION

Because of the limitations described in both the traditional etiological-categorical approach and the descriptive-developmental approach, it is obvious that neither provides a complete definition. We present, then, ASHA's definition of language disorders as an alternative:

> A language disorder is the abnormal acquisition, comprehension or expression of spoken or written language. The disorder may involve all, one, or some of the phonologic, morphologic, semantic, syntactic, or pragmatic components of the linguistic system. Individuals with language disorders frequently have problems in sentence processing or in abstracting information meaningfully for storage and retrieval from short and long term memory. (ASHA, 1980, pp. 317–318)

According to the definition, impairment is in language comprehension (understanding), expression (formulation), or a combination of both. These deficits may be noted in listening and speaking or in reading and writing. Children who have language disorders may have difficulty in processing linguistic information, organizing and storing it, or retrieving it from memory. In short, ASHA's definition informs us about three important guidelines for considering language disorders: the components of language that might be impaired, the modalities that might be impaired, and the processes that might be impaired.

SUMMARY

In this chapter we have described the nature of language and its subsystems. After defining language, we went on to explain the various approaches to language acquisition. The discussion began with the behavioral approach and proceeded through the approaches of the psycholinguistic/syntactic, semantic/cognitive, and the pragmatic. Lacking a full-blown model, we integrated the several approaches to language acquisition by suggesting that normal language acquisition is a temporal process emphasizing different dimensions of language development at different stages of chronological development. Apropos is the comment of Owens (1984), who concluded his monograph on language development by saying, "A teacher or speech-language pathologist has to rely upon many sources of information" (p. 334). These sources of information equate with the various approaches to language development. On a practical level, this means that the speech-language pathologist "should be a behaviorist, a pragmatist, a cognitivist, a linguist, a developmentalist, and an optimist in order to put together an effective means of teaching language to children" (Schiefelbusch, 1978, p. 461).

A discussion of language disorders followed, with a review of two different approaches to language disorders: the etiological-categorical and the descriptive-developmental. Each approach was shown to have advantages as well as disadvantages. Unable to reconcile the differences, we presented an alternative, ASHA's approach to defining language disorders, attempting to summarize those impairments in the linguistic system that account for language disorders.

The following eleven chapters will elaborate and detail the preliminary discussions and definitions presented here. As you study them, do not hesitate to refer to the terms and definitions outlined in this introductory chapter. This will significantly contribute to a better understanding of communication acquisition and its disorders.

STUDY QUESTIONS

1. List at least five ways of communicating that you have used. Be specific.
2. What is the relationship of speech to language? Is language part of speech or speech part of language?
3. a. Define each of the following systems of language:
   (i) phonology
   (ii) morphology
   (iii) syntax
   (iv) semantics
   (v) pragmatics
3. b. How do each of the above subsystems fit into Bloom and Lahey's model of form/content/use?
4. Discuss the strengths and weaknesses of each of the following perspectives in language acquisition:
   a. the behavioral perspective
   b. the psycholinguistic/syntactic perspective
   c. the semantic/cognitive perspective
   d. the pragmatic perspective
5. Compare and contrast the etiological-categorical classification of language disorders with the descriptive-developmental approach. What are the contributions and limitations of each approach?

REFERENCES

The ASHA Committee on Language, Speech and Hearing Services in the Schools. (April, 1980). Definitions for communicative disorders and differences, *ASHA, 22,* 317–318.

The ASHA Committee on Language. (June, 1983). Definition of language, *ASHA, 25,* 44.

Bates, E. (1976). *Language and context: The acquisition of pragmatics.* New York: Academic Press.

Bates, E., Benigni, L., Bretherton, I., Camaioni, L., & Volterra, V. (1979). *The emergence of symbols: Cognition and communication in infancy.* New York: Academic Press.

Berko Gleason, J. (2001). *The development of language.* Boston: Allyn & Bacon.

Bernstein, D. K. (1978). *Semantic development of congenitally blind children.* Unpublished doctoral dissertation, City University of New York.

Beukelman, D. R., & Mirenda, P. (1992). *Augumentative and alternative communication: Management of severe communication disorders in children and adults.* Baltimore: Paul H. Brookes.

Bloom, L. (1970). *Language development: Form and function of emerging grammars.* Cambridge, MA: MIT Press.

Bloom, L., & Lahey, M. (1978). *Language development and language disorders.* New York: Macmillan.

Bohannon, J., & Bovillian J. (2001). Theoretical approaches to language acquisition. In J. Berko Gleason (Ed.), *The development of language* (5th ed.). Boston: Allyn & Bacon.

Bowerman, M. (1974). Discussion summary—Development of concepts underlying language. In R. Schiefelbusch & L. Lloyd (Eds.), *Language perspectives—Acquisition, retardation and intervention.* Baltimore: University Park Press.

Bowerman, M. (1978). The acquisition of word meaning: An investigation in some current conflicts. In N. Waterson & C. Snow (Eds.), *The development of communication.* New York: Wiley.

Braine, M. (1963). The ontogeny of English phrase structure: The first phrase. *Language, 39,* 1–13.

Brown, L., Nietupski, J., & Hamre-Nietupski, S. (1976). The criterion of ultimate functioning and public school services for severely handicapped students. In M. A. Thomas (Ed.), *Hey, don't forget about me!* Reston, VA: The Council for Exceptional Children.

Brown, R., & Bellugi, U. (1964). Three processes in the child's acquisition of syntax. *Harvard Educational Review, 34,* 133–151.

Brown, R., & Fraser, C. (1964). The acquisition of syntax. In U. Bellugi & R. Brown (Eds.), *The acquisition of language. Monographs of the Society for Research in Child Development, 92.*

Bruner, J. (1974/1975). From communication to language: A psychological perspective. *Cognition, 3,* 225–287.

Cairns, H. (1996). *The acquisition of language.* Austin, TX: Pro-Ed.

Chomsky, N. (1957). *Syntatic structures.* The Hague: Mouton.

Chomsky, N. (1959). A review of Skinner's "Verbal Behavior." *Language, 35,* 26–58.

Chomsky, N. (1965). *Aspects of the theory of syntax.* Cambridge, MA: MIT Press.

Chomsky, N. (1981). *Lectures on government and binding: The Pisa lectures.* Dordecht, the Netherlands: Foris.

Chomsky, N. (1999). On the nature, use and acquisition of language. In W. Ritchie & T. Bhatia (Eds.), *Handbook of child language acquisition.* New York: Academic Press.

Cromer, R. (1974). The development of language and cognition: The cognitive hypothesis. In D. Foss (Ed.), *New perspectives in child development.* New York: Penguin Education.

Cruickshank, W. (1976). *Cerebral palsy: A developmental disability.* Syracuse, NY: Syracuse University Press.

Dore, J. (1975). Holophrases, speech acts, and language universals. *Journal of Child Language, 2,* 21–40.

Fillmore, C. (1968). The case for case. In E. Bach & R. Harmes (Eds.), *Universals in linguistic theory.* New York: Holt, Rinehart & Winston.

Glennon, S., & DeCoste, D. (1997). *Handbook of augmentive and alternative communication.* San Diego, CA: Singular.

Halliday, M. (1975). *Learning how to mean: Explorations in the development of language.* New York: Edward Arnold.

Hansson, K., & Nettelbladt, U. (1995). Grammatical characteristics of Swedish children with SLI. *Journal of Speech-Hearing Research, 38,* 559–598.

Hobbs, N. (1978). Classification options: A conversation with Nicholas Hobbs on exceptional child education. *Exceptional Children, 44,* 494–497.

James, S. (1990). *Normal language acquisition.* Boston: Allyn & Bacon.

Johnston, J., & Schery, T. (1976). The use of grammatical morphemes by children with communication disorder. In D. Morehead & A. Morehead (Eds.), *Normal and deficient language* (pp. 239–258). Baltimore: University Park Press.

Kamhi, A. (1990). Language disorders in children. In M. Leahy (Ed.), *Disorders of communication.* London: Whurr.

Leonard, L. (1992). The use of morphology by children with specific language impairment: Evidence from three languages. In R. Chapman (Ed.), *Processes in language acquisition and disorders* (pp. 186–201). Chicago: Mosby-Yearbook.

Leonard, L. B., & Loebb, D. F. (1988). Government binding theory and some of its applications: A tutorial. *Journal of Speech and Hearing Research, 31,* 515–524.

McCormick, L., & Schiefelbusch, R. (1990). *Early language intervention* (2nd ed.). Columbus, OH: Merrill/Macmillan.

McCormick, L., & Schiefelbusch, R. L. (1984). *Early language intervention.* Columbus, OH: Merrill/Macmillan.

McDonald, E. T., & Chance, B., Jr. (1964). *Cerebral palsy.* Englewood Cliffs, NJ: Prentice Hall.

McGinnis, M. (1963). *Aphasic children: Identification and education by association method.* Washington, DC: Alexander Graham Bell Association for the Deaf.

McLean, J., & Snyder-McLean, L. (1978). *A transactional approach to early language training.* Columbus, OH: Merrill/Macmillan.

McLean, J. & Snyder-McLean, L. (1999). *How children learn language.* San Diego, CA: Singular Publishing.

Menyuk, P. (1964). Syntactic rules used by children from preschool through first grade. *Child Development, 35,* 533–546.

Miller, J. (1981). *Assessing language production in children.* Baltimore: University Park Press.

Mowrer, O. (1954). The psychologist looks at language. *American Psychologist, 9,* 660–694.

Myklebust, H. (1954). *Auditory disorders in children: A manual for differential diagnosis.* New York: Grune & Stratton.

Mysack, E. (1971). Cerebral palsy speech syndromes. In L. E. Travis (Ed.), *Handbook of speech pathology and audiology.* Englewood Cliffs, NJ: Prentice Hall.

Naremore, R. (1980). Language disorders in children. In T. Hixon, L. Schriberg, & J. Saxman (Eds.), *Introduction to communication disorders.* Englewood Cliffs, NJ: Prentice Hall.

Naremore, R. (1995). *Language intervention with school-aged children.* San Diego, CA: Singular.

Nelson, K. (1973a). Some evidence of the cognitive primacy of categorization and its functional basis. *Merill-Palmer Quarterly, 19,* 21–39.

Nelson, K. (1973b). Structure and strategy in learning to talk. *Monographs of the Society for Research in Child Development, 38.*

Nelson N. W. (1998). *Childhood language disorders in context: Infancy through adolescence.* Boston: Allyn & Bacon.

Newport, E. (1976). Motherese: The speech of mothers to young children. In J. Castellan, D. Pisoni, & G. Potts (Eds.), *Cognitive theory* (Vol. 2). Hillsdale, NJ: Lawrence Erlbaum Associates.

Osgood C. (1963). On understanding and creating sentences. *American Psychologist, 18,* 735–751.

Owens, R. E. (1984) *Language development: An introduction.* Columbus, OH: Merrill.

Owens, R. E. (1990). Communication, language, and speech. In G. Shames & E. Wiig (Eds.), *Human communication disorders* (3rd ed.). Columbus, OH: Merrill/Macmillan.

Owens, R. E. (2001). *Language development: An introduction* (5th ed.). Boston: Allyn & Bacon.

Phillips, J. (1973). Syntax and vocabulary of mothers' speech to young children: Age and sex comparisons. *Child Development, 44,* 182–185.

Piaget, J. (1952). *The origins of intelligence in children.* New York: International Universities Press.

Piaget, J. (1954). *The construction of reality in the child.* New York: Basic Books.

Piaget, J. (1964). Three lectures. In R. Ripple & U. Rockcastle (Eds.), *Piaget rediscovered.* Ithaca, NY: Cornell University Press.

Rees, N. (1978). Pragmatics of language. In R. Schiefelbusch (Ed.), *Bases of language intervention.* Baltimore: University Park Press.

Rees, N. (1980). Learning to talk and understand. In T. J. Hixon, L. D. Shriberg, & J. H. Saxon (Eds.), *Introduction to communication disorders.* Englewood Cliffs, NJ: Prentice Hall.

Rice, M. (1983). Contemporary accounts of the cognition-language relationship: Implications for language clinicians. *Journal of Speech and Hearing Disorders, 48,* 347–359.

Schiefelbusch, R. (1978). Summary and interpretation. In R. Schiefelbusch (Ed.), *Bases of language intervention.* Baltimore: University Park Press.

Schiefelbusch, R. L., & Bricker, D. D. (Eds.). (1981). *Early language: Acquisition and intervention.* Baltimore: University Park Press.

Schlesinger, I. (1977). The role of cognitive development and linguistic input in language acquisition. *Journal of Child Language, 4,* 153–169.

Searle, J. (1965). What is a speech act? In M. Black (Ed.), *Philosophy in America.* New York: Allen & Unwin; Cornell University Press.

Sinclair-deZwart, H. (1973). Language acquisition and cognitive development. In T. E. Moore (Ed.), *Cognitive development in the acquisition of language.* New York: Academic Press.

Skinner, B. R. (1957). *Verbal behavior.* New York: Appleton-Century-Crofts.

Snow, C. (1972). Mothers' speech to children learning language. *Child Development, 43,* 549–566.

Staats, A. W. (1963). *Complex human behavior.* New York: Holt, Rinehart & Winston.

Westby, C. (1980). Assessment of cognitive and language abilities through play. *Language, Speech and Hearing Services in Schools, 111,* 154–168.

CHAPTER 2

Deena K. Bernstein
Lehman College
City University of New York

Sandra Levey
Lehman College
City University of New York

Language Development

A Review

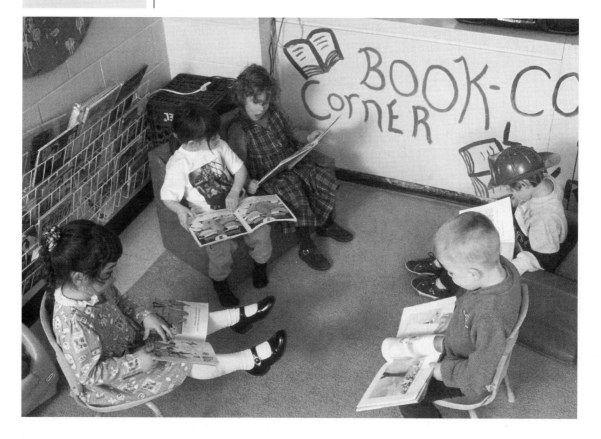

■ Describe the prelinguistic abilities of young children
■ Explain the role of the environment in language development
■ Describe the development of form, content, and use in preschool and school age children
■ Trace the development of literacy skills

O
B
J
E
C
T
I
V
E
S

The acquisition of speech, language, and communication is a complex process. It begins in infancy and continues to change throughout life. In Chapter 1 we discussed the nature of speech, language, and communication and showed how they are different but interdependent. This chapter presents a general overview of language development from birth through the school-age period. We include a review of the linguistic forms, meanings, and communicative functions acquired by children and adolescents. The following aspects of language development are its focal points:

1. The cognitive and social prerequisites for language acquisition
2. The prelinguistic development of infants and toddlers
3. The growth of phonological, morphological, syntactic, semantic, and pragmatic development from toddlerhood through the school-age years
4. The development of literacy skills

For a more detailed discussion of language development, the reader is referred to Berko Gleason (2001), James (1990), McLaughlin (1998), McLean and Snyder-McLean (1999), Nelson (1998), and Owens (2001).

LANGUAGE DEVELOPMENT: AN OVERVIEW

Children come to the language acquisition process biologically equipped to learn language. However, they are not passive (Sokolov & Snow, 1994; Karmiloff-Smith, 1995; Hirsh-Pasek & Golinkoff, 1997). The literature shows that active learning begins early in children's development. For example, by 1 to 4 months, infants are able to detect intonational changes in speech patterns (Jusczyk, 1992), and they can recognize the connection between mouth movements and the sounds connected with these movements by 18 to 20 months (Kuhl & Meltzoff, 1997). Caretaker input, social interaction, play, and cognitive development all play a role in language development.

The preschool period, from 2 to 5 years of age, is a period of rapid growth in all areas of language: phonology (sequencing speech sounds to produce words, phrases, and sentences), syntax (sentence structure), semantics (meaning), and pragmatics (language use). Children begin to produce two-word utterances at age 2, but by age 5, they are producing lengthy sentences that contain information about the past and the future. Children have a 200- to 300-word vocabulary at 24 months and a vocabulary of approximately 2,000 words by age 5. They have mastered most sounds by 4 years of age. By 3 to 4 years of age, children are able to adjust their messages to accommodate to a listener's knowledge, to a listener's status (child versus adult), and to use more polite forms to make requests.

Language development continues through the school-age years. These years are characterized by growth in all aspects of language: form (phonology, morphology, and syntax), content (semantics), and use (pragmatics). In addition, there is an increased awareness of language, which is necessary to develop more abstract language abilities.

During the school-age years, children also master new forms and learn to use these forms as well as existing structures to communicate more effectively. They learn to clarify messages and to monitor communications that indicate the success or failure of their communicative efforts. They expand the range of their communicative functions as they learn to use language in the classroom. In this environment, children must negotiate their turns by seeking recognition from the teacher and responding in a highly specific and precise manner to teachers' questions. During the school-age years, children also develop metalinguistic skills that enable them to think and talk about language. Metalinguistic skills help them master two important language skills: reading and writing.

Learning to read and write requires that children build on their previous language skills, such as their knowledge that speech sounds (phonemes) correlate with written letters (graphemes), and then they begin to communicate in this new mode. It is important for the reader to keep in mind that (1) children's rate of language development shows variation due to differences in intellect, learning style, ethnicity, and socioeconomic factors (Owens, 2001); (2) the later stages of language development depend on the earlier ones; (3) language growth is a gradual process; and (4) phonological, morphological, syntactic, semantic, and pragmatic acquisition in spoken language are related to the acquisition of written language. Knowledge of these later areas of development is vital to our understanding of older children who exhibit deficits in reading and writing (Beck & Juel, 1995; Butler, 1999; Catts, 1991, 1996; Greene, 1996; Henry, 1993; Rubin, Patterson, & Kantor, 1991; Wallach, 1984) (see also Chapters 5 and 9).

In the next section we will focus on some of the underpinnings of language acquisition, including children's cognitive development and their interaction with the environment.

COGNITIVE DEVELOPMENT

Early **cognitive development** involves a process by which children construct and reconstruct a representation of the entities and the events around them (Witt, 1998). Initially egocentric (centered around themselves), this egocentrism disappears as children become more aware that they are separate from the world, that they are not the cause of all activities, and that objects have properties separate from their own perception of their activity with these objects. Cognitive development is also tied to linguistic interaction with adults, siblings, and to activities in the environment.

According to Piaget (1954), children are viewed as having psychological structures (schema or schemata) that allow them to process information. These schemas change in response to the environment (adaptation). When confronted by a novel object or action, the child can either fit that novel event into a preexisting schema (assimilation), or will be required to change the existing schema if that novel event does not fit into the preexisting schema (accommodation). Thus, children assimilate novel events into preexisting schema or accommodate preexisting schema to meet the demands of new situations. Equilibrium (cognitive balance) is the goal and is achieved through assimilation or accommodation.

Piaget (1954) specified the following cognitive stages that begin at birth and continue until maturity (Table 2.1).

The sensorimotor period is divided into six stages. At stage 1 (birth to 1 month), children demonstrate accommodation or modification of a scheme (sucking) in response to environmental stimuli. In response to environmental experience, infants become more efficient at locating the nipple.

At stage 2 (1 to 4 months), there is an increase in eye–hand coordination, visual tracking of moving objects, and localization to sound. Primitive anticipation appears: the infant is now able to identify a wider set of signals that are associated with an event. For instance, a child will perform sucking-like movements when held by the mother, prior to presentation of the nipple. At an earlier stage of cognitive development, children begin sucking only when the nipple is placed in their mouths.

At stage 3 (4 to 8 months), children are (and will remain for a long time) egocentric, the cause of all actions. Imitation appears at this stage and represents the child's attempt to understand and to interact with the world. Children are now able to anticipate the path of a moving object and to reach for an object, even if it is partially hidden, and to manipulate this object.

At stage 4 (8 to 12 months), children are able to anticipate events; to establish a goal with a means to obtain that goal (means–end behavior); to imitate a wider set of actions; to understand that an object remains the same even when it is viewed from

TABLE 2.1	Piaget's Stages of Cognitive Development		
	Stage	Age (years)	Characteristics
	Sensorimotor period	(0–2)	Children become aware of the world and, at the end of this stage, use words to refer to entities, properties, and actions.
	Preoperational thought	(2–7)	Children become aware of space, time, and quantity concepts and relationships.
	Concrete operations	(7–11)	Children develop logical thought processes.
	Formal operations	(11–15)	Children develop logical abstract thought.

a different perspective, such as upside-down or empty (object constancy); to understand that actions have a cause (causality); and to remember that an object exists even when it is removed from sight (object permanence). Increased but limited short-term memory is evident (Owens, 2001), and egocentrism is decreased.

At stage 5 (12 to 18 months), children experiment, explore, and use earlier established schemes or patterns of behaviors to solve new problems. In this manner, older schemes are modified. Children are now interested in producing new behaviors. Symbolic behaviors appear with the appearance of first words.

At stage 6 (18 to 24 months), children solve problems through thought rather than through physical means. They produce labels for objects or actions, even when the referent is not immediately present. Deferred imitation may also appear; that is, children can observe an action, store it in memory, and reproduce this action later.

Summary

Children's early cognitive development begins with the gradual awareness of entities and events in the world and culminates in the ability to represent entities and events through a mental representation. It is at this time that children produce their first words. This milestone represents the symbolic representation of these entities and events.

The next section presents the role of the environment in language development, with a focus on child–adult interaction. Although children may possess the genetic underpinnings for language development (Berko Gleason, 2001), language acquisition depends in no small measure on the interaction of the child with people and events in the environment.

THE ROLE OF THE ENVIRONMENT IN LANGUAGE DEVELOPMENT

Recent literature describes the role of the environment in language acquisition, specifically the influence of adult–child interaction (Sokolov & Snow, 1994). Caretaker–child interaction differs from the language used between adults and adult–older child interaction in a number of ways: shorter sentences, simplified syntax, focus on objects or activities on which the child is focused or engaged, repetition of their own utterances, repetition of the child's utterances, a higher pitch, exaggerated intonation patterns, increased pause duration between separate utterances, and a greater number of questions and commands (James, 1990; Owens, 2001). Adult-to-child speech efforts are also characterized by focus on the here-and-now. In fact, it was found that 90 percent of maternal input to younger children is focused on events and objects in the immediate environment (Ninio & Snow, 1996).

As noted previously, cognitive development is dependent on interaction with others and on interaction with the environment. Children assimilate or interpret events such as parental responses to their cries or demands. Children receive specific input relative to language from adults, and they attend to this information (Sokolov and

Snow, 1994). The adult-to-child communication patterns presented in Table 2.2 are hypothesized to facilitate language development.

The style of adult-to-child interaction differs from culture to culture (Sokolov & Snow, 1994) and two basic interactive approaches are proposed by Snow, Perlmann, and Nathan (1987). In the first interactional style, parents provide *discourse frames* for children by being responsive to children's actions, gestures, and vocalizations, thus providing children with a rich source of information about the language system through contingent input. In the second approach, parents present children with predictable texts, based on the repeated presentation of familiar materials, allowing children to recognize and to internalize the structure of these texts, found in book reading or story telling. Whichever approach is used, children benefit by gaining information about language.

The influence of adult input to children is found in the difference between the first words produced by English-speaking children and Chinese-speaking children.

TABLE 2.2 **Adult-to-Child Interaction Patterns**

Adult Pattern	Description	Example
Expansion	Verbal responses that increase the length or complexity of the child's utterance	*Child:* That doggie. *Adult:* Yes, that's a doggie or Yes, that's a big doggie.
Expatiations	Verbal responses that add new but relevant information to the child's utterance	*Child:* It fell down. *Adult:* Yes, it fell down because it was too close to the end of the table.
Vertical structuring	Questions are posed to fill in the pieces of an utterance; the adult then produces the entire utterance	*Child:* That moose holding up a hammer. *Adult:* What would happen if he dropped it? *Child:* It would fall on his toe. *Adult:* If moose dropped the hammer, it would hit his toe.
Prompts	Comments and questions that extend what the child has said	*Child:* He was scared of that monster. *Adult:* What did he think the monster would do to him?
Repetition	Repeating the child's utterance	*Child:* Big bird eating. *Adult:* Big bird eating.
Recast	Providing a model of the adult form of the child's utterance	*Child:* That my ball. *Adult:* That's my ball.

Adapted from Gillam (1999) and Strapp (1999). Copyright Gillam, R.B. (2000). Used by permission.

For example, nouns are more prevalent in adult-to-child interaction by English-speaking adults (Owens, 2001), whereas adult-to-child interaction by Mandarin Chinese-speaking adults consists mainly of verbs (Tardif, 1995; Tardif, Shatz, & Naigles, 1997). Consequently, the first words produced by English-speaking children are mainly nouns (Gentner, 1982; Nelson, 1973), but the first words produced by Mandarin Chinese-speaking children are nouns and verbs. Similar results were found for Korean-speaking children, whose parents use more words for activities than words for objects (Choi, 2000; Choi & Gopnik, 1995). These differences suggest that adult-to-child speech plays a significant role in some aspects of language development.

Summary

During the first year of life, children learn about people, objects, and events in the world. They develop concepts about entities and about their ability to manipulate the world. These developments are a result of their cognitive abilities as well as a result of their interaction with the environment. In the following section we will focus on the acquisition of communicative abilities by infants and toddlers.

INFANT AND TODDLER EARLY COMMUNICATION

Infants possess innate abilities that prepare them for learning language. Some investigators argue that there is a connection between the sounds produced in infancy and early words. This view assumes that babbling is related to later speech production and constitutes a form of practice that contributed to language development (Stoehl-Gammon & Cooper, 1984). During babbling, the child stores the associations between oral–motor movements and sounds. Later in development, the child is able to draw on this behavior to produce meaningful speech.

Infants are capable of producing intentional communication. This means that they are able to use communication to indicate specific wants and needs. In infancy, intentionality is signaled by the use of gesture and/or vocalization, coupled with eye contact and by persistent attempts to communicate a request (James, 1990).

The sounds produced by infants from birth to 1 month of age consist of crying and vegetative sounds, such as clicks and burps (McLaughlin, 1998). Vowel-like sounds are also produced, termed *quasi-resonant nuclei* (Oller, 1978). At this stage of development, infants are able to discriminate between their mother's and another mother's voice and between utterances in a foreign language and their mother's language (Jusczyk, 1992).

Between 1 and 6 months of age, cooing, laughter, squealing, and growling appear. Cooing consists of vocalic sounds, sometimes produced in combination with the back consonants, /k/ and /g/, in consonant–vowel (CV) forms. In addition, infants are able to detect changes in intonation and to detect and to recognize the occurrence of the same syllable in different utterances.

By 4 months of age, infants are able to match some vocalizations with corresponding facial shapes, and show a preference for infant directed speech (e.g., exaggerated intonation patterns, slower speech production, and higher pitch). They are also able to follow their mother's eye gaze or direction of pointing (Owens, 2001).

At 4 to 6 months of age, marginal babbling appears, and consists of vowels, CV (/ba/) and VC forms (/ab/) followed by reduplicated babbling, which appears at 6 to 8 months of age. Reduplicated babbling consists of the alternation of consonants and vowels (*babababab*). Vocal play also emerges at this stage, and there is an increase in the variety of sounds that the child produces. Infants at this stage are now able to distinguish between words produced in their native language and words produced in a foreign language, based on the difference in prosodic features.

Variegated babbling appears at 8 to 10 months of age. This consists of strings of alternating consonants and vowels (*babigabadidu*). Babbling now corresponds to the intonation patterns of the adult language, but a decline occurs in the ability to detect phonetic contrasts and phonetic cues in foreign languages (Werker & Tees, 1984). This change correlates with the emergence of first words, and suggests that discrimination has become more focused on the language spoken in the infant's environment.

At 8 to 12 months of age, echolalia appears. This is characterized by a parrot-like imitation of another's speech (McLaughlin, 1998). For example, the child may attempt to imitate the adult's utterances as well as the adult's tonal quality and gestures. At 9 to 12 months of age, jargon emerges. Jargon consists of strings of syllables that mirror the stress patterns of adult speech, but these speech efforts are unintelligible.

Sounds that are consistent relative to a specific context emerge at 9 to 10 months of age. At this stage, children may produce one sound to indicate a request and a distinctly different sound to indicate refusal or rejection. These sounds are labeled *phonetically consistent forms* (PCFs), *vocables,* or *performatives* (James, 1990). PCFs or performatives are the consistent production of sounds to match a particular request within a context, such as *ah* to request being picked up by an adult and *uh* to request food items. While children produce sounds or sound sequences to communicate their intentions, sometime these are paired with gestures or with pointing.

Summary

During the first year of life, children are actively accumulating information about language. They are able to perceive differences between voices and sounds, learn to produce sounds, use eye gaze, vocalizations, and gestures to communicate their intentions, and will now begin to produce words to represent their knowledge of the world. Interaction with adults, siblings, and the environment provides them with information about language and how to use language intentionally to communicate.

The development of the ability to use language to represent meaning is described in the next section.

SEMANTIC DEVELOPMENT

Semantics is the component of language concerned with meaning. Meaning can be conveyed through language at the word, sentence, and discourse levels, with discourse defined as a continuous stretch of speech, such as conversation. The meaning of some words can also be derived from the nonlinguistic context.

Vocabulary Development

Children's first words are produced at around 12 months of age. Their early word meanings consist of labels for familiar entities, action, and properties in the child's environment. An investigation of English-speaking children's first words (Nelson, 1973) revealed that the majority of them are nouns, such as *mommy* and *ball* (65 percent), followed by action words such as *go* and *up* (13 percent), modifiers such as *hot* and *mine* (9 percent), personal-social words such as *bye-bye* and *no* (8 percent), and function words such as *what* (4 percent). Nelson, Hampson, and Shaw (1993) also found that many of these first words could also be considered either nouns or verbs (*drink*).

Children's early word meanings often do not correspond to adult meanings. For example, children may use the word *dog* to label other four-legged animals (sheep, cows, pigs, and horses). The use of a word to extend beyond the category for that word is called *overextension*. Notice that in the case above, the overextension that is produced by the child is related to the target word in terms of perceptual similarity (shape or movement). A child may also use the label *hat* to refer to a hat, a scarf, a ribbon, and a hairbrush. This overextension is related to the target word in terms of its function (Peccei, 1999). Some researchers hypothesize that children produce overextensions because the target word has not yet been acquired and the child chooses the word that best fits that target. Another explanation offered is that children use overextension as a device for requesting the correct label for the target. In either case, overextension is a frequent pattern in acquisition until around 3 years of age. As children develop their semantic abilities, their meanings will more closely resemble the adult target.

Young children have an expressive vocabulary of one or more words at 12 months, a 4- to 6-word vocabulary at 15 months, a 20-word vocabulary at 18 months, and a 200- to 300-word vocabulary at 24 months. Children's receptive vocabulary generally exceeds their expressive vocabulary. For example, when children have an expressive vocabulary of 10 words, they are usually able to comprehend at least 50 words.

Relational Meaning

In addition to acquiring lexical knowledge that specifies referents, children acquire meanings that code relationships among people, objects, and events. Later, these relationships are coded in children's simple sentences. The semantic relations that appear when children are at the one-word stage are shown in Table 2.3.

As children develop cognitively, the relationships they map and the forms they use to express these relationships become increasingly complex. The study of early semantic development by Brown (1975) revealed that children consistently produced certain semantic roles. These are presented in Table 2.4.

TABLE 2.3	**Relational Words: One-Word Utterances**

Category	Meaning	Example
Existence	The child notes an object	Points or says *that* or *what that?*
Nonexistence	The child notes that an entity is absent	Says *no* or *gone*
Disappearance	The child notes that an entity has disappeared	Says *gone* or *allgone*
Recurrence	The child requests reappearance or notes that an entity reappears	Says *more*

Adapted from R. E. Owens, *Language Development.* Copyright © 2001 by Allyn & Bacon. Reprinted/adapted by permission.

TABLE 2.4	**Semantics Roles Underlying Children's Early Language**

Semantic Role	Definition/Example
Nomination	Labeling an animate or an inanimate object: *doggie, ball*
Existence	Noting the existence of an animate or an inanimate entity: *mommy, that shoe*
Agent	Recognition that an animate initiated an activity: *daddy throw*
Object	Recognition that an inanimate is receiving the force of an action: *cut bread*
Possession	Recognition that an object belongs to or is in the frequent presence of someone: *mommy shoe*
Location	Recognition of a spatial relationship between two objects: *doggie bed*
Experiencer	Recognition that animate was affected by an event: *baby fall*
Attribution	Recognition of properties not inherently part of the class to which the object belongs: *baby cry*
Denial	Rejection of a proposition: *no bed*
Nonexistence	Recognition of the absence of an object that was once present: *cookie all gone*
Rejection	Prevention or cessation of the occurrence of an activity or the appearance of an object: *no more throw*
Instrument	awareness that an inanimate was causally involved in an activity: *car bump*
Recurrence	awareness of the potential for marking the reappearance of an object or reenactment of an event: *more cookie*
Notice	recognition that an object has appeared or some event has occurred: *hello daddy*

Adapted from R. E. Owens, *Language Development.* Copyright © 2001 by Allyn & Bacon. Reprinted/adapted by permission; and J. S. Peccei, *Child Language.* Copyright © 1999 by Routledge. Reprinted by permission.

Summary

Early language development is characterized by children's representation of the environment through gesture, vocalization, and later by their use of single words. These achievements are a result of children's growing knowledge of the world, of the people with whom they interact, and of their ability to manipulate entities and events in the world.

The following section discusses toddlers' pragmatic development. Children's increase in social awareness will be evidenced in the uses to which they put their developing language skills.

PRAGMATIC DEVELOPMENT

Children at the one-word stage use language to communicate three main functions: regulating others' behavior, establishing joint attention, and social interaction (James, 1990). Children between 1 and 2 years of age increase the variety of communicative intents to include regulation intents (gaining attention, requests, and calling), statement intents (naming, description, and giving information that is beyond the here and now), exchange intents (descriptions of activities, intent to carry out an action, refusal, and protest), conversational intents (imitation, answer, conversational responses, and questions) (McShane, 1980).

Children's early attempts to communicate their intentions have also been described by Halliday (1975). According to this researcher, the function of toddlers' early communicative intentions are (1) the *instrumental* function, used to obtain a goal and to have wants and needs met (the child holds out a cup and says *more*); (2) the *regulatory* function, used to control others' behaviors (the child gives a ball to an adult to request play and says *ball*); (3) the *interaction* function, used to obtain joint attention (the child calls *mama*); and (4) the *personal* function, used to express feelings or attitudes (the child says *yum* while eating a cookie) (Halliday, 1975). Dore (1978) discussed the early communicative intentions produced by infants and toddlers at the prelinguistic and the one-word utterance stage. He labels these primitive speech acts as shown in Table 2.5. Whichever taxonomy one uses, it is now clear that babies understand that their words will produce responses from others; they have become active communicators.

We now turn our attention to toddlers' productions of sounds in words. These productions, which appear between 12 and 24 months, reflect children's acquisition of the sound system.

PHONOLOGICAL DEVELOPMENT

Children produce their first words with recognizable meaning between 1 and $1\frac{1}{2}$ years of age. Toddlers' abilities to make themselves understood is often limited by their difficulty in producing sounds and the sound sequences that constitute words.

TABLE 2.5	Primitive Speech Acts		
	Speech Act	**Nonlinguistic Aspect**	**Example**
	Requesting action	Gesture, attends to adult	Cannot reach a toy, utters *uh, uh* while reaching for the toy.
	Protesting	Resists, attends to adult	Cries and resists being dressed
	Requesting answer	Addresses adult, gesture	Holds out a toy and produces label with a rising intonation, awaits adult response
	Labeling	Attends to entity	Touches doll's nose and says *nose*
	Answering	Addresses adult	Adult points to a picture of a cow and asks, "What's that?"; the child answers *moo*
	Greeting	Attends to adult or entity	Child says *hi* when sees adult
	Repeating	Attends to preceding utterance	Adult says *book*; child says *book*
	Practicing	Not addressed to adult	Child practices words or phrases
	Calling	Addresses adult and expects a response	Child calls *Mama* from another room

Adapted from R. E. Owens, *Language Development*. Copyright © 2001 by Allyn & Bacon. Reprinted/adapted by permission.

Unfamiliarity with the child's manner of speaking or with the nonlinguistic context often makes it difficult to recognize /gɔgi/ for *doggie* or /dus/ for *juice*.

Children's acquisition of speech sounds is orderly, but a great deal of variability is shown by them in their acquisition of particular sounds. Figure 2.1 shows the age at which most children acquire specific consonants.

In the process of learning the sound system of a language, children often simplify the adult word targets. The simplifications children use as they attempt to produce adultlike speech are called **phonological processes**. Phonological processes may consist of substitution of one sound for another (*tat* for *cat*), the omission of a sound or a syllable (*nana* for *banana*), the distortion of a sound (a sound produced incorrectly), or the addition of a sound (*buhlack* for *black*).

Toddlers' productions of words are often characterized by the following phonological processes: reduplication, unstressed syllable deletion, final consonant deletion, and cluster reduction (Owens, 2000). These are defined in Table 2.6, where examples of the processes are given.

The phonological processes listed in Table 2.6 are part of the typically developing child's speech, and may persist for many years. Researchers believe that the presence of phonological processes in children's speech may be due to either their difficulty in perceiving the adult target or to their limited ability to produce the adult target, and its presence often interferes with their speech intelligibility.

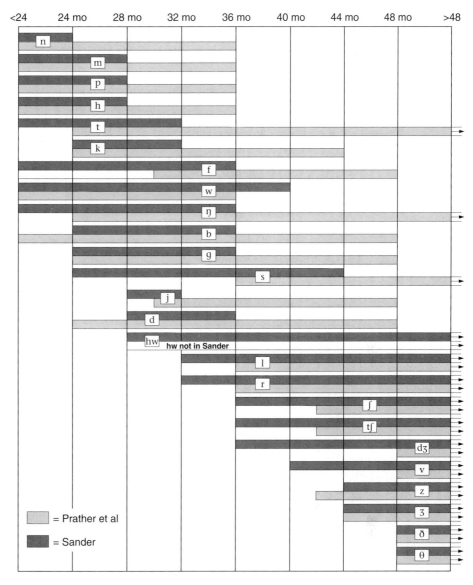

FIGURE 2.1

Normative Articulation Data

The left-hand margin of each bar represents the age at which 50 percent of the children in a normative study used the specified sound correctly. The right-hand margin shows the age at which 90 percent of the children used the sound correctly.

Adapted from Bernthal, J. E. & Bankson, N. W., *Articulation and Phonological Disorders.* Copyright © 1998 by Allyn & Bacon. Reprinted/adapted by permission; and Prather, Hedrick, and Kern (1975). Articulation development in children aged two to four years. *Journal of Speech and Hearing Disorders,* *40,* 186. © American Speech-Language-Hearing Association. Reprinted with permission.

TABLE 2.6 | **Common Phonological Processes of Toddlers**

Process	Example
Reduplication: the first syllable of a word is repeated and is substituted for subsequent syllables in the word.	*Cracker* becomes *caca* /kækæ/.
Final consonant deletion: the final consonant of a word is deleted (CV/ CVC).	*Bed* becomes *be* /bɛ/.
Cluster reduction: one or more consonants from a target consonant cluster is deleted.	*Please* becomes *pease* /piz/.
Deletion of unstressed syllables: a simplification.	*Giraffe* becomes *raffe* /ræf/.

Adapted from R. E. Owens, *Language Development.* Copyright © 2001 by Allyn & Bacon. Reprinted/adapted by permission.

Summary

In this section we presented a brief overview of cognitive development during the first 18 months of life and the environmental contributions to the early language learning processes. We focused on the use to which infants and toddlers put their prelinguistic and their developing language skills in order to communicate their intentions. In addition, we presented some data on children's production of sounds and on their early word productions. Lastly, we focused on children's early semantic and pragmatic development, which allows them to communicate their meanings and their intentions in social contexts.

In the next section we will present data on the development of children's language during the preschool period. We will see that children's vocabulary grows, they learn new word meanings, their utterances increase in length and complexity, and they begin to use more sophisticated ways to express their intentions.

PRESCHOOL LANGUAGE DEVELOPMENT: AN OVERVIEW

As children advance from simple one- and two-word utterances, their utterances become longer and more complex. They gradually elaborate the way they say things by adding more detail and by adding and filling in words and word endings that were missing in their early utterances. Whereas children at 18 months are producing such utterances as *mama, milk, close it, sock off,* and *more juice,* as their language abilities grow, their language samples consist of two- and three-word utterances that include articles *(a, the)*, prepositions *(in, on)*, pronouns *(I, he)*, auxiliary verbs *(is, are)*, noun endings (such as *-s* to indicate plurality), and verb endings (such as *-ed* to indicate past tense). Examples of such utterances include *want a cookie, block in box, he is bad, more cookies,* and *door opened.*

In the preschool period, children's vocabulary continues to grow and they learn many new word meanings. They learn new concepts and how to code these concepts linguistically. As they develop cognitively, they begin to refer to objects, actions, people, and events that are displaced in terms of time and place, and they transform their ideas into sentences by using a variety of sentence types.

During this period children also learn more complex ways to use language socially and begin to develop discourse skills, such as participating in conversations; giving instructions; providing descriptions about objects, events, and people; and relating personal experiences and simple stories. Lastly, during this period they learn about the nature of print. The emergence of preliteracy skills during the preschool years lays the foundation for their development of reading and writing.

It is important to note that children's development of language during this period is related to their cognitive development. We now turn our attention to this area and its relationship to play skills and language development.

Cognition, Play, and Language

According to Piaget (1954), the preoperational stage of development occurs between 2 and 7 years of age. Symbolic functioning appears and is represented by symbolic play and further language development.

Patterson and Westby (1998) provide a description of symbolic or pretend-play development that occurs during this period. At around 18 months, play consists of activities that are familiar to children, such as pretending to sleep or to drink. This period is followed, at 19 to 22 months, by the extension of these activities to another entity or person, with children pretending to feed a doll or imitating adult activities. At 24 months of age, children begin to perform sequences of familiar activities, such as baking a cake, and between 24 and 30 months, they include dolls in their pretend activities, ascribing needs to the doll (hungry, tired, or sick) and placing the doll in the role of agent (walking the doll rather than carrying it).

The scope of play expands at about 30 months as children begin using a wider set of less frequently occurring activities in their play activities: going to the store, going to the doctor, or going to visit a relative are play sequences that are often observed. Play behaviors that are episodic and consist of multischeme sequences emerge at about 3 years of age. These multischeme sequences may include going to the store to buy groceries, cooking and serving dinner, or having a birthday party. Ascribing emotional states to dolls (or stuffed toys) and talking for a toy appears at 3 to $3\frac{1}{2}$ years of age. By $3\frac{1}{2}$ to 4 years of age, children begin to take on different roles in play activities. These roles expand to include fantasy characters, police and fire fighters, and more familiar family roles. Their play may involve imaginary friends, or they may take a multifaceted role, such as a mother who goes to work. By 5 years of age, children do not need props to engage in play, and they can use language alone to maintain play activities. Their play consists of complex sequences that include dialogue.

Patterson and Westby (1998) argue for a relationship among cognition, pretend play, and language development. They assert that the emergence of first words co-occurs with the emergence of pretend (symbolic) play because pretend play demonstrates a child's ability to separate an object from an immediate context. Thus, a child may use a block to represent a train or a telephone and a word to represent an object or action that is removed from the immediate context. Over time, as children develop cognitively, their play becomes increasingly sophisticated.

In the next section we present the development of preschool children's language form, focusing on their development of syntactic, morphological, and phonological skills.

The Development of Syntax and Morphology

Children begin to produce two-word utterances at about 18 months of age. This stage is characterized by utterances such as *see boy, see, sock, push it, close it, allgone milk, I sit, I see, boot off, mama come, milk cup, dry pants, change diaper, more juice, other bib,* and *do it* (O'Grady, 1997). Children at this stage are remarkably accurate in producing the correct syntactic form. For example, children place modifiers in the correct position preceding common nouns (*big doggy*) and preceding indefinite pronouns (*big one*). They do not make errors by placing the modifier preceding a definite pronoun (**big he*) (P. Bloom, 1990).

As children advance from simple two-word utterances, their utterances become longer and more complex. They elaborate their utterances by adding more details, such as words and suffixes (inflectional and derivational morphemes) that were missing in their early utterances. Words take the form of articles (*a, the*), prepositions (*in, on*), pronouns (*I, he*), and auxiliary verbs (*is, are*). Inflectional morphemes take the form of the plural -*s* attached to nouns to indicate plurality, the possessive *'s* to indicate possession, the present progressive -*ing* attached to verb stems to indicate present and ongoing action, and the past-tense marker -*ed* to indicate prior activity. The inclusion of these forms acts to expand young children's utterances, making their utterances more adultlike and less telegramatic. They progress from producing utterances such as "More milk" at 12 to 18 months to utterances such as "I want more chocolate milk" at 24 to 36 months.

Young children's sentences frequently are produced with subject drop, or omission of pronouns in the initial position in utterances—for example, *want cookie, give cookie,* and *go car*. Subject drop will persist until children's mean length of utterance (MLU) is increased (Valian, 1991), their preference for a strong–weak stress pattern is lost (Gerken, 1991), or they are able to produce verb tenses (Hyams, 1992).

By age 4, most children's syntax is adultlike (Gopnik, 1997), but language continues to develop and to be refined throughout childhood and adulthood. Children learn how to transform their ideas into sentences, and they begin to use a variety of sentence types. Their utterances contain expanded noun phrases ("Gimme *the big red ball*") and verb phrases ("He pushed me *down the steps*"). Utterances also consist of negative sentences ("I *won't* do it"), yes/no questions ("*Can* you cut the cake?"), and *Wh-* questions ("*What* will I do later?"). Causal constructions ("He didn't get a prize *because* he was bad"), conditional constructions ("*If* I do my homework, I'll get to watch TV"), and temporal constructions ("*When* he comes, he'll get a surprise") are also evident.

Brown's Stages

Brown's pioneering work, *A First Language (1975),* demonstrated that children's acquisition of syntactic structures is not as much a function of their chronological development as it is a function of the average number of morphemes per utterance that they produce. This measure is called **mean length of utterance** (MLU). In a longitudinal study of three children, Adam, Eve, and Sarah, Brown found that utterance length and the mastery of grammatical forms varied greatly with age. For example, Sarah and Adam progressed from MLU of less than 2.0 to MLU of 4.0 in fifteen months. It took Eve less than eight months to make this progress. Major linguistic changes take place as MLU increases. These changes are characterized by certain MLU stages, outlined in Table 2.7.

Stage I is characterized by single-word utterances and early multiword combinations that follow semantic rules. Examples of utterances during this period include *More* and *Mommy.* Later in this stage, children produced two-word utterances such as *Drink milk, Gimme juice,* and *Push car.*

Stage II is characterized by the appearance of grammatical morphemes. Children expand and modify their linguistic productions by including morphological endings such as *-ing,* the plural *-s,* and the prepositions *in* and *on.* Utterances such as "Jimmy eat*ing,*" "Put ball *in,*" and "See cat*s*" are characteristic of this stage. At Brown's Stage II (at approximately 2 to $2\frac{1}{2}$ years of age), American English-speaking children begin filling out their short, immature sentences by incorporating one or more of the fourteen grammatical morphemes studied by Brown. Grammatical morphemes begin to emerge in Stage II, but many are not mastered (used correctly 90 percent of the time) until after Stage V.

The fourteen morphemes studied by Brown are obligatory, meaning that their use is required. The absence of a particular morpheme in a child's utterance at a certain stage of development may mean that either it has not yet been acquired, or it

TABLE 2.7	Brown's Stages			
Linguistic Stage	MLU	Approximate Chronological Age (months)	Characteristics	
I	1.0–2.0	12–26	Use of semantic rules	
II	2.0–2.5	27–30	Morphological development	
III	2.5–3.0	31–34	Development of a variety of sentence types: negative, imperative, interrogative	
IV	3.0–3.75	35–40	Emergence of complex constructions: coordination, complementation, relativization	
V	3.75–4.5	41–46		
VI	4.5+	47+		

Adapted from Brown (1975).

may indicate a developmental delay. Table 2.8 lists the order of emergence of these fourteen grammatical morphemes.

The three children studied by Brown (1975) were remarkably consistent with each other in the order in which morphological endings and function words were acquired. These results were confirmed in a later study of morphological development of twenty-one children (de Villiers and de Villiers, 1978). A more recent study of morphological development in forty-two children (Lahey, Liebergott, Chesnick, Menyuk,

TABLE 2.8	**Order of Emergence of 14 Grammatical Morphemes***		
Grammatical Morphemes		**Examples**	**Age of Mastery (months)**
1. Present progressive verb ending *-ing*		Mommy push*ing*. Johnny throw*ing*.	19–28
2. Preposition *in*		Put *in* box.	27–30
3. Preposition *on*		Put *on* table.	27–30
4. Plurals (regular) (*-s*)		Eat cookie*s*. More block*s*.	24–33
5. Past irregular verbs (*came, fell, broke, went*)		He *went* outside. Johnny *broke* it.	25–46
6. Possessive noun (*'s*)		Jimmy*'s* car. Mommy*'s* coat.	26–40
7. Uncontractible copula (*be* as the main verb: *am, is, are, were, was*)		He *was* bad. They *are* good.	27–39
8. Articles (*a, the*)		Billy throw *the* ball. Give me *a* big one.	28–46
9. Past regular (*-ed*)		He jump*ed*. She push*ed* me.	26–48
10. Third-person singular regular		He cook*s*. Johnny goe*s*.	26–46
11. Third-person singular irregular		He *has* books. She *does* work.	28–50
12. Uncontractible auxiliary (*be* verbs preceding another verb: *am, is, are, was, were*)		The boys *are eating*. The baby *is crying*.	29–48
13. Contractible copula		I*'m* good. She*'s* nice.	29–49
14. Contractible auxiliary		I*'m* eating. She*'s* jumping. They*'re* playing.	30–50

*Used correctly 90% of time in obligatory contexts.
Adapted from Brown (1975).

& Adams, 1992) found that variability among children was higher until MLU reached 3.5 or 4.0, or until children were 35 months of age. In addition, the order of acquisition differed somewhat from earlier studies: the uncontractible copula ranked higher and the irregular past ranked lower in comparison to Brown's (1975) results. In addition, mastery of certain morphemes was found to be slower than previously described.

A burst of syntactic development occurs in Stage III. Utterance length continues to grow as children begin to use simple declarative sentences, imperatives, *wh-* questions, and simple negative sentences. During this period, children begin to use a variety of sentence types. Examples of utterances characteristic of this stage include "Jimmy hit the ball," "Will I eat?" "The boy is not eating," and "Push the truck."

Stage IV is marked by the emergence of complex constructions, although the mastery of syntax continues beyond this stage. Children exhibit the use of noun- and verb-phrase elaborations as well as compound and complex sentences. Examples of utterances produced at Stage IV and beyond include "Daddy is cooking and Mommy is writing," "The first boy is nice," "Jill wants to buy the dress with the green band," "She likes to eat chocolate ice cream," and "I want to push the red truck."

Pronoun Acquisition

Learning the English pronominal system is a very complex process (Rispoli, 1998; Oshima-Takane, Takane, & Shultz, 1999; Dale & Crain-Thoreson, 1993; Ricard, Girouard, & Decarie, 1999; Bloom, Barss, Nicol, & Conway, 1994). In the case of *I* and *you,* the child must learn to understand that the referent changes, depending on the changing role of speaker and listener in a communicative interaction. Learning also requires understanding that a pronoun may refer to a previously mentioned word or an entity—for example, "Sue bought a dress; *it* was expensive." The meaning of a sentence that contains a pronoun often cannot be understood without referring to a preceding sentence. This use of a pronoun in reference is known as **anaphoric reference** and is discussed more fully later in this chapter.

Some pronouns appear in Brown's Stage II, whereas others emerge much later. In general, the earliest pronouns to emerge usually involve the child as subject *(I, mine, my, me).* Other subjective pronouns emerge later *(he, she, they).* Objective pronouns *(him, her, them)* follow and are acquired earlier than possessive pronouns *(his, her, theirs).* Reflexive pronouns *(himself, herself, themselves),* the last to emerge, are usually not mastered until after age 5. Table 2.9 presents the general order of pronoun acquisition.

Adjective and Noun Suffixes

During the preschool years, children acquire some additional suffixes for adjectives and nouns. The adjectival comparative *-er* and the superlative form *-est* emerge between 3 and 5 years of age (McLaughlin, 1998). Children add these forms to adjectives to create the words *nicer, biggest,* and *smallest.* Comparatives and superlatives that are exceptions to the rule *(better, best)* usually take longer to acquire. Derivational noun suffixes are usually understood by children by age 5 and mastered somewhat

TABLE 2.9	Development of Pronouns within Brown's Stages
Brown's Stages	**Pronouns**
I	I, mine
II	My, me
III	He, she, we, you, your
IV	They, his, hers
V	Their, our, ours, theirs
V+	Herself, himself, themselves

Adapted from Haas and Owens (1985) and Owens (1988). Reprinted by permission.

later. Thus, by age 5, children understand and produce such words as *hitter* and *teacher* (which contain the derivational noun suffix *-er)*, whereas they acquire words that contain the derivational *-ist* morpheme somewhat later *(pianist, cyclist).*

Phrase and Clause Development

Whereas words are made up of morphemes, sentences are composed of phrases and clauses. There are two major types of phrases: noun phrases and verb phrases. **Noun phrases** must contain a noun and may contain optional elements that modify the noun, such as a determiner *(the)* or adjectives *(big, pretty).* The **verb phrase** must contain a verb and may contain other optional elements, such as adverbs *(fast, slowly)* and another noun phrase *(in the morning, at school, a cookie).* An example of a sentence that contains all of these elements is "The little dog slowly ate the big cookie in the kitchen." There are four types of noun phrase modifiers:

1. *Determiners* include articles *(a* and *the)*, possessive pronouns *(my, your)*, demonstratives *(this, that)*, and qualifiers *(any, some).* They are always the first element in a noun phrase *(the* boy, *my* book, *some* toys).
2. *Adjectivals* include adjectives *(little, big)*, ordinals *(first, last)*, and quantifiers *(two, few).* They modify nouns *(two* dresses, *big* boy).
3. *Initiators* include *all, only, both,* and *just,* which limit or quantify nouns and must precede a determiner *(only* the boy, *all* the girls).
4. *Postmodifiers* follow the main noun. They may include prepositional phrases (the toy *on the floor* is broken) and clauses (the boy *who came to my house).*

Although noun phrases emerge at Brown's Stage II, the greatest surge in their development occurs at Stage IV, when sentences that contain seven words may be produced. At this stage, semantics, pragmatics, syntax, and morphology have become more adultlike (Norris, 1998). Early modifier types are determiners and adjectivals; initiators and postmodifiers appear later in development. By late Stage IV, nounphrase elaboration appears in both subject and object positions and includes the use of almost all the modifier types mentioned previously.

Verb phrases must contain a main verb and may contain some optional elements. In the sentence, "The girl is pushing the boy," *is pushing the boy* is the verb phrase. It contains the auxiliary verb *is,* the main verb *push,* and the optional present progressive form *-ing.* Optional elements of verb phrases include progressive constructions (is eat*ing*), modals (words that indicate mood or attitude (*may, must*), and perfective constructions (used to specify a single-occurring, nonhabitual action, e.g., *has seen, has eaten*). Verb-phrase elaboration emerges at Brown's Stage II (with the marking of the present progressive) and continues through Stage V. Modals emerge at Stage IV, and both the contracted and perfective ("I *have* eat*en* dinner") constructions at Stage V (Norris, 1998).

In contrast to a phrase, a **clause** is a group of words that contains both a subject and a predicate. Some clauses can stand alone and can function as simple sentences ("Billy walks," "Mary ate"). Sentences that are made up of two or more main clauses are called compound sentences ("John drank and Mary ate"). These structures usually emerge at Brown's Stage IV (Norris, 1998). Complex sentences are made up of one main clause and one subordinate clause ("The dress *that we bought yesterday* was pretty"). The embedding of subordinate clauses appears late in language development, usually at early Stage V.

Generally, intransitive clauses (clauses containing a verb that cannot take a direct object, such as "The girl walked") appear in children's declarative sentences before transitive clauses (clauses that take a direct object, such as "The boy drank milk"). Equative clauses, containing a copula and complement ("Sam is the teacher") emerge last (Dever, 1978). The interaction between syntax and verb identity may affect the difficulty with acquisition of transitive clauses. The first verbs produced by young children describe simple actions (Bloom, Lightbown, & Hood, 1975), such as *eat, read, do,* and *fix.*

Gleitman and Gleitman (1994) point out that verb learning occurs when children become aware of syntactic (sentence) structure. In terms of the nature of verbs, the verb *hit* is a two-argument verb (expressing a relationship between two things) and, consequently, requires a transitive clause: for example, "Daddy hit the ball." In contrast, the verb *cries* is a one-argument verb and is found in intransitive structures: for example, "Mary cries." These factors may explain acquisition in terms of argument structure requirements and the stages of verb acquisition.

Sentence Development

One of the most basic syntactic rules states that every sentence must contain a noun phrase and a verb phrase. Thus the only required syntactic elements of a sentence are a subject and a predicate. By the end of Brown's Stage II or early Stage III, children have mastered this rule, and can understand and produce simple, active declarative sentences such as "The boy hit the ball." Children then begin to modify this basic sentence pattern. They produce a variety of sentence types, including the negative, interrogative, and imperative sentence forms. The emergence of the adultlike form of sentence types is evident within Brown's Stage III. Table 2.10 presents the acquisition of sentence forms within Brown's stages of development. A more detailed account of the development of each sentence type follows.

TABLE 2.10   Acquisition of Sentence Forms within Brown's Stages of Development

Stage	Negative	Interrogative	Embedding	Conjoining
Early I (MLU: 1–1.5)	Single word—*no, all gone, gone;* negative + X	Yes/no asked with rising intonation on a single word; *what* and *where*		Serial naming without *and*
Late I (MLU: 1.5–2.0)	*No* and *not* used interchangeably	*That* + X; *What* + noun phrase + (doing)?	Prepositions *in* and *on* appear	*And* appears
Early II (MLU: 2.0–2.25)		*Where* + noun phrase + (going)?		
Late II (MLU: 2.25–2.5)	*No, not, don't,* and *can't* used interchangeably; negative element placed between subject and predicate	*What* or *where* + subject + predicate	*Gonna, wanna, gotta,* etc., appear	
Early III (MLU: 2.5–2.75)				*But, so, or,* and *if* appear
Late III (MLU: 2.75–3.0)	*Won't* appears; auxiliary forms *can, do, does, did, will,* and *be* develop	Auxiliary verbs begin to appear in questions (*be, can, will, do*)		
Early IV (MLU: 3.0–3.5)			Object noun phrase complements appear with verbs such as *think, guess, show*	Clausal conjoining with *and* appears (some children cannot produce this form until late V); *because* appears
Late IV (MLU: 3.5–3.75)	Adds *isn't, aren't doesn't,* and *don't*	Begins to invert auxiliary verb and subject; adds *when, how, why*		
Stage V (MLU: 3.75–4.5)	Adds *wasn't, wouldn't, couldn't,* and *shouldn't*	Adds modals; stabilizes inverted auxiliary	Relative clauses appear in object position; multiple embeddings by late V; infinitive phrases with same subject as the main verb	Clausal conjoining with *if* appears
Post-V (MLU: 4.5+)	Adds indefinite forms *nobody, no one, none,* and *nothing;* has difficulty with double negatives		Relative clauses attached to the subject; embedding and conjoining appear within same sentence above an MLU of 5.0	Clausal conjoining with *because* appears with *when, but,* and *so* beyond MLU of 5.0; embedding and conjoining appear within same sentence above an MLU of 5.0

From Owens, 1988; reprinted by permission.

The Development of Negative Sentence Forms

L. Bloom (1991) found that children at the one- and two-word utterance stage express three types of negation: (1) **nonexistence** (*Allgone juice*—when there is no more juice in the cup), (2) **rejection** (*No milk*—as the child rejects the offer of milk), and (3) **denial** (*Not a book*—as mother points to a truck and says, "This is a book"). Three phases of negative construction development have been described (Bellugi, 1967; L. Bloom, 1991; Peccei, 1999). Table 2.11 illustrates the development of the negative sentence form.

In Phase I, the negative element is placed outside of the sentence (*No bed*). Drozd (1995) describes the use of presentence *no* as a metalinguistic exclamatory negation. In this case, the child is responding to an adult utterance ("Do you want to go to bed?"), and repeating most of this adult utterance (*No bed*). O'Grady (1997) proposes a trigger for the child's utterance. When adults frequently say, "No, don't touch that," the position of the negative (*no*) cues the child to produce this negative element in sentence-initial position (*no touch*).

In Phase II, children transfer the *no* marker to its correct position before the verb ("I no want milk"). The negative form, *not*, also appears in this phase ("He not big"). In Phase III, when MLU is greater than 4.0, the negative contractible forms *can't* and *don't* emerge ("I don't have a cookie").

Indefinite negative words such as n*obody*, *no one*, and *nothing* present the young language learner with difficulty. Young children often say, "I want anything," when they mean, "I want nothing" (Seymour & Roeper, 1999). Older, school-aged children might say, "I don't got no books," and even adults might say, "I don't see nobody." Although these sentences may be judged to be ungrammatical, double negatives are considered grammatical in many other languages and dialects (Peccei, 1999).

The Development of the Interrogative Sentence Form

There are two types of questions: **yes/no questions** ("Do you want a cookie?") and *wh-* **questions,** which begin with *who, what, when, where, why,* or *how*). Yes/no questions require that the listener simply answer the question with either a *yes* or a *no* word. *Wh-* questions are more complicated because they require that the listener provide additional information. For example, *where* questions demand information about location, *when* questions demand temporal information, and *who* questions demand information about people.

TABLE 2.11	Development of the Negative Sentence	
Phase	**Description**	**Example**
I	The negative marker appears outside the sentence.	*No* the girl running.
II	The negative marker occurs before the verb.	The girl *not* running.
III	The auxiliary is added and completes the transformation to the adult form.	The girl is *not* running.

To form correct yes/no questions, children must learn to invert the subject and the auxiliary verb ("Is the boy eating?"). To form correct *wh-* questions, they must learn to (1) transpose the subject and the auxiliary verb and (2) add the *wh-* form at the beginning of the sentence ("What is the boy eating?"). Children go through four phases as they develop the ability to formulate questions (L. Bloom, 1991; Klima & Bellugi, 1966).

Phase 1—use of rising intonation and some *wh-* forms (MLU 1.75 and 2.25). In this first phase, children typically ask yes/no questions by adding a rising intonation to the end of their utterances. Examples of such question forms are "Johnnie eat?," "Baby drinking?," and "Go outside?". To ask *wh-* questions, young children simply attach a *wh-* word to an assertion and produce questions like "Where doggie?" and "What dat?" These *wh-* questions are used in routines in which children generally ask for the names of objects, actions, or locations, such as the location of an object that has disappeared. *Where* and *what* questions are the more prominent *wh-* questions used during this phase. At this phase, children do not respond appropriately to any of the *wh-* questions.

Phase 2—use of a greater variety of *wh-* questions (MLU 2.25 to 2.75). Children in this phase continue to ask yes/no questions by using rising intonation. Children ask *wh-* questions by adding the *wh-* form at the beginning of the question but fail to use the auxiliary verb. Children are able to provide appropriate answers to *what, who,* and *where* questions. Examples of *wh-* questions that characterize this period are

Where my truck?

Why you pushing it?

What the man doing?

Phase 3—limited use of inversion (MLU 2.75 to 3.5). Auxiliary + verb inversion appears when children's MLU is at 3.5 morphemes (O'Grady, 1997). In this phase, children regularly invert the subject and verb to produce yes/no questions but fail to do so in all *wh-* questions. Examples of questions that characterize this period are

Will I go?

What the boy is riding?

Phase 4—use of inversion in positive *wh-* questions (MLU 3.5+). In this last stage, children invert the subject and the auxiliary verb when asking positive *wh-* questions but still have difficulty with negative *wh-* questions. Examples of *wh-* questions of this period are

What is the boy eating?

Where are you going?

Why I can't do that?

What, where, and *who* questions are mastered before *why, how,* and *when* questions (L. Bloom, 1991; Ervin-Tripp, 1970). In the case of the former, the *wh-* words that introduce the questions can be recovered from a sentence—for example, "John (*who*) ate pizza (*what*) in his house (*where*)"—whereas the words *why, how,* and *when* require additional information that must be recovered from context or discourse—for example, "Why did John do it?," "When will you go?" Thus, *what, where,* and *who* forms code cognitively simpler ideas involving objects, people, or places (Norris, 1998), whereas *when, why,* and *how* forms involve the need to consider intentionality and planning. The order of acquisition of questions is summarized in Table 2.12.

Bloom, Merkin, and Wooten (1982) hypothesize an interaction between *wh-* questions and verbs. They argue that young children, between 22 and 36 months of age, use questions with the verbs *do, go,* and *happen* because these verbs have a general use within a wide range of activities, such as doing things, going places, and things that are happening. In contrast, the later-occurring *why* and *how wh-* questions are used with descriptive verbs with a more limited range of use, such as *sing* and *fix.*

The Development of Imperative Sentence Forms

The imperative sentence requests, demands, commands, or insists that a listener perform some action. At the prelinguistic level, infants request and demand by pointing and gesturing. As they develop into toddlers, they begin to employ the imperative form to request, demand, and command. At Brown's Stage I, children produce forms that sound like imperatives because they often omit the subject (subject drop), even when it is required (*touch doggy*).

In imperative sentences, the subject *you* is understood and not included in the surface form of the sentence, and the verb is uninflected. Examples of imperative

TABLE 2.12	Order of Acquisition of *Wh-* Questions

Type	Example
What	What is the girl eating?
Where	Where is the ball?
Who	Who is pushing the truck?
When	When will you go?
Why	Why is it dark?
How	How did it break?

From S. Ervin-Tripp, "Discourse agreement: How children answer questions," In J. R. Hayes (Ed.), *Cognition and the development of language,* Copyright © 1970 by John Wiley & Sons, Inc. Reprinted by permission of John Wiley & Sons, Inc.

sentences are "Gimme milk," "Push the truck," and "Pass the butter, Please." True imperatives begin to appear at Brown's Stage III, when the omission of the subject in the surface form reflects the mastery of the rule of subject deletion in imperatives.

The Development of Complex Sentences

Children begin to combine more than one semantic/syntactic relation in a single utterance when their MLU increases beyond 3.0. Their utterances reflect the elaboration or specification of agent–action–object interactions, and sentence construction advances from a linear ordering of words to a hierarchical ordering within and among sentence elements. Children learn to use complex sentences that allow the expression of old functions and new ideas with increasing clarity (Tyack & Gottsleben, 1986).

Coordination

The complex construction that emerges first in children's language is **coordination.** There are two types of coordination constructions: sentential coordination and phrasal coordination. In **sentential coordination,** two events are combined into one sentence by the conjunction *and* ("John went to the doctor *and* his sister stayed home"). In **phrasal coordination,** the connective *and* is also used, allowing the speaker to delete a redundant element. In the sentence, "Jane went to the movies and ate popcorn," the word *and* allows for the deletion of *Jane* from the second phrase ("Jane went to the movies and _ _ _ _ ate popcorn"). Lund and Duchan (1993) suggest that semantic and cognitive complexity affect children's learning of complex sentence structures such as coordinated structures. Children must determine the grammatical relations within sentences, and the deletion of one or more elements in the sentence.

The earliest use of coordination by children is in stereotypic phrases (*bread and jam, milk and cookie*) that are present in young children's utterances as responses to routine questions such as, "What do you want to eat?" Both types of coordination are acquired at the same time (Bloom, Lahey, Hood, Lifter, & Fiess, 1980). Children $2\frac{1}{2}$ to 3 years of age use both sentential and phrasal coordinations appropriately when the communicative context is set up to elicit them: sentential coordination for events at different times and places; phrasal coordination for events at the same time and place (Owens, 2001).

L. Bloom (1991) focused on semantic considerations in the acquisition of coordinated sentences and found the following order of acquisition of *and* coordinations:

1. **Additives**—the use of *and* to connect two propositions that go together ("Mother is baking a cake and Daddy is reading").
2. **Temporal**—the use of *and* to designate a sequential ordering of events ("Mommy will mix the batter and put it in the oven").
3. **Causal**—the use of *and* to indicate that one event led to another ("She put a bandage on and it made her feel better").
4. **Adversative**—the use of *and* to indicate a contrast relationship ("This goes in here and that goes there"). Often the connective used in this instance is *but.*

Complementation

There are several types of complement structures in English. **Complementizers** in English consist of words such as *that* (i.e., "I said *that* I would call him"). Other examples of sentences with complement constructions are "I want *to buy a red lolli- pop*," "Show me *where this one goes*," and "Look at *what she's doing*." In each of these sentences, the main portion of the sentence is coupled with a clause that modi- fies the verb.

Bloom, Lifter, and Hafitz (1980) studied complement constructions and found that the order of emergence is based on the semantics of the verb. The first comple- ments to emerge in children's speech contain state verbs, verbs that express a feeling or intention. *Like, want,* and *need* are state verbs and take the complement *to* ("I want to go home" and "I like to get dirty"). The next complement to emerge is at- tached to notice verbs, such as *see, look,* and *watch*. These verbs are followed by the complement *what* ("Look at what he's doing").

The third complement to emerge is attached to knowledge verbs such as *know* and *think*. These are followed by the complement *that* or *what* ("I know what to do," or "I think that one is good").

The last complement to emerge is attached to speaking verbs, such as *ask, tell,* or *promise*. Speaking verbs require the complement construction *to* plus a verb. Sen- tences such as "Ask Mary to come inside" or "John promised to leave" are examples of sentences with speaking verb complements. Bloom, Lifter, and Hafitz (1980) con- cluded that the acquisition of complement constructions is a function of semantic constraints: these verbs are used to qualify the degree of certainty or uncertainty of a proposition (i.e., "I know what to do" versus "I *think* I know what to do").

Relativization

Complex sentences can be formed by adding **relative clauses,** which restrict or qual- ify the meaning of another portion of the sentence. Relative clauses usually begin with complementizers (*that*) or relative pronouns (*who, which, whom, whose*). Relative clauses are of two types: objective and subjective. Objective relative clauses modify the object of the sentence, as in "That picture is about some birds *that got all smeared up.*" An example of a sentence with a subject relative clause is "The girl *who lives down the block* is my cousin."

Children are reported to produce sentences that contain objective relative clauses before subjective relative clauses, such as "The book [that you want] is on the table" (Menyuk, 1977). The objective relative clause develops after 5 years of age, whereas the relative clause that is part of the subject phrase of the sentence is rare even at 7 years of age. O'Grady (1997) argues that interpretation of relative clause constructions requires determining (1) the role of a gap (a missing noun phrase) and (2) the reference of this gap. Preschool children interpret the sentence "The lion [that the horse kisses _ _ _ _ _ _ _] knocks down the duck" as "The lion [that _ _ _ _ _ _ kisses the horse] knocks down the duck." In this example, the broken lines mark the gap, or the missing noun phrase *the lion*. In the example above, children have difficulty determining the subject of the action *kisses*, but have less difficulty with sentences such as "The dog [that _ _ _ _ _ _ jumps over the pig] bumps into the lion." In both examples, children identify the first noun as the subject of the relative clause.

Summary

Children's morphological and syntactic development shows a great deal of growth during this period. The ability to produce and to understand more complex syntactic forms continues to grow through the later stages of language development.

In a previous section, we noted the use of phonological processes used by toddlers. We will now turn our attention to the simplifications and changes that preschoolers make in their attempts to produce adult word targets.

PRESCHOOL CHILDREN'S PHONOLOGICAL PROCESSES

The phonological patterns of preschool children can be classified into two basic categories (Bernthal & Bankson, 1998): whole-word processes (simplifications of words, syllables, or contrasts between sounds) and segment-change processes (changes in sounds). Examples of these processes follow.

Whole-Word Processes

Children frequently simplify words by reducing them to either the basic consonant–vowel (CV) syllable or to CVCV structure. Four processes that accomplish this simplification are reduplication, final consonant deletion, cluster reduction, and unstressed syllable omission (found in Table 2.5). Additional processes that affect word production consist of the following:

> **Epenthesis** occurs when children insert a segment in a word. An example is the production of /bəlæk/ for *black.*
>
> **Metathesis** consists of the reversal of two segments in a word. An example is the production of /bæksɪt/ for *basket.*

Segment-Change Processes

A number of rule-governed segment changes are common in the speech of preschoolers. These changes are classified according to the place or manner of production of the speech sounds. Among these processes are *fronting, stopping,* and *gliding.*

> **Fronting**—This process occurs when children replace palatal and velar sounds (made in the back of the mouth) with alveolar sounds (made in the front of the mouth). Examples are the production of /tʌp/ for *cup* or /dʌn/ for *gun.* Fronting of velars is usually suppressed by $2\frac{1}{2}$ to 3 years of age, and velar consonants are usually established in children's speech by age four at the latest.
>
> **Stopping**—Instead of producing fricatives (sounds that are made by passing air through a narrow constriction, thereby creating a hissing sound) or affricates

(sounds that combine a popping sound and a fricative), children substitute a plosive (a popping sound). The use of the stopping process results in productions such as /dut/ for *juice* or /bæn/ for *van*. Stopping begins to disappear for most fricatives and affricates by 2½ to 3 years of age.

Gliding—Children substitute glides (sounds that are produced during the movement of articulators from one vowel position to another) for liquids (sounds with vowel-like quality of little air turbulence). Examples of gliding are the production of /wæbɪt/ for *rabbit* or /jaɪt/ for *light*. This process may persist for many years.

Assimilation Processes

Another group of processes are those in which two phonemes within a word become alike: *consonant harmony* and *prevocalic voicing*.

Consonant harmony—a process in which consonants within a word become more alike in terms of place or manner of articulation. An example of consonant harmony is the production of /gɔgi/ for *doggy*.

Prevocalic voicing—a process in which unvoiced consonants are affected by the following vowel and take on the voicing feature of the vowel. The result is the production of /dʌb/ for *tub*.

Unstressed syllable deletion, final consonant deletion, velar fronting, consonant assimilation, reduplication, and prevocalic voicing should disappear by three years of age. Cluster reduction, epenthesis, gliding, and stopping may persist after 3 years of age.

Phonological Processes: Language Differences

Some of the phonological processes found in typically developing 3- to 4-year-old Spanish-speaking children of Puerto Rican descent consist of the following examples (Goldstein & Iglesias, 1996).

- Word-final /s/ and /n/ may be deleted: /pæ/ for *pan*
- The glide /j/ is produced as the voiced alveo-palatal affricate /ʤ/: /ʤo/ for *yo*
- The labiodental fricative /f/ becomes a bilabial fricative /Φ/ in initial and medial positions in words: /kaΦɪ/ for *coffee*

Some phonological processes found in speakers of African American English (AAE) consist of the following examples (Goldstein, 2000).

- Devoicing of final consonants: /pɪk/ for *pig*
- Diphthongs often neutralized to vowel form: /aɪ/ for /a/
- Final stops devoiced and followed by glottal stop: /bætɪ/ for *bad*
- Final stops devoiced: /bæt/ for *bad*
- Final consonant deletion of nasals and stops: /pæ/ for *pan*
- Stopping in word-initial position: /d/ for /ð/: /de/ for *they*
- Intervocalic production of /f/ for /θ/ v for /ð/: /brəvɚ) for *brother*
- Final production of /f/ for /θ/ and v for /ð/: /bæf/ for *bath*

- Postvocalic liquids deleted: /mo:/ for *more*
- Substitution of /k/ for /t/ in initial consonant clusters: /skrit/ for *street*
- Metathesis: /æks/ for *ask*
- Initial unstressed syllable deletion: /baut/ for *about*

Children's development of phonological and speech production skills plays an essential role in their ability to communicate, especially with unfamiliar listeners. Some phonological difficulties appear only when children produce longer sentences, possibly as a result of the increased demands on sound sequencing when producing longer sentences.

Summary

Children's development of linguistic form can be traced in the directions of (1) lengthier utterances and (2) increased phonological, morphological, and syntactic complexity. It is important to note that the elaboration of children's linguistic form is the result of their need to express more complex ideas in a greater variety of social situations.

Attention now turns to children's semantic development during the preschool years, with emphasis on their understanding and use of words in producing sentences and in discourse.

PRESCHOOL SEMANTIC DEVELOPMENT

Semantics is the component of language concerned with meaning. Without meaning, there would be no point to language. People talk in order to express meaning, and they listen in order to discover the meaning of what others say. Meaning can be conveyed through language at the word, sentence, and discourse levels. The meaning of some words can also be derived from the nonlinguistic context.

Lexical Meaning

The most familiar sense of meaning is **lexical meaning.** It is concerned with the meaning of words and the characteristics of the category to which a word belongs. The preschool period is one of rapid lexical growth. Vocabulary increases markedly during the second year of a child's life (Golinkoff, Mervis, & Hirsh-Pasek, 1994). At 3 years of age, preschool children have an expressive vocabulary of 900 to 1,000 words. By age 4, their expressive vocabulary is 1,500 words, and at 5, over 2,000 words (Owens, Metz, & Haas, 2000).

As children develop, they become better able to define words. For example, during the late preschool period and into the early school years, children's word definitions are concrete, and consist primarily of a referent's appearances and function. Later in development, children's definitions are more abstract and include synonymy (i.e., words with similar features, such as *sick* and *ill*), explanation (i.e., giving the reason for an action), and specifications of categorical relationships (i.e., placing entities in categories, such as *dog* and *bird* in the category *animal*). Lexical growth is a gradual process and continues for many years.

Relational Meaning

In addition to acquiring lexical knowledge that specifies referents, children acquire meanings that code relationships among people, objects, and events. The **relational meanings** that were coded at the early stage of language development also appear in the language of preschool children. These relationships are now conveyed at the sentence level (also called *intrasentence meaning*).The early relational meanings (or semantic content categories) of existence, nonexistence, and recurrence that are evident in children's early language are coded during this period, not with single words but with multiword combinations and simple sentences (see Table 2.13). As children develop cognitively, the semantic relations expressed by them include the coding of concepts of space, time, causation, and sequencing of action using more complex linguistic forms and a variety of sentence types.

Contextual Meaning: The Role of Discourse

Context affects many aspects of language, including language meaning. The **linguistic context,** or discourse, provides information necessary to derive intrasentence meaning. The influence of the linguistic context on meaning can be understood by examining the following sentence:

He bought it.

It is not possible to derive the meaning of this sentence without knowing something about the previous linguistic context, which supplies the information of who *he* refers

TABLE 2.13 | **Semantic Relations (Intrasentence Meanings) Expressed by Two- to Four-Year-Olds**

Semantic Relation	Age	Example
Coordination	2.0	My car . . . truck.
Sequence	2.0	Bye-bye, Mommy, Daddy, Joey.
Causality (logical)	2.0	I can't do it. It too long.
Reasons	2.4	You hit me because you don't like me.
Temporality	2.8	Now I wash my hands, then I eat. When he goes to school he goes on the bus.
Conditionality	3.4	I wear this while walking.
Temporal sequence	3.5–4.0	I will make a tree after I finish this.

Adapted from Miller (1981).

to and what *it* is. Within the context of the following discourse, however, the meaning of *he* and *it* becomes clear:

> *Tom:* John saw a red Jaguar at a car dealer yesterday.
>
> *Susan:* What happened?
>
> *Tom:* He bought it.

In the discourse, the pronouns *he* and *it* are used to refer to something that had already been identified linguistically. The use of a pronoun to refer to a previously mentioned referent is called **anaphoric reference**. Anaphoric reference, as well as other linguistic devices, helps bind discourse so that its meaning is better understood. Collectively, these are called **cohesive devices** because they provide the glue for intersentence meaning. Table 2.14 defines some cohesive devices and gives examples of each. Although there is limited information about preschool use of coherence devices, researchers have concluded that the ability to use pronouns anaphorically is a developmental achievement related to their linguistic, cognitive, and social awareness (Cairns, 1996; Chien and Wexler, 1990).

Contextual Meaning: The Role of the Nonlinguistic Context

In addition to the linguistic context, the **nonlinguistic context** gives clues about the meaning of words whose referents shift with the perspective of the speaker and the timing of the utterance. Consider the sentence, "I want you to go there tomorrow." The meanings of *I, you, there,* and *tomorrow* depend on who is speaking, who is lis-

TABLE 2.14 | **Cohesive Devices**

Type	Definition	Example
Personal pronouns	Substitute for noun	*I, you, she, it,* etc.
Demonstrative pronoun	Deictic (pointing) words	I'll take *this/that* one.
Anaphoric reference	Pronoun used to refer to a previously established entity	Mary is happy. *She* passed the test.
Cataphoric reference	Pronoun used to refer to a coming event	*Here* comes a surprise.
Verb ellipsis	Deletion of information available in the discourse	Do you like cake? I do *(like cake)*
Nominal ellipsis	Deletion of information that is available in the discourse	Where is he? *(He is)* here!
Conjunctions	Conjoining elements	*and, or, but*
Lexical cohesion	Synonyms referring to previously mentioned entity	A lion appeared. The *beast* roared.
Comparative references	Comparison between entities	*Bigger than . . .*

Adapted from Halliday and Hasan (1976).

tening, where the speaker is when the sentence is uttered, and when the sentence is spoken. Words whose meaning shifts as the nonlinguistic context changes are called **deictic terms.** Thus *I, you, here, there, today,* and *tomorrow* express the deictic relationship of person, place, and time, respectively.

Studies have examined children's development of person, place, and time deixis. In general, pronoun deixis (*I/you, me/my,* and *my/you*) is acquired before the contrasts *this/that, these/those, here/there,* which refer to spatial concepts (McLaughlin, 1998). Last to emerge is temporal deixis (*today, tomorrow*). Children may have difficulty in the difference between *this* and *that* at 4 years of age, and some deictic contrasts present difficulty even for 7-year-olds (Owens, 2001).

Semantics: Language Differences

Goldstein (2000) points out that lexical differences exist among dialects, with similar words having different meanings. For example, the word *bomba* means *balloon* in some dialects of Spanish but means *bomb* in others. Stockman (1999) summarized the four types of meaning relationships that can exist among different dialects and languages: (1) identical words (no differences), (2) different words and different referents for these words, (3) different words for the same referents, or (4) different referents for the same forms. These differences should be considered when evaluating children with different cultural and linguistic backgrounds.

Summary

The acquisition of words, their meanings, and the links between them is a process that requires time. During the preschool period, children acquire new words and gradually develop an understanding of the nature of words, sentences, and their relationship. The meanings that children learn are the result of their encounters with the physical and social world and are dependent on their cognitive and social development.

Attention is now turned to children's pragmatic development during the preschool years, with emphasis on the expansion of their repertoire of linguistic use.

PRESCHOOL PRAGMATIC DEVELOPMENT

As noted earlier in the chapter, language is learned within a social context. As children interact with their caretakers (and later with their peers), the uses to which they put language continually multiply. The intentions they code increase, and they learn to become more aware of social settings and the interactors within those social settings.

During the preschool period, children learn to describe objects and events removed from the immediate context. They relate personal experiences and they use language effectively to convey their wants and needs. In addition, they become more aware of the general conditions governing cooperative conversations. They learn to take turns in a conversation, to stick to the conversational topic, and to contribute new and relevant information to the discourse. Although these abilities emerge in the preschool period, they continue to grow through the years as children mature cognitively and socially.

The Elaboration of Communicative Functions

In addition to the early communicative functions outlined in a previous section (also see Table 2.5), children expand their repertoire of language use. Dore (1978) explored children's use of language during the preschool years. He found that the communicative intentions coded by 2- to 5-year-olds included:

1. Requesting information by asking a variety of questions ("Can I go now?," "Is he eating candy?," "Where are you going?," "Why can't I have it?")
2. Responding to requests by answering questions or supplying information ("It's in my closet," "I wasn't the one who broke the cup," "I don't want to")
3. Describing events, objects, or properties("There's a red truck," "He's building it slowly," "That's a truck with a crane")
4. Stating facts, feelings, attitudes, and beliefs ("It happened yesterday," "I feel sick," "I don't like her," "Ghosts are not real")

The internal cognitive and social changes that take place in children influence the ways they use language. For example, young preschoolers use language to direct themselves and to instruct others, as well as to report on present and past experiences (Hulit & Howard, 1997). Older preschoolers, however, add more complex communicative functions; they use language to reason, to think, and to solve problems (Tough, 1979). Consider the following scripts.

Ari (age 5):   If the roof isn't strong enough, he'll fall in.

Eli (age 5):   I think the tape will fix it. Yep, I'll get the tape.

Sheri (age 5$\frac{1}{2}$):   If you put the block here and I put my block there, it will hold everything up.

In the later preschool years, children also use language to tease, to annoy, to complain, to criticize, and to threaten. These communication functions are observed not only as they interact with caretakers and siblings, but also as they interact with their peers. Consider the following utterances produced by 5-year-olds.

Teasing: You're a fatso.

Annoying: I'll do it again and again.

Complaining: You always give the big one to him.

Criticizing: Your picture is yucky.

Threatening: Give it back or I'll tell Mommy.

During this period, we see children expressing a wide variety of communicative intentions with expanding linguistic forms.

Conversation Skill Development

In general, children learn language within a conversational context. Preschool children acquire many conversational skills, but much of their conversation concerns the here and now. Their conversations are very short, and the number of turns they take in a conversation are limited.

Topic maintenance in preschoolers usually occurs only when the communicative partner's previous utterance consists of a topic-sharing response to the child's prior utterances (Bloom, Rocissano, & Hood, 1976). Young children ($2\frac{1}{2}$ to 3) are good at introducing new conversational topics in which they are interested, but they have difficulty sustaining that topic beyond one or two turns. Although they learn to acknowledge their communicative partner, they often fail to wait for their conversational turn and to build a bridge for the next speaker's turn.

Between 3 and 4 years of age, children seem to gain a better awareness of the social aspects of conversation. They begin to adapt their language to the needs of their listeners. With the realization that other people's perspective must be taken into account (called *presuppositional ability*) comes language that is adapted to the listener. That is not to say that preschoolers are always successful in getting their messages across. They are often unable to reformulate their messages in response to a facial expression of miscomprehension and must be asked specifically to clarify their messages. The most common way preschoolers clarify or repair their messages is simply to repeat what they have said (McLaughlin, 1998).

> *Child (age $3\frac{1}{2}$) to mother:*   He took it away from me.
>
> *Mother:*   What?
>
> *Child:*   He took it away from me.
>
> *Mother:*   What?
>
> *Child:*   He took it away from me (in a louder voice).
>
> *Mother:*   Who did what?
>
> *Child:*   John took away my book!

The inability to respond to a nonspecific request for clarification is characteristic of preschoolers. The ability to respond more appropriately does not develop until the school-age years (Owens, 2001).

Lastly, during the preschool period children begin to manifest the ability to understand and to use indirect requests. Consider the sentence, "It's awfully hot in here." While this sentence might be a statement, it is usually uttered when a request for action is intended by a speaker (for the listener to open the window). The ability to understand and to to use indirect requests advances as children mature socially and linguistically. Between 3 and 4 years of age, children seem to gain a better awareness of the social benefit of using indirect requests (Ervin-Tripp, 1980; Ninio & Snow, 1996; Wells, 1985). A typical indirect request of a 4-year-old is "Mommy, can I have a cookie, please?"

In the next section we will examine children's development of a different discourse skill: their ability to tell narratives.

Narrative Development

The narrative is a form of discourse. Narratives differ from conversations in that a listener response is not required. When producing a narrative, the speaker produces a monologue throughout and must presuppose the information needed by the listener. The speaker must present all the information in an organized way and must introduce and organize sequences so that events are related and lead to some conclusion.

There are a number of different types of narratives. Narratives include sharing and recounting of personal events and experiences, self-generated stories, telling and retelling of familiar tales, and the retelling of stories from movies, books, and television shows.

Research has shown that 2-year-olds incorporate dialogue that accompanies familiar everyday routines into their speech. This type of narrative is called a *script* and is used by young children to talk about events that occurred to them (Owens, 2001; Tiegerman-Farber, 1995). However, it is not until the age of 4 that they are able accurately to describe event sequences, called a *plan* (Karmiloff-Smith, 1986).

Narratives contain principles and structure that give them cohesiveness (McLaughlin, 1998). Around $3\frac{1}{2}$ years of age, preschool children produce **proto-narratives**, which are stories about recent events. The organizational structure is a set of unrelated elements (**heaps**), which emerges at 30 months of age.

In general, two types of strategies are used by preschool children for organizing their narratives: *chaining* and *centering*. Children of 3 years of age use **chaining** (a narrative that relates to a central topic with no particular temporal order) when producing a narrative. At around 4 years of age, children produce narratives with increased organization that follow a central theme (**centering**). By age 5, 75 percent of typically developing children use both strategies. Below are examples of typically developing preschoolers retelling a story and recounting a birthday experience.

> *Child (age 3) retelling a story:*   There was this magician. He had a hat and rabbits came from the hat. The end.

> *Child (age 5):*   I had a birthday party. All the children came to my party. Everybody sang "Happy Birthday to You." I got presents. We ate cake.

By the time that they enter school, children acquire the basic elements of narratives and can share their experience and recount familiar events sequentially. In the school-age years, as their linguistic abilities and knowledge of the world develops, they learn to understand and produce more complex narrative forms.

Summary

In our review of pragmatic development we have seen that preschool children elaborate their use of language to suit a variety of social contexts and begin to gain competence in their use of different discourse skills (e.g., conversations, narratives). During this period they also begin to learn that language is not only spoken, but that meanings can be conveyed in words and sentences using print or written language.

The next section presents the research in this area of preschool language development.

EMERGENT LITERACY

Recent research has begun to highlight the importance of the preschool years in laying the foundation for children's development of reading and writing abilities (Butler, 1999; Snow, Scarborough, & Burns, 1999). There are strong indications that listening/ speaking and reading/writing share, at least in part, a common linguistic base, although they differ in other ways. The importance of this information for speech-language pathologists and educators who work with preschool children lies in the fact that delays in the comprehension and the formulation of oral language foreshadow difficulties in reading and writing that will appear during the school years (Butler, 1999).

The term that has often been used for the knowledge that preschoolers acquire about print before learning to read is called **emergent literacy.** Studies of emergent literacy have taken numerous directions. Some investigators have concluded that during the preschool period children:

- Master the convention of print (how to hold a book, awareness that the organization of English print is from left to right and top to down, scribble writing)
- Learn to name and write letters
- Recognize that print represents meaningful ideas
- Acquire an understanding of the structure of written language (that stories are organized in a particular way)
- Develop a print-related vocabulary (understanding and using words such as *read, write, story, page*)
- Acquire the rudimentary skills of phonological awareness (that words consist of discrete units)

Other researchers have focused on the print literacy environment of the young child, particularly in the child's home. They have found that the availability of print in the home (books, posters, magazines, postcards, and nameplates) as well as print artifacts (crayons, pencils, and markers) have a positive correlation with literacy acquisition. Most of the literacy events that occur in the lives of preschool children are embedded in ongoing real-life family experiences. Caretakers use techniques such as semantic contingency (staying on a topic introduced by a child), scaffolding (structuring the linguistic and nonlinguistic context to facilitate the child's success), and routines (highly predictable situations that occur frequently) to help facilitate an appreciation for literacy experiences (Snow, Perlmann, & Nathan, 1987). Justice and Ezell (2000) found that book reading by parents significantly enhanced children's early literacy development.

Most research has focused on literacy socialization in middle-class mainstream families, regardless of ethnicity. Not all families, however, are alike even when they have similar cultural and sociolinguistic histories (Heath, 1996). There may be culturally based differences in literacy events, parental guidance, and the preliteracy expectations of parents for their preschool children (Nelson, 1993). In spite of the diverse approaches to literacy activities found in different cultures, the outcome is the same: children can develop literacy abilities (Heath, 1996).

In sum, children develop literacy skills and absorb a wealth of knowledge about print before learning to read. Family literacy events assist them in developing an understanding of this form.

Phonological Awareness

During the preschool period, children begin to develop an awareness of the sound structure of words. They learn (1) that words are composed of segments, (2) that these segments have distinctive features, the phonetic properties that act to provide contrasts between sounds (e.g., the voicing difference that distinguishes /p/ and /b/), and (3) that letters represent sounds in words (Ball, 1997; Snowling, Hulme, Smith, & Thomas, 1994; Torgesen 1999). These skills allow the child to segment syllables into words (*ba-na-na*), to rhyme (What rhymes with *cat*? Do *cat* and *bat* rhyme?), to blend sound segments (What word is /k/-/æ/-/t/?), to segment sounds in words (What is the first/last sound in *cat*?), to manipulate sounds (Delete the first sound in the words *smart/mart, spark/park*, and *stop/top*), to match words on the basis of initial phonemes (What words have the same first sound: *toy, take*, or *chair*?), to produce alliteration (*big bad bugs bite boys*), and to choose a target word from a set based on the difference in final or beginning sounds (*doll, dog*, or *toy*?). While some phonological awareness skills appear in the preschool period, development continues into the school-age years.

Preschoolers are able to engage in sound play, repair speech errors, recognize rhyme, and segment syllables (Kamhi & Catts, 1991). Later developing phonological skills include segmenting sounds in words and matching words on the basis of initial phonemes. The relationship of phonological awareness and reading has been discussed by many researchers (Torgesen, 1999; Bryant, Bradley, MacLean & Crossland, 1989; Jorm & Share, 1983) and a correlation between deficits in phonological awareness and reading difficulties has been found (Ball, 1997; Snyder & Downey, 1997; Swanson, Mink & Bocian, 1999; Westby, 1998; Shaywitz, Fletcher, Holahan, & Shaywitz, 1992). The deficits in phonological awareness evidenced in children with language learning and reading difficulties are discussed more fully in Chapters 5 and 9.

Summary

Children's language development is indeed a multifaceted and complicated process. Although there are common developmental patterns, there are variances in children's language acquisition that account for their respective differences. Children have unique predispositions from birth and different cognitive, social, cultural, and linguistic experiences. In a similar vein, the rate of learning linguistic forms differs among children.

Children's utterances are observed to increase in length and complexity during the preschool period. From a MLU of 2.0 and continuing beyond a MLU of 4.0, children learn several linguistic subsystems simultaneously. They master the phonological system, develop grammatical morphemes, and are able to understand and produce a variety of sentence types. They acquire more abstract meanings and the ability to map these onto linguistic structures. They elaborate their use of language to suit a variety of social contexts and to describe events and personal experiences as well as sequences and outcomes. Finally, they begin to gain knowledge about print, even though they may not actually learn how to decode print until they are formally taught to do so in school. Although each component of language was discussed separately, language form (phonology, morphology, and syntax), content (semantics), and use (pragmatics) are interrelated in development.

In the next section we examine language development in the school-age years. We focus on the children's increased ability to produce complex sentences, to increase their vocabulary, and to develop their conversational skills. Lastly, we will turn our attention to the development of reading and writing abilities during this period.

SCHOOL-AGE LANGUAGE DEVELOPMENT: AN OVERVIEW

Although children's language has reached a measure of complexity by age 5, much communicative development is yet to come. Vocabulary continues to grow throughout the school years (McGhee-Bidlack, 1991; Johnson & Anglin, 1995). Children begin to use nonliteral language such as jokes, riddles, and metaphors in middle childhood (Bernstein, 1986, 1987; Nippold, Leonard, & Kail, 1984) and to comprehend sentences that contain verbs such as *promise* or *ask* (Chomsky, 1969; Eisenberg & Cairns, 1994).

During the school-age years, the cognitive and social changes that take place in children influence the ways that they use language. They expand their pragmatic and discourse skills, their conversational abilities become refined, and they are better able to plan, organize, and sequence their ideas into more coherent and cohesive complex narratives. Lastly, during this period, children also develop the ability to think and talk about language (called *metalinguistic ability*) and master language in another mode by learning to read and write. Although language development continues as children mature cognitively and socially, a good deal of language learning has already been mastered by the time the child enters first grade.

Syntactic and Morphological Development

In the realm of morphology and syntax, school-age language development consists of simultaneous expansion of existing forms and acquisition of new ones. Children continue to expand their sentences by elaborating noun phrases and verb phrases. They expand their understanding and use of conjoined sentences with the addition of *therefore, although,* and *unless,* which are used to join clauses ("I went to the store, although my brother was supposed to go"). Correct interpretation of the words *if* and *although* may not occur until age 11, and *unless* may not be understood completely until age 15 (McLaughlin, 1998).

Children's use of embedding expands with their comprehension of more syntactically complex embedded sentences; their understanding will depend on the place and type of embedding used. Embeddings may occur in the center of the sentence or at the end; the two clauses of the embedded sentence may share the same subject or object—called **parallel embedding**—or they may not—called **nonparallel embedding.** The comprehension of embedded sentences progresses from the easiest to the most difficult, reflecting the child's cognitive development. Table 2.15 outlines the order in which various types of embedded sentences are acquired.

TABLE 2.15	**Development Sequence of Embedded Sentence Comprehension**

Type	Example
Parallel center embedding—same subject (*girl*) serves both clauses.	The girl who bought the dress went to the party.
Parallel ending embedding—same object (*gift*) serves both clauses.	He gave me a gift that I don't like.
Nonparallel ending embedding—the object of the main clause (*boy*) is the subject of the embedded clause.	She hit the boy who ran away.
Nonparallel central embedding—the subject of the main clause (*cat*) is the object of the embedded clause.	The cat that was chased by the dog ran up a tree.

Adapted from Abrahamsen & Rigrodsky (1984), Lahey (1974), and Owens (1996).

Several morphological structures emerge during the early school-age years. Gerunds, which are verbs to which *-ing* has been added to produce a form that fulfills a noun function (e.g., *to fish* becomes *fishing;* "Fishing is fun"), emerge after Stage V (Owens, 2001). Derivational morphemes first appear in the late preschool years with the adjectival comparative *-er* (*bigger*) emerging between 4 and 5 years of age and *-est* (*biggest*) emerging between 5 and 6 (Norris, 1998). The derivational suffix *-er* (*farm + er*), used to change a verb to a noun, emerges in the late preschool years. The derivational morpheme *-ist* emerges at 7 years of age, and the derivational suffixes *-ful, -less, -ly, -ness, -al,* and *-ance* emerge during the school-age years (Wiig & Semel, 1984).

By the end of second grade, children comprehend irregular noun and verb agreement ("The fish are eating" versus "The sheep is sleeping"), the implicit negative form ("Find the one that is neither red nor blue"), and several verb tenses, such as the past participle (*had eaten*) and the perfect (*has been eating*).

Although children 5 to 7 years of age are able to use most elements of noun and verb phrases, they frequently omit them. Even at age 7, they will omit some elements (articles) while expanding others, such as double negatives. In addition, school-aged children may still have difficulty with some prepositions, verb tense, and plurals (Menyuk, 1969). Lastly, irregular past tense verbs that form past tense by vowel and (sometimes) consonant change present adolescents and even adults with difficulty (Nelson, 1998) (e.g., *lie–lay–lain* and *swim–swam–swum*)(McLaughlin, 1998).

During the preschool years, reversible passive sentences ("The boy was hit by the ball") are difficult for children to understand and produce because the passive sentence violates the child's strategy of determining *who did what to whom* from the word order. Children do not fully comprehend passives until $5\frac{1}{2}$ years of age, and full passives are not produced until around $7\frac{1}{2}$ to 8 years of age (Owens, 2001).

Other linguistic forms are acquired during the school-age years, such as the ability to distinguish between mass and count nouns. **Mass nouns** are nonindividual, homogeneous substances such as *water, sand,* and *money.* **Count nouns** are heterogeneous individual objects such as *a glass, a toy,* or *a house.* Mass nouns differ from count nouns in that the former cannot accept the plural morpheme -*s* (apple*s* versus sand*s*). Mass nouns take different quantifying modifiers (*much* and *little*) than those (*many* and *few*) taken by count nouns.

By early elementary school, children have learned most of the correct noun forms, so that constructions like *monies* and *mens* are rare. Early on, children discover a way around the quantifier question by using *lots of* with both types of nouns; however, children are able to use the correct quantifier (*some* and *any*) with mass nouns (*salt* or *sand*) by age 4 (Owens, 2001). *Many* then appears with plural count nouns, as in *many houses. Much* is usually learned by late elementary school, although even nine-year-olds may have difficulty with this form. Full mastery is not accomplished until adolescence (McLaughlin, 1998), when children attach the correct quantifier to the noun (*much* + a mass noun).

Syntax and Morphology: Language Differences

There are differences between the morphological and syntactic rules of Spanish and English (Goldstein, 2000). Spanish is a subject-drop language; therefore, the sentence "Tengo un gato" [have a cat] is considered grammatical. In contrast to English, with fixed word order, word order in Spanish is not fixed, e.g., "Los niños tienen dos gatos" [The boys have two cats] or "Tienen dos gatos los niños" [Have two cats the boys]. Unlike English, articles and adjectives agree with nouns, e.g., *el perro* [the dog] but *los perros* [the dogs]. These differences are often reflected in the English utterances of Spanish-speaking children when attempting to master English morphology and syntax.

According to the rules of African American English (AAE), certain inflectional morphemes need not necessarily be produced (possessive -*s*, plural-*s*, regular past -*ed*, and third-person -*s*) (Goldstein, 2000; Haynes and Shulman, 1998). Statements may not be reversed to form questions ("What it is?"); double negatives ("Nobody don't never like me") and pronominal appositions ("Daddy he mad") are also produced. MLU differences also are present among different languages and dialects. For example, a Standard American English (SAE) speaker might produce eight morphemes in the sentence, "Two cats are in John's house" (*two, cat, -s, are, in, John, -'s,* and *house*), but an AAE speaker might produce the same sentence with five morphemes, e.g., "Two cat in John house" (*two, cat, in, John,* and *house*) (Seymour and Roeper, 1999). These differences between AAE and SAE may lead an educator to believe that an AAE speaker has a language disorder rather than a language difference.

Because the rules of AAE require that redundant and repetitive information be avoided, certain morphemes (i.e., plural -*s*, possessive *'s,* and the auxiliary verb *are*) are omitted because this information is signaled by the preceding words (i.e., *two* + *cat* and *John* + *house*). Although both speakers may be typically developing children of the same age, an educator or a therapist may incorrectly judge the lower MLU to indicate a language delay. Because MLU differences can be found between SAE and AAE speakers, as well as speakers of other languages, speech-language pathologists must be cautious when using only MLU to determine language development for children with dialectal differences or for those children whose first language is not SAE. For a more detailed discussion of differences in language development, the reader is referred to Taylor and Leonard (1999), Haynes and Shulman (1998), Goldstein (2000), and also Chapter 8.

Summary

During the school-age years, children add new morphological and syntactic structures to their linguistic repertoire and expand and refine existing forms. These developments enable them to express increasingly more complex relationships and to use language more creatively.

In the next section, we will discuss semantic development during the school-age years. The focus will be on two aspects of meaning: vocabulary growth and the development of nonliteral meaning.

SCHOOL-AGE SEMANTIC DEVELOPMENT

During the school-age years, children increase the size of their vocabulary and the specificity of their word definitions. By 6 years of age, children's expressive vocabulary is at 2,600 words and receptive vocabulary is between 20,000 and 24,000 words (Owens, 2001). However, adding lexical items is only a portion of the change that occurs in a child's vocabulary growth.

During the school-age years, children's ability to add new dimensions to their existing lexicon also increases. Differences between the abilities of older and younger school-age children become evident when defining words. Whereas preschoolers define words narrowly in terms of their own experience, school-aged children define words using more socially shared meanings (McLaughlin, 1998). Their definitions not only include the meaning of a word learned in early childhood (*block*), but also new (and in some cases nonliteral) meanings of this word ("Walk around the block," "Don't block the entrance," "A block of text"). In high school, adolescents' definitions are abstract and/or represent a concept of function modified by perceptual attributes. The definitions of upper-high-school students (as well as of adults) tend to be descriptive, having concrete terms of reference to specific instances used to modify a concept, and contain synonyms, explanations, and categorizations (Johnson & Anglin, 1995).

Vocabulary knowledge is highly correlated with general linguistic competence and academic aptitude. Acquiring a broad vocabulary allows a child not only to understand and to express more complex ideas with greater facility but also to achieve a higher degree of competence in reading and writing.

The Development of Nonliteral Meaning

Nonliteral meaning adds richness and depth to language by communicating indirectly what would otherwise be communicated directly. Consider the meaning in the metaphor, "Her eyes were ice," or in the proverb, "The early bird catches the worm." Metaphors, proverbs, and jokes are examples of nonliteral language—with meaning that goes beyond the words of the sentence. The understanding and use of nonliteral meaning depend on the ability to disregard literal interpretation and to rely on non-referential, abstract, general meaning.

Metaphoric Language

Studies dealing with children's comprehension and use of nonliteral language have focused on **metaphors,** which use a likeness to stand for a word, a referent, or an idea ("He has a heart of stone"). When metaphoric language is marked by the connective *as* or *like,* it is called a **simile** ("It is as light as air").

The ability to comprehend metaphoric language emerges early and continues to develop with time (Bernstein, 1987; Nippold, 1985, 1991, 1998; Nippold, Leonard, & Kail, 1984). Although 3-year-old children may have some understanding of metaphor, they are unable to identify and to explain metaphors until about 7 years of age (Kogan & Chadrow, 1986; Vosniadou, Ortony, & Reynolds, 1984).

Metaphor comprehension requires the understanding that language can associate domains. For example, 5- to 7-year-old children have difficulty equating the physical and psychological domains and will interpret the metaphor, "She is a cold person," in physical terms—that is, the person is cold because of temperature or location in a cold place (Owens, 2001). Children do so because they do not understand the psychological meaning of words such as *sweet, cold,* or *bright* until they are 7 to 8 years of age (Westby, 1998). Children are able to understand cross-sensory metaphors ("Her perfume was bright as sunshine"), which associate perceptual domains, more easily than metaphors that associate the psychological-physical domains ("The prison guard was a hard rock") (Winner, Rosentiel, & Gardner, 1976).

Similarity metaphors, in which objects are compared based on shared features ("The stars are a thousand eyes"), are comprehended more easily than proportional metaphors, in which three objects are mentioned and a fourth must be inferred to complete a proportion ("My head is like an apple without a core"). Performance on each of the more difficult metaphor types increases with age. Billow (1975) suggested that the precise understanding and use of metaphors are related to children's cognitive development.

Idioms

Figurative, nonliteral expressions that express complex ideas in colorful and concise ways are called **idioms.** Included in different idiomatic types are semantically based idioms that can be assigned to various categories (foods—sour *grapes;* animals—dark *horse;* colors—in *the red*). Idiom comprehension develops and improves throughout childhood, adolescence, and into the adult years (Nippold, 1988, 1991; Nippold & Martin, 1989; Nippold & Taylor, 1995). Although preschoolers comprehend the nonliteral meaning of some idioms, their literal interpretation predominates through childhood and even adolescence (Nippold & Martin, 1989).

Proverbs

Another form of nonliteral language, proverbs, are more abstract than metaphors. In a **proverb,** the domain that is the topic is never mentioned. Wise sayings that express truths are such proverbs as "Don't put all your eggs in one basket," or "A stitch in time saves nine." Preadolescents are generally unable to interpret proverbs, and it is not until adolescence or adulthood that proverbs, are understood (Owens, 2001).

Humor

We often infer information about children's semantic knowledge (or lack of knowledge) from the riddles and jokes they understand and tell. The source of humor in riddles and in jokes is largely semantically based. Humor in riddles and jokes can depend on understanding words that sound the same but are spelled differently (*bear/bare*) or words that sound the same and are spelled the same way but have more than one meaning (*glasses, tie*). The comprehension of humor often depends on perceiving the incongruity among the meanings of homonyms or multiple-meaning words (*bank*) (Bernstein, 1986). Children's understanding of jokes and riddles depends on their metalinguistic skills and their ability to comprehend four types of linguistic ambiguity (Westby, 1998): (1) phonological ambiguity ("Why did the clock go to the doctor? Because he was tick."), (2) lexical ambiguity ("What happened to the girl's feet? She had bare feet."), (3) surface-structure ambiguity, based on a figurative versus literal interpretation of a word ("Tell me, how long are trains? Six letters."), and (4) deep-structure ambiguity, based on two diverse meanings for a phrase ("Call me a cab. You're a cab."). Phonological ambiguity is understood at 6 or 7 years of age, followed by the understanding of lexical ambiguity. The comprehension of surface-structure and deep-structure ambiguity occurs later in development.

Summary

In this section, current trends in the study of children's later semantic development were presented. We examined children's development of vocabulary and their understanding and use of nonliteral meaning as evidenced by their comprehension and use of figurative language and humor. These areas of semantic development are assessed during a language evaluation and may be targeted for remediation if found deficient.

The next section traces the expansion of school-age children's use of language in social contexts.

SCHOOL-AGE PRAGMATIC DEVELOPMENT

The development of pragmatics in the preschool years sets the stage for later changes. During the school years, children learn to be skilled conversationalists and more effective communicators as they become increasingly sensitive to what their listeners need to know. Throughout the school years, children increase their range of communication functions and learn how to become good conversational partners, how to make indirect requests, and how to process the language of the classroom. During this period, children learn to organize and plan narratives and can relate stories in a coherent and cohesive manner. Last, they add various means of conveying their intentions, including greater use of indirect expressions.

Expansion of Communicative Functions

In addition to the wide variety of communicative functions that preschoolers use, the changing world of the school-age child requires using language in a wider variety of social contexts. Children's social-emotional and cognitive skills enable them to expand their repertoire of language use. White (1975) maintained that the school-age child displays the following communicative abilities:

1. Gaining and holding adults' attention in a socially acceptable manner
2. Directing and following peers
3. Using others, when appropriate, as resources for assistance or for information
4. Expressing affection, hostility, and anger, when appropriate
5. Expressing pride in themselves and their accomplishments
6. Role-playing
7. Competing with peers in storytelling

The Development of Narratives

By the time children are in school, they exhibit a story-telling talent; that is, they can communicate information through coherent and cohesive units called narratives. **Narrative** is a form of discourse. It is an uninterrupted stream of language modified by the speaker to capture and hold the listener's interest and attention (Owens, 2001). Narratives differ from conversations in a number of ways. When producing a narrative, the speaker produces a monologue throughout and must presuppose the information needed by the listener. In addition, the speaker must present all the information in an organized way, and introduce and organize the sequences of events so that the elements of the narrative are related and lead to some conclusion.

As toddlers, children are exposed to narratives, or stories, in picture books and on television and, as noted previously, they are able to produce narratives by age 4. By first grade, demands are placed on children to relate narratives, to participate in show-and-tell, to relate vacation activities or holiday experiences, or to retell a story heard previously. Later, these activities appear in the form of written assignments such as "My Summer Vacation," "How I Spent the Holidays," or a synopsis of a book.

A perspective on the natural structure of narrative is seen in the work of Stein and Glenn (1979). Stein and Glenn (1979) describe a model of story structure that follows certain rules. According to this model, stories have an internal structure. They contain statements that are logically connected to reflect causal and temporal relationships, and contain principles that promotes structure and cohesion. Stein and Glenn maintain that stories are made up of various categories, units, and rules. Category definitions and the rules of the story grammar model are shown in Table 2.16.

When competent storytellers structure their information, a full understanding of the story is ensured. When children hear stories in which the information sequences are inverted (for example, they are told the consequence unit before the initiating event), they remember the events less well than if the story is told to them in the order given by the model. If children are given individual narrative statements and asked to make up a story, the sequence of their stories correlates highly with the sequence

TABLE 2.16	**Story Grammar Model**

Initiating Event	Action or occurrence that influences the main characters (rain, storm, earthquake): the perception of an event (thunder), a physiological state (hunger, thirst, fatigue)
Internal Response	A character's emotional status relative to the initiating event; a reference to motivation or purpose
Plan	The character's strategy for solving a problem or obtaining a goal
Attempt	The actions used to solve the problem or to obtain the goal
Consequence	Success or failure in the attempt to solve the problem or to obtain the goal
Resolution	The character's feelings, thoughts, or actions in response to the consequences; success or failure of the protagonist
Ending	The conclusion of the story: a summary of the story or a moral

From Introduction to Language Development, 1st edition, by McLaughlin © 1998. Reprinted with permission of Delmar a division of Thomson Learning. Fax 800-730-2215.

predicted by the story grammar model. In addition, when asked to retell a story, children are most likely to include the setting unit, initiating event, and the consequence unit.

Although children use the schematic knowledge of story grammars to understand stories and to formulate narratives, there are developmental differences between the abilities of younger and older children (Westby, 1998). The following characteristics are more likely found in the stories of 10-year-olds:

1. Greater detail in setting information
2. Goal directed episode: centering (central character) and chaining (one activity the cause of another); story grammar components appear for initiating event, response, and consequence
3. Complete episodes: character goals and intentions described; story grammar components present for initiating event, internal response, plan, attempt, and consequence
4. In general, less extraneous detail

By the late elementary school period, children's narratives consist of elaborated stories that contain:

1. Multiple episodes: story with "chapters," and each chapter consisting of minimal story grammar structure
2. Complex episodes: multiple plans and multiple attempts because of obstacles to obtaining a goal
3. Embedded episodes: one episode embedded in another

School-aged children also include reference to emotional states, double meanings, mystery, attitude statements, and story evaluations in their narratives (Crais & Lorch, 1994). The older adolescent storyteller not only utilizes the above abilities, but also employs argumentation and dramatization, and includes asides and morals in the narrative (Larson & McKinley, 1995).

Conversational Skills

Children learn language within a conversational context. Although preschool children acquire many conversational skills, much of their conversation centers on the here-and-now. However, they must learn about the conventional routines of conversation, such as taking turns (being a sender or a receiver), clarifying or repairing their message, and maintaining a topic. These skills are refined during the school-age years.

Two processes enable the child to become a more effective communicator, neo-egocentrism and decentration. **Neo-egocentrism** is the ability to take the perspective of another person. (This ability has also been called *presuppositional ability*.) In general, as a communication task becomes more difficult, the young child is less able to take a speaker's perspective. As the child matures cognitively and socially and gains greater facility with language structure, she can concentrate more effectively on her audience. Being able to shift perspective enables her to consider what the listener knows (and needs to know) when she constructs a message. This ability is refined during the school years. Being neo-egocentric also allows the child greater facility in the use of deictic terms. You will recall that the understanding and use of these terms depend on the nonlinguistic context—the perspective of the speaker and the listener. The acquisition of deictic terms begins in the preschool period and advances during the school years.

Decentration is the ability to consider several aspects of a problem simultaneously. This cognitive achievement allows the child to move from one-dimensional descriptions of objects and events to coordinated, multiattributional ones. The child recognizes that many dimensions can be used to describe an object or an event and adjusts her messages accordingly (Owens, 1996). Whereas a younger child's descriptions are more personal and do not consider the information that must be available to the listener, a school-age child's messages are more accurate because the child considers the listener's perspective and provides more extensive information. By the time children reach Piaget's concrete operational stage, they perceive the needs of their listeners and make undifferentiated adaptations in their communication to satisfy those needs. In settling peer disputes, children give reasons for disagreements involving their own feelings and beliefs about an event or an action. In the stage of formal operations, children adapt to their listeners' needs in a differentiated manner by negotiating, justifying, and stating reasons for their positions. Table 2.17 summarizes the different communication strategies used by children in Piaget's preoperational, concrete, and formal operational stages. Note the differences between older and younger children's communicative strategies.

Clarification

Successful conversation involves coordinated interaction between speakers and listeners, and when misunderstandings occur, speakers must repair their messages. During the school-age years, children repair and clarify their messages using a variety of

TABLE 2.17 Communication Strategy Development: An Overview

Cognitive Stage	Strategy	Examples
Preoperational (ages 2–7)		
Early	Self-oriented perception Nonadaptation to listener	*Context:* Jim and John in sandbox. John wants to play with the pail and shovel. Jim is playing with it.
		John: Gimme pail and shovel.
Late	Perception of listener Nonadaptation to listener	*Context:* Sue and Jean are in the yard. Sue has been riding the bike for five minutes.
		Jean: Now *I* want to ride the bike!
Concrete (ages 7–11)	Perception of listener Undifferentiated adaptation to listener	*Context:* Bill and Sam are on the playground.
		Bill: Please, pretty please, can I try your baseball glove?
		Context: Linda borrowed Stacy's pen.
		Linda: I'm sorry I broke your pen.
Formal (ages 11–14)	Perception of listener Differentiated adaptation to listener needs	*Context:* Jason and Peter are on the playground.
		Jason: If you'll let me try your mitt, I'll let you try my head-to-head football game. (Jason takes the game out of his pocket.)
		Context: Lisa has returned from school. Her mother is upset.
		Lisa: I know you're upset, but the English teacher assigned a composition about El Salvador for tomorrow, and I stopped off at the library to get some books to do the research.

strategies (Konefal & Folks, 1984). Whereas 6-year-olds will elaborate some elements in their repetitions and provide more information to a listener, 9-year-olds are capable of addressing the source of the communicative breakdown and can produce background, context, and can define terms to provide additional clarification (Owens, 2001). Nine-year-olds not only elaborate their repetitions, they also seem capable of addressing the perceived source of communication breakdown. Last, they are sensitive to cues that indicate the failure of the communicative attempt and can talk about the process of conversational repair (Brinton, Fujiki, Loeb, & Winkler, 1986, Crais & Lorch, 1994; Hulit & Howard, 1997).

Topic Maintenance

Much of the control of conversation during the young school-age years is exercised by adults who ask children many questions. As noted previously, preschool children maintain a topic by repeating the information in the adult utterance, but older children provide additional information in their responses (Brinton & Fujiki, 1984).

During the school-age years, approximately 60 percent of children's peer interactions are effective. This is because children of this age have developed metalinguistic skills, or the ability to reflect on effectiveness of the language used in conversation. The greatest change occurs during the years from late elementary school to adulthood (Brinton & Fujiki, 1984; Nelson, 1993). A related decrease in the number of different topics introduced or reintroduced occurs. Thus, the school years bring a growing adherence to the concept of conversational relevance and topic maintenance. Although 8-year-olds can sustain a topic through a number of conversational turns, their topics tend to be concrete. Discussions involving abstract topics usually are not sustained until age 11 (Owens, 2001).

Code Switching

When they talk to their peers, 8-year-olds speak differently than when addressing infants or adults. When speaking with infants, school-age children tend to reduce the length and complexity of their utterances, appearing to understand that very young children require a different form of interaction. Among adults, school-age children vary their codes for parents and for those outside the family. In general, parents are usually the recipients of demands, whining, and short (less conversational) narrative (Owens, 2001). It is not surprising that parents are often shocked when their child, who talks to them with language that is less than polite and informative, is described by other adults as charming, entertaining, and interesting.

During the later school age years, conversation becomes more demanding. It is an important medium for adolescents' social interaction. During conversation, adolescents add information during their turn and can shade from one topic to another (Larson & McKinley, 1995). During this period, the adolescent can make transitions between formal and informal language, relying more on formal registers with not only adults, but their peers as well (unless particularly close to the peer). Modification of the verb phrase is key in switching between informal and formal codes ("Pass me my pen," as opposed to "Would you pass me my pen?")—a skill that the adolescent masters. Lastly, conversation directed to peers by adolescents usually involves more expressed feelings than conversation directed toward adults (Larson & McKinley, 1995).

Indirect Requests

Another dimension of pragmatic development that occurs during the school-age years is the ability to use indirect requests. The development of indirect requests is particularly noteworthy because it represents the child's growing awareness of both socially appropriate requests and the communication context (Hulit & Howard, 1997).

Indirect requests are first produced in the preschool years; the proportion of their occurrence to direct requests increases between the ages of 3 and 5 (Garvey, 1977). This proportion does not change markedly between ages 5 and 6 (Levin & Rubin, 1982). In general, the 5-year-old gets what she wants by asking for it *directly*. By age 7, however, she gains greater facility with indirect forms (Garvey, 1975; Grimm, 1975). Flexibility in the use of indirect requests continues to increase with age. For example, Ervin-Tripp (1980) found that the proportion of hints ("That sweater would go so nicely with my new skirt") increases from childhood through adulthood.

Pragmatics: Language Differences

Researchers have shown that cultural differences can affect pragmatic skills (Taylor, 1999). For example, African American English (AAE) speakers view direct or personal questions as inappropriate and tolerate interruption in conversation. AAE speakers are said to prefer indirect eye contact to direct eye contact while listening to a speaker, whereas Spanish language users view lack of eye contact as inappropriate. Finally, hand shaking with persons of the opposite sex is not customary for Asians and Asian Americans.

In addition to cultural nonverbal communication differences, Haynes and Shulman (1998) report that narratives vary in different cultures. For example, when producing stories, Spanish-speaking children use articles and nouns *(a girl . . .), pronouns (he . . .)*, ellipsis ("She went to school, ate her lunch"), and demonstratives (*this*) for cohesion (Owens, 2001). On the other hand, AAE narrative style employs anecdotes that are more personal, and prosody is used more often than semantic or syntactic cues for cohesion. For more information on cultural and linguistic differences, see Chapter 8.

Summary

In our review of pragmatic development, we have seen that children elaborate their use of language to suit a variety of social contexts and begin to gain competence in their use of different discourse skills (i.e., conversations, narratives).

In the next section, we will focus on a child's ability to think about language independent of the basic requirements of comprehension and production. These metalinguistic skills support the ability to meet the linguistic needs of the school-aged child, such as the demands of the classroom.

Language in the Classroom

The language of the classroom differs from that used in informal social interactions. In the classroom, children are expected to process the language of the teacher and the language of the textbooks. As grade levels increase, so does the complexity of the language that the students are expected to process (Nelson, 1986; Chapter 5).

Children with language abilities commensurate with the linguistic demands of the classroom do well in school. However, children who have linguistic deficits have difficulty in the classroom that can affect them emotionally and socially (Gerber, 1981; Nelson, 1985, 1993).

The language of the classroom differs in several ways from that used in informal social interaction and the language of the home. Children of preschool age receive their major linguistic input from caretakers and can rely on the familiarity of the home context to help them understand what is expected of them. Because language at home depends heavily on context, children can act appropriately by following familiar routines, even if they understand only a little of what is presented to them linguistically. In addition, interactions between children and caretakers during the preschool years are dyadic; if children misunderstand the language directed to them, their caretakers repair the message.

Language in the classroom, however, is highly **decontextualized,** that is, it is not presented in the context that is related to the topic discussed. This removes the contextual cues that the child can rely on to better understand classroom language. In addition, in school, as children advance through the grades, teachers use longer sentences, more complex syntactic structures, more rapid speaking rates (Cuda & Nelson, 1976; Nelson, 1986, 1993), and the number of opportunities to obtain clarification is decreased (McLaughlin, 1998). Lastly, textbook language is expository, more varied in content, and less predictable (Westby, 1998). Table 2.18 describes the characteristics of expository texts.

Because of the increased linguistic demands of the classroom, children with language deficits cannot derive maximal benefit from classroom instruction. In

TABLE 2.18 Characteristics of Expository Texts

Text Pattern	Text Function	Key Words
Description	The text tells what somethings is.	Is called, can be defined as, is, can be interpreted as, is explained as, refers to, is a procedure for, is someone who, means
Collection/enumeration	The text gives a list of things that are related to the topic.	An example is, for instance, another, next, finally, such as, to illustrate
Sequence/procedure	The text tells what happened or how to do something or make something.	First, next, then, second, third, following this step, finally, subsequently, from here . . . to, eventually, before, after
Comparison/contrast	The text shows how two things are the same or different.	Different, same, alike, similar, although, however, on the other hand, contrasted with, compared with, rather than, but, yet, still, instead of
Cause/effect explanation	The text gives reasons for why something happened.	Because, since, reasons, then, therefore, for this reason, results, effects, consequently, so, in order to, thus, depends on, influences, is a function of, produces, leads to, affects, hence
Problem/solution	The text states a problem and offers solutions to the problem.	A problem is, a solution is

From Communicative refinement in school age and adolescence, C. E. Westby (1998). In W. O. Haynes and B. B. Shulman (Eds.), *Communication development: Foundations, processes, and clinical applications.* Baltimore, MD: Lippincott Williams & Wilkins. Copyright © 1998 Lippincott Williams & Wilkens. Reprinted by permission.

educational settings, the speech-language pathologist can provide the classroom teacher with strategies to help support the academic success of children with language difficulties (see Chapters 7 and 9).

THE DEVELOPMENT OF METALINGUISTIC ABILITIES

During the preschool period, children view language as a means of communicating. They do not focus on the manner in which language is conveyed. During the school-age years, children begin to reflect on language as a decontextualized object. This ability is called **metalinguistic ability** and enables children to think and to talk about language—that is, to treat language as an object of analysis and to use language to talk about language. The development of metalinguistic abilities is most obvious during middle childhood, between 5 and 8 years of age.

van Kleeck (1982) identified three important aspects of metalinguistic development: (1) recognizing that language is an arbitrary conventional code, (2) recognizing that language is a system of units and rules for combining those units, and (3) recognizing that language is used for communication.

1. Language is an arbitrary conventional code. Understanding that language is an arbitrary conventional code includes understanding that words are arbitrary labels, separate from the objects or events they represent. Young children do not recognize the arbitrary nature of language; thus, they tend to treat words as though they were part of their referents. For example, a 4-year-old might say that the word *jet* is a big word because jets are big and that *ant* is a short word because ants are short. In contrast, a 7-year-old is likely to say that the word *jet* is a small word because it does not have many letters.

Evidence of the arbitrary nature of language can also be seen in children's ability to recognize ambiguity—that is, that words and sentences can have more than one meaning. An example of ambiguity detection involves the recognition that the sentence, "The duck is ready to eat," could mean either (1) the duck (that is in the field) is ready to eat some grass or (2) the duck (which has been cooked) is ready to be served for dinner. Surface- and deep-structure ambiguity, such as in sentences that allow for more than one interpretation ("She fed her dog biscuits"), are not understood until 11 or 12 years of age (Westby, 1998).

Children's awareness of the arbitrary nature of words is reflected in rhyming and word play. In this case, children are able to understand that words are composed of segments and that these segments can be manipulated. Another metalinguistic skill that depends on the awareness that language is an arbitrary code is the ability to understand that different sentence forms can convey the same meaning. This ability is called **recognizing synonymy**. An example of recognizing synonymy would be realizing that the following sentences describe the same event: "The girl chased the boy," "The boy was chased by the girl," and "It was the girl who chased the boy." Children are unable to recognize synonymy until the early to middle elementary school years (Tunmer, Pratt, & Herriman, 1984).

2. Language is a system of units and rules. The awareness that language is a system of units is demonstrated by children's ability to break down larger linguistic units into smaller parts. This ability allows the child to divide the sentence, "The dog chased the cat," into five words. It also enables the child to break down the word *cat* into three phonemes. The ability to segment words into their component sounds is a result of the child's phonological awareness. It is characterized by the ability to rhyme, to segment words into syllables and sounds, to manipulate sounds, and to blend sounds (Goswami & Bryant, 1990). Three-year-old children are able to break words into syllables but not into segments, but six-year-old children are able to accomplish both tasks. Researchers have found a strong relationship between early rhyming abilities and later phonological awareness (Ball, 1997; Blachman, 1991; Bryant, MacLean, & Bradley, 1990; Catts, 1996; Hatcher, Hulme, & Ellis, 1994; MacLean, Bryant, & Bradley, 1987; Shaywitz, Fletcher, Holahan, & Shaywitz, 1992; Snyder & Downey, 1997; Swanson, Mink, & Bocian, 1999; Torgesen, Wagner, & Rashotte, 1994; Westby, 1998).

The recognition that linguistic rules must be used to combine syntactic units also emerges during the early school years (Owens, 2001). This is illustrated by children's awareness that the utterance, "The cat chasing the dog," is ungrammatical, and that to make it grammatically acceptable one must either add an auxiliary verb (*is* or *was*), change the progressive form to the third-person singular (*chases*), or use the past tense of the verb chase (*chased*).

3. Language is used for communication. As noted in a previous section, preschool-age children demonstrate some awareness of the social rules for language use at age 3 to 4, but it is not until the early elementary school years that they can judge the adequacy and appropriateness of their messages—what constitutes good communication. They can judge if an utterance is appropriate for a specific listener or setting and are aware that they should be polite to achieve their goals.

Metalinguistic abilities emerge about the same time children are learning to read, and it has been suggested that metalinguistic awareness and reading development are related (Blackman & James, 1985; Catts, 1996; Saywitz & Cherry-Wilkinson, 1982; Tunmer & Bowey, 1984; van Kleeck, 1995). However, research has also shown that some language-disordered children demonstrate deficits in metalinguistic abilities (Kamhi & Koenig, 1985; van Kleeck, 1995; Wallach & Butler, 1994), and that metalinguistic and language processing deficits underlie reading disabilities (Brady & Shankweiler, 1991; Catts, 1996; Catts & Kamhi, 1987; Fletcher et al., 1994; Vellutino, Scanlon, Small, & Tanzman, 1991). Silliman and Diehl (Chapter 5) and Seidenberg (Chapter 9) suggest that speech-language pathologists need to assess metalinguistic abilities in school-age children suspected of having a language disorder or a reading disability.

Reading Development

Reading is a complex process that is not totally understood by development and educator professionals. However, it is now recognized that literacy is built on a foundation of intact language skills, and that there is a relationship between phonological awareness, verbal memory and retrieval, and learning to read.

It is beyond the scope of this chapter to detail reading models and the cognitive processes that underlie this area of development. However, because reading is a language-based process and language pathologists target linguistic intervention in their therapy with children who have language learning or reading disabilities, their understanding of the links between oral language, reading, and reading difficulties is crucial.

Five stages of reading development have been proposed by Chall (1983). At the prereading stage, from birth to 5 or 6 years of age, children establish the understanding that print has meaning. They also learn to perceive the differences or the contrasts between sounds, to recognize and discriminate between the letters of the alphabet, and to scan print. By 4 years of age, children are able to recognize their names in print and some words in signs and labels (Dickinson, Wolf, & Stotsky, 1993). The word *stop* and the *M* symbol for McDonald's restaurant are recognized at an early age.

The first stage of reading development, from 5 to 7 years of age, consists of learning phoneme–grapheme correspondence rules. However, often there is a lack of correlation between sounds and written segments, such as the association of the grapheme *a* with at last three different sounds (*hat, came,* and *lawn*). This makes the mastery of some sound–letter correspondences difficult for children. Early on, children concentrate on decoding single words in simple stories. At this stage, children rely on the visual configuration of a word in order to recognize it. They pay particular attention to the first letter of the word and to word length while ignoring the order of the letters. Children at this stage learn letter–sound correspondence rules, recognize their importance, and are able to sound out novel words by using the phonetic approach. In addition, they learn that text provides messages and does more than just describe pictures (Ferreiro & Teberosky, 1982).

First-grade readers begin to use text to analyze unknown words. Whenever they read a word incorrectly, it is because they do not know that particular word. Instead, they substitute another word that makes sense in that context. Torgesen (1999) presents three facts regarding context: (1) skilled readers do not rely solely on context (Share & Stanovich, 1995), (2) poor readers rely on context more than good readers (Briggs, Austin, & Underwood, 1984), and (3) context is not adequate for word identification.

The second stage of reading development, from 7 to 9 years of age, involves consolidating the knowledge gained in the earlier stages. Children learn to use their knowledge of decoding skills and of story structure to increase their understanding of written materials. They are able to recognize words based on orthographic configuration or spelling patterns and are able to use information about the phonological composition of words to aid them in decoding. However, at this stage, many children with reading difficulties are unable to make use of phonological material or the composition of words to aid them in coding.

In the third stage, from 9 to 14 years of age, decoding abilities are automatized and children are now able to focus on the comprehension of reading material (Kamhi & Catts, 1991).

The fourth stage, from 14 to 18 years of age, finds that lower-level skills are firmly established. Adolescents must now use higher-order skills, such as inference and the recognition of the author's viewpoint, to assist them in comprehending the written material. The final stage, from 18 years of age and up, finds readers able to deal with multiple points of view. Since vocabulary skills are now well developed, the ability to read critically and to understand more abstract written materials increases.

Phonological Decoding

Investigators now believe that stage theories offer an oversimplification of reading development because (1) children follow different paths and (2) not all words are read with the same approach at each stage (Catts & Kamhi, 1999; Share & Stanovich, 1995). For example, readers are confronted by unfamiliar words at all stages of development. Therefore, the strategies used for unfamiliar words may require different strategies than are used for familiar words. A self-teaching theory of reading development, based on phonological decoding, has been proposed to explain the development of word-recognition skills by children.

This self-teaching mechanism begins with early decoding of the correspondence between sounds and letters. These correspondences become associated with particular words as children become aware of spelling regularities. Consequently, high-frequency words (e.g., cat) are recognized quickly, but low-frequency words require the phonetic decoding skills developed earlier (i.e., sound–letter correspondences). Children may use partial decoding to identify unfamiliar words. For example, they use the first letter or letters to establish sound identity. Next, they rely on contextual information to confirm their decoding judgments. Later in development, children develop the awareness of morphology and use language-based units to decode new words (Catts and Kamhi, 1999). This theory points to the need for early and frequent exposure to print in order to familiarize children with sound–letter correspondences.

Reading Processes

Theoretical positions that attempt to explain the processes involved in reading follow two major approaches: the bottom-up approach (perceptual and phonemic processes) and the top-down approach (cognitive processes). These processes are viewed as being interactive, with a third- or fourth-grade reader using the bottom-up strategy for reading words in isolation and the top-down strategy for text (Owens, 2001).

The Bottom-Up Approach

The **bottom-up approach** defines reading as the "translation of written elements into language" (Perfetti, 1984, p. 41). Bottom-up theories emphasize lower-level perceptual and phonemic processes and their influence on higher cognitive functioning. According to this view, knowledge of the perceptual features of letters and of their correspondence to sounds assists in word recognition and decoding. The bottom-up theory assumes that the child must learn to decode print into language. That is, the child must be able to divide each word into phonemic elements and learn the alphabetical letters (graphemes) that correspond to these phonemes. Only when this process is automatic can the child give sufficient attention to the meaning of the text. If the child gains automaticity processing at the visual and auditory levels, the other stages of processing written materials will be more easily acquired.

According to the bottom-up theory, each word acts like a switchboard that activates the visual, auditory, and semantic features of that word. If the reader has enough information from these features, the information is automatically presented to the other parts of the system for processing. In sum, the bottom-up theory of reading emphasizes that lower-level processes (perceptual and phonological stages) critically influence all further stages of processing.

The Top-Down Approach

In contrast to the bottom-up theories, theories that subscribe to the **top-down approach** emphasize the cognitive task of deriving meaning from print. This approach has been termed the problem-solving model (Owens, 2001). Higher cognitive functions, such as concepts, inferences, and levels of meaning, influence the processing of lower-order information. The reader generates hypotheses about the written material based on her world knowledge, the content of the material in the text, and the syntactic structures used. Sampling of the reading confirms or disconfirms the hypotheses.

The Interactive Approach

The interactive approach to explaining the reading process incorporates portions of both bottom-up and top-down models (Rumelhart, 1977; Stanovich, 1980). According to this view, top-down and bottom-up processes provide information to the reader simultaneously, at various levels of analysis. This information is then synthesized. The processes are interactive and relative reliance on each varies with the skills of the reader and the material that is being read.

It has been proposed that by third or fourth grade, children rely on a bottom-up strategy when reading isolated words and a top-down strategy when reading text. Context supports the more rapid, top-down processes; when such support is lacking, the slower, bottom-up processes are used. Although variations on bottom-up and top-down models of reading abound, all researchers agree that learning to read requires the integration of multiple sensory, perceptual, linguistic, and conceptual processing strategies.

Writing Development

Phonological abilities also play a role in writing development (Lewis, O'Donnell, Freebairn, & Taylor, 1998). Consistent with reading development, phonological awareness is considered a strong predictor of spelling success (Nation & Hulme, 1997). The awareness of the correspondence between sounds and letters is necessary for translating the speech sounds (phonemes) to written letters (graphemes). Learning to spell also involves morphological knowledge (Kamhi & Hinton, 2000). For example, children must learn that the past -*ed* morpheme has different phonological realizations, such as *pitched* (/t/), *dragged* (/d/), and *ticketed* (/ɪd/).

The development of writing abilities follows five stages (Henderson & Beers, 1980; Owens, 2001): the preliterate stage, the letter-name stage, the within-word stage, the syllable juncture stage, and the derivational constancy stage. Written language is initially represented by drawing, followed by scribbling, followed by attempts to represent letters, followed by inventive spelling, and culminating in conventional writing patterns.

In the preliterate stage, children draw, scribble, begin to write some letters, and talk about the writing project at hand. Writing and drawing are differentiated by 3 years of age (Owens, 2001). In the letter-name stage, children use invented spellings. In this stage, children rely on phonological knowledge, with each written letter representing a speech sound. The sound that children hear is matched to the letter, and their writing reflects this match. Initially, children represent the entire word with the first letter and pay little attention to the other letters of the word. For example, DRLM or DBC may represent *daddy* or MBRS may represent *mommy* (Owens, 2001). This is similar to the initial stage of reading, in which the child pays attention to only the first letter.

Next, children represent syllables, often without vowels. For example, *girl* might be written as GRL or *boy* as BY. In the final stage of inventive spelling, phonemic spelling, children are aware of the alphabet and the correspondence of graphemes to phonemes. Words such as *cat, it,* and *me* are spelled correctly, but words such as *knife, night,* or *soup* are not. Examples of spelling development are also shown in the attempts to spell *dragon* by different children at different grades: MPRMRHM (kindergarten), GAGIN (first grade), and DRAGUN (second grade). The sentence YUTS A LADE YET FEHEG AD HE KOT FLEPR is an example of invented spelling that represents the sentence, "Once a lady went fishing and she caught Flipper" (Temple, Nathan, Temple, & Burris, 1993). Finally, children are aware of the sound–symbol correspondence and can produce sentences like HE HAD A BLUE CLTH to represent "He had a blue cloth" (Owens, 2001).

In the letter-name stage, children are not concerned with finding a sound–letter match, but in the within-word pattern stage, they rely on standard orthographic patterns to write. They also begin to recognize the correct spelling of grammatical endings and sound–spelling differences. In addition, better-developed aspects of a child's spelling, handwriting, and sentence structure will often deteriorate when new levels of complexity are introduced, such as changes from print to script or the introduction of greater complexity.

At the syllable juncture stage, children are aware of stress patterns in words, and at the derivational constancy stage they attend to root forms of words. The formal instruction of school brings mastery of the conventional spelling system. In addition, during the school-age years, children begin to pay attention to format, spacing, and punctuation when producing a written piece of work. In the third or fourth grade, their increased syntactic knowledge allows them to write using complex clauses and phrases, and to revise and proofread their written work. By the end of elementary school, the complexity of typically developing children's written language surpasses that of their spoken language (Gillam & Johnson, 1992).

Summary

In the school-age years, language development increases significantly. By kindergarten, children have acquired much of the mature language user's form. Development continues as children add new forms and gain new skills in transmitting messages. During the school-age years, children expand their sentences, their vocabulary, and they master nonliteral language. Their conversational abilities increase with their social skills and they become good story tellers. Once children have gained a working knowledge of spoken language, most of them adapt to the new mode of written language (reading and writing) with relative ease. Their metalinguistic abilities enable them to decontextualize language and use their knowledge to understand language in the classroom. However, for children with language learning difficulties, the school years pose special problems. Their needs must be met by a variety of specialists who assess their skills and integrate programming so that they can fully benefit from classroom instruction (see Chapters 5, 7, and 9). We conclude this chapter with a quotation from Rees (1980):

> For professionals in the area of communication disorders, it is recognized that only the most complete understanding possible of the nature and growth of child language will suffice as basic information with which to approach clinical problems. Normal language development provides not only the base of reference against which to evaluate the communicative functioning of the clinical subject, but also guidelines for assessment and intervention. (p. 38)

Information about language development in typically developing children provides the speech-language pathologist with a framework for understanding the assessment and remediation of language disorders in children. Because new knowledge is continuously emerging about the stages, strategies, and processes of normal language development, what we "do today will be replaced tomorrow by wiser principles and improved techniques" (Rees, 1980, p. 38).

STUDY QUESTIONS

1. Describe the prelinguistic abilities of young children.
2. Explain the importance of environmental interaction in language acquisition.
3. What are the major communicative intents coded by young children?
4. Outline the semantic relations found in preschool children and give examples of each.
5. Describe the phonological processes observed in preschoolers' language and explain which phonological processes should disappear by 3 years of age.
6. What are the main characteristics of each of Roger Brown's stages of language development?
7. Describe the literacy events that support emergent literacy.
8. Compare the pragmatic skills of preschool and school-aged children.
9. Trace narrative development from the preschool years through the school-age years. What major changes take place?
10. List the metalinguistic abilities that are related to the development of reading and (a) briefly describe the bottom-up and top-down theories of reading, (b) explain the stages in the development of reading abilities.
11. Describe the development of writing abilities.
12. Trace the syntactic achievements of the preschool-age years.

REFERENCES

Abrahamsen, E., & Rigrodsky, S. (1984). Comprehension of complex sentences in children at three levels of cognitive development. *Journal of Psycholinguistic Research, 13,* 333–350.

Ball, E. W. (1997). Phonological awareness: Implications for whole language and emergent literacy programs. *Topics in Language Disorders, 17,* 14–26.

Bankson, N. W., & Bernthal, J. E. (1998). Analysis and interpretation of assessment data. In J. E. Bernthal and N. W. Bankson (Eds.). *Articulation and phonological disorders* (4th ed.), (pp. 270–298). Boston: Allyn & Bacon.

Beck, I., & Jeul, C. (1995). The role of decoding in learning to read. *American Educator, 19*(2), 8–13.

Bellugi, U. (1967). The acquisition of negation. Doctoral dissertation, Harvard University.

Berko Gleason, J. (2001). *The development of language* (5th ed.). Boston: Allyn & Bacon.

Bernstein, D. K. (1986). The development of humor: Implications for assessment and intervention. *Topics in Language Disorders, 4,* 65–73.

Bernstein, D. K. (1987). Figurative language: Assessment strategies and implications for intervention. *Folia Phoniatrica, 39,* 130–144.

Bernthal, J. E., & Bankson, N. W. (Eds.). (1998). *Articulation and phonological disorders* (4th ed.). Boston: Allyn & Bacon.

Billow, R. (1975). A cognitive developmental study of metaphor comprehension. *Developmental Psychology, 11,* 415–423.

Blachman, B. (1991). Phonological awareness: implications for prereading and early reading instruction. In S. Brady and D. Shanweiler (Eds.), *Phonological processes in literacy* (pp. 29–36). Hillsdale, NJ: Erlbaum.

Blackman, B., & James, S. (1985). Metalinguistic abilities and reading achievement in first grade children. In J. Niles and R. Lalid (Eds.), *Issues in literacy: A research perspective* (pp. 280–286). Thirty-fourth Yearbook of the National Reading Conference.

Bloom, L. (1991). *Language development from two to three.* Cambridge, UK: Cambridge University Press.

Bloom, L., Lahey, M., Hood, L., Lifter, K., & Fiess, K. (1980). Complex sentences: Acquisition of syntactic connectives and the semantic relations they encode. *Journal of Child Language, 7,* 235–261.

Bloom, L., Lifter, K., & Hafitz, J. (1980). Semantics of verbs and the development of verb inflection in child language. *Language, 56,* 386–412.

Bloom, L., Lightbown P., & Hood, L. (1975). Structure and variation in child language. *Monographs of the Society for Research in Child Development, 40.*

Bloom, L., Merkin, S., & Wooten, J. (1982). *Wh*-questions: Linguistic factors that contribute to the sequence of acquisition. *Child Development, 53,* 1084–1092.

Bloom, L., Rocissano, L., & Hood, L. (1976). Adult-child discourse: Developmental interactions between information processing and linguistic interaction. *Cognitive Psychology, 8,* 521–552.

Bloom, P. (1990). Syntactic distinctions in child language. *Journal of Child Language, 17,* 343–356.

Bloom, P., Barss, A., Nicol, J., & Conway, L. (1994). Children's knowledge of binding and coreference: Evidence from spontaneous speech. *Language, 70*(1), 53–71.

Brady, S., & Shankweiler, D. (Eds.). (1991). *Phonological processes in literacy.* Hillsdale, NJ: Lawrence Erlbaum.

Briggs, A., Austin, R., & Underwood, G. (1984). Phonological coding in good and poor readers. *Reading Research Quarterly, 20,* 54–66.

Brinton, B., & Fujiki, M. (1984). Development of topic manipulation skills in discourse. *Journal of Speech and Hearing Research, 27,* 350–358.

Brinton, B., Fujiki, M., Loeb, D., & Winkler, E. (1986). Development of conversational repair strategies in response to request for clarification. *Journal of Speech and Hearing Research, 39,* 75–82.

Brown, R. (1975). *A first language: The early stages.* Cambridge, MA: Harvard University Press.

Bryant, P., Bradley, L., MacLean, M., & Crossland, J. (1989). Nursery rhymes, phonological skills and reading. *Journal of Child Language, 16,* 407–428.

Bryant, P., MacLean, M., & Bradley, L. (1990). Rhyme, language, and children's reading. *Applied Psycholinguistics, 11*(3), 237–252.

Butler, K. (1999). From oracy to literacy: A millennial perspective. *Topics in Language Disorders.* Frederick, MD: Aspen Press.

Cairns, H. S. (1996). *The acquisition of language* (2nd ed.). Austin, TX: Pro-Ed.

Catts, H. W. (1991). Early identification of reading disabilities. *Topics in Language Disorders, 12*(1), 1–17.

Catts, H. W. (1996). Defining dyslexia as a developmental language disorder: An expanded view. *Topics in Language Disorders, 16*(2), 14–25.

Catts, H. W., & Kamhi, A. G. (Eds.). (1999). *Language and reading disabilities.* Boston: Allyn & Bacon.

Chall, J. (1983). *Stages of reading development.* New York: McGraw-Hill.

Chien, Y., & Wexler, K. (1990). Children's knowledge of locality conditions in binding as evidence for the modularity of syntax and pragmatics. *Language Acquisition, 1,* 225–295.

Choi, S. (2000). Caregiver input in English and Korean: Use of nouns in book-reading and toy-play contexts. *Journal of Child Language, 27,* 69–96.

Choi, S., & Gopnik, A. (1995). Early acquisition of verbs in Korean: A cross-linguistic study. *Journal of Child Language, 22,* 497–529.

Chomsky, C. (1969). *The acquisition of syntax in children from 5 to 10.* Cambridge, MA: MIT Press.

Crais, E. R., & Lorch, N. (1994). Oral narratives in school age children. *Topics in Language Disorders, 14*(3), 13–28.

Cuda, R. A., & Nelson, N. (1976, November). Analysis of teacher speaking rate, syntactic complexity, and hesitation phenomena as a function of grade level. Paper presented at the Annual Convention of the American Speech-Language-Hearing Association, Houston, TX.

Dale, P. S., & Crain-Thoreson, C. (1993). Pronoun reversals: Who, when, and why? *Journal of Child Language, 20,* 573–589.

de Villiers, J. G., & de Villiers, P. A. (1978). *Language acquisition.* Cambridge, MA: Harvard University Press.

Dever, R. (1978). *TALK: Teaching the American language to kids.* Columbus, OH: Merrill/Macmillan.

Dickinson, D., Wolf, M., & Stotsky, S. (1993). Words move: The interwoven development of oral and written language. In J. Berko Gleason (Ed.), *The development of language* (3rd ed.) (pp. 225–257). Columbus, OH: Merrill/Macmillan.

Dore, J. (1978). Requestive systems in nursery school conversations: Analysis of talk in its social context. In R. Campbell and P. Smith (Eds.), *Recent advances in the psychology of language: Language development and mother-child interaction* (pp. 271–292). New York: Plenum Press.

Drozd, K. F. (1995). Child English pre-sentential negation as a metalinguistic exclamatory sentence negation. *Journal of Child Language, 22*(3), 583–610.

Eisenberg, S., & Cairns, H. S. (1994). The development of infinitives from three to five. *Journal of Child Language, 21,* 713–734.

Ervin-Tripp, S. (1970). Discourse agreement: How children answer questions. In J. R. Hayes (Ed.), *Cognition and the development of language* (pp. 79–107). New York: Wiley.

Ervin-Tripp, S. (1980). Lecture, University of Minnesota, May 14, 1980.

Ferreiro, E., & Teberosky, A. (1982). *Literacy before schooling.* Exeter, NH: Heinemann.

Fletcher, J., Shaywitz, S., Shankweiler, D., Katz, L., Liberman, I., Stuebing, K., Francis, D., Fowler, A., & Shaywitz, B. (1994). Cognitive profiles of reading disabilities: Comparison of discrepancy and low achievement definitions. *Journal of Educational Psychology, 86,* 6–23.

Garvey, C. (1975). Requests and responses in children's speech. *Journal of Child Language, 2,* 41–63.

Garvey, C. (1977). The contingent query: A dependent act of communication. In M. Lewis & L. Rosenblum (Eds.), *Interaction, conversation, and the development of language.* New York: Wiley

Gentner, D. (1982). Why nouns are learned before verbs: Linguistic relativity versus natural partitioning. In S. A. Kuczaj II (Ed.), *Language development. Vol 2: Language, thought and culture* (pp. 301–334). Hillsdale, NJ: Erlbaum.

Gerber, A. (1981). Problems in the processing and use of language in education. In A. Gerber and D. N. Bryen (Eds.), *Language and learning disabilities* (pp. 75–112). Baltimore: University Park Press.

Gerken, L. (1991). The metrical basis for children's subjectless sentences. *Journal of Memory and Language, 30,* 431–451.

Gillam, R. (1999). Communicative patterns that facilitate language development. http://www.utexas.edu/ftp/courses/gillam/commpat.html

Gleitman, L. R., & Gleitman, H. (1994). A picture is worth a thousand words, but that's the problem: The role of syntax in vocabulary acquisition. In B. Lust, M. Suñer, and J. Whitman (Eds.), *Heads, projections, and learnability* (pp. 291–299). Hillsdale, NJ: Lawrence Erlbaum.

Goldstein, B. (2000). *Cultural and linguistic diversity resource guide for speech-language pathologists*. San Diego, CA: Singular.

Goldstein, B., & Iglesias, A. (1996). Phonological patterns in normally developing Spanish-speaking 3- and 4-year-olds of Puerto Rican descent. *Journal of Communication Disorders, 29*(5), 367–387.

Golinkoff, R. M., Mervis, C. B., & Hirsh-Pasek, K. (1994). Early object labels: The case for a developmental principles framework. *Journal of Child Language, 21,* 125–155.

Gopnik, M. (1997). *The inheritance and innateness of grammars*. Oxford, UK: Oxford University Press.

Goswami, U., & Bryant, P. E. (1990). *Phonologic skills and learning to read*. Hillsdale, NJ: Erlbaum.

Greene, J. (1996). Psycholinguistic assessment: The clinical base for identification of dyslexia. *Topics in Language Disorders, 16*(2), 45–72.

Haas, A., & Owens, R. (1985, November). Preschooler's pronoun strategies: You and me make us. Paper presented at the American Speech-Language-Hearing Association Annual Convention, Washington, DC.

Halliday, M. (1975). *Learning how to mean: Explorations in the development of language*. New York: Edward Arnold.

Halliday, M., & Hasan, R. (1976). *Cohesion in English*. London: Longman.

Hatcher, P. J., Hulme, C., & Ellis, A. W. (1994). Ameliorating early reading failure by integrating the teaching of reading and phonological skills: The phonological linkage hypothesis. *Child Development, 65,* 41–57.

Haynes, W. O., & Shulman, B. S. (Eds.). (1998). *Communication development: Foundations, processes, and clinical applications* (pp. 361–386). Baltimore: Williams & Wilkins.

Heath, S. B. (1996). What no bedtime story means: Narrative skills at home and school. In D. Brenneis and R. K. S. Macaulay (Eds.), *The matrix of language* (pp. 12–38). Cumnor Hill: Westview Press.

Henderson, E. H., & Beers, J. W. (Eds.). (1980). *Developmental and cognitive aspects of learning to spell: A reflection of word knowledge*. Newark, DE: International Reading Association.

Henry, M. (1993). Morphological structure: Latin and Greek roots and affixes as upper grade code strategies. *Reading and Writing: An Interdisciplinary Journal, 5,* 227–241.

Hirsh-Pasek, K., & Golinkoff, R. M. (1997). *The origins of grammar: Evidence from early language comprehension*. Cambridge, MA: MIT Press.

Hulit, L. M., & Howard, M. R. (1997). *Born to talk: An introduction to speech and language development*. New York: Macmillan.

Hyams, N. (1992). A reanalysis of null subject in child language. In J. Weissenborn, H. Goodluck, and T. Roeper (Eds.), *Continuity and change in development* (pp. 249–268). Hillsdale, NJ: Erlbaum.

James, S. (1990). *Normal language acquisition.* Boston: Allyn & Bacon.

Johnson, C. J., & Anglin, J. M. (1995). Qualitative development in the content and form of children's definitions. *Journal of Speech and Hearing Research, 38,* 612–625.

Jorm, A. F., & Share, D. L. (1983). An invited article: Phonological recoding and reading acquisition. *Applied Psycholinguistics, 4*(2), 103–147.

Jusczyk, P. W. (1992). Developing phonological categories from the speech signal. In C. A. Ferguson, L. Menn, and C. Stoehl-Gammon (Eds.), *Phonological development: Models, research, implications* (pp. 17–64). Timonium, MD: York Press.

Justice, L. M., & Ezell, H. K. (2000). Enhancing children's print and word awareness through home-based parent intervention. *American Journal of Speech-Language Pathology, 9*(3), 257–269.

Kamhi, A. G., & Catts, H. W. (1991). *Reading disabilities: A developmental language perspective.* Boston: Allyn & Bacon.

Kamhi, A. G., & Hinton, L. N. (2000). Explaining individual differences in spelling ability. In K. G. Butler (Ed.), *Topics in Language Disorders, 20*(3), 37–49.

Kamhi, A. G., & Koenig, L. (1985). Metalinguistic awareness in language disordered children. *Language, Speech and Hearing Services in Schools, 16,* 199–210.

Karmiloff-Smith, A. (1986). Some fundamental aspects of language development after age 5. In P. Fletcher and M. Garman (Eds.), Language *acquisition studies in first language development* (2nd ed.) (pp. 455–474). New York: Cambridge University Press.

Karmiloff-Smith, A. (1995). *Beyond modularity: A developmental perspective on cognitive science.* Cambridge, MA: MIT Press.

Klima, E., & Bellugi, U. (1966). Syntactic regularities in the speech of children. In J. Lyons and R. Wales (Eds.), *Psycholinguistic papers* (pp. 183–208). Edinburgh: Edinburgh University Press.

Kogan, N., & Chadrow, M. (1986). Children's comprehension of metaphor in the pictorial and verbal modality. *International Journal of Behavioral Development, 9,* 285–295.

Konefal, J., & Folks, J. (1984). Linguistic analysis of children's conversational repairs. *Journal of Psycholinguistic Research, 13,* 1–11.

Kuhl, P. K., & Meltzoff, A. N. (1997). Evolution, nativism, and learning in the development of language and speech. In M. Gopnik (Ed.), *The inheritance and innateness of grammars* (pp. 7–44). Oxford, UK: Oxford University Press.

Lahey, M. (1974). The role of prosody and syntactic markers in children's comprehension of spoken sentences. *Journal of Speech and Hearing Research, 17,* 656–668.

Lahey, M., Liebergott, J., Chesnick, M., Menyuk, P., & Adams, J. (1992). Variability in children's use of grammatical morphemes. *Applied Psycholinguistics, 13,* 373–398.

Larson, V. L., & McKinley, N. (1995). *Language disorders in older students, preadolescents and adolescents.* Eau Claire, WI: Thinking Publication.

Levin, E., & Rubin, K. (1982). Getting others to do what you want them to: The development of children's requestive strategies. In K. Nelson (Ed.), *Children's language* (Vol. 4). New York: Gardner Press.

Lewis, B. A., O'Donnell, B., Freebairn, L. A., & Taylor, H. G. (1998). Spoken language and written expression-interplay of delays. *American Journal of Speech-Language Pathology, 7,* 77–84.

Lund, N., & Duchan, J. (1993). *Assessing children's language in naturalistic contexts.* Englewood Cliffs, NJ: Prentice Hall (originally published 1983).

MacLean, M., Bryant, P., & Bradley, L. (1987). Rhymes, nursery rhymes, and reading in early childhood. Special issue, Children's reading and the development of phonological awareness. *Merrill-Palmer Quarterly, 33*(3), 255–281.

McGhee-Bidlack, B. (1991). The development of noun definitions. A metalinguistic analysis. *Journal of Child Language, 18,* 417–434.

McLaughlin, S. (1998). *Introduction to language development.* San Diego, CA: Singular.

McLean, J., & Snyder-McLean, L. (1999). How children learn language. San Diego, CA: Singular.

McShane J. (1980). *Learning to talk.* New York: Cambridge University Press.

Menyuk, P. (1969). *Sentences children use.* Cambridge, MA: MIT Press.

Menyuk, P. (1977). *Language and maturation.* Cambridge, MA: MIT Press.

Miller, J. F. (1981). *Assessing language production in children: Experimental procedures.* Baltimore: University Park Press.

Nation, K., & Hulme, C. (1997). Phonemic segmentation, not onset-time segmentation, predicts early reading and spelling skills. *Reading Research Quarterly, 32,* 154–167.

Nelson, K. (1973). Structure and strategy in learning to talk. *Monographs of the Society for Research in Child Development, 38.*

Nelson, K., Hampson, J., & Shaw, L. K. (1993). Nouns in early lexicons: Evidence, explanations, and implications. *Journal of Child Language, 20,* 61–84.

Nelson, N. W. (1985). Teacher talk and children listening—Fostering a better match. In C. Simon (Ed.), *Communication skills and classroom success: Assessment of language-learning disabled children* (pp. 65–104). San Diego, CA: College-Hill.

Nelson, N. W. (1986). Individual processing in classroom settings. *Topics in Language Disorders, 6,* 13–27.

Nelson, N. W. (1993). *Childhood language disorders in context: Infancy through adolescence.* New York: Macmillan.

Nelson, N. W. (1998). *Childhood language disorders in context: Infancy through adolescence* (2nd ed.). Boston: Allyn & Bacon.

Ninio, A., & Snow, C. E. (1996). *Pragmatic development: Essays in developmental science.* Boulder, CO: Westview.

Nippold, M. A. (1985). Comprehension of figurative language. *Topics in Language Disorders, 3,* 1–20.

Nippold, M. A. (1988). Figurative language. In M. A. Nippold (Ed.), *Later language development: Ages nine through nineteen* (pp. 179–210). Austin, TX: Pro-Ed.

Nippold, M. A. (1991). Evaluating and enhancing idiom comprehension. *Language, Speech and Hearing Services in Schools, 22*(3), 100–105.

Nippold, M. A. (1998). *Later language development: The school-age and adolescent years* (2nd ed.). Austin, TX: Pro-Ed.

Nippold, M. A., Leonard, L., & Kail, R. (1984). Syntactic and conceptual factors in children's understanding of metaphors. *Journal of Speech and Hearing Research, 27,* 197–205.

Nippold, M. A., & Martin, S. T. (1989). Idiom interpretation in isolation versus context: A developmental study with adolescents. *Journal of Speech and Hearing Research, 32,* 59–66.

Nippold, M. A., & Taylor, C. L. (1995). Idiom understanding in youth: Further examination of familiarity and transparency. *Journal of Speech and Hearing Research, 2,* 426–443.

Norris, J. A. (1998). Early sentence transformations and the development of complex syntactic structures. In W. O. Haynes and B. B. Shulman (Eds.), *Communication development: Foundations, processes, and clinical applications* (pp. 263–310). Baltimore: Williams & Wilkins.

O'Grady, W. (1997). *Syntactic development.* Chicago: The University of Chicago Press.

Oller, D. (1978). Infant vocalizations and the development of speech. *Allied Health and Behavior Sciences, 1,* 523–549.

Oshima-Takane, Y., Takane, Y., & Shultz, T. R. (1999). The learning of 1st and 2nd pronouns in English: Network models and analysis. *Journal of Child Language, 26,* 545–575.

Owens, R. (1988). *Language development and communication disorders in children* (2nd ed.). Columbus, OH: Merrill/Macmillan.

Owens, R. E., Jr. (1996). *Language development: An introduction* (3rd ed.). Columbus, OH: Merrill/Macmillan.

Owens, R. E., Jr. (2001). *Language development: An introduction* (5th ed.). Boston: Allyn & Bacon.

Owens, R. E., Jr., Metz, D. E., & Haas, A. (2000). *Introduction to communication disorders: A life span perspective.* Boston: Allyn & Bacon.

Patterson, J. L., & Westby, C. E. (1998). The development of play. In W. O. Haynes and B. B. Shulman (Eds.), *Communication development: foundations, processes, and clinical applications* (pp. 135–163). Baltimore: Williams & Wilkins.

Peccei, J. S. (1999). *Child language* (2nd ed.). London: Routledge.

Perfetti, C. (1984). Reading acquisition and beyond: Decoding includes cognition. *American Journal of Education, 93,* 40–60.

Piaget, J. (1954). *The construction of reality in the child.* New York: Basic Books.

Rees, N. (1980). The nature of language. In T. Hixon, L. Shriberg, & J. Saxman (Eds.), *Introduction to communication disorders* (pp. 2–41). Englewood Cliffs, NJ: Prentice Hall.

Ricard, M., Girouard, P. C., & Decarie, T. G. (1999). Personal pronouns and perspective taking in toddlers. *Journal of Child Language, 26,* 681–697.

Rispoli, M. (1998). Patterns of pronoun case error. *Journal of Child Language, 25,* 533–554.

Rubin, H., Patterson, P., & Kantor, M. (1991). Morphological development and writing ability in children and adults. *Language, Speech and Hearing Services in the Schools, 22*(4), 228–236.

Rumelhart, D. (1977). Toward an interactive model of reading. In S. Dornic (Ed.), *Attention and performance VI* (pp. 573–606). Hillsdale, NJ: Lawrence Erlbaum Associates.

Saywitz, K., & Cherry-Wilkinson, L. (1982). Age related differences in metalinguistic awareness. In S. Kuczaj (Ed.), *Language development: Vol. 1. Language, thought and culture* (pp. 249–250). Hillsdale, NJ: Lawrence Erlbaum Associates.

Seymour, H. N., & Roeper, T. (1999). Grammatical acquisition of African American English. In L. B. Leonard and O. L. Taylor (Eds.), *Language acquisition across North America: Cross-cultural and cross-linguistic perspectives* (pp. 109–152). San Diego, CA: Singular.

Share, D. L., & Stanovich, K. E. (1995). Cognitive processes in early reading development: Accommodating individual differences into a model of acquisition. *Issues in Education, 1,* 1–57.

Shaywitz, B. A., Fletcher, J. M., Holahan, J. M., & Shaywitz, S. E. (1992). Discrepancy compared to low achievement definitions of reading disability: Results from the Connecticut longitudinal study. *Journal of Learning Disabilities, 25*(10), 639–648.

Silliman, E. R., & James, S. (1997). Assessing children with language disorders. In D. K. Bernstein and E. Tiegerman-Farber (Eds.), *Language and communication disorders in children* (pp. 197–271). Boston: Allyn & Bacon.

Snow, C. E., Perlmann, R., & Nathan, D. (1987). Why routines are different: Toward a multiple-factors model of the relation between input and language acquisition. In K. E. Nelson, and A. van Kleeck (Eds.). *Children's language, vol. VI* (pp. 65–97). Hillsdale, NJ: Erlbaum.

Snow, C., Scarborough, H., & Burns, M. S. (1999). What SLPs need to know about early readings. *Topics in Language Disorders, 20,* 48–58.

Snowling, M. J., Hulme, C., Smith, A., & Thomas, J. (1994). The effects of phoneme similarity and list length on children's sound categorization performance. *Journal of Experimental Child Psychology, 58,* 160–180.

Snyder, L. S., & Downey, D. M. (1997). Developmental differences in the relationship between oral language deficits and reading. *Topics in Language Disorders, 17,* 27–40.

Sokolov, J. L., & Snow, C. E. (1994). The changing role of negative evidence in theories of language development. In C. Gallaway and B. J. Richards (Eds.), *Input and interaction in language acquisition* (pp. 38–55). Cambridge, UK: Cambridge University Press.

Stanovich, K. (1980). Toward an interactive-compensatory model of individual differences in the development of reading fluency. *Reading Research Quarterly, 16,* 32–71.

Stein, N., & Glenn, C. (1979). An analysis of story comprehension in elementary school children. In R. Freedle (Ed.), *New directions in discourse processing* (pp. 53–120). Norwood, NJ: Ablex.

Stockman, I. (1999). Semantic development of African American children. In L. B. Leonard and O. L. Taylor (Eds.), *Language acquisition across North America: Cross-cultural and cross-linguistic perspectives* (pp. 61–106). San Diego, CA: Singular.

Stoehl-Gammon, C., & Cooper, J. (1984). Patterns of early lexical and phonological development. *Journal of Child Language, 11,* 247–271.

Strapp, C. M. (1999). Mothers', fathers', and siblings' responses to children's language error: Comparing sources of negative evidence. *Journal of Child Language, 26,* 373–391.

Swanson, H. L., Mink, J., & Bocian, K. M. (1999). Cognitive processing deficits in poor readers with symptoms of reading disabilities and ADHD: More alike than different? *Journal of Educational Psychology, 91*(2), 321–333.

Tardif, T. (1995). Nouns are not *always* learned before verbs, but why? Evidence from Mandarin Chinese. *Proceedings of the Twenty-Sixth Annual Child Language Research Forum*, Stanford University, 26, 224–230.

Tardif, T., Shatz, M., & Naigles, L. (1997). Caregiver speech and children's use of nouns versus verbs: A comparison of English, Italian, and Mandarin, *Journal of Child Language*, 24, 535–565.

Taylor, O. L. (1999). Cultural issues and language acquisition. In O. L. Taylor & L. B. Leonard (Eds.). *Language acquisition across North America* (pp. 21–37). San Diego, CA: Singular.

Taylor, O. L., & Leonard, L. B. (1999). *Language acquisition across North America*. San Diego, CA: Singular.

Temple, C., Nathan, R., Temple, F., & Burris, N. A. (1993). *The beginnings of writing* (3rd ed.). Boston: Allyn & Bacon.

Tiegerman-Farber, E. (1995). *Language and communication intervention in preschool children*. Boston: Allyn & Bacon.

Torgesen, J. K. (1999). Assessment and instruction for phonemic awareness and word recognition skills. In H. W. Catts & A. G. Kamhi (Eds.). *Language and reading disabilities* (pp. 128–153). Boston: Allyn & Bacon.

Torgesen, J. K., Wagner, R., & Rashotte, C. (1994). Longitudinal studies of phonological processing and reading. *Journal of Learning Disabilities, 27*, 276–286.

Tough, J. (1979). *Talk for teaching and learning*. Portsmouth, NH: Heinemann.

Tunmer, W., and Bowey, J. (1984). Metalinguistic awareness and reading acquisition. In W. Tunmer, C. Pratt, and M. Herriman (Eds.), *Metalinguistic awareness in children: Theory, research and implications* (pp. 144–168). New York: Springer-Verlag.

Tunmer, W., Pratt, C., & Herriman, M. (Eds.). (1984). *Metalinguistic awareness in children: Theory, research and implications*. New York: Springer-Verlag.

Tyack, D., & Gottsleben, R. (1986). Acquisition of complex sentences. *Language, Speech, and Hearing Services in Schools, 17*(3), 160–175.

Valian, V. (1991). Syntactic subjects in the early speech of American and Italian children. *Cognition, 40*, 21–81.

van Kleeck, A. (1982). The emergence of linguistic awareness: A cognitive framework. *Merrill-Palmer Quarterly, 28*, 237–265.

van Kleeck, A. (1995). Learning about print before learning to read. In K. Butler (Ed.), *Best practices 11. The classroom as an interaction context* (pp. 3–23). Gaithersburg, MD: Aspen.

Vellutino, F. R., Scanlon, D., Small, S., & Tanzman, M. (1991). The linguistic bases of reading disability: Converting written to oral language. *Text, 11*, 99–133.

Vosniadou, S., Ortony, A., & Reynolds, R. E. (1984). Children's comprehension of metaphor in the pictorial and verbal modality. *International Journal of Behavioral Development, 9*, 288–295.

Wallach, G. (1984). Who shall be called "learning disabled"? Some new directions. In G. Wallach and K. Butler (Eds.), *Language learning disabilities in school age children* (pp. 1–14). Baltimore: Williams & Wilkins.

Wallach, G., & Butler, K. (1994). *Language learning disabilities in school age children and adolescents*. New York: Macmillan.

Wells, G. (1985). *Language development in the preschool years*. New York: Cambridge University Press.

Werker, J., & Tees, R. (1984) Cross-language speech perception: evidence for perceptual reorganization during the first year of life. *Infant Behavior and Development, 7*, 49–64.

Westby, C. E. (1998). Communicative refinement in school age and adolescence. In W. O. Haynes and B. B. Shulman (Eds.), *Communication development: foundations, processes, and clinical applications* (pp. 311–360). Baltimore: Williams & Wilkins.

White, B. (1975). Critical influences in the origins of competence. *Merrill Palmer Quarterly, 22*, 243–266.

Wiig, E.H., & Semel, E. M. (1984). *Language assessment and intervention for the learning disabled* (2nd ed.). New York: Merrill/Macmillan.

Winner, E., Rosentiel, A., & Gardner, H. (1976). The development of metaphoric understanding. *Developmental Psychology, 12*, 189–297.

Witt, B. (1998). Cognition and the cognitive-language relationship. In W. O. Haynes and B. B. Shulman (Eds.), *Communication development: Foundations, processes, and clinical applications* (pp. 101–133). Baltimore: Williams & Wilkins.

PART II

Language Assessment and Intervention

3

Interactive Teaming

The Changing Role of the Speech-Language Pathologist

Ellenmorris
Tiegerman-Farber
Adelphi University

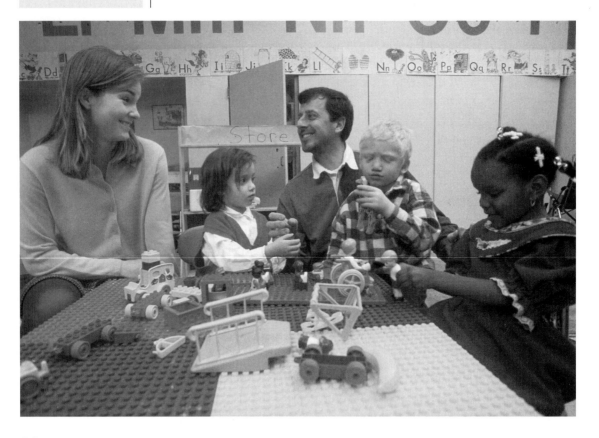

- Discuss why parents need to become part of the collaborative decision-making process
- Explain why inclusion requires individualized programming
- List the barriers to successful collaboration
- Discuss how the makeup of the collaborative team determines the role that it plays in educational reform
- Explain why collaborative teaming requires that speech-language pathologists, parents, and teachers change their roles and responsibilities
- Articulate the difference between consultation and collaboration as service delivery models

In this chapter, the interactive teaming approaches described as consultation and collaboration are service delivery models that can be used to provide services for children with disabilities. The difference between the two models relates to the way in which parents and professionals interact with each other to solve child-based learning problems. The chapters that follow in this part present much more detail about the changing role of the speech-language pathologist (SLP) as a teacher consultant, parent trainer, and collaborative team member. As special education law (Public Law 99-457) has introduced programming for infants and preschoolers, language development has become a critical component in the evaluation and treatment of young children with disabilities. No other professional has the knowledge, training, and expertise of the speech-language pathologist to meet this educational challenge. Most children with developmental disabilities have language and communication disorders (LCD) (Tiegerman-Farber & Radziewicz, 1998). The importance of language in early childhood development has shifted the role of the speech-language pathologist from related service provider to classroom teacher in some programs. It is a very exciting time for the field of speech-language pathology as our professional skills become more important to all aspects of educational programming. Interactive teaming in its various forms has become a part of the school reform movement in many schools nationwide. The interactive models take into consideration a number of issues that occur in special education.

1. Cultural and linguistic differences between professionals and families require the use of models that facilitate and enhance effective communication.
2. With the reauthorization of the Individuals with Disabilities Education Act (IDEA) there is an increased focus on the provision of services within inclusive environments and natural settings.
3. To maximize the efficiency and effectiveness of service provision, professionals need to use models that facilitate the coordination of multiple services provided to children with disabilities.
4. Special education has become family focused, which requires the inclusion of parents within the decision-making process. Consultation and collaboration are used during assessment, educational/clinical programming, and annual review of the child's progress.
5. Public Law 99-457 emphasizes the importance of early intervention.

With the increased emphasis on inclusive programming in schools and natural settings, the speech-language pathologist will be required to utilize both of these models to meet the needs of culturally and linguistically diverse children and families. The dynamic interface between professionals and parents must be learned "on the job," because few teacher-training internships facilitate this type of professional interaction (Ogletree, 1999). The speech-language pathologist will also be working more frequently with children, teachers, and parents in special and regular education classrooms; this change in responsibilities requires the development of new professional competencies. The speech-language pathologist and the classroom teacher have different academic training experiences and professional perceptions of their roles (Harn, Bradshaw, & Ogletree, 1999). Professionals with different backgrounds and training must learn to work together cooperatively to identify child-based learning problems and to develop appropriate intervention strategies. This chapter will discuss how interactive teaming provides a mechanism for professionals to share their expertise with each other and with parents to maximize opportunities for parents and children in more diverse settings (Chisholm, 1994).

CHANGES IN SPECIAL EDUCATION LAW

Education for All Handicapped Children Act (EAHCA)

The Education for All Handicapped Children Act, Public Law 94-142, was passed in 1975 after many years of advocacy from parents and service organizations. Up until this point most children with disabilities were not being educated in local public schools. PL 94-142 guaranteed children with disabilities a free and appropriate public education (FAPE) to the maximum extent possible with peers without disabilities. PL 94-142 established national procedures and safeguards for parents to ensure that children with disabilities had the same opportunities to an education as children without disabilities.

After the passage of PL 94-142, many researchers and educators argued that the law did not mandate services for children from birth to five years and therefore did not go far enough. Issues related to early identification and intervention focused on the dramatic needs of infants and preschoolers with disabilities. The significance of the educational problem was highlighted by the fact that technological advancements that enabled the earlier diagnosis of many disorders did not then result in educational intervention. Services to infants and preschoolers were not then mandated in educational settings and, as a result, voluntary agencies (e.g., United Cerebral Palsy, the Association for Children with Down's Syndrome, and the Association for Children with Learning Disabilities) developed and expanded to address this need. However, the types and levels of services varied from community to community across the United States; some communities provided extensive services and some provided none for children below the age of 5 years. Clearly, identification required intervention, but it was not until 1986 that Public Law 99-457 was passed.

Essentially, PL 99-457 addresses two groups of children with disabilities: preschoolers and infants. It extends to the first group—preschool children ages three and four—all federal requirements, rights and protections currently applicable to school-aged children with disabilities (5 to 21 years of age). Such requirements include an individualized education plan (IEP), adherence to least restrictive environment (LRE) guidelines, and due process provisions including educational committees (Committee on Special Education, Committee on Preschool Special Education/Individual Family Service Plan) that allow parents the right to challenge educational decisions. In addition, PL 99-457 amended the Education for All Handicapped Children Act to develop and implement comprehensive, coordinated, multidisciplinary, interagency programs of early intervention services for infants and toddlers and their families. This policy explanation is based on the recognized need:

1. To enhance the development of infants and toddlers with disabilities and to minimize their potential for developmental delay
2. To reduce the educational costs to our society, including our nation's schools, by minimizing the need for special education and related services after infants and toddlers reach school age
3. To minimize the likelihood of institutionalization of individuals with disabilities and to maximize their potential for independent living in society
4. To enhance the capacity of families to meet the special needs of their infants and toddlers with disabilities

Since the passage of PL 94-142, programs were developed nationally to provide educational and therapeutic services to children who were either not receiving an education or were not receiving adequate services. In the reauthorization of PL 94-142, the 101st Congress changed the name of the Education for All Handicapped Children Act (EHCA) to Individuals with Disabilities Education Act (IDEA). In addition, the term "handicap" was replaced by "disability." Although the development of public education programs for children with disabilities addressed a critical need, it simultaneously presented a range of related challenges that now require attention and resolution. One of these issues relates to *how* decisions are made about a child's developmental needs.

Early Intervention

Part H of PL 99-457 requires an Individual Family Service Plan (IFSP) for children from birth through two years. Early intervention programs provide an important role in the lives of families of infants and toddlers with developmental disabilities. Families receive a comprehensive range of services, including direct therapeutic and developmental services in school-based programs, and early childhood as well as home settings. Early intervention services require a collaborative relationship between family members and professionals within the early intervention system (Dinnebeil & Hale, 1999). The IFSP focuses on the needs of the *family* as well as the needs of the child. For instance, if a parent needs counseling in order to function more appropriately with the infant or toddler, the IFSP includes such counseling services. If a parent has economic hardships and has no means of getting to the counseling services, the IFSP will provide for transportation. The early intervention system emphasizes the role of the parent as the front-line service provider and educator for the child. The early intervention system that has evolved presents a change in focus from the needs and strengths of the child to the needs and strengths of the child within the family. This enlarged view of the child as part of a family system reflects an ecological view of child development (Wehman, 1998). Bronfenbrenner (1977) conceptualized this ecological view to consider the child as a member of a family unit, which in turn is a member of a larger interactive community. The philosophy that generated PL 99-457 supports a family-centered approach that emphasizes that the needs of the child and the needs of the family are intertwined and interdependent (Mahoney & Bella, 1998).

With the development of the early intervention system, the role of the speech-language pathologist changed dramatically; differences in speech and language skills were often the first warning signs recognized by parents (Sanger, Maag, & Shapera, 1994). Because language is the means of communicative exchange, the speech-language pathologist is the primary professional to teach parents, teachers, and peers to facilitate the language learning process. The implementation of PL 99-457 has dramatically changed how services are provided, where they are provided, and by whom (Bailey, Aytch, Odoms, Symons, & Wolery, 1999). Previously, diagnostic teams for children aged 5 to 21 years focused on the child's needs; after PL 99-457, however, the needs of families of children were also considered during the assessment process.

With this program extension to younger children, a more encompassing ecological perspective became necessary. Public Law 99-457 also requires an Individual Education Plan (IEP) for preschool children as they transition from the early intervention to the preschool system. Federal law emphasizes the need for states to develop a seamless system for children and families. As a result, transition planning and programming must be detailed within the child's IFSP and (preschool) IEP. Parental involvement is a significant part of the early intervention and preschool process. States have different designations for the school district committees that evaluate preschool and school-age children with disabilities. In New York State, the Committee on Preschool Special Education (CPSE) must generate a plan (IEP) that is acceptable to the family. The speech-language pathologist is skilled in assessing the speech and language behaviors of the child as well as the communicative interactions of parents and caregivers, and can provide insights into enhancing and developing these skills within the family. For the young child, most early learning is mediated through language; therefore, it is vital that families participate in an intervention program along with the speech-language pathologist. It is interesting to note that the majority—83 percent—of children in New York State identified with a developmental disability in 1998–1999 received speech-language services. With the early intervention system shifting to a family-centered approach, the speech-language pathologist needs to interact with parents and teachers on a more interpersonal basis in school and home (Gallagher, 1999).

There has been an explosion of information regarding the communication behaviors of children below the age of 5 years. The American Speech-Language-Hearing Association (ASHA) published a position statement in 1990 on the role of the speech-language pathologist in service delivery to infants, toddlers, and their families. This position statement clarifies the changing roles and responsibilities of the speech-language pathologist as including:

1. Screening and identification
2. Assessment and evaluation
3. Design, planning, direct delivery, and monitoring of treatment programs
4. Case management
5. Consultation with and referral to agencies and other professionals that provide services to this young population and their families

These roles should be assumed as part of a comprehensive program that is family centered and is also coordinated with other services that families and their children may need or receive (Figure 3.1). The SLP provides comprehensive services to children, teachers, and parents across a continuum of settings from therapy room to classroom (Meyer, 1997). Diversity has been introduced in to the required competencies and professional competencies of the speech-language pathologist. The issue of diversity has become a part of who we are as professionals and not just what we do. The speech-language pathologist has become an integral member of the multidisciplinary team serving families and their infants or toddlers (ASHA, 1990). In addition, the complex needs of culturally and linguistically diverse families has also required the development of specialized courses and training for speech-language pathologists and other professionals. Many academic programs are just now including courses on early intervention and cultural diversity within the graduate curriculum (Jones & Blendinger, 1994). For professionals already in the field, these new competencies and skills will have to be learned "on the job," which creates significant difficulties for

Children	Team	Document	Settings	Role/Responsibility/Model
5–12 years	CSE	IEP	Therapy room/school/center Special education classroom Regular education classroom Job training site Camp Home	Evaluation team collaboration Teacher-consultant Co-teacher–collaboration Parent trainer consultation Private therapist Related service provider
3–5 years	CPSE	IEP	Therapy room/school/center Special education classroom Camp Home Daycare/nursery school	Teacher consultant Trainer–consultation Private therapist Evaluation team–collaboration Related service provider Co-teacher–collaboration
Birth–3 years	IFSP	IFSP	Therapy room/school/center Developmental group Daycare Home Hospital Early intervention classroom	Related service provider Evaluation team–collaboration Teacher consultant Co-teacher–collaboration Private therapist

FIGURE 3.1

The Role of the Speech-Language Pathologist

schools and clinics attempting to integrate children with disabilities. As a result, the educational field will require several years to develop staff development programs to "teach" speech-language pathologists and other professionals the necessary competencies to be part of a school-wide reform program (Midkiff & Lawler-Prince, 1992). This training effort has its own set of problems within schools, early childhood programs, and camps attempting to integrate children with disabilities. At the present time the speech-language pathologist is being encouraged to work closely with other professionals in diverse settings outside the traditional therapy room. The limited preservice training emphasizes the need for public schools and community centers to develop staff training programs "yesterday" (Little & Robinson, 1997).

THE PROCESS BEGINS . . .

Although this chapter discusses consultation and collaboration as service delivery models, it is important to make a distinction between them at this point for the sake of clarity.

Consultation can be defined as a structured series of interactions that occur between two individuals to bring about changes in a target person. This occurs when a speech-language pathologist works with a special education teacher to identify strategies that will facilitate the generalization of language learning goals for a specific child into the environment of the classroom. Consultation provides the mechanism for the speech-language pathologist to provide support and instructional advice about addressing the needs of a child with language and communication disorders within either special education or regular classrooms. In consultation, the professionals communicate, cooperate, and coordinate their instruction to facilitate the evaluation, planning, and implementation of learning goals, but the speech-language pathologist functions as an advisor (Tiegerman-Farber & Radziewicz, 1998).

Collaboration is defined by joint decision making. Members of the team function as equal contributors and share the responsibility for decision making. "Collaboration is an interactive process that enables people with diverse expertise to generate creative solutions to mutually defined problems. The outcome is enhanced, altered and produces solutions that are different from those that the individual team members would produce independently" (Idole, Paolucci-Whitecomb, & Nevin, 1986). The collaboration team may include the regular education teacher, the special education teacher, the occupational therapist, the parents, the psychologist, and the speech-language pathologist.

Interactive teaming that includes consultation and collaboration is used at all stages of educational and clinical decision making, from evaluation to intervention to reevaluation. Figure 3.2 describes the mandated process used by schools to make decisions about the needs of a child and his family and whether or not they receive special education services. PL 94-142 describes the assessment responsibilities of a multidisciplinary team, called the Committee on Special Education (CSE) and the Committee on Preschool Special Education (CPSE) in New York State, which consists of professionals and parents in an interactive process of dialogue and decision

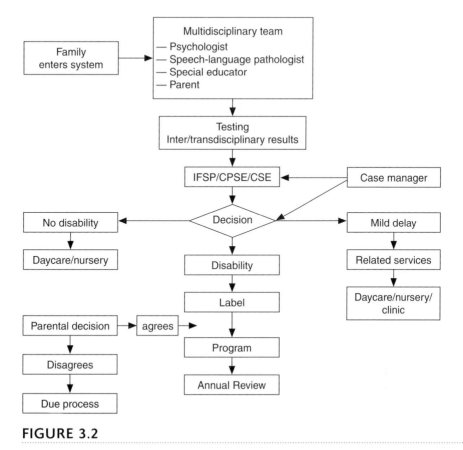

FIGURE 3.2

CSE/CPSE/IFSP Evaluation Process

making. The collaborative model is used by this multidisciplinary team from the initial point of assessment through the intervention process. Notice that the speech-language pathologist is an integral member of the multidisciplinary team. Intervention that involves the actual provision of services to the child may include consultation and/or collaboration. Interpersonal dynamics and financial resources will often determine whether either or both models are used by professionals and parents within specific programs and schools.

PL 94-142 requires child assessment by means of a **multidisciplinary** team consisting of several different professionals. In the **interdisciplinary team model,** different professionals work independently to assess then exchange information. Although treatment goals may be planned jointly, the delivery of services is often isolated. With a **transdisciplinary team model,** different professionals work together across discipline boundaries, with the purpose of integrating their findings into a transdisciplinary treatment plan. This model of assessment and intervention is considered most appropriate for families and children. The needs of the family and the child determine the necessary members of the team. Cooperation among all team members is of paramount importance. Inherent within the interactive team is interdependence among team members; each member can attain her goals only if the other team members achieve theirs. In addition, team members should have knowledge of early child development, assessment procedures, and intervention techniques (McCollum & Hughes, 1988). Although parents have a knowledge base different from professionals, they must also become members of the team and participate in the process; this issue will be discussed further in the latter part of the chapter.

Family Assessment Is Different

In order for an assessment to be complete, the team must acknowledge the importance of the family and conduct a family-focused assessment, in which both family and professionals consider the child within the context of the family. Traditionally only the needs and strengths of the child were considered; now the needs and strengths of the family must be brought to the forefront. When family strengths are considered, parents feel competent; when family needs are met, they feel empowered. The family-oriented assessment is inclusive of the child's strengths and needs, while the eco-behavioral focus provides a community context to the provision of services. The family of a child with an autism spectrum disorder living in an urban versus a rural area requires very different support services; consider the following scenarios presented by parents.

I live in a very rural area of Alabama and the closest school is 50 miles away. It is impossible to find specialists such as a speech-language pathologist, occupational therapist and physical therapist to provide services in my home on a regular basis. In addition, given my son's adaptive/physical requirements I want him to be with other children who have special needs. I have agreed to place my child on a bus for an hour so that he can attend a full day self contained program which I try to visit on a weekly basis.

I live in an apartment building in Los Angeles. I am just learning English along with my child. My husband and I work several jobs during the week. I do not want social workers and professionals coming to my home; it is intrusive to my family. Besides my parents do not speak any English and I do not want to explain myself here. I want my daughter to receive her services in a half day special education program and then bussed to a day center in the afternoon so I can pick her up at 7 p.m. It has been difficult to find a good day care program to accept my daughter since she has a disability.

The family assessment approach interfaces community institutions with parents in order to enhance a family's ability to function well and to facilitate development of the child with a disability (Briggs, 1998). The family assessment model meets the challenge of implementation of Part H of PL 99-457, which directs agencies to support and enable parents to be aware of and choose from a wide range of creative intervention options for families.

Several factors must be considered when shifting the focus from child-centered assessment to family assessment. One must remember that although assessment of the infant is assured through law, it is up to the family to decide *if* they want an assessment to be performed. If the family understands that they are respected by the professional team and that their needs as well as their child's needs are considered important, they are more likely to be committed to the assessment process. The assessment must be conducted by personnel trained to utilize appropriate methods and procedures and is based on information provided by the family through a personal interview. The assessment must incorporate the family's description of its resources, priorities, and concerns (Wehman, 1998).

Several important questions need to be considered before the assessment process begins. What strategies should be used in this assessment process? When is the best time for a family assessment to be done? How can the team prevent the family from viewing the assessment process as intrusive? Who should perform the family assessment? What if the team identifies a family need that the family does not recognize? Why is an assessment of family strengths important? Figure 3.2 indicates that the multidisciplinary team may consist of a school psychologist, a speech-language pathologist, a special education teacher, and a parent. Professional members of the team need to explain to the parent not only the results of their particular assessment but also how their results fit in with the total picture of the child within the context of the family and its needs. If effective family assessment is to be achieved:

1. The child needs to be evaluated by a multidisciplinary team with the parents as members of the team—in the child's primary or natural language.
2. Professionals should use a range of multicultural assessment instruments, but only after the child has been in an experimental/diagnostic classroom and has had an opportunity to interact with members of the evaluation team, including the parents.
3. There should be multiple observations of the child. Observational analysis and discussion will facilitate a product that reinforces common goals across discipline areas. In the school setting, the classroom represents the most natural context.
4. Parent–child analyses should be part of the diagnostic protocol. The diagnostic team might observe the child with the family, enabling the team to acquire information for a family assessment, as well as information on the quantity and quality of family–child interactions.

What Is Collaboration?

Coufal (1993) notes that interactive teaming defines how participants interact with each other as equal contributors in a decision-making process to generate common or shared goals. This suggests that all of the "stakeholders"—psychologist, speech-language pathologist, special education teacher, and parent—share goal decision making, status, accountability, and resources in an ongoing working relationship (Dinnebeil & Rule, 1994). This may be difficult for the psychologist, speech-language pathologist, special educator, and parent to do initially, given traditional professional expectations. The process of "coming together" requires a reevaluation and re-creation of roles, responsibilities, and relationships. In order to do this, interactive teams must pay close attention to interactional variables such as communication skills, problem-solving skills, and conflict-resolution strategies. The formation and development of an interactive team involves a learning process that includes a set of competencies. Members of the team must consider the following communicative competency skills (Crais, 1993):

1. Willingness to listen to others
2. Being supportive of someone else's ideas
3. Being receptive to input
4. Managing differences of opinion and conflict
5. Accepting and integrating suggestions of others
6. Expressing opinions and conflict
7. Expressing opinions and ideas without criticism
8. Acknowledging and using the ideas of others
9. Being flexible

These interactive behaviors contribute to the effectiveness and the efficiency of decision making. By developing these behaviors and adopting a collaborative style, the participants ultimately create and generate an effective working relationship that will benefit the child. In addition, as schools and clinics attempt to develop inclusive programming, the need to identify an effective process for decision making becomes more important (Slavin, Madden, Dolan, & Wasik, 1996). Parents, teachers, and speech-language pathologists must believe that a shared effort will result in a better outcome than an individual effort. The social and psychological dynamics of contributing to group decision making create a premium on maintaining positive communicative relationships (Friend & Bursuck, 1996).

In order to achieve inclusive programming for children with language and communication disorders, a school must engage in levels of collaborative teaming (Figure 3.3). Before implementing inclusion within any classroom, there need to be school as well as community-based discussions (Epstein, 1995). Part of the challenge in the development of inclusive programming within a school involves supportive networking before, during, and after changes are made within the classroom. Collaborative teams consisting of representatives from the various stakeholder groups must be provided with the opportunity to discuss the significant issues related to inclusion and general school changes that will occur (Gitlin, 1999). Each level of teaming provides direction and scaffolding for the next. A decision-making hierarchy allows for a more focused analysis of issues from a macro to a micro level: community to school to classroom. As a result, decisions are based on the recommendations of the prior level. This ensures continuity as well as a progression in decision making as issues and problems become the pragmatic realities of individual teachers, parents, and children. Successful educational reform requires partnerships and alliances sharing ideas and problem solving about changes that will affect the personal lives of and interpersonal relationships between professionals, parents, and children (Tiegerman-Farber & Radziewicz, 1998). Figure 3.3 indicates that collaborative teams must be developed to address community-based, school-based, and classroom-based reforms. These teams solve problems not only within their group, but also across groups.

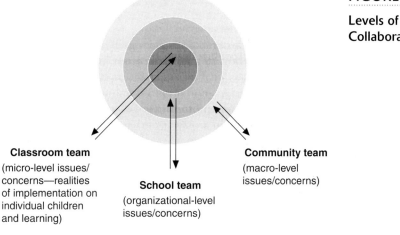

FIGURE 3.3

Levels of
Collaboration

Classroom team
(micro-level issues/
concerns—realities
of implementation on
individual children
and learning)

School team
(organizational-level
issues/concerns)

Community team
(macro-level
issues/concerns)

- The reality of educational change occurs on a daily basis in the classroom in terms of learning outcomes for children with and without disabilities.
- How well has each level of collaboration identified issues occurring on a daily basis for children with the inclusion classroom?
- Remember that there is a learning curve for committee effectiveness.

Collaborative Teaming: Community

This *community*-based team should have a broad representation consisting of community leaders, regular education teachers, special education teachers, speech-language pathologists, administrators, and parents of children with and without disabilities. The purpose of the team is to develop a clear mission statement about inclusion that will be discussed, negotiated, and formulated with community issues in mind. Because the school exists within a specific multicultural environment, the community as a whole needs to understand the mission of inclusion as well as the reforms that will result from this new program model. This team should also identify community issues and barriers that are likely to arise as educational reform continues (Buysse & Wesley, 1999). If the community does not support the mission and goals of inclusion programming, the school will have a difficult time achieving physical, social, and instructional interactions between children with and without disabilities. In any collaborative team the process of resolving philosophical differences and conflicts is of critical importance, and collaborative decision making should include the following steps:

1. Identifying the problem
2. Identifying ways to deal with the problem
3. Thinking about the possible results of each recommendation
4. Generating a responsible proactive decision
5. Evaluating the decision and its results

6. Reconsidering the decision
7. Being flexible

Collaborative Teaming: School-Based

The collaborative team within a school must take into consideration the concerns and issues of the community in order to implement the goals related to the mission statement (Lazar, Broderick, Mastrilli, & Slostad, 1999). Will the community support the school's mission? How will the community support the school? The school-based collaborative team should consist of an administrator, a special education teacher, a speech-language pathologist, a regular teacher, and parents of children with and without disabilities. The school-based collaborative team needs to consider:

1. The requirements necessary to implement the mission statement within the school as an educational environment. Here, too, the collaborative challenge involves supportive networking between the school and community before, during, and after inclusive programming has been developed.
2. A timeline for programmatic development that includes community updates on progress.
3. A proposal for procedural changes reflecting the educational reforms that must take place.
4. The process of change and how long-range changes will be accomplished by classroom-based collaborative teams.

Also, the strategies to achieve classroom inclusion require school modifications and problem solving regarding:

1. Financial costs of programming changes
2. Hiring of new staff
3. The number of children with and without disabilities in the inclusion classroom
4. Organizational changes within the classroom
5. Space allocation problems
6. Necessary classroom resources, such as supplies and materials
7. Fears and concerns of parents, teachers, and children

Collaborative Teaming: Classroom-Based

The classroom-based collaborative team should consist of the special education teacher, regular education teacher, speech-language pathologist, and parents of children with and without disabilities. This team has the most complicated responsibilities because there are short-term as well as long-term problems that will require discussion, negotiation, and resolution within the parameters of the classroom. Successful inclusion will not be accomplished if the stakeholders cannot come to consensus about the educational benefit of inclusion for children with and without disabilities (Gable, Korinek, & Laycock, 1997). This collaborative team will attempt to achieve physical, social, and instructional interactions between children with and without disabilities. Inclusion requires the identification and removal of barriers, including personal and instructional concerns (Gable & Hendrickson, 1997). The collaborative classroom team must learn how to make decisions by means of a group process; this involves a major reevaluation of interpersonal relationships, responsibilities, and educational decision making.

Identifying the Problem

The collaborative team will be faced with many problems that must be discussed, reviewed, and resolved (Gable, Korinek, & Laycock, 1997). Part of the difficulty involves the fact that members of the team will have different degrees of training and past experiences concerning collaboration. The team will need time to coalesce and understand the individual needs of members, as well as the combined mission of the team. The development of group thinking or team decision making represents an ongoing learning experience for the individual members of the team. The collaborative process and collaborative decision making involve a learning experience for all of the members who contribute their time, knowledge, and expertise (Gable & Manning, 1999). At times, collaborative teaming is frustrating and all too human in its problems and decisions. Over time, however, the team will develop its own personality and style; no two collaborative teams are the same, nor should they be.

Identifying Ways to Solve the Problem

The collaborative team may decide that it can generate recommendations to resolve each of the problems, or it may identify specialists and consultants who can address these problems. Given the time frame established by the community to implement an inclusion program, the team may not have the schedule or the resources to investigate minutely each and every issue. The amount of time spent in preplanning is obviously a critical factor in the ability of parents, teachers, and administrators to implement a program successfully. Intensive discussions related to problems and concerns may short-circuit a whole host of implementation difficulties. It is important for the team to attempt to anticipate obstacles that may arise later, but it may not always be feasible to do this, given the time constraints. The purpose here should be to attempt to identify as many problems as possible and then discuss the implications and the personnel who will be necessary to address these issues on a long-term basis (Epstein, 1995).

Possible Results and Recommendations

In the process of generating recommendations for program implementation, it is important for the team to discuss the results of such recommendations (Tiegerman & Radziewicz, 1998). What are the implications for introducing children with mild language and communication disorders into the regular classroom? What are the implications for introducing children with LCD and who have physical disabilities into the regular classroom? What are the implications for introducing children with severe LCD into the regular classroom? With each of these decisions, what kinds of resources, services, and personnel need to be identified to meet the challenge of the committee's goals and recommendations? What are the prerequisites to inclusion? What are the barriers to inclusion? Each change in educational programming that moves a step closer to inclusive programming will create dramatic results for parents, teachers, and children (Bahr, Vellerman, & Ziegler, 1999). It is important to focus on the fact that children will be grouped differently; they will have different classroom experiences and peers. The educational curriculum within the classroom will be different. Educational outcomes and child performances will reflect a different philosophy of instruction. The number and types of children, along with their teachers, will be different. The very nature of classroom interaction and procedural instruction will change. The collaborative team needs to consider how parents, professionals, and administrators will respond to each and every one of these changes (Tiegerman-Farber & Radziewicz, 1998). How can members of the staff and leaders within the community assist the collaborative team to support these changes through open discussion and consciousness raising?

Responsible Decision Making

It is important for the collaborative team to take into consideration the community context and the multicultural diversity of the educational environment. The attitudes of parents and professionals must be taken into consideration by the team when it generates its recommendations (Dinnebeil & Hale, 1999). Responsible decision making requires the collaborative team to link planning and program implementation to the needs of the community. The generation of a decision that is not going to be accepted by professionals and parents will only serve to create a confrontational division between the school and the community. During the process of decision making, the collaborative team should report on a regular basis to the key participants and players: parents, professionals, and administrators (Blosser & Kratcoski, 1997). It may also be important to consider discussions with children as classroom programs and procedures begin to change. Because it is the child's environment that will be changed within the classroom, incorporating children may be as important to success as empowering parents within the process. Children make decisions about their peers, just as parents make decisions about whether they will allow their children to remain within specific school settings (Tiegerman-Farber & Radziewicz, 1998). Making responsible decisions suggests a process of open discussion and inclusion of ideas as well as people.

Addressing Cultural and Linguistic Diversity

Today most schools in metropolitan environments have a multicultural and multilinguistic diversity of children (Jones & Blendinger, 1994). These differences *already* exist within classrooms. The major problems in education do not necessarily involve the infusion of children with disabilities into regular classrooms. The existing problems in education relate to the development of educational programming for stylistically different learners. The introduction of a child with a disability just adds an additional difference. The problem of diversity within regular classrooms is a preexisting condition. Cultural differences and linguistic diversity create a stress and strain on schools struggling to deal with the demands of parents and professionals who are clamoring for educational excellence, safe schools, and outcome-based instruction (Bruskewitz, 1998).

How Collaboration Is Achieved

The inclusion classroom as an ecological environment is different from the traditional classroom. The goals are different, the teachers are different, the instructional process is different, learning is different, child outcomes are different, and the curriculum is different. The inclusion process stimulates a synergy of change focused within one small space—the classroom. The agents of change, the collaborators, must all share a common focus and commitment to create the necessary changes.

The purpose of a collaborative model is to provide the interactive team with a representational structure that can be used to highlight why specific interactions operate or do not operate effectively. Chess (1986) described a "goodness of fit concept" that can be used as a starting point by a collaborative team to make decisions about assessment, language goals, instructional procedures, and placement needs within the least restrictive setting. Tiegerman-Farber and Radziewicz (1995) described decision making as an interactional process among individuals that helps the regular and special education teachers and the speech-language pathologist to understand the characteristics and behaviors of effective collaboration (Figure 3.4). If we look more closely at the "goodness of fit" model, we realize that members of the collaborative team—teachers and speech-language pathologists—need to be aware of the other person's perception of the child. Once these baseline perceptions are discussed and agreed upon, joint expectations arise. These joint expectations manifest themselves in mutual goals, parity, shared participation, and accountability, all of which are inherent in collaboration. The consequence of this matching is the inclusion of families from the beginning of the referral process through the placement of the child with a disability in the least restrictive environment. The stakeholders must develop a common focus and commitment to engage in interactive dialogue to "set the ground rules." In order to do this, several operating principles or guidelines for group decision making can be highlighted by using the "goodness of fit" model:

- Co-equality and co-participation
- Reciprocity
- Commonality in goals

THE CHANGING ROLE OF THE SPEECH-LANGUAGE PATHOLOGIST

Co-equality and Co-participation

Within the collaborative process, the roles of the teacher (regular or special education) and the speech-language pathologist will be different within the inclusion classroom; the two professionals will have to learn to work as partners.

FIGURE 3.4

Professional Collaboration—Working toward a Shared Vision of the Inclusive Classroom

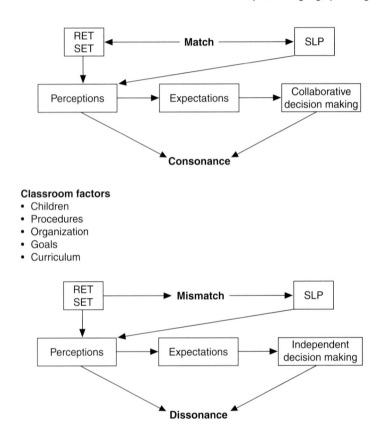

Match = consonance

Mismatch = dissonance

RET = Regular education teacher
SET = Special education teacher
SLP = Speech-language pathologist

1. A regular education teacher and a special education teacher may spend all of their time together when schools utilize a full inclusion model and children with disabilities receive their related services in the classroom.
2. A special (or regular) education teacher and a speech-language pathologist may spend part of their time working together in the classroom when schools utilize a modified inclusion or push-in model. The speech-language pathologist provides individual speech-language services to children from the class and also works with these same children in class to generalize their language skills to a more natural setting with peers.
3. The teacher and the speech-language pathologist need to spend time together brainstorming about: (a) classroom space, (b) the number of regular education students and children with disabilities, (c) the specialty needs of the children with disabilities, (d) the individual learning needs of all of the children, (e) strategies

to facilitate child-to-child learning experiences. The teaching team needs to develop an educational plan for the classroom as a whole, as well as for each child individually.

4. The learning process in an inclusion classroom will be different:
   (a) The teacher and the speech-language pathologist will have a different working relationship, which affects individual and group learning: team teaching, consultation as well as direct intervention in the classroom.
   (b) The speech-language pathologist will use instructional techniques to facilitate language for the child with a disability in a group setting.
   (c) The child with a disability will have the opportunity to interact with typical peers in a variety of academic and social activities. This will change the structure and the organization of classroom learning.
   (d) The physical classroom environment will be organized differently.
   (e) Parents of children with and without disabilities will have more opportunities to meet, to socialize, and to learn from each other.
   (f) The process for and content of learning will be based on a curriculum that includes language and communication goals.
   (g) Children teaching children will become an important means of implementing the curriculum.

Who the teachers are and how each professional functions within the inclusion classroom often present many challenging changes for professionals. The teacher and the speech-language pathologist need to be provided with intensive in-service instruction and support over a long period of time. As children with LCD are introduced into the general education classroom, the regular education teacher and the speech-language pathologist need to receive formal instructional training on the possible organizational changes that need to occur within their classrooms (O'Shea, Williams, & Sattler, 1999). They also need time to discuss their concerns and feelings about changes in their roles and responsibilities. The teacher needs to know about children with developmental disabilities and what the educational and behavioral implications are for integrating them within the classroom. He needs to know what to expect from the child with LCD in terms of communication and social skills. He also needs to know about management strategies, about the kinds of procedures and techniques that can be used to integrate the child with a language-communication disorder into ongoing classroom activities (Gable & Manning, 1999).

Co-teaching

Co-teaching or team teaching is a collaborative process. It may provide one educational mechanism for beginning the inclusion process (Beck & Dennis, 1997). This would mean that the relationship between the speech-language pathologist and the special education or regular education teacher would change immediately. The role of the speech-language pathologist would change from that of providing direct services to children with LCD in a separate room to providing services to *all* children in the same classroom. The fact that there will be two professionals within the inclusion classroom presents instructional and interpersonal challenges for professionals who have been trained in different discipline areas (Bruskewitz, 1998). The regular education teacher, the special education teacher, and the speech-language pathologist have highly specialized and divergently different foundations for knowledge. They approach the teaching experience from different vantage points; their academic coursework has been different, their teaching experiences have been different, and the settings within which they have worked are different. Perhaps the first and most immediate problem involves an understanding of the new working relationship that must be created (Hammond & Warner, 1996).

The speech-language pathologist can assist the classroom teacher to develop an understanding of the individual needs of children with LCD within the classroom. The speech-language pathologist has a set of specialty skills that includes management techniques, task analysis skills, and instructional procedures that can facilitate language learning for *all* of the children in the inclusion classroom—children who have been classified with LCD are not the only ones with individual needs. The speech-language pathologist can also assist in facilitating interactions between the classroom teacher and the children with LCD, as well as between child peer groups (Norris, 1997).

The classroom teacher can contribute to the inclusion classroom by providing instructional techniques and activities for the speech-language pathologist with the typical children in the classroom. The classroom teacher is uniquely skilled in developing academic curriculum goals that provide a level of motivation and skill development for typical children. Each professional has something to share with her colleagues. Each professional has something to contribute to the transdisciplinary curriculum and to the integration of students within the classroom. The professional differences create a strength in the inclusion classroom. Each professional contributes her expertise to an educational curriculum that could not have been developed by either separately. Figure 3.4 indicates that when there is co-equality and co-participation, collaborative decision making will be enhanced. Co-teachers need to acknowledge their academic and professional differences as a starting point as they work side by side in the classroom. Dynamic collaborative decision making through dialogue exchange creates a new classroom product and exciting interpersonal experiences (Trivette, 1998). When there is a mismatch between professionals, collaborative decisions cannot be generated; co-teachers need to analyze the interactional dialogue by evaluating their perceptions and expectations concerning classroom factors. From these shared perceptions come a set of shared expectations. If the collaborative process is operating correctly, these expectations are based on clear communication, active listening and responding, effective brainstorming, and creative integration of ideas. Consequently, good decision making results in consonance between professionals (Gitlin, 1999). If, on the other hand, the two professionals do not communicate clearly, listen to each other, and/or maintain a good rapport, there will be no attainment of shared perceptions or expectations. When a state of dissonance arises, the result will be independent decision making rather than shared problem solving.

Consultation

Consultation within the classroom provides a different interactive relationship between the speech-language pathologist and the special and/or regular education teacher.

The speech-language pathologist provides related services either within the classroom or within a separate setting, but her relationship with the teacher is different than the one she would have within a collaborative model. By means of teacher consultation, the speech-language pathologist provides instructional advice about procedures and techniques to facilitate the generalization of language goals for a specific child from an individual therapeutic setting to a more natural social setting with classroom peers. In both collaboration and consultation, the speech-language pathologist has a case-load of children who require speech-language therapy (Figure 3.5). One difference between the models is that in collaboration the decision-making process is developed together, and shared while the primary setting is the classroom. In consultation, the speech-language pathologist assumes a different role and has a different relationship with the teacher: the speech-language pathologist assumes an advisory position but the classroom teacher remains the primary facilitator within the classroom.

Reciprocity

Many special education teachers are concerned that with the development of inclusive classrooms, they will lose their jobs. Special education teachers express the frustration that their skills and training are being phased out of the educational system.

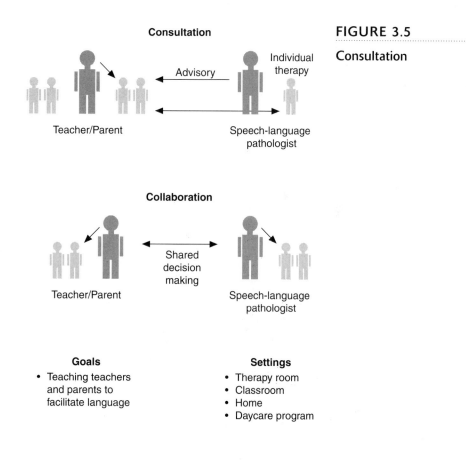

FIGURE 3.5

Consultation

Many regular education teachers, on the other hand, describe an inability to meet the challenge of inclusive instruction. These teachers claim that they are poorly prepared to work with children with LCD in a regular classroom. Some regular education teachers express negative attitudes about children with LCD because of the necessary changes that must occur as these students are integrated. Many regular education teachers pinpoint behavioral disruptions and that children with LCD will demand an inordinate amount of time and will take away valuable instructional time from the other children. Most teachers express feelings of incompetence, fear, anger, and frustration about being coerced into inclusion classrooms (Volk & Stahlman, 1994). Professional change must include a process of personal growth. Professionals need to talk about their feelings, their fears, and their concerns (Hudson & Glomb, 1997). If teachers do not have control over their classrooms, what do they have control over? Professionals need to speak to each other and see themselves within a supportive environment. The inclusion classroom must be supportive of professional change for the speech-language pathologist, the special education teacher, and the regular education teacher.

The reciprocity of interpersonal exchange allows the regular teacher, the special education teacher, and the speech-language pathologist to work toward recognizing how they can support each other in their personal and professional growth. They must each come to realize that they have an investment in the classroom. Co-teaching and/or teacher consultation cannot occur without the commitment of each professional; in fact, school reform will never be successfully achieved unless both professionals are working together (Walther-Thomas, 1997). Professionals must learn how to talk to each other about children, curriculum, and management issues. They must learn that co-teaching and teacher consultation cannot succeed with "territorial" thinking. In the movement to provide services within the least restrictive environment (LRE), co-teaching and teacher consultation team teaching needs to take place between the regular education teacher and the speech-language pathologist, between the regular education teacher and the special education teacher, and between the special education teacher and the speech-language pathologist.

Co-teaching and teacher consultation require mutual support and respect, as well as an understanding that professionals will work as interdependent partners within the classroom (Winton, 1998). Reciprocal exchange between professionals suggests that the classroom is really a bridge that spans across a professional divide: each professional from her side builds towards and reaches a common meeting place in the middle. Ultimately, inclusion within the regular classroom can only be achieved when the bridge between professionals provides a firm foundation for all children, with and without LCD, to walk across.

THE CHANGING ROLE OF THE PARENT

The inclusion classroom leads to a recognition of the unique characteristics of families and the role of parents as members of the collaborative team. The inclusion classroom encourages a culturally sensitive, family-centered process of educational decision making (Buysee & Wesley, 1999). The collaborative team must include the parent as an equal decision maker. Developmental information, knowledge, and input concerning the child can be effectively shared by parents. Information networking across discipline boundaries should include parent input to develop an appropriate common focus to the understanding of the needs of the family. The parent as caregiver has highly specialized concerns, insights, and priorities regarding his or her child. Historically, the role of parents has changed within the educational system as children receiving services have become younger; it is now necessary to incorporate parents into the decision-making process.

Co-equality and Co-participation

Parents provide critical information about family issues and cultural concerns (Dinnebeil, 1999). The parent serves as the primary caregiver and mediator of change in the child's home environment. The parent can contribute to child learning and educational generalization. Parents play a role in the identification of the child's communication needs and of events that critically affect developmental changes within the child. Although the parent may not have clinical knowledge, a parent's insights and knowledge provide valuable information that can be used by professionals to determine educational objectives and priorities (Broderick & Mastrilli, 1997).

As a member of the collaborative team, the parent participates as a respected *equal* contributor in the decision-making process. A parent's insights can provide information that is helpful in prioritizing and organizing IEP goals (Hoover-Dempsey & Sandler, 1997). The collaborative team needs to incorporate the feelings and concerns of the parent when establishing short-term and long-term classroom goals. By being a member of the team, parents in turn become supportive of the educational process. They have invested in the outcome and success of the inclusion experience (see Figure 3.6). Having contributed to the goals and decisions related to the child and the classroom, the parent can continue to plan and collaborate on the daily educational changes required for inclusion. School reform can only be achieved if the parent is recognized as a partner in classroom learning and generalization (Briggs, 1998). Specific modifications are required to create successful collaborative relationships with parents (Tiegerman-Farber & Radziewicz, 1998):

1. Successful collaboration requires that parents become part of school teams.
2. Successful collaboration develops a process for parent advocacy:
   - Changes in how parents and teachers interact
   - Changes in how parents contribute to decision making in the classroom
   - Changes in child outcomes by incorporating parent input into problem-solving solutions
3. Successful collaboration involves teaching parents about educational issues. Parent education programs must be scheduled with working parents in mind:
   - Parents need to know about laws and procedures—teach advocacy skills.
   - Parents need to know about child development and disorders.
   - Parents need to know about instructional techniques and procedures.
4. Successful collaboration establishes parent–teacher teams for each classroom.

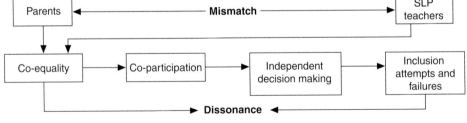

Match = consonance

Mismatch = dissonance

Variables
- Commitment
- Communication
- Time
- Schedules
- Attitudes
- Beliefs
- Classroom access
- Roles
- Responsibilities

FIGURE 3.6

Decision-Making Process

The inclusion of parents in the collaborative process is critical. Parents must be part of the decision-making team.

5. Successful collaboration acknowledges the primary role of parents in inclusive classrooms.
6. Successful collaboration requires educational modifications and accommodations for parents to participate in their child's learning: observing in the classroom and videotapes.

The inclusion of parents in team decision making is an investment; it ensures that parents will maintain a working relationship with professionals at home to generalize educational behaviors across different contexts (McBride, Sharp, Hains, & Whitehead, 1995). Parental empowerment requires that parents be recognized as decision makers and, therefore, serve as acknowledged members of their child's learning. It is not enough for parents to participate if they cannot contribute substantively as decision makers to the process. It has been suggested (Pogorzelski & Kelly, 1993) that parents should become active members in committees that deal with district-wide educational issues, not just "bake sales."

Reciprocity

The term *reciprocal exchange* suggests an ongoing relationship that involves modification over time. Part of the process that occurs between equal partners—parent and professional—involves such an exchange of information. Parents and professionals need to work together when making decisions about child change and educational needs. A mutual respect for each other and differences in perspectives create a healthy tension between parent and professional (Lazar & Slostad, 1999). Reciprocal exchange does not mean that the speech-language pathologist or teacher "hears what the parent has to say." Reciprocal exchange does mean that the speech-language pathologist and teacher listen and incorporate what the parent has to say into the ongoing educational programming provided for the child (Coufal, 1993).

It is interesting to note that, historically, the issue of parent participation has related specifically to parents of children with disabilities. The legal cases concerning advocacy, least restrictive environment, and educational placement all involved families of children with disabilities (Yell, 1995). Collaboration provides the opportunity to change traditional relationships and ideas within the classroom by presenting a benefit for parents of regular education students as well. Because the classroom will include an integration of children with and without LCD, parents of regular education students may also seek to expand their relationships with professionals. Just as the inclusion classroom provides a commingling of experiences for children, it could also provide a collaborative experience for parents of children with and without LCD (Arllen, Gable, & Hendrickson, 1996).

Parent–Teacher–Speech-Language Pathologist Teaming

Inclusion cannot be successfully achieved without collaborative interaction between parent, teacher, and speech-language pathologist. It was noted earlier that collaboration requires co-equality and co-participation among members of the team. This suggests that the parent has as much to say as professionals about the process of learning, the procedural aspects of instruction, and the academic components of curriculum development. A great deal of parent–teacher–speech-language pathologist planning and programming must occur prior to the establishment and during the implementation of the inclusion classroom (Dinnebeil and Rule, 1994). This suggests that parent–teacher–speech-language pathologist teaming requires an innovative working relationship; the collaborative variables of time and communication must be addressed if the team outcomes are to be successful (see Figure 3.6).

Parent–teacher–speech-language pathologist teams need to delineate their roles, rules, and responsibilities during their meetings. Teams also need to establish specific times and goals for all of their meetings by means of a formalized process. This will obviously have an effect on scheduling, because it may be difficult for teams to meet during the day. The school should make a clear commitment to flexible hours and after-school meetings to facilitate interactions among the parent, teacher, and speech-language pathologist. The goals of collaboration require changes in schedules, working hours, and commitments from all of the collaborators involved with the process. Perhaps the greatest benefit will be a break from traditional ideas and notions about roles, rules, and responsibilities (Waggoner and Griffith, 1998). The more flexibility that parents and professionals have for creative solutions, the greater will be the probability that the goals of inclusion will be accomplished through the collaborative process.

Consultation

Consultation provides the mechanism for the speech-language pathologist to assume an advisory role with parents in school or in the home (see Figure 3.5). Here, the decision making is not shared but advisory and supervisory in nature. The primary function of consultation is for the speech-language pathologist to teach the techniques and procedures so that the parent can become an agent of change for the child to generalize language skills to natural settings. The starting point for parent education begins with formalized instructional programming (Tiegerman-Farber & Radziewicz, 1998). If parents are going to be taught to facilitate their children, they must receive some kind of educational instruction. Schools must assume the responsibility of developing parent-training programs. Schools must also determine how to teach and what to teach parents; again, the speech-language pathologist can assume the role of the consultant with school educators to develop parent-training programs and goals that are culturally and linguistically sensitive to the needs of diverse families (Dinnebeil, 1999). Parent training provides a knowledge base that empowers parents to advocate effectively. The child with LCD presents a constellation of problems. Early intervention, parent education, respite services, therapeutic services, and counseling services underscore the need for a broad-based comprehensive approach to facilitating family involvement. Many children with LCD continue to have language learning problems as they grow older. Although many children with LCD are eventually mainstreamed or included within regular classrooms, parent educators need to help families address their fears and concerns about a life-cycle continuum of services and a life-long commitment to advocacy (Lazar, Broderick, Mastrilli, & Slostad, 1999).

Parent Education Variables

McDade and Varnedoe (1987) discuss several variables that should be included in the content of a parent-education program. Language facilitative techniques include training parents to provide positive feedback for children's communicative attempts. This stresses the importance of communication and deemphasizes the attention parents often pay to structural and syntactic aspects of their children's speech. Parents are also taught to use expansions and comments to facilitate children's language. In this parent-training program, parents are trained individually during thirty-minute weekly sessions for eight to ten weeks. Parent–child dyadic interactions are video-taped to determine initial parent-training goals. Parents are released from parent training once they demonstrate that they can exhibit a set of target behaviors. The researchers noted that there are limitations in the use of video equipment that involve additional time and space.

Fitzgerald and Karnes (1987) describe the RIP (Regional Intervention Programs for Parents and Preschools) service delivery system, which has been used in the treatment of families with young at-risk children with development disabilities. Parental involvement is central to the RIP model (Timm & Rule, 1981). Parents function as change agents, as case managers for other parents, and as evaluators of program's success. Parental participation has two operational phases, a treatment phase and a generalization phase. In the treatment phase, parents work individually with their own children at home and at the RIP site. When this phase has been completed, they give their time and skills to train other, newer parents, conduct interviews, collect and analyze data, and teach in the classroom. The RIP model uses trained parents as the cornerstone of the operation of the program, effectively addressing the problem of generalization of skills to other contexts and agents. The level of involvement of parents is both an advantage and disadvantage. Although the success of the program relates to the role of the parents, many parents do not want to be taught by other parents, nor do they want the responsibilities of teaching their own children.

The research presents multiple examples of parent training and education programs. There is general agreement that parent involvement is critical to the success of school reform and the successful achievement of inclusion. The reality, however, is that few public schools have committed time and resources to developing and implementing programs for parents. Whereas children with LCD have entered the "schoolhouse doors," parents with and without LCD have not. One reason that parents nationally have advocated for school reform and vouchers is the growing frustration that they do not have access to classrooms and educational decision making. Few schools have incorporated the clear results of many research investigations emphasizing that parents must be equal partners. Interestingly enough, this appears to be less of a problem for speech-language pathologists, given our historically close working relationship with parents. Speech-language pathologists, like parents, have never been acknowledged as significant facilitators to classroom learning, because "language" was taught in a therapy room by a related service provider. However, speech-language pathologists are no longer *just* related service providers, because language has finally been recognized as critical to all aspects of educational learning. The speech-language pathologist may be the key professional to the successful integration of parents and children with LCD into the regular classroom.

CONCLUSION

This chapter has discussed some of the issues underlying decision making and interactive teaming. Interactive teaming provides the mechanism for diverse individuals to come together to develop inclusive programming. Interactive teaming involves a learning process for all of the members who embark on the inclusion mission.

Parents and professionals who have had the opportunity to be part of an interactive process have indicated the remarkable changes that have occurred as members of a team working together to develop a mission and a program. Eventually, the team has a life force of its own and proceeds through a series of changes as each member learns about the process and commits to the mission. The diversity and the difference of each individual contribute to the collective creativity of the team. The resulting creative product reflects a synergy that could not have been achieved by members individually. Interactive teaming reflects what the inclusive process is all about; differences can be a force for creative change when they are focused to accomplish a mission or goal. We all learn together and from each other. The "inclusion whole" becomes greater than the sum of its parts. Each stakeholder contributes to the creation of the inclusion classroom. It is important to stress that inclusion, although an opportunity for all, remains the final step in an educational journey. The speech-language pathologist has a significant role to play in the child-based decision making that will ultimately benefit each and every child within the classroom. It is important to caution that inclusion is an option for every child but not necessarily an academic and/or social benefit. This is a controversial issue in education; many professionals do not support a full-inclusion model that does not allow for a continuum of educational options for children with LCD. The interactive team must also discuss who will benefit and how each child will benefit from an inclusive classroom experience. Clearly, interactive teaming provides the pathway to educational reform.

STUDY QUESTIONS

1. Describe the changing role of the speech-language pathologist in educational decision making.
2. Discuss why parents should be advocates for their children.
3. Explain the difference between consultation and collaboration in terms of the provision of services for children with developmental disabilities.
4. Discuss the educational problems related to inclusion of children with disabilities for teachers and parents within the regular educational classroom.
5. What does responsible decision making mean?
6. Co-equality and co-participation are part of the collaborative process; explain what these terms mean.

REFERENCES

American Speech-Language-Hearing Association, ASHA (1990). The roles of speech-language pathologists in service delivery to infants, toddlers, and their families. *ASHA,* 32 (suppl. 2), 4.

Arllen, N., Gable, R. A., & Hendrickson, J. M. (1996). Accommodating students with special needs in general education classrooms. *Preventing School Failure, 41,* 7–13.

Bahr, R. H., Velleman, S. L., & Ziegler, M. A. (1999). Meeting the challenge of suspected developmental apraxia of speech through inclusion. *Topics in Language Disorders, 19*(3), 19–35.

Bailey, D. B., Aytch, L. S., Odom, S. L., Symons, F., & Wolery, M. (1999). Early intervention as we know it. *Mental Retardation and Development Disabilities, 5,* 11–20.

Beck, A., & Dennis, M. (1997). Speech-language pathologists' and teachers' perceptions of classroom-based interventions. *Language, Speech, and Hearing Services in Schools, 2,* 146–153.

Blosser, J., & Kratcoski, A. (1997). PAC's: A framework for determining appropriate service delivery options. *Language, Speech, and Hearing Services in Schools, 2,* 99–107.

Briggs, M. H. (1998). Families talk: Building partnerships for communicative change. *Topics in Language Disorders, 18*(3), 71–84.

Broderick, P. C., & Mastrilli, T. (1997). Attitudes concerning parent involvement: Parent and teacher perspectives. *Pennsylvania Educational Leadership, 16,* 30–36.

Bronfenbrenner, U. (1977). Toward an experimental ecology of human development. *American Psychologist, 32,* 512–531.

Bruskewitz, R. (1998). Collaborative intervention: A system of support for teachers . . . teachers; students—Psychology. *Preventing School Failure, 42*(3), 129.

Buysse, V., & Wesley, P. (1999). Community development approaches for early intervention. *Topics in Early Childhood Special Education, 19*(4), 236.

Chess, S. (1986). Early childhood development and its implications for analytical theory and practice. *American Journal of Psychoanalysis, 46,* 122–148.

Chisholm, I. M. (1994). Preparing teachers for multicultural classrooms. *Journal of Educational Issues of Language Minority Students, 14,* 43–67.

Coufal, K. (1993). Collaborative consultation for speech/language pathologists. *Topics in Language Disorders, 14*(1), 1–14.

Crais, K. (1993). Families and professionals as collaborators in assessment. *Topics in Language Disorders, 14*(1), 29–40.

Dinnebeil, L. A. (1999). Defining parent education in early intervention. *Topics in Early Childhood Special Education, 19*(3), 161.

Dinnebeil, L. A., & Hale, L. (1999). Early intervention program practices that support collaboration. *Topics in Early Childhood Special Education, 19*(4), 225.

Dinnebeil, L. A., & Rule, S. (1994). Variables that influence collaboration between parents and service coordinators. *Journal of Early Intervention, 18,* 349–361.

Epstein, J. L. (1995). School/families/community partnerships: Caring for children we share. *Phi Delta Kappan, 76,* 101–102.

Fitzgerald, M. T., & Karnes, D. E. (1987). A parent-implemented language model for at risk and developmentally delayed preschool children. *Topics in Language Disorders, 7*(3), 31–46.

Friend, M., & Bursuck, W. D. (1996). *Including students with special needs.* Boston: Allyn & Bacon.

Gable, R. A., & Hendrickson, J. M. (1997). Teaching all the students: A mandate for educators. In J. Choate (Ed.), *Successful inclusive teaching: Detecting and correcting special needs* (2d ed.) (pp. 2–17). Boston: Allyn & Bacon.

Gable, R. A., Korinek, L., & Laycock, V. (1997). Collaboration in the schools: Ensuring success. In J. Choate (Ed.), *Successful inclusive teaching: Detecting and correcting special needs* (2d ed.) (pp. 50–71). Boston: Allyn & Bacon.

Gable, R. A., & Manning, M. L. (1999). Interdisciplinary teaming: Solution to instructing heterogeneous groups of students. *The Clearing House, 72*(3), 182–185.

Gallagher, T. M. (1999). Interrelationships among children's language, behavior, and emotional problems. *Topics in Language Disorders, 19*, 1–15.

Gitlin, A. (1999). Collaboration and progressive school reform. Educational change; School management and organization; reformers. *Educational Policy, 13*(5), 630.

Hammond, A., & Warner, C. (1996). Physical educators and speech-language pathologists: A good match for collaborative consultation. *Physical Educator, 53*(4), 181.

Harn, W. E., Bradshaw, M. L., & Ogletree, B. T. (1999). The speech-language pathologist in the schools: Changing roles. *Intervention in School & Clinic, 34*(3), 163.

Hoover-Dempsey, K. V., & Sandler, H. M. (1997). Why do parents become involved in their children's education? *Review of Educational Research, 67*(1), 3–42.

Hudson, P., & Glomb, N. (1997). If it takes two to tango, then why not teach both partners to dance? Collaboration instruction for all educators. *Journal of Learning Disabilities, 30*, 442–448.

Idole, L., Paolucci-Whitecomb, P., & Nevin, A. (1986). *Collaborative consultation.* Rockville, MD: Aspen.

Individuals with Disabilities Education Act of 1997 (IDEA), 20 U.S.C. Section 1400 et seq.

Jones, L. T., & Blendinger, J. (1994). New beginnings: Preparing future teachers to work with diverse families. *Action in Teacher Education, 16*, 79–88.

Lazar, A., Broderick, P., Mastrilli, T., & Slostad, F. (1999). Educating teachers for parent involvement. Parent-teacher relationships and education—Parent participation. *Contemporary Education, 70*(3), 5–6.

Lazar, A., & Slostad, F. (1999). How to overcome obstacles to parent-teacher partnerships. *The Clearing House, 72*(4), 206–210.

Little, M. E., & Robinson, S. M. (1997). Renovating and refurbishing the field experience structures for novice teachers. *Journal of Learning Disabilities, 30*, 443–441.

Mahoney, G., & Bella, J. M. (1998). An examination of the effects of family-centered early intervention on child and family outcomes. *Topics in Early Childhood Special Education, 18*(2), 83.

McBride, S. L., Sharp, L., Hains, A. H., & Whitehead, A. (1995). Parents as co-instructors in preservice training: A pathway to family-centered practice. *Journal of Early Intervention, 19*, 343–355.

McCollum, J., & Hughes, M. (1988). Staffing patterns and team models in infancy programs. In J. Jordan, J. Gallagher, P. Hutinger, & M. Karnes (Eds.), *Early childhood special education: Birth to three* (pp. 129–146). Arlington, VA: The Council for Exceptional Children.

McDade, H., & Varnedoe, D. (1987). Training parents to be language facilitators. *Topics in Language Disorders, 7*, 19–30.

Meyer, J. (1997). Models of service delivery. In P. E. O'Connell (Ed.), *Speech, language, and hearing programs in schools: A guide for students and practitioners* (pp. 241–286). Gaithersburg, MD: Aspen.

Midkiff, R. B., & Lawler-Prince, D. (1992). Preparing tomorrow's teachers: Meeting the challenge of diverse family structures. *Action in Teacher Education, 14*, 1–5.

Norris, J. (1997). Functional language intervention in the classroom: Avoiding the tutoring trap. *Topics in Language Disorders, 17,* 49–68.

Ogletree, B. T. (1999). Practical solutions to the challenges of changing professional roles: Introduction to the Special Issue. *Intervention in School & Clinic, 34*(3), 131.

Pogorzelski, G., & Kelly, B. (1993). *Inclusion: The collaborative process.* Buffalo, NY: United Educational Services.

Sanger, D., Maag, J., & Shapera, N. (1994). Language problems among students with emotional and behavioral disorders. *Intervention in School and Clinic, 30*(2), 103–108.

Slavin, R. E., Madden, N. A., Dolan, L. J., & Wasik, B. A. (1996). *Every child, every school: Success for all.* Thousand Oaks, CA: Corwin.

Tiegerman-Farber, E., & Radziewicz, C. (1995). Match-mismatch: A clinical intervention model. In E. Tiegerman-Farber (Ed.), *Language and communication intervention in preschool children* (pp. 129–153). Boston: Allyn & Bacon.

Tiegerman-Farber, E., & Radziewicz, C. (1998). *Collaborative decision making: The pathway to inclusion.* Upper Saddle River, NJ: Prentice Hall.

Timm, M. A., & Rule, S. (1981). RIP: A cost effective parent-implemented program for young handicapped children. *Early Development and Care, 7,* 147–163.

Trivette, C. M. (1998). How much is enough: Training issues regarding family-centered practices. *Journal of Early Intervention, 21,* 111–113.

Volk, D., & Stahlman, J. (1994). "I think everybody is afraid of the unknown": Early childhood teachers prepare for mainstreaming. *Day Care and Early Education, 21*(3), 13–17.

Waggoner, K., & Griffith, A. (1998). Parent involvement in education. *Journal for a Just & Caring Education, 4,* 65.

Walther-Thomas, C. S. (1997). Co-teaching experiences: The benefits and problems that teachers and principals report over time. *Journal of Learning Disabilities, 30,* 395–407.

Wehman, T. (1998). Family-centered early intervention services: Factors contributing to increased parent involvement and participation. *Focus on Autism & Other Developmental Disabilities, 13*(2), 80.

Winton, P. (1998). Socially valid but difficult to implement: Creative solutions needed. *Journal of Early Intervention, 21,* 114–116.

Yell, M. (1995). Least restrictive environments, inclusion, and students with disabilities: A legal analysis. *Journal of Special Education, 28*(4), 389–404.

4

Early Communication Assessment and Intervention

Nancy B. Robinson

California State University, Chico

Michael P. Robb

University of Connecticut at Storrs

A Dynamic Process

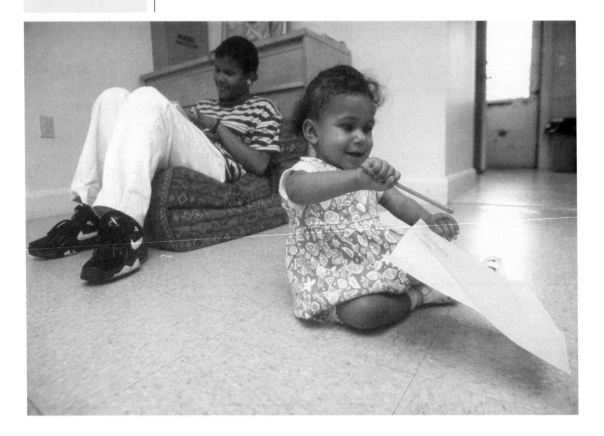

- Describe infant behaviors that provide indices for assessment and intervention at the prelinguistic and emergent language levels
- Implement assessment and intervention processes that include selection of appropriate informal and formal methods
- Discuss current best practice in early language intervention and selection of appropriate strategies for individual children
- Identify policy and legislation that defines professional practice for SLPs in early intervention settings
- Describe family-centered and culturally competent approaches to early assessment and intervention with infants, toddlers and families
- Discuss the roles of early intervention team members and the collaborative approaches to assessment and intervention for infants and toddlers

In a chapter designed to introduce students to the processes involved in communication assessment and intervention with infants and toddlers, one may question what early communication, speech, and language abilities are found among the youngest of humans. In fact, the term "infant" originates from a Latin term meaning, "one unable to speak." The literal interpretation implies a being without communication abilities, a view that has been challenged in recent decades, beginning with Chomsky's (1965) proposal that language is an "innate property of the human mind" and that the human enters life in the earliest days with preprogrammed linguistic ability. Since the development of the nativist proposals articulated by Chomsky, recent theorists have proposed a more generalized ability in the infant that predisposes the human to the development of spoken language and highly specific prelinguistic skills that lead to interaction with caregivers and the environment (Kent & Hodge, 1991). Infants are now assumed to enter the world with a tremendous degree of organization and predilection for language acquisition rather than specific linguistic programming (Paul, 1999).

This chapter focuses on three major areas: early prelinguistic communication; emergent speech and language abilities in the first years of life; and most importantly, assessment and intervention strategies for early intervention specialists, particularly speech-language pathologists, to enhance language development with infants and toddlers at high risk of communication disorders.

Several strands of research lend support to the efficacy of early intervention to enhance language development, including health and education disciplines of psychology, psychiatry, nursing, medicine, early childhood special education, occupational therapy, physical therapy, speech-language pathology, nutrition, and others. Continuity and predictive relationships between early prelinguistic behaviors in infants and emerging language behaviors in toddlers were found in the last two decades (Bates, Benigni, Bretherton, Camaioni, & Volterra, 1979; Bates, Bretherton, & Snyder, 1988; Snow, 1979). Researchers in medicine and psychology also found that parent–child interaction patterns in infancy are related to later developmental outcomes (Brazelton & Als, 1979). The role of the environment to influence developmental outcomes for young children, particularly language, is further supported in recent research that investigated long-term outcomes for children in various SES groups.

Theories of language development during infancy continue to be influenced by many fields and most recently, neurobiology. Bates (1999) summarized research and evidence from neurobiology that challenges the nativist position and illuminates our understanding of the critical nature of infant development related to processes that support and lead to speech, language, and communication behavior in the early years of life. Bates argues that the neurobiological underpinnings of language are based on adaptations of general properties and functions of the brain. Second, she identifies results of research with adults and infants with focal brain injury that reinforces the notion that the infant's brain is highly plastic, with the ability to permit language learning through alternatives in brain development. Although Bates argues that specific localization in the brain for language functions is not supported in research, infant humans begin life with highly differentiated brain functions, perhaps with certain regions biased toward information processing that are important for language development. The findings reported by Bates and her colleagues strengthen the assumptions that the infant's interactions with caregivers in the environment are critical to maximize language development. Early intervention professionals are faced with the challenge of early identification of young children at risk of communication disorders. Locke (1994) emphasized the "cascading effect" of even subtle impairments in the ability to process and learn auditory information in young children. The importance of early identification, assessment, and intervention is thus clearly supported.

Recent research increases our understanding of risk factors that may lead to limitations in communication, speech, and language development in young children and underscores the urgent need for early identification and intervention when brain development is rapid with a degree of "plasticity." The goal of this chapter is to introduce to the student a foundation of behaviors that describe the infant's developing linguistic and communication system. The specification of prelinguistic behaviors and stages of development that are now considered predictive of later language development and risk factors for communication disorders is aimed at preparing professionals to better assist these children and families at a critical time in early life. The chapter is divided into five sections, beginning with policy guidelines for early communication intervention. The second section of the chapter describes known risk factors that are related to poor developmental outcomes in young children, particularly delays in language development. The third section examines traditional and dynamic approaches to early language assessment and intervention. The fourth section provides an organizational framework for dynamic processes of assessment and intervention and includes suggested methods and tools to implement comprehensive and collaborative intervention for children at risk of communication disorders. Finally, the fifth section applies suggested processes for assessment and intervention to three case studies for demonstration and student discussion. Families and children in the United States are increasingly of diverse cultural and linguistic backgrounds. Throughout the chapter, changing societal demographics and practices recommended to support families and children in a multicultural society are included. Further, the chapter is based on the principle that early intervention requires a team of professionals, with the central member being the family. Processes and practices in early communication assessment are applicable for all early intervention professionals and are targeted specifically for the speech-language pathologist (SLP).

POLICY GUIDELINES FOR THE SLP IN EARLY INTERVENTION

The involvement and role of the SLP in early intervention was defined more clearly with the passage of Public Law 99-457 in 1986. Since the reauthorization of the Individuals with Disabilities Act (IDEA) in 1997, the need for early intervention continues to be strongly supported. Recent American Speech-Hearing-Language Association (ASHA) initiatives focusing on the identification of newborn infants at risk for hearing loss are one example of policies that recognize that the first years of life are critical for language learning.

The policy statement issued by ASHA in 1989 remains current to support the role of SLPs in early intervention settings. Passage of reauthorization of IDEA in 1997 strengthened the legal requirements for early intervention and the role of the SLP to assist young families and children.

> Families and their infants and toddlers (birth–36 months) who are at-risk or have developmental disabilities present a broad spectrum of needs that the appropriately certified and/or licensed speech-language pathologist is uniquely qualified to address. These include delays and disabilities in communication, language, and speech, as well as oral-motor and feeding behaviors. Speech-language pathologists, and independent practitioners, assume various roles in addressing these needs of families and their infants. (p. 116)

This ASHA position statement describes possible roles of SLPs in early intervention to include (1) screening and identification, (2) assessment and evaluation, (3) design, planning, direct delivery, and monitoring of treatment programs, (4) case management, and (5) consultation with, and referral to, agencies and other professionals. The intention is that the SLP is expected to assume these multiple and changing roles within a community-based, family-centered program, as part of an early intervention team. Although brief in content, the position statement embodies considerable thought and broad implications about the way we interact with families and their infants at risk for communicative disorders (Catlett, 1991).

CHILDREN AT RISK FOR COMMUNICATION/LANGUAGE DELAYS

When genetic heritage and prenatal life are favorable, the infant's roots are securely anchored and normal development should occur (Kopp, 1990). Unfavorable genetic or prenatal factors set the stage for vulnerabilities, that is, the child becomes "at risk" for developmental delays. Since the inception of PL 99-457, attention has been directed toward identifying and intervening with the at-risk infant. There are two basic forms of risk: biological and environmental. Biological risks stem from genetic conditions as well as from exposure to *teratogenic* factors (e.g., viral infections, and drug use). Environmental risk generally refers to adverse rearing conditions (e.g., maternal depression, abuse, and environmental toxins).

The following describes biological and environmental factors that place infants at risk for communicative disorders. The list is not meant to be all-inclusive. Many other sources have reviewed well-known biological risks that can be identified early in life, such as Down syndrome, cerebral palsy, cleft lip and palate, and so on. The present review highlights recent information regarding risk factors that are increasingly identified among newborn infants. The risk factors range from minor to significant involvement.

Biological Risks

Illegal Substances

When considering the perinatal effects of illegal or illicit substances, the basic tenets of maternal–fetal physiology and pharmacology apply (Dattel, 1990). Illicit drugs tend to be of low molecular weight, passing freely between the mother and child within minutes of ingestion. Because of the rapid transfer across the placental barrier, the drug concentration received by the fetus is usually 50 to 100 percent of maternal levels. The effects of drugs on the fetus are also linked to embryological development. For example, most of the body organs and the structures comprising the face and head are formed within the first trimester of pregnancy. Brain development continues throughout pregnancy. So it is not only a matter of which drug and how much of the drug is ingested by the mother, but when the drug was taken during the pregnancy. Unfortunately, incidence and prevalence data are difficult to establish. The substance being abused is often illegal; thus, parental disclosure of drug use is rare. In addition, identifying and isolating a specific drug used by a parent is problematic because of the mixture of over-the-counter drugs (e.g., caffeine, alcohol). Recent estimates place the number of infants exposed in utero to one or more illegal drugs at between 625,000 and 729,000 per year (about 15 to 18 percent) (National Institute on Drug Abuse, 1995).

Cocaine and Methamphetamines

The effects of cocaine (including crack) and methamphetamines (ecstasy, ice, speed) on the central nervous system include increased respiratory and heart rate, restlessness, and excitement. The drugs suppress the mother's appetite, and she is often sleep deprived. Developmental outcomes of infants exposed to any of these drugs include shorter body length, smaller head circumference, and lower birthweight than infants delivered to drug-free women. If these drugs are taken later in the pregnancy, the infant runs a greater risk of being born addicted to the drug and may experience withdrawal symptoms including cardiovascular problems, seizures, and difficulty sucking, swallowing, and feeding (McElhatton, Bateman, Evans, Pughe, & Thomas, 1999). Because the brain continues to develop throughout pregnancy, it is also possible that the infant may show cognitive impairments.

Marijuana

Studies of marijuana use by pregnant women are inconclusive because the drug is often taken in conjunction with other drugs, notably alcohol and tobacco. Marijuana used during pregnancy is associated with a variety of adverse outcomes, including prematurity, low birthweight, decreased maternal weight gain, complications of pregnancy, difficult labor, congenital abnormalities, increased chance of stillbirth and perinatal mortality, poor neonatal assessment scores, and limited verbal and memory abilities (Fried & Watkinson, 1990). Use of marijuana following birth has also been shown to have an adverse effect on infants who are breastfed. Howard and Lawrence (1998) found infants exposed to breastmilk that contained the active ingredient in marijuana (delta-9-tetrahydro cannabinol) to be lethargic and to feed less frequently and for shorter periods of time.

Commonly Used Teratogens

The term *teratogen,* translated literally from its Greek roots, means "monster maker" (*teratos* = monster; *gen* = derived from). The practical application of the term is reserved for substances that produce anomalies when the developing embryo is exposed to them (Shprintzen, 1997). Alcohol, nicotine, and caffeine are teratogenic agents that are capable of interfering with the development of a fetus.

Alcohol

People have been brewing and fermenting alcoholic drinks since the dawn of time. Alcohol is the most widely used, and abused, drug in the United States. Nearly 100,000 Americans die each year as a result of alcohol abuse, and alcohol is a factor in more than half of the country's homicides, suicides, and traffic accidents (National Institute on Alcohol Abuse and Alcoholism, 1997). On average, three of every five women of childbearing age consume alcoholic beverages (ASHA, 1991). Because alcohol can interfere with essentially any developmental process in the embryo, the variation in both the physical and behavior features of the infant can be quite dramatic (Shprintzen, 1997). Jones and Smith (1974) were the first to describe fetal alcohol syndrome (FAS), resulting from excessive prenatal exposure to alcohol. FAS is a pattern of altered tissue and organ development that involves cardiovascular problems, craniofacial abnormalities (e.g., cleft lip and/or palate), limb defects, growth deficiency, and poor fine and gross motor coordination (Gerber, 1990). It is still unknown how much alcohol is necessary to produce the symptoms of FAS. Children who demonstrate subtle signs of prenatal alcohol exposure are said to show fetal alcohol effects (FAE). The FAS syndrome appears in 3 per 1,000 live births and FAE occurs in 10 per 1,000 live births (Shprintzen, 1997). Reported communication problems include delayed language and problems with speech articulation, fluency, voice, and swallowing (ASHA, 1991; Sparks, 1989).

Nicotine

Nicotine is a stimulant that causes a short-term increase in blood pressure, heart rate, and the flow of blood from the heart. An estimated 28 percent of reproductive-age women smoke cigarettes, which equates to more than 14 million women ages 18–44 who are smokers. Approximately 90 percent of the nicotine inhaled is absorbed into the mother's body (Dattel, 1990). Smoking during pregnancy, specifically the ingestion of nicotine, raises the risk of miscarriage or premature labor. However, the primary danger associated with smoking is low birthweight, accounting for at least 20 percent of all low-birthweight infants born in the United States. Nicotine depresses the mother's appetite at a time when she should be gaining weight, and smoking reduces the ability to absorb oxygen. The fetus, being deprived of both nourishment and oxygen, may not grow as it should. Documented effects of nicotine ingestion on the infant include impaired neurological and intellectual development, and a higher risk of sudden infant death syndrome (SIDS). A recent report by Fergusson, Woodward, and Horwood (1998) found that children exposed to maternal smoking during pregnancy showed high rates of conduct disorder, alcohol abuse, substance abuse, and depression later in life.

Caffeine

Caffeine acts as a stimulant to the central nervous system and is commonly found in tea, coffee, carbonated soft drinks, and chocolate. Caffeine is a substance commonly used during pregnancy. At least 80 percent of pregnant women ingest caffeine in some form daily (Dattel, 1990). As with other chemicals, caffeine freely crosses the placental barrier between mother and child. However, because caffeine is broken down much more slowly than some other substances, its potential influence on the developing child is greater. To date there has been no definitive evidence to suggest a link between caffeine use and poor developmental outcome in human infants (Hatch & Bracken,1993). However, results from animal studies have shown that significant amounts of caffeine during pregnancy are related to an increase in birth defects and a decrease in fetal weight (Narod, Sanjose, & Victora, 1991). As a general rule, pregnant women are advised to limit their caffeine intake.

Other Health Risks

Two medical conditions that have been shown to adversely impact communication development are middle-ear infections and infection with the virus that causes acquired immunodeficiency syndrome (AIDS).

The rapid and short onset of signs and symptoms of inflammation in the middle ear is termed acute otitis media (Bluestone, 1990). Acute otitis media occurs in almost every child at some time during the first few years of life. Many infants experience multiple episodes of acute otitis media; some spend months, with fluid discharge (of effusion) in both ears (Paradise, Rockette, Colburn, Bernard, Smith, Kurs-Lasky, & Janosky, 1997; Teele, Klein, Chase, Menyuk, & Rosner, 1990). Considerable data show that, although otitis media with effusion (OME) produces only a temporary hearing loss, it is the persistent or recurrent nature of OME that produces a fluctuating hearing loss. It is a fluctuating hearing loss that poses a challenge for young children attempting to acquire speech and language (Gravel & Wallace, 2000). Teele et al. (1990) found that children who experienced OME during the first three years of life were later found to have lower scores on tests of cognitive ability and on follow-up speech and language tests at 7 years of age. Further, Shriberg, Friel-Patti, Flapsen, and Brown (2000) have suggested that children aged 12–18 months who experienced OME with an accompanying mild hearing loss were at a 33 percent risk for developing delayed speech and language by 3 years of age.

In 1981 the Centers for Disease Control (CDC) reported an outbreak of a rare form of cancer among homosexual men residing in New York and California, known medically as Kaposi's sarcoma. About a year later, the CDC linked the illness to blood and termed the illness AIDS (Acquired Immune Deficiency Syndrome). In 1985, the human immunodeficiency virus (HIV) was discovered to be the cause of AIDS. The HIV has since come to encompass large numbers of heterosexuals, intravenous drug abusers, persons with hemophilia, and other recipients of contaminated blood products (Cohen, 1990). As of 1999, the cumulative number of AIDS cases reported to the CDC was 733,374. Adult and adolescent AIDS cases total 724,656, with 604,843 cases in males and 119,810 cases in females. Most infants with HIV contracted the virus by perinatal exposure. The first reports of pediatric AIDS were in 1983, and presently there are over 2,000 pediatric HIV cases and approximately 270 AIDS cases in the United States. Central nervous system involvement is prominent in children with HIV, and only recently are reports surfacing regarding the communicative outcome in infected children. The primary pediatric communication disorders appear to be in the areas of language comprehension, although reports of unusual voice disorders such as hysterical aphonia and elective mutism have also been noted (Zuniga, 1999).

Environmental Risks

Socioeconomic Status

In families experiencing economic hardships, poor living conditions, unstable family life, and/or inadequate alternative childcare resources, parenting itself may be disturbed, resulting in a child with an insecure attachment (Lyons-Ruth, Connell, & Grunebaum, 1990; Shaw & Bell, 1993). Such attachment difficulties place the child at risk for psychopathology during the school years (Rutter, 1979). Low socioeconomic status also appears to be predictive of lower mental development scores, impoverished language development, placement in special classes, and school failure (Bryant & Ramey, 1987).

Maternal Influences

Aside from the drug-related maternal influences that place a child at risk for communication delay, there are environmental risks as well. Maternal anxiety can produce a variety of psychological changes, changes in heart rate, the constriction of blood vessels, and decreases in gastrointestinal motility. Generally, the greater the anxiety, the more severe the response, which ultimately affects the developing fetus. Child-rearing practices also place an infant at risk. Specifically, parental rejection and lack of involvement are two parenting factors that have been identified as salient (Lyons-Ruth et al., 1990). Shaw and Bell (1993) believe that, during infancy, these parenting behaviors are expressed as a lack of parental responsiveness, as parents who were hostile and/or uninvolved consistently fail to respond to the infant's needs. The developmental outcome of these children is often revealing of poor cognitive abilities.

Lead

Around the beginning of the 1900s it was recognized that women employed in the lead trades often gave birth to infants who were small, weak, and neurologically damaged (American Academy of Pediatrics, 1987). Lead had crossed the placental barrier, resulting in retarded intrauterine growth and postnatal failure to thrive. In the United States, thanks to regulations limiting the amount of lead in gasoline, house paint, and other consumer products, current exposure to lead has been dramatically reduced. However, it is now thought that many women of child-bearing age who were exposed to lead as children (e.g., in soil and drinking water) have sufficient amounts of lead accumulated in their bones to threaten the health of their babies many years later (Gonzalez-Cossio, Peterson, Sanin, Fishbein, Palazuelos, Aro, Hernandez-Avila, & Hu, 1997). Noted developmental outcomes of lead exposure include lowered IQ, behavioral problems, language learning difficulties, and school failure.

Nutrition and Diet

Meeting the nutritional needs of infants is well recognized as essential for infants' healthy growth and development (American Academy of Pediatrics, 1993). Proper nutrition during the first year of life plays a vital role in the future growth and development of a child. In addition to meeting nutritional needs, positive feeding experiences can enhance fine motor skills and provide social interaction during infancy (McKinney, Ashwill, Murray, James, Gorrie, & Droske, 2000). The growth rate during infancy is more rapid than any other time during the life cycle. An infant's birth weight may double by 6 months and triple by 1 year of life. Providing adequate calories, protein, vitamins and minerals to support optimal growth is essential. Both the American Academy of Pediatrics and the American Dietetic Association recommend breastfeeding as the preferred method of feeding during the first year of life (American Dietetic Association, 1997). Worldwide, malnutrition contributes to nearly 7 million child deaths every year (UNICEF, 1998). Where it does not kill, poor nutrition can leave children physically impaired (stunted growth), with a weakened immune system, and intellectually impaired.

This section addressed several prevalent risk factors described in recent studies of infants and toddlers born in the United States. Table 4.1 summarizes the foregoing discussion, identifying risk factors and predicted developmental outcomes related to each risk factor. The reader should keep in mind that a single risk factor alone cannot clearly predict a specific outcome, given the mediating effects of the infant's own resiliency and the caregiving environment.

EARLY LANGUAGE ASSESSMENT AND INTERVENTION

We now turn to assessment and intervention for very young children with delays in communication and language development. Communication assessment and intervention are inseparable processes, particularly with infants and toddlers and the relatively rapid developmental period that is taking place. The need to assess known risk factors quickly and accurately, and to provide effective intervention in support of optimal communication and language development requires a dynamic interaction between assessment and intervention processes. Recently, the term *dynamic assessment* has been applied with somewhat older children at the primary and elementary school-age levels to describe a test–teach–retest approach for specific linguistic targets such as emergent spelling, phonemic awareness, vocabulary, syntax, and concept development. Butler (1997) described the historic development of assessment prac-

TABLE 4.1	Selected Risk Factors Related to Adverse Developmental Outcomes	
	Risk Factor	**Possible Outcome**
	Biological risks	
	Cocaine/crack	Low birthweight, shorter body length, smaller head circumference, tremulousness
	Methamphetamines, "ice"	Cognitive, social, behavioral differences
	Marijuana	Prematurity, low birthweight, congenital abnormalities
	Alcohol	Low birthweight, shorter length, fetal alcohol syndrome
	Smoking/nicotine	Neurological impairment, respiratory distress
	Caffeine	Possible decrease in fetal weight and birth defects
	Otitis media	Conductive hearing loss, delayed phonetic development
	HIV infection	Central nervous system disorder, death
	Environmental influences	
	Socioeconomic status	Low mental development, psychopathology
	Maternal influences (e.g., stress)	Low mental development
	Lead	Mental retardation
	Nutrition	Low mental development, learning disorders

tices in speech and language pathology and current trends to sample a child's linguistic skills in "real-life" contexts, particularly related to reading and writing. She points out that the strengths of the approach are based on the collection of assessment data and intervention planning simultaneously. While infants and toddlers do not possess emerging literacy and linguistic skills, prelinguistic interactions with caregivers provide a context to gather assessment data and to demonstrate intervention strategies in a dynamic process. This section of the chapter includes a comparison of traditional approaches to infant assessment and dynamic approaches that include both assessment and intervention strategies, applied specifically to early language development.

Models of Assessment: Traditional and Dynamic Approaches

The two most commonly applied models of assessment are developmental models and naturalistic models. Developmental models are the traditional approach and rely almost exclusively on age-expected or normative criteria. Developmental assessment tools include age-expected behaviors and represent a *static* form of assessment in which the individual infant is assessed against a given set of age-referenced criteria. Developmental assessment tools can be normative, such as the Bayley Scales of Infant Development (Bayley, 1993), or criterion referenced, such as the Hawaii Early Learning Profile (Furuno, O'Reilly, Inatsuka, Hosaka, Allman, & Zeisloft-Falboy, 1987).

Wetherby and Prizant (1992) voiced dissatisfaction with many of the available developmental instruments because of their limited scope and difficulty in thoroughly evaluating preverbal communication behaviors, and they advocate for a *naturalistic* approach. Naturalistic assessment involves viewing the infant's communication skills in commonly occurring settings and contexts such as play and daily routines (Crais, 1995). Far fewer assessment instruments are based on a naturalistic model. Naturalistic approaches and dynamic assessment are closely aligned due to the emphasis on the child's performance in natural contexts and the *process* of determining communication skills. Dynamic assessment can be viewed as a specific application of naturalistic assessment with specific strategies to determine the child's optimal performance when provided with adult support and intervention. A comparative listing of assessment tools that are based on a developmental/traditional model and naturalistic/dynamic approach is given in Table 4.2.

Given the rapid sequence and complexity of developmental processes in the first year of life, we agree with Wetherby and Prizant (1992) that developmental assessment models are often too limited in their examination of the infancy period. Naturalistic and dynamic approaches allow much needed flexibility, which is particularly important when confronted with children with special needs. On the other hand, a naturalistic approach may not provide the milestone information necessary to evaluate the child's communication abilities compared to his same-age peers.

Dynamic Assessment

Recent emphasis on dynamic assessment in speech and language pathology has relevance for assessment with infants and toddlers and is consistent with emphases in the field of early intervention on processes of communication demonstrated by the child and the social interactive context with caregivers. As Butler (1997) stated, assessment is an essential precursor to intervention and should lead to effective intervention. However, standardized tests measure what a child already knows, and are static. In contrast, dynamic assessment provides a sample of the child's performance in the context of interaction with a more knowledgeable partner. Cues and support from the examiner are permitted to determine the extent of the child's emerging language competence and the degree of scaffolding required from adults. When applied with school-age children with language-learning disabilities, the dynamic assessment process is implemented in a test–intervene–test cycle and attention is paid to the strategies that best support the child to display learning abilities. Swanson (cited in Butler, 1997) asserted that dynamic assessment strategies for children with language-learning disabilities contributed to improved information-processing abilities by improving access to previously stored information. While the principles of dynamic assessment appear to have relevance for younger children, Butler cautions that dynamic assessment techniques are more appropriate for use with children with metacognitive abilities.

What similarities are found in dynamic assessment and the dynamic processes recommended for use with infants and toddlers? Butler (1997) outlines the compo-

TABLE 4.2 | **Early Language and Communication Assessment Tools for Infants and Toddlers**

Developmental/Traditional Assessment Tools	Naturalistic/Dynamic Assessment Tools
Minnesota Child Development Inventory (Ireton & Thwing, 1974)	Assessing Prelinguistic and Linguistic Behaviors (Olswang et al., 1987)
Preschool Language Sale—3 (Zimmerman, Steiner, & Pond, 1992)	Neonatal Behavioral Assessment Scale, 2d ed. (Brazelton, 1984)
Battelle Developmental Inventory (Newborg, Stock, & Wnek, 1984)	Assessment of Mother–Child Interaction (Klein & Briggs, 1987)
The Language Development Survey (Rescorla, 1989)	MacArthur Child Development Inventories, Infant and Toddler forms (Fenson et al., 1993)
Reynell Developmental Language Scales (Reynell, 1985).	Parent–Child Interaction Assessment (Comfort & Farran, 1994)
Bayley Scales of Infant Development (Bayley, 1993)	Communication and Symbolic Behavior Scales (Wetherby & Prizant, 1993)
Infant-Toddler Language Scale (Rossetti, 1990)	Communication Matrix (Rowland, 1996)
Receptive-Expressive-Emergent Language Scale—2 (Bzoch & League, 1991)	Integrated Developmental Experiences Assessment (Norris, 1992)
Clinical Linguistic and Auditory Milestones Scale (Capute & Accardo, 1978)	Assessment Evaluation and Programming System (Bricker, 1993)
Hawaii Early Learning Profile (Furuno et al., 1987)	Syracuse Assessments for Birth to Three (Ensher et al., 1997)
Sequenced Inventory of Communicative Development—Revised (Hedrick, Prather, & Tober, 1984)	Communication Play Protocol (Adamson & Bakeman, 1999)
Early Language Milestone Scale (Coplan, 1993)	Transdisciplinary, Play-Based Assessment (Linder, 1993)
Mullen Scales of Early Learning (Mullen, 1997)	
Infant/Toddler Checklist for Communication and Language Development (Wetherby & Prizant, 1998)	

nents and purposes of dynamic assessment to evaluate the child's communicative and learning competence in the following areas:

- Address the child's knowledge base.
- Evaluate the child's attention abilities.
- Evaluate the child's encoding of perception and memory, storage, and retrieval.
- Evaluate the child's strategy selection and application.
- Evaluate the child's degree of self-regulation.

- Evaluate the child's analysis of stimuli presented during the assessment process.
- Evaluate the child's ability to modify learning strategies.

Dynamic Assessment Approaches Applied to Early Intervention

The principles and procedures of dynamic assessment are generally designed for children with the ability to observe and modify their own learning performance, as stated by Butler. However, the principles of determining the child's true knowledge and degree of scaffolding required to demonstrate emergent abilities are applicable and found in recent assessment practices with infants and toddlers. Key applications include the following:

1. Use of parent report to determine the child's performance in natural contexts of daily activities in familiar environments
2. Observation of child and parent or primary caregiver in interactive contexts
3. Interview data to determine child's communication abilities in ideal settings
4. Demonstration by examiner to determine level of scaffolding required for child to demonstrate emergent abilities

Billeaud (1998) described *serial assessment* of infants and toddlers in natural environments as a method that includes observations of children in 1) routine daily activities, 2) interactions with familiar people, 3) manipulation of objects; and 4) development of play. Videotaping is recommended to allow the SLP to interact freely with the parent and child and to provide documentation for intervention and monitoring of progress. Billeaud further suggests that the assessment process be used as a period of *trial intervention* in the context of play to gather information about the child's typical and preferred means of communication. To extend Billeaud's guidelines, the SLP can further determine the types of strategies that optimally stimulate the child to communicate at higher developmental levels. There are clear differences between the naturalistic method of assessment recommended by Billeaud and the steps identified to conduct dynamic assessment with older children who comprehend basic language concepts and display some degrees of verbal language. However, there are similarities in the steps used to observe *habitual* or typical communication patterns and to provide appropriate scaffolding to elicit optimal communication behavior.

Play-based assessment is particularly appropriate to conduct a dynamic assessment approach. Using play as the context, the child is assessed in a transdisciplinary or multidisciplinary team. Differences in the two team models will be discussed in a later section of the chapter. Play schemes are varied to elicit many aspects of communicative behavior, particularly expressive language. Linder's (1993) model for transdisciplinary play-based assessment allows for the early intervention team to gather assessment data through observation of other professionals interacting with the child and family members. The Communication and Symbolic Behavior Scale (Weatherby & Prizant, 1993) is one tool based on naturalistic assessment procedures and applicable for use in a dynamic assessment approach. Specific activities are constructed in the context of play with the child in order to determine his or her response to natural and novel bids for communication.

The application of a dynamic process of assessment and intervention is particularly appropriate for infants and toddlers at risk of communication delays and disorders. A traditional model of assessment involves several stages, including (1) screening, (2) diagnosis, (3) determination of eligibility for services, and (4) progress evaluation following a period of intervention (Ensher, 1989). Sparks (1989) advised that assessments with infants and toddlers be serial, addressing the child, the family, and their interactions. Assessment tools are developed with this approach in mind, for collection of information regarding the child's strengths and weaknesses for purposes of intervention planning. With current policy and practice guidelines leading to a family-centered, dynamic process that incorporates many domains of development and a systems approach to considering family resources, a reconceptualization of communication assessment for infants and toddlers is needed.

Practices and principles that are described by Billeaud (1998) include the following:

1. Early intervention provides optimal opportunities for infants and toddlers with risk of developmental delays to develop communicative competence for school success.
2. Families are the primary members of the early intervention team and require support to provide optimal environments over the long term.
3. Early intervention for communication delays and disorders requires collaboration and teamwork across a variety of professionals and agencies involved with individual families.
4. Family diversity requires a range of early intervention models and approaches by SLPs and other professionals.
5. Specific knowledge and skills are needed to provide effective early intervention services with infants, toddlers at risk of communication delays and disorders, and their family members.

Efficacy of Early Identification and Language Intervention

The importance of early identification and early intervention for children at risk for communication disorders is the primary thesis of this chapter. Recent literature is rich with findings that support the rationale for early identification and early intervention. For example, Oller, Eilers, Neal, and Schwartz (1999) identified the early predictive power of delayed onset of canonical babbling to identify children at risk for delayed speech and language development. While it is well established that delayed onset of babbling is a common characteristic of infants who are deaf or hard of hearing, Oller et al. provide new insight regarding the potential role of babbling in language development in other children at risk of delayed development. In their study of 3,400 infants, late onset of canonical babbling (reduplicated sequences of CV units) at 10 months of age was related to smaller productive vocabularies at 18, 24, and 30 months of age compared to the control group. The authors speculate that delayed onset of canonical babbling may assist in predicting apraxia, dysarthria, specific phonological disorders, and perhaps more general speech and language disorders. McCathren and Yoder (1999) also reported predictive relationships between a number of specific characteristics of vocalization and later language development (expressive vocabularies) among children with identified developmental delays during infancy and in one-year follow-up when subjects were 17 to 24 months of age.

A further implication of interest related to canonical babbling in infants is that parents tend to respond to this type of babbling as if true speech were produced. As Snow (1979) identified twenty years earlier, parents treat all infant behavior as if meaningful communication occurred. The closer approximation to verbal language creates a setting for critical parent–child interaction at the babbling stage. It follows that delayed onset of canonical babbling may create a situation where parents are less likely to interact verbally with their infants and thus reduce environmental input at a critical language learning point. Thus, while delayed onset of babbling is critical information, it is not the entire picture in the complexities of precursors to potential delays in language development in young children.

Paul (1999) challenged the interpretations presented by Oller et al. (1999), emphasizing the multiple variables that affect language development in infants and toddlers. Further, she questions the assumption that babbling is a necessary precursor of speech, citing Bliele (1997), who reported only modest and transient delays in speech and language development in children who were tracheostomized and prevented from babbling as infants. She cautions that use of delayed onset of canonical babbling as a clinical indicator of children at risk of delayed speech and language development may result in excessive numbers of false positives, children who are referred needlessly. She argues for a more comprehensive view of risk factors for speech and language delays and early preventative measures that emphasize monitoring of development combined with parent education and language stimulation for young children with late onset of babbling and early vocabularies.

As Robertson and Weismer (1999) point out, evidence supporting the efficacy for early language intervention with infants and toddlers is scant. They point out that the "watch and see policy" advocated by Paul (1999) and more active intervention approaches lack clear guidelines in research. Treatment methods studied in infants and toddlers are based on interactive approaches. These authors reported positive increases in a number of linguistic and social skills with late-talking toddlers.

Early Language Intervention Approaches

Iacono (1999) reviewed language intervention with early-childhood populations within a framework of early intervention, emphasizing the reciprocal relationship of the wider context of early intervention and language intervention. She describes the development of research that demonstrated effectiveness of early intervention as *first-generation research* and refers to *second-generation research* as the more specific questions asked in the later part of the 1990s to determine the effectiveness of certain components of early intervention. Specific areas of second generation research include parental involvement; program structure, intensity, duration, and timing; location of the intervention; and training of the interventionists. The increasing specificity of effectiveness research in early intervention parallels the development of research in early language intervention, which is becoming increasingly specific regarding the type of intervention strategies implemented with children with communication delays and special needs.

Iacono (1999) provided a comprehensive review of historical developments in early language intervention that has moved from highly structured and didactic to naturalistic and play based. Research in parent–child interaction and IDEA resulted in current best practice guidelines for team models of early language intervention. Current models have historical foundations in behavioral, psycholinguistic, and sociolinguistic theory and can be understood on a continuum of structure and intrusiveness. Key features of early language intervention models are highlighted in Table 4.3, with high structure/most intrusive to low structure/least intrusive approaches arranged from left to right. Similarities are found in the use of natural environments and daily routines in all approaches; however, the degree of structure and adult directives vary. Specific features of each model can be compared related to several variables including, (1) directives by adults, (2) plan for intervention, (3) location or contexts, and (4) method of intervention.

Iacono (1999) further compared the key features of each model and discussed outcomes of each model documented in research. The movement toward naturalistic

TABLE 4.3 High-Structure/Intrusive to Low-Structure/Nonintrusive Models of Early Language Intervention

Direct Instruction	Milieu Teaching	Enhanced Milieu Teaching	Responsive Interaction	Conversation-Based Interventions
SLP identifies specific linguistic goals	Child-oriented focus with environmental arrangement	Child-oriented with focus on organizing the environment to increase communication opportunities	Child-oriented with focus on organizing the environment to increase communication opportunities	Intervention is child oriented; child discovers properties of language
Intervention based on incremental steps	Specific language structures are targeted in "arranged play"	Specific language structures are targeted in "arranged play"	Generalized child communication gains are targeted	All language domains are interrelated; no specific objectives
Intervention conducted in pull-out settings	Intervention conducted in typical child routines	Intervention in natural environments and typical routines	Intervention in natural environments and typical routines	SLP relys on rich learning environments in natural settings
Drill, practice, and reinforcement methods of teaching to achieve mastery	Adult-directed requests (mand-model) for child response and incidental teaching procedures	Incidental teaching approaches in responsive conversational style	Adult follows child's lead and provides linguistic models in response to child's behavior	Adult–child interaction to achieve reciprocal communication

intervention within a context that is familiar for young children is largely supported by current research. Iacono summarized best practices in early language intervention that are found to be effective to support language development in children who are developing typically and those with communication delays and disorders. They include the following.

> *Environmental arrangement.* Design of the environment is recommended to be of high interest, with relevant activities and objects that will engage the child. A variety of techniques are recommended to "sabotage" the environment, such as placing materials in view but just out of reach, in clear plastic containers; and offering choices of materials and activities to engage the child's attention focus.

> *Responsive interaction.* Environments are arranged to engage the child in typical, relevant activities, with adult interaction following the child's lead and building on the establishment of joint attention to expand the child's communication and turn-taking. Specific incidental teaching techniques are used within the context of naturally occurring activities that are the focus of the child's attention. According to Jones and Warren (1991), "Incidental teaching occurs when a child initiates interaction with the teacher in the form of a request, question, comment or other communicative behavior" (p. 49).

> *Prelinguistic milieu intervention.* Modifications of milieu teaching for prelinguistic interventions include the initial uses of requests and comments. Strategies taken from milieu teaching also include following the child's lead, environmental arrangement, and embedding modeling in routines and social interactions.

> *Augmentative and Alternative Communication (AAC).* Incorporation of AAC into play-based intervention is recommended to provide opportunities for children at risk of severe communication delays to communicate in meaningful contexts. Strategies to implement AAC interventions may include precise behavioral objectives and methods and naturalistic procedures to promote the child's use of AAC in communication interactions with peers and adults.

The Effects of "Input"

McCathren, Yoder, and Warren (1995) investigated the role of directives in early language intervention. **Directives** are described as adults' verbal behaviors that communicate to the child the expectation that they do, say, or attend to something. These authors identified three types of directives employed: (1) **follow-in directives** which follow the child's lead; (2) **redirectives,** which initiate a new topic; and (3) **introductions,** or directives given to an unengaged child. The use of directives is a key feature of naturalistic language intervention approaches, including those under the category of milieu and conversational approaches discussed by McDonald (1985) and by Mahoney and Powell (1984). Generally, extensive use of directives by the adult is not encouraged in naturalistic language intervention because of the assumption that the child's spontaneous communication will be inhibited. The exception to the caution against heavy use of directives is follow-in directives, which actually follow the child's focus of attention and attempt to expand communication behavior from the foundation of the child's perspective. The importance of the work by McCathren et al. is their specific identification of the facilitative effect of follow-in directives on language development in young children. Follow-in directives set the stage for the child to learn salient vocabulary and language concepts, and are further reported to affect language development outcomes at later points in time through increased expressive semantic and syntactic development.

Conclusions drawn from this review of the effects of parent interaction on early language development are important because they help to define specific aspects of language that are most effectively facilitated by specific types of directives:

1. Milieu approaches, using follow-in directives, are most effective to facilitate vocabulary and early semantic relations.
2. Directives that are not based on the child's focus of attention are not facilitative of language development.
3. Directives that change the topic (redirectives) or direct the child's attention to new stimuli (introductions) are not positively related to language development outcomes.
4. Although the importance of follow-in directives is established in promoting language development, cultural variation is not accounted for and requires further research.
5. The use of redirectives and introductions has validity in some cases, particularly with children with behavioral problems.

ORGANIZATIONAL FRAMEWORK FOR INFANT ASSESSMENT AND INTERVENTION

In an earlier version of this chapter, a model to organize assessment and intervention strategies in early communication and language development was proposed, the Communication Assessment Model for Infants (CAMI) (Robinson & Robb, 1997). When evaluated in light of recent literature, the CAMI provides a dynamic process and allows the SLP to move easily between assessment and intervention in working with families and infants and toddlers at risk of language and communication delays. Best practice in early intervention requires that families be at the center of all professional intervention. The CAMI is organized around six strands: (1) family preferences, (2) developmental processes, (3) individual differences, (4) communicative contexts, (5) early intervention teams, and (6) intervention strategies. Each of these strands includes recent policy and practice in early intervention with infants and toddlers with communication delays and disorders. Together, these strands provide the clinician with a structural plan for observations, data gathering, interviews with family members, and specific test procedures required for comprehensive assessment and intervention planning.

As shown in Figure 4.1, the CAMI establishes a blueprint for the clinician to plan initial assessment questions and select assessment tools for individual children and

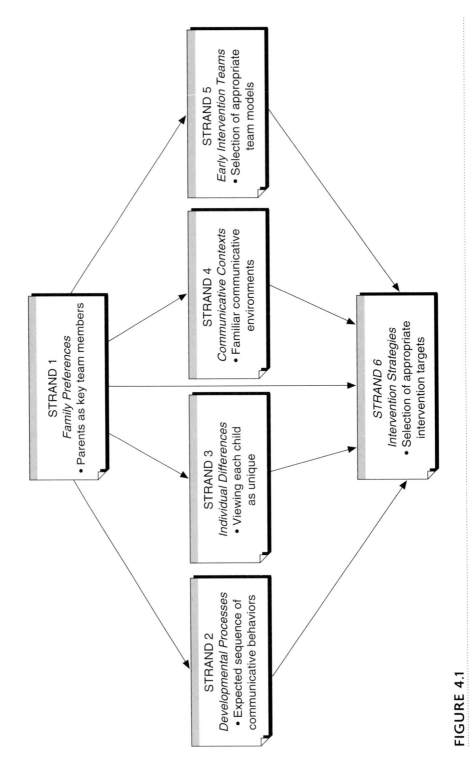

FIGURE 4.1

Six Strands of the Communication Assessment Model for Infants

families. The family preferences strand is always the beginning point, as the information gathered and shared at this level will drive the subsequent assessment and intervention activities. Each strand is distinct, yet interdependent, and each has a direct bearing on intervention strategies. Implicit in the CAMI is the flexibility for the SLP to conduct brief assessments of the infant's current status and to immediately implement or demonstrate intervention to support further communication/language development.

Strand 1: Family Preferences

The field of early intervention is changing rapidly, as professionals move from direct intervention with children to collaborative roles with family members. In many ways, early intervention services are changing with reorganization of health care. According to Cochrane, Farley, and Wilhelm (1990), "The field of early intervention is evolving from discipline specific, child-centered services, to a family oriented context within which professionals from many disciplines address the educational, medical, psychological, and therapeutic needs of handicapped infants and their families" (p. 373). To meet these new challenges, professionals must acquire competency-based training in family support skills. Such training should include communication with families, case management, interdisciplinary teaming, family intervention, and family-centered values and ethics.

The unique characteristics of families in the United States today call for SLPs to cultivate highly developed sensitivity to cultural and individual strengths and preferences (Turnbull & Turnbull, 1990; Hanson, Lynch, & Wayman, 1990). Diverse cultural groups have differing views that range from seeing the child with a disability as a "good luck omen" to viewing the disability as a shameful event, caused by wrongdoing in previous generations. Direct questioning by the professional may be aversive to families from some cultures, and the subject of disability within the family must be approached very gradually. In Hawaii, for example, a "talk story" format of interaction is preferred to build a relationship before focusing on concerns about the child. In addition to the need for sensitivity to cultural styles of interaction, professionals also need to be attuned to individual family styles (e.g., single parents, extended-family caregivers, foster families, working parents, and teen parents).

The importance of sensitivity to individual family preferences is clearly important in early communication and language assessment. Because the initial contact with families begins the assessment and intervention process, the success of that first meeting has implications for the continuing parent–professional relationship and, ultimately, intervention outcomes for the child (Gradel, Thompson, & Sheehan, 1981). During the initial family contact, the SLP needs to acknowledge that family members play a key role in the team. The initial meeting helps the SLP determine the primary caregiver's primary concerns about the child, strengths in parent–child interactions, and appropriate assessment tools.

Strand 2: Developmental Processes

Development implies a high degree of continuity and stability in behavior change within and between children across time (Dunst & Rheingrover, 1982). The approach used most often to evaluate the development of a child is to organize the child's changing behavior as a function of stage intervals occurring at a specific chronological age. A **stage model of development** is a description of measurable aspects of behavioral development (Brainerd, 1978). In the typical stage model of development, as shown in Figure 4.2, the sequence of development is based on one behavior serving as the antecedent for the next behavior. The antecedent must occur in order for the ensuing behavior to develop. For the most part, a stage model of development is conceptually similar to the previously described developmental assessment model.

There are at least two primary drawbacks to using a stage model in evaluating a young child. First, an important characteristic of stage models is that the particular stages are assumed to occur in an invariant sequence, yet the determination of stages seems to be quite arbitrary, because stage models are constantly being revised. For example, a group of researchers in 1950 may have identified three stages in a child's development of walking; twenty years later another group of researchers may have identified five stages. Thus, the more we learn about development, the more stages we seem to require. The second drawback relates to ascribing an age expectancy to each stage. Chronological age often misrepresents readiness skills and expectant behavior. To post norms based on age is often a matter of convenience and practicality, and deviations should be weighed accordingly, because early- and late-maturing children do not display similar characteristics at the same chronological age. Thus, although a developmental assessment instrument may be useful as a gauge to compare individual children, caution is warranted. One needs to be careful not to adhere too closely to specific age expectations. That is not to say that stages are not important in infant assessment protocols, as stage models play an important role in determining a general guide for the SLP.

We believe that a more appropriate approach to describing a child's ongoing development is through the use of a process model. A **process model of development** allows for overlapping of behavior, as well as for the individual differences displayed by infants. For the most part, a process model of development is conceptually similar to previously discussed dynamic and naturalistic models. Although the advantages

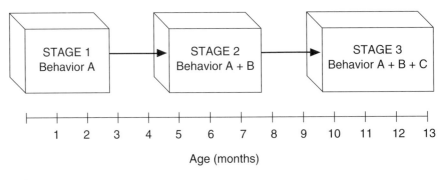

FIGURE 4.2

Stage Model of Behavioral Development

of applying a process model to early communication seems clear, surprisingly few commercial instruments are available that adhere to such a philosophy.

Vocal Stages and Processes

A child's early vocal development is usually described with respect to a stage model of development (Stoel-Gammon & Cooper, 1984; Stark, 1980). Several versions of this model have been published, but they differ somewhat in the number of stages recognized, the particular characteristics of each stage, and the age period covered. However, most models recognize approximately five major stages, referenced according to chronological age (refer to Figure 4.3). These include:

1. Reflexive and cry vocalizations. Usually thought to occur during the first month of life.
2. Cooing or gooing. The basic syllable shapes (V, CV) and consonants /k/ and /g/ are identified between ages 2 and 3 months.
3. Reduplicated or canonical babbling. The same CV syllable shape is produced in repetitive strings and occurs by 6 months of age.
4. Variegated or nonreduplicated babbling. The variety of sounds and syllable strings produced increases markedly by 8 months of age.
5. Single word production. Occurs around 12 months of age.

Oller et al. (1999) provide a stage model of phonological development based on multiple longitudinal studies conducted since the 1970s. Oller et al. outline the stages of early phonological development as follows:

- Phonation stage: quasivowels, glottals
- Primitive articulation stage: gooing
- Expansion stage: full vowels, raspberries, marginal babbling
- Canonical stage: well-formed canonical syllables, reduplicated sequences

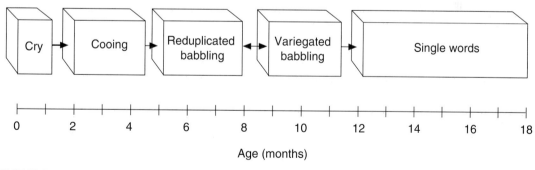

FIGURE 4.3

Schematic Representation of a Traditional Stage Model of Vocalization Development

The various stage assignments, according to chronological age, are based on the work of Holmgren et al. (1986), Koopmans van-Beinum and van der Stelt (1986), Oller (1980), Proctor (1989), and Stark (1980). The two-way arrow between reduplicated and variegated babbling stages indicates co-occurring behaviors.

Stages of development serve as a useful general framework for organizing early vocalization behaviors (Proctor, 1989). However, because stages are descriptive and somewhat impressionistic, they can become obsolete and their inadequacies more obvious (Shatz, 1983). For example, recent research (Mitchell & Kent, 1990; Smith, Brown-Sweeney, & Stoel-Gammon, 1989) suggests that because reduplicated and variegated babbling were found to co-occur, they are not separate stages of vocal development. Futhermore, the notion of a discrete single-word stage has been criticized due to the apparent mixture of identifiable word forms, as well as nonword (e.g., jargon) forms (Robb, Bauer, & Tyler, 1994). A guideline when using the stage model is to allow for overlap or individual differences from one child to the next.

Gestural Stages and Processes

Stages of gestural development appear to follow a sequence similar to that found in vocal development, as the infant moves from early reflexive activity to intentional control over planned sequences of behavior. Gestural communication proceeds from the infant's first year of life and continues well beyond the emergence of verbal language. Individual differences occur and are expected in the specific gestures used. Furthermore, there seems to be a direct relationship between motor development and the infant's ability to use precise gesturing toward caregivers.

The earliest gestures are found during the first month of life, when the neonate displays engagement and disengagement cues, signaling readiness to interact or to "take a break" from interaction. Brazelton, Koslowski, and Main (1974) described both subtle and potent forms of engagement and disengagement cues of young infants that let caregivers know how to adjust and respond during daily care and play routines. Engagement cues are those that convey to caregivers that the infant welcomes interaction; these nonverbal behaviors include facial brightening, eye widening, smiling, open hands, smooth movements of extremities, head turning toward the caregiver, and reaching toward the caregiver. Disengagement cues are signals that the infant is ready for a break from interaction; these behaviors include whimpering, hiccoughs, increased rate of sucking, frowns, yawning, leg kicking, and immobility. Sensitive and trained caregivers who respond to engagement cues by interacting with the infant and to disengagement cues by giving the baby a break from interaction can assist their newborns to express their own communicative behaviors.

During the early months of life, the infant displays increasing mastery over discrete facial expressions and movements of arms, legs, and fingers, to express pleasure, anticipation, hunger, and readiness to play. As infants become accustomed to daily caregiving routines, they display to caregivers a range of gestural responses, including lifting legs in diapering routines, grasping adults' hands or facial parts, whole-body orientation toward the parent, and exploring the mother's clothing during feeding.

An infant's reciprocal imitation of facial and hand gestures begins to emerge by 6 months of age (Moore & Meltzoff, 1978). For example, an infant will attempt to restart games such as pattycake and peekaboo by reaching toward the adult's hands or the cloth hiding the adult's face. By 9 months of age, gestures play a key role in the emergence of verbal language, particularly during the period of intentional communication. Transitions from nonintentional to intentional communication are aided by a range of vocal, gestural, and gaze patterns that differ across individual children. Common patterns are found, however, in the sequence of increased refinement and range of meanings expressed. Infants typically display intentional gesturing during the use of preverbal requests for a specific item or action from the adult. These are called *protoimperatives*. Intentional communication sequences (e.g., giving, showing) that indicate the child's desire to gain adult attention related to a specific object or environmental event (protodeclaratives) are also evident at this stage (Crees, 1999; Bates, Bretherton, Snyder, Shore, & Volterra, 1980; Bates et al., 1979; Harding & Golinkoff, 1979; Snyder, Bates, & Bretherton, 1981). Table 4.4 reveals the sequence of intentional communication behavior in protoimperatives at nine months of age.

Proto imperative and proto declarative sequences are observed before the systematic use of pointing in communication. With the development of intentional forms of communication comes the development of reference, which is the ability to differentiate one entity from many and to note its presence (Owens, 1992). Reference coincides with the age period of approximately 11 months. Bates et al. (1979) have taken the position that showing and giving gestures are precursors to pointing, as the child learns how to conduct referential communication acts. Bates has termed the gestures observed during the intentional period and their rapid ritualization the gesture complex. The role of the gesture complex in establishing reference has been found to be strongly correlated with the subsequent emergence of verbal naming.

Social Interaction Stages and Processes

As noted in Chapter 2, caregiver–child social routines are important in the development of prelinguistic and early linguistic communication. During the first months of infancy, children take a responsive role in interactions with caregivers; toward the end of the first year they gain more intentional control. The growth-fostering aspect of social interaction with caregivers is often referred to as social scaffolding, providing a context for the development of social, emotional, psychological, and cognitive

TABLE 4.4	Sequence of Intentional Communication Behavior in Protoimperatives at 9 Months of Age	
	Communicative Behavior	**Example**
	1. Gaze alternation	Mother and cookie are not in same line of vision. The child looks back and forth from the cookie to the adult, indicating that he expects adult intervention.
	2. Repair of failed message	If initial signaling (gaze and/or gesture) fails to result in adult action, child repeats and expands signaling (reaching toward object, looking back at adult, vocalizing loudly).
	3. Ritualization of previously instrumental gestures	True reaching toward the object becomes abbreviated grasping motion, and vocalization for the cookie may become insistent "mmmm" sound.

development (Brazelton & Als, 1979; Brazelton, et al., 1974; Bruner, 1983). Through daily caregiving routines, games, and other interactions with caregivers, infants have repeated opportunities to experience the effect of their actions on caregivers and the home environment. The role of the caregiver is a supportive and structural responsibility. The caregiver's ability to make adjustments in timing, verbal stimulation, presentation of objects, changing positions in space, and introducing a variety of activities and experiences contributes to the infant's growing world of referents.

Social interactions develop over the first year of life, expanding from early face-to-face interactions with caregivers to intentional and referential communication in less specific environmental contexts. Key elements in this developmental process include the dyad, the infant's state control, mutuality, reciprocity, synchronicity, and turn taking. The dyad refers to the interactive pair of infant and caregiver. Mother–infant dyads are observed most often, but sibling–infant, father–infant, relative–infant, and baby sitter–infant are all viable caregiving dyads that may play an important role in fostering the infant's communication development. Infant state control refers to the neonate's mastery over smooth movement from sleep to wake states. Brazelton and Als (1979) described progressive states, including deep sleep, drowsiness, quiet alert, and crying. Neonates repeatedly cycle through these states during the first month of life, demonstrating increased physiological and neurological maturity. The quiet alert state is the optimal state for the infant to interact with caregivers. As the infant matures in state regulation, longer periods of the quiet alert state are observed. Other terms applied to parent–infant communication include mutuality, reciprocity, synchronicity, and turn–taking. These terms, defined in Table 4.5, refer to qualities of interaction between caregivers and infants that are considered to enhance communication development with young infants over the first year of life.

The supporting role of caregivers is significant to provide multiple opportunities for infants to practice and refine the vocal, gestural, and social communication behaviors. For the SLP and other early intervention professionals, understanding the developmental processes underlying prelinguistic and early linguistic communication is critical to providing appropriate services.

Strand 3: Individual Differences

The third strand of the CAMI involves the notion of individual differences. The possibility that children may follow different paths or strategies in language acquisition was noticed as early as the 1960s, when the prevailing emphasis in the field was on universal aspects of development (c.f. Vihman & Greenlee, 1987). Since then, there have been numerous accounts of variation across subjects in the acquisition of syntax and single-word vocabulary, pragmatic development, and phonological development (Bates, Thal, Whitesall, Fenson, & Oakes, 1989; Stoel-Gammon & Cooper, 1984; Vihman & Greenlee, 1987). However, individual differences in language acquisition are not limited to vocal/verbal forms of communication. Concomitant aspects of communication development also vary considerably from child to child (DeWeerth, van Geert, & Hoijtink, 1999). Among these aspects are intentional acts (Bates et al., 1988; Harding & Golinkoff, 1979), turn taking (Mahoney & Powell, 1984), and gesturing (Bates et al., 1989).

TABLE 4.5	Social Scaffolding Qualities in Caregiver–Infant Interaction

Quality	Definition
Mutuality	Both partners in the interactive dyad are aware and attentive to each other, accepting any contribution to the interaction made by the other partner (Brazelton, Koslowski, & Main, 1974).
Reciprocity	Adaptive modifications are made within the dyad by both partners in response to communicative behavior of the other partner. Reciprocity can be observed in repair strategies by both the mother and child that serve to continue, or to "repair" the interaction. Infants learn to repair interactions through repeated signaling to reengage caregivers (Brazelton, Koslowski, & Main, 1974).
Synchronicity	Building on sensitivity and awareness of the other partner, synchronous dyads include mutuality and reciprocal interaction. Mutual sensitivity to the emotional and attention state of the other partner is coupled with continuous adjustments in timing and intensity of stimulation (Clark & Siefer, 1983).
Turn taking	A turn is defined as any single communicative act, verbal or nonverbal, that is directed toward another person. Turn taking is considered one of the primary social interaction skills learned in infancy. Parents initially take more turns, but infants later take a more active role in social games and routines. Turns between parents and infants become more balanced as each partner learns to respond contingently to the other (Kaye & Charney, 1981).

Given the complexities of communication development and varied opportunities for learning, variability in rate of learning is to be expected. As noted in Chapter 2, we can generally conclude that children exhibit a high degree of variability in the individual competence each brings to communication development. For the SLP, accepting that a child displays individual differences helps in recognizing the uniqueness of a child's development, specifically the approach he takes to acquire language. The differing rates and styles of language development increasingly found among typically developing infants support the need to approach developmental assessment of infants and toddlers with language/communication delays with caution. The CAMI acknowledges these differences and incorporates them into the assessment paradigm.

Strand 4: Communicative Contexts

Language development occurs within familiar contexts (see Chapter 2). Developmentally, children go through a gradual process of decontextualization, in which utterances are no longer bound to limited contexts. Snyder et al. (1981) have described the process of decontextualization in relation to a child's acquisition of first words and early word combinations. Young children first exhibit utterances that are bound to specific contexts, such as saying "Daddy go" only when Daddy is walking out the front door at home. Later, the same child may generalize such utterances to other people, in other locations, and possibly in picture contexts (i.e., decontextualization). When assessing infants, clinicians need to be aware that familiar routines at home may be the only contexts that elicit vocalizations and communicative intent. Situational variables, such as degree of structure (low/high), environment (familiar/unfamiliar), persons (familiar/unfamiliar), age of communicative partner (adult/peer/younger child), and communicative function (request, comment, showing off, greeting, etc.) influence the communicative and linguistic performance of young children.

For children with language and communication delays, the relationship between familiar context and communicative behavior takes on additional significance. Kennedy, Sheridan, Radlinski, and Beeghly (1991) recently studied the relationships between play behavior and subsequent language development in a small sample of children with developmental delays. Using play as the context for assessments, symbolic play behavior and early language skills were compared for six children ranging in age from 2 years 9 months to 3 years 4 months. Although relationships among language comprehension, expression, and symbolic play schemes were similar to those found in typically developing children of similar language development skills, wide fluctuations in play and language behavior were found. Observed differences in language skills demonstrate that children with language and communication delays may be more sensitive to context, structure of assessment situation, and the demands placed on them (Donahue & Pearl, 1995).

Strand 5: Early Intervention Teams

The next strand of the CAMI involves selecting an appropriate early intervention team. Three types of team models are identified in the literature and in practice: the multidisciplinary, interdisciplinary, and transdisciplinary models (Campbell, 1987; McCormick & Goldman, 1978). Although clear differences exist among the models in the patterns of interactions with families and in the delivery of early intervention services, early intervention professionals actually use variations and combinations of all three team models. The three models can be outlined as follows.

> *Multidisciplinary model.* Professionals from multiple disciplines work independently to provide services to an individual child and family. For example, in the case of a speech and language delay related to a child born with cleft lip and/or palate, the child's parents may see multiple medical specialists, an audiologist, SLP, genetic counselor, hospital social worker, and other professionals over the course of many months, in relatively separate interactions. Parents and children are involved in a number of different assessments and interventions, as each professional interacts individually with the family.

> *Interdisciplinary model.* This model involves a greater degree of interaction among disciplines and more coordinated service delivery with families and young children. For example, in an interdisciplinary model, parents of an infant with health and developmental needs related to prenatal drug exposure and positive HIV status may interact with medical, social work, public health nursing, speech-language pathology, physical therapy, occupational therapy, and psychology professionals. Rather than interact with families individually throughout the iden-

tification, assessment, and intervention process, professionals meet together to discuss findings of individual assessment and, most often, to synthesize individual findings into a single report intended to be comprehensive to family members. Similar to the multidisciplinary model, interdisciplinary services are provided through professionals interacting individually with families and children.

Transdisciplinary model. The third model of teamwork requires a great deal more communication between team members, as coordinated interactions with families and children with disabilities are the primary goal of this model. Transdisciplinary approaches move beyond single-discipline interactions with families at all levels of identification, assessment, and intervention with young children and their caregivers. For example, a child with early communication and language delays related to combined biological and environmental risks, such as a very-low-birthweight infant born to a teenage mother, may have maximum contact with the SLP and minimal contact with other related disciplines. In this case, the SLP relies on the input and consultative roles of professionals from other disciplines, such as the physical therapist (PT), the occupational therapist (OT), the social worker, and others, to provide comprehensive services with the young mother, infant, and other family members involved.

The transdisciplinary model is often considered the preferred model for increasing communication and collaboration among disciplines and for maintaining continuity in services to families (Briggs, 1993). However, individual family and child needs, as well as the particular needs of the program (staffing, location, etc.), may necessitate the use of multidisciplinary and interdisciplinary models at times. For example, children who are identified at birth as having been exposed to drugs require confidentiality to prevent possible stigma. A multidisciplinary model may be required to identify these children; however, a transdisciplinary model may best serve them when planning intervention. Because the transdisciplinary model calls for a primary care provider to maintain contact with the parent and child, the intervention should be more confidential and meaningful to family members.

Collaborative Team Models

The three types of team models described above apply to interactions of team members within teams, or intrateam processes. Also critical to the coordination of services for families and young children are the interactions across teams, or interteam processes. Professionals in early intervention services are increasingly urged to develop collaboration across disciplines and service systems, in order to create more effective transitions and services with families. For example, families with high-risk newborns born prematurely are faced with interactions with multiple teams in the hospital, home, and early intervention center. Interactions with each of these teams are made in very rapid succession in the child's early months of life. The importance of coordination and collaboration across teams is defined as best practice in providing family-centered care and links across one team of providers to the next. Wyly, Allen, Pfalzer, and Wilson (1996) describe collaborative team models within the context of the neonatal intensive care unit with the following key components:

- Establishing partnership with family members at the outset
- High-risk infant interventions
- Transition information and support to early intervention services
- Continuity of care from hospital, home, center-based services
- Communication between hospital, home, and center-based team members

As noted in Chapter 3, the role of the speech pathologist has increasingly become one of a consultant and collaborative team member especially in early intervention settings. Billeaud (1998) identifies the primary role of the SLP on the early intervention team as a partner with the family members involved, under the broad goal of IDEA which is to empower the family to enhance the child's development. The natural opportunity available to SLPs is to build partnerships with family members in the assessment, planning, and intervention phases of early intervention.

In addition to skills to support family members to take part in the team process of assessment and intervention, SLPs are also team members with other disciplines. The degree of contact between the SLP and other disciplines can vary widely, related to the intervention model and setting where services are provided. The role of the SLP and relationship to the family and other professionals will vary widely, from one-time contacts in the assessment process to consultative contacts, intensive short-term services, intermittent assessment, or follow-up. Iacono (1999) described the recent trend for the SLP to change from a direct intervention role to that of consultant to the family and other professional team members involved in the child's early intervention plan, or Individualized Family Support Plan. Briggs (1993) identified the importance of open communication skills to be effective team members and outlined the characteristics of effective teams:

1. There is a mission, purpose, and goals that members understand and accept.
2. There are sufficient resources available.
3. Members have appropriate training, skills, and experience.
4. There is an open communication system that encourages diversity, manages conflict, and seeks feedback.
5. Sufficient time is devoted to examining team norms, values, beliefs; and to fostering growth of individuals and the team as a whole.
6. An effective problem-solving strategy is utilized.
7. High standards are established internally, and a method for evaluating individual roles, responsibilities, and performance is instituted.
8. A climate of trust and personal, as well as professional support, is established.
9. One leader is identified or the responsibility is shared appropriately among the members.
10. Organizational support is provided to ensure success of the team process and product.

While recognizing the barriers to becoming an effective team, Briggs identifies the transdisciplinary model as the standard of best practice in early intervention for five key reasons: (1) flexibility in disciplinary boundaries results; (2) role overlap promotes true collaboration; (3) a single coordinator improves efficiency; (4) interdependency on all members rather than one member; (5) family are full members who ultimately make decisions.

Systems theory, an approach that places the early intervention team in the context of the larger ecological system that includes family, child, service providers, program, and policy levels, is a wider context to examine the role of team relationships within and across services and society. Briggs (1997) has defined and discussed a multilayered systems model that includes the family, child, core intervention team, administration, and policy makers related to early intervention programs. She emphasizes the need for SLPs and other early intervention professionals to learn to work across boundaries of their agencies and communities within which they function. The interrelatedness of all levels of the system influences the roles and effectiveness of our interventions with families.

Strand 6: Intervention Strategies

The last strand of the CAMI involves the design of intervention strategies for infants and toddlers. However, intervention begins in the assessment phase and is not the last component in the sequence of the implementation of assessment. Indeed, in a dynamic model of assessment and intervention, the SLP moves between assessment and intervention in an ongoing process to determine a child's communicative strengths and needs, and to determine intervention strategies to promote communication and language development.

The selection of intervention strategies is guided by assessment information and individual characteristics of children and families. As the clinician moves through the assessment process, beginning with identification of family concerns, intervention goals may become evident. For example, a parent may identify increased vocalization and "talking" as intervention targets. Keeping this intervention target in mind, information regarding developmental processes, individual differences, communicative contexts, and roles of team members will allow the SLP and parent to refine the initial target and develop collaborative goals. At each stage in the assessment process, linkages to intervention can be developed. The intervention goals are then based on a synthesis of shared information, between parents, the SLP, and other team members.

Intervention Planning

Bailey (1988) outlined a process of developing collaborative goals and objectives for early intervention personnel and families. An **intervention goal** is a long-term statement that includes an outcome statement for a given time frame (e.g., 6 months to 1 year). **Intervention objectives** are specific, short-term goals that include (1) the precise behaviors to be accomplished, (2) a description context for the behaviors expected of the individual, and (3) specific criteria to evaluate the attainment of the objective. The development of precise intervention goals, as recommended in the earlier part of the 1990s, has changed to more general intervention targets, or **benchmarks.** Benchmarks represent skills to be achieved by within a specific timeframe, such as three months. The determination of benchmarks is related to many variables, beginning with family preferences and professional assessment, as required in the process of developing Individualized Family Support Plans (IFSPs). However, the specific nature of the linguistic targets or benchmarks will vary, related to the intervention strategy selected. Direct, behavioral intervention strategies may target specific communication behaviors such as "increased vocalization to request objects," whereas naturalistic approaches may have broader targets such as "increased imitation of vocalization."

As the student will discover in the case studies presented in the final section of this chapter, individual child characteristics, family preferences, and professional findings influence the selection of intervention approaches. The theoretical bases for early language intervention were discussed in an earlier section of this chapter. This section continues that discussion with specific strategies for intervention. Two primary types of intervention approaches are used in practice and described in the literature: naturalistic and direct (McCormick, Loeb, & Schiefelbusch, 1997). Differing theory and principles underlie the two types of intervention. Naturalistic approaches are based on a developmental, cognitive, and social model, and direct approaches are based on a behavioral model incorporating reinforcement principles. Major types and features of naturalistic and direct early language intervention approaches that are consistent with recent research and best practice outlined by Iacono (1999) are described below.

Naturalistic Communication Intervention

Naturalistic approaches to language and communication are based on the assumptions that (1) young children learn to communicate using speech and language in a variety of daily routines and activities with caregivers; and (2) intervention is best conducted within the context of familiar environments. Based on the work of Hart and Risely (1975), naturalistic approaches to language intervention have their basis in "incidental teaching" techniques that rely primarily on a time-delay procedure (withholding desired items briefly) in order to elicit further communicative attempts with children with developmental delays. Since that time, the many forms and procedures of naturalistic approaches to intervention to support young children with language delays have more commonly been referred to as *milieu approaches*. Other terms that are used to refer to similar methods of embedding language intervention within naturally occurring activities and routines include (1) transactional teaching, (2) pragmatic intervention, (3) child-oriented teaching, (4) interactive modeling (Wilcox, Kouri, & Caswell, 1991), (5) social partnership (MacDonald & Carroll, 1992), and (6) enhanced milieu teaching (Kaiser & Hester, 1995). A more complete review of the past development of naturalistic/milieu intervention approaches was provided by Warren and Gazdag (1990), who defined several common elements, including incidental teaching, social routines, turn taking, and environmental arrangement.

Conversational Approaches

The notion of "balanced" turns between adult and child were incorporated into conversational forms of language intervention by MacDonald and Gillette (1985) and Mahoney and Powell (1984). Turn-taking interventions are planned primarily as play sessions between the parent and child, with the focus on achieving a balanced turn ratio between partners. MacDonald and Carroll (1992) have more recently proposed a social partnership model that is designed to support parents to learn that communication "develops even from the [child's] simplest actions and sounds." Parents are encouraged to respond to any child behavior that might be communicative, treating each child behavior as one conversational "turn." The effects of the social partnership model are reported to increase levels of child imitation, vocalization, and communicative turn taking in the context of interaction with parents.

MacDonald and Carroll (1992) have extended earlier work to support verbal language between children and caregivers to intervention with infants and toddlers. The ECO model has specific applications to children with communication disorders and families in daily routines. The context of play interactions is recommended for assessment and intervention processes with young children and family members. In the ECO approach to intervention, parents are supported to learn that communication "develops even more from the [child's] simplest actions and sounds" and to respond to any child behavior that might be construed as communication. Similar to findings in the work by Yoder et al., MacDonald and Carroll have reported that parents demonstrated qualitative changes in communication behavior directed toward their children that included actions and words more closely matched to the child's play.

Responsive Interaction

Adults use responsive interactions to follow the child's lead and comment, request, and expand the child's attention and communication within the context of social interactions and play. Within environments that are arranged to engage the child in typical, relevant activities, adult interaction follows the child's lead and builds on the establishment of joint attention to expand the child's communication and turn taking.

Milieu Teaching

Milieu approaches are the most well-known methods of naturalistic language intervention and incorporate incidental teaching strategies. The concept and application of incidental teaching has remained central to the application of naturalistic interventions, as SLPs, parents, and other members of the team are required to become skilled in observation and identification of "teachable moments" with young children. For example, an infant who is reaching toward her bottle provides caregivers the opportunity to hold the bottle momentarily and comment, "Yes, that's Ana's milk!," thus engaging the baby's attention and providing a verbal label for her behavior. The importance of joint attention between caregiver and child and responsiveness to the child's focus of attention are stressed in naturalistic intervention as the key starting points. Specific incidental teaching techniques are used within the context of naturally occurring activities and focus of the child's attention. According to Jones and Warren (1991), "Incidental teaching occurs when a child initiates interaction with the teacher in the form of a request, question, comment or other communicative behavior" (p. 49).

Enhanced Milieu Teaching

The application of naturalistic intervention approaches was originally demonstrated within the context of early language development in preschool children with developmental delays (Halle, Baer, & Spradlin, 1981). Strategies taken from milieu teaching include following the child's lead, environmental arrangement, and embedding modeling in routines and social interactions. Bruner (1983) identified the importance of familiar names and social routines such as peekaboo, due to their defined structure, repetition, and opportunities for young children to experience anticipation, response, initiation, and conclusion. Bruner described the adult's use of naturally occurring games, interactions, and routines as teaching opportunities with the child as "scaffolding." The application of naturalistic or milieu approaches are by nature embedded within daily routines and familiar activities for young children. In application, authors range from carefully planned environments and activities to naturally occurring events; agreement is stated that young children demonstrate increased generalization of language and communication behaviors when familiar routines are used for the context of intervention such as play, mealtimes, bath, and so on (Kaiser & Hester, 1995). Norris and Hoffman (1990) have described specific steps that caregivers can structure and respond to child communication through selection of toys, expansion of child behavior, and natural consequences.

Prelinguistic Milieu Intervention (PMT)

Modifications of milieu teaching for prelinguistic interventions with infants and toddlers in stages of prelinguistic communication and emergent language development have been reported in recent years (Norris & Hoffman, 1990; MacDonald & Carroll, 1992; Yoder, Warren, Kyoungram, & Gazdag, 1994). Yoder et al. described the application of a modified milieu approach combined with linguistic mapping to teach intentional requesting to young children with Down syndrome. Intervention techniques were implemented in a play setting while adults employed time delay, joint attention, and environmental arrangement to elicit requesting behaviors with young children. In addition, linguistic mapping was employed as adults verbally labeled the child's actions and focus of attention. As children increased intentional requesting (nonverbal gestures to signal requesting), Yoder et al. found that adults also increased verbal labeling (mapping) of the child's actions. The effect of increased child communicative behavior on increased adult responsiveness was described as a transactional effect. As children increased in their intentional communication behaviors, adults increased responsive communication toward the children.

Through the increased modification and demonstration of naturalistic intervention approaches to communication and language intervention with young children, researchers have demonstrated positive effects for the parent–child dyad and the reciprocal communication between child and caregiver, rather than a single focus on the increase in child behavior that was reported in earlier research.

Direct Communication Intervention

Direct intervention models are based on learning principles as defined in behavioral psychology. Applications of direct intervention strategies are often incorporated in naturalistic settings with a high degree of structure. The reader is referred to McCormick et al. (1997) for a detailed overview of direct intervention strategies, including modeling, reinforcement, shaping, chaining, fading, and prompting-cueing strategies. The beginning SLP often feels more comfortable pursuing direct intervention over naturalistic techniques because of the highly structured nature of direct intervention. However, direct intervention approaches are not easily applied with infants and toddlers who have communication and language delays; play-based and naturalistic methods are better aligned with this age group. Drash and Tudor (1990) reported that direct intervention approaches are effective to develop contingency awareness in infants and toddlers with severe disabilities.

AAC Applications

Incorporation of AAC into play-based intervention is recommended to provide opportunities for children at risk of severe communication delays to communicate in meaningful contexts. Strategies to implement AAC interventions may include precise, behavioral objectives and methods as well as naturalistic procedures to promote the child's use of AAC in communication interactions with peers and adults. The need for access to communication by children with severe communication disabilities (e.g., cerebral palsy, cognitive disabilities, and autism, to name a few) is becoming increasingly clear, and technology advances create opportunities for very young children to have alternative means to develop communication and language skills. The importance of prelinguistic communication skills such as imitation, social interaction, symbolic play, and intentional communication have been identified as components of skills required for use of AAC systems and devices (Adamson & Bakeman, 1999; Crees, 1999; Romski & Sevcik, 1999; Yoder & Warren, 1999). Research in the use of AAC for assessment and intervention with infants and toddlers has just begun. The next decade will surely give us greater insights in this exciting area.

APPLICATIONS OF ASSESSMENT AND INTERVENTION APPROACHES: THREE CASE EXAMPLES

Example 1: Early Infancy

The CAMI allows for assessment of infants and toddlers across several periods of development. Case examples are provided in this section to apply the processes of assessment and intervention discussed thus far. The first case focuses on the period of early infancy. Early infancy is characterized by basic physiological responses to the external world and development of primary relationships with caregivers.

Kwan was born three months prematurely and weighing only 949 grams, placing her within the very-low-birthweight range. Her condition at birth was such that she required breathing assistance with a respirator and feeding with a gavage tube. She remained in the hospital for three months, going home at her term gestational age of nine months. Her weight at discharge had improved, at nearly 1500 grams. At the time of discharge, Kwan was medically stable, having overcome irregular breathing patterns. She was discharged with a gastrostomy tube for feeding. Kwan's mother, a twenty-year-old single parent, cared for her with the help of her own mother and sister in the home that the three adults shared. Kwan's mother and her family had immigrated to a large urban area on the U.S. mainland from Taiwan ten years earlier. Kwan's mother and grandmother were referred to the early intervention program through the public health nurse, and a home visit was scheduled for an assessment. Kwan's mother expressed concern because her baby did not seem to make many movements or vocal sounds (except prolonged crying every day between 6:00 and 9:00 p.m.). Kwan's mother reported that she had difficulty handling Kwan, as she cried often and stiffened when picked up out of her crib.

Family Preferences

Because Kwan's mother is young and offers only a small amount of information about her daughter's early development, professionals may mistakenly assume that her limited knowledge in some way contributes to Kwan's fussiness and slow development. However, the characteristics that Kwan brings to the caregiving interaction contribute to her mother's frustration. Further questioning of Kwan's mother and grandmother about their primary concerns for Kwan's development reveal deeply concerned caregivers. With the help of Kwan's grandmother, Kwan's mother has spent many hours watching her daughter in the hospital and learning how to feed and care for her. The grandmother carries on most of the home chores so that Kwan and her mother can be together. Further, the grandmother and Kwan's mother have different concerns about the baby and these must be incorporated in the assessment plan. Kwan's mother sincerely wants to learn skills to better handle and soothe her daughter, and the grandmother feels the baby would grow better with formula fed through a bottle rather than a gastrostomy tube. Their concerns and awareness of Kwan will guide assessment and intervention. As the clinician observes and gathers further information about Kwan's early development, Kwan's family members can be encouraged to participate actively, as primary informers about Kwan's interactive cues and feeding behaviors at home.

Developmental Processes

Based on information gathered from the brief report provided by Kwan's mother and grandmother, certain questions emerge regarding Kwan's development thus far. Knowing her multiple risks at birth, assessment of Kwan's physiological, sensory, and motor development are needed. The following questions can now be formulated to systematically determine her developmental status and communication development:

1. To what extent does Kwan respond to voices and familiar sounds and voices?
2. What are Kwan's sleep and waking patterns, and how does she transition?
3. What are Kwan's overall muscle tone and movement patterns when she is placed in prone, supine, and feeding positions?
4. What primitive reflexes are observed in Kwan's repertoire at this time?
5. When Kwan is placed in close proximity to her caregivers, what social responses (e.g., brightened gaze, smile, open mouth, arm thrust, foot movement, or other generalized response to caregivers) are observed?
6. What is Kwan's regular intake at each feeding, and how steady is her weight gain?

As these questions indicate, the focus of assessment at this point is to gather further information about critical developmental processes that are typically observed in infants at one month of age. Communication development is clearly not the only concern for Kwan. With her history of very low birthweight, a number of developmental processes are affected. Developmental tools available include the Minnesota Infant Development Inventory, a subtest of the Minnesota Child Development Inventory (MCDI) (Ireton & Thwing, 1974) and the Hawaii Early Learning Profile (HELP) (Furuno et al., 1987). Both of these tools can be administered through parent report and supplemented with direct observation. Although only limited items assess developmental processes in very young infants, these instruments allow for flexibility and parent report in administration.

Individual Differences

With information regarding the developmental status of Kwan's communication behavior, we gather a more complete picture of Kwan's individual communication patterns.

> Kwan's mother reported that her daughter is beginning to recognize familiar people when she is awake, generally after a feeding and in her swing. Kwan's mother is not sure if her own voice or face are more effective in getting Kwan to gaze in her direction. When observed at home, Kwan did not localize to sounds readily but exhibited a "whole body" response when her mother said her name. Her mother reported that Kwan's waking from sleep in midmorning is more gradual than other times. At other times, Kwan has difficulty waking, sleeping on and off throughout the day, fussing and quickly developing an agitated cry before her mother can get to the room to pick her daughter out of bed. According to the mother, preparation of the gastrostomy tube, formula, and attaching the tube takes more time than Kwan is willing to wait. Her intake of formula is quite good, as the entire 4 ounces are absorbed rapidly through the tube. Kwan does show some reflexive sucking activity near the beginning of feeding, and her family wants to begin bottle feeding. Observations of Kwan's muscle tone and motor development showed low muscle tone and weak startle reflexes in response to loud sounds.

Further report by Kwan's mother and grandmother and direct observation by the SLP will provide a record of sleeping, feeding, and waking times so that we can understand the best times to play with Kwan and support her responsive interactions with her family. Two different types of assessment tools are now helpful, the Neonatal Behavioral Assessment Scales (NBAS), Second Edition (Brazelton, 1984) and the Bayley Scales of Infant Development (BSID) (Bayley, 1993). The first instrument, the NBAS, requires extensive training to administer and a very clear method to assess sleep, wake, and activity behaviors in very young infants. The BSID, on the other hand, is a standardized test with limited reliability for use with young infants. However, the early items on the BSID will identify Kwan's gaze, reach, and preferred motor positions, and will highlight individual differences and strengths. From what we know about her individual preferences thus far, Kwan requires support to adjust to environmental stimulation throughout the day. For example, her intense crying periods in the evening may be a result of increasing stimulation throughout the day that results in potent disengagement cues including body arching, hands at sides, and inconsolable crying.

Communicative Contexts

Kwan's communicative contexts can be determined through her daily caregiving routines. The individual engagement and disengagement behaviors that she displays are intimately tied to the context of the caregiving environment. Observations of parent–child interaction help the clinician and caregiver determine the specific contexts for Kwan's early behavioral signals (i.e., communicative behavior). Tools that are useful at this point in assessment are the Parent-Child Interaction Assessment (Comfort & Farran, 1994) and Assessment of Mother-Child Interaction (Klein & Briggs, 1987). Information from these assessments will enable the SLP and parent to determine optimal methods to respond to Kwan's readiness to engage and interact in prelinguistic "conversations."

Early Intervention Teams

With a baby who is medically at risk, multiple contacts with a range of health care and social service professionals are unavoidable. Thus, a team approach is needed to support Kwan and her family. To minimize the fragmentation the family may experience, a primary care coordinator, or case manager, is recommended. At the hospital level, this person may be the primary care nurse assigned to Kwan's mother or perhaps the SLP or other professional responsible for early assessment and parent education in the neonatal intensive care unit. After the family goes home, the public health nurse often becomes the case manager. At the point when Kwan's family contacts an early intervention program, they will have made several transitions between several different service systems and professionals.

The SLP can build a partnership with Kwan's family by taking a key role in coordinating recommendations from other disciplines that affect Kwan's intervention plan. Based on the assessment information gathered thus far, it is clear that concerns about Kwan's motor development, feeding, general health, hearing, vision, and communication will involve at least the following disciplines: speech language pathology, audiology, physical therapy, occupational therapy, nursing, nutrition, pediatrics, and early intervention specialists. In this case, the SLP is the obvious professional to coordinate contacts and recommended interventions with Kwan's family, due to the central nature of her families' concern about Kwan's limited interactions. The team model that most applies in this situation is a combination of transdisciplinary and interdisciplinary approaches, as individual disciplines will continue to have direct involvement with Kwan's family.

Intervention Strategies

Kwan's family identified three primary areas of concern at the outset of the assessment process: difficulty in soothing her when crying, feeding with a bottle, and a general lack of noncry vocalization. As the SLP and other team members conduct an assessment, these areas of concern can guide assessment and intervention goals. At least three possible goals can be generated for Kwan: (1) develop alternative techniques for Kwan's mother to soothe her daughter, (2) increase Kwan's tolerance for oral feeding, and (3) increase social interaction times between Kwan and her family members. Several researchers in infant development provide effective strategies to enhance the infant's self-regulation and tolerance of external stimuli, shown in Table 4.6. The underlying principle for all the approaches is to continually monitor infant engagement and disengagement cues, adjusting caregiver behaviors in direct response to infant cues. Adjustments of caregiver behavior may include simply taking a break in the interaction, allowing the infant to brace her feet against the caregiver's hand,

TABLE 4.6 | Communication Intervention Goals, Strategies, and Models for Kwan

Intervention Goal	Intervention Strategy	Intervention Model
Develop alternative techniques for Kwan's mother to soothe her daughter.	Demonstrate holding, wrapping, and soothing techniques with Kwan and her mother.	Swaddling, self-regulation, and slow movements (Cole, 1996).
Increase Kwan's tolerance for oral feeding.	Provide pacifier or nipple on bottle to increase oral tolerance; gradually increase amounts of formula by mouth.	Consult physician and OT regarding feeding techniques and plan for increasing oral feeding (Ahman, 1986).
Increase social interaction times between Kwan and her family members.	Encourage Kwan's mother and grandmother to respond to vocal, visual, and gestural behaviors during Kwan's awake/alert times.	Support parent-child interaction (Hanson & Krentz, 1986; McCollum & Yates, 1994).

or providing a small toy for the infant to grasp. Of course, strategies must be individualized for each infant, and the parent and SLP must discover the appropriate techniques through trial and error. Table 4.6 also provides more extensive guidelines that may be applied and modified for individual infants.

Example 2: Middle Infancy

In middle infancy, the child becomes a more active participant in the world around her. She sleeps less, sits upright, and vocalizes often. The following example applies the CAMI components to a child in middle infancy.

Lucy was referred at the age of 7 months for an evaluation of her general developmental status, particularly in communication, as her mother reported that "Lucy's muscles are weak and do not allow her to make sounds like my other children." Lucy's mother reported that her pregnancy was normal but that Lucy was born in a "breech" position and was diagnosed as having cerebral palsy shortly after birth. Lucy's mother reported that an earlier developmental assessment of Lucy performed at 3 months of age indicated that her cerebral palsy is considered "spastic hemiplegia" affecting the right side of her body. Reportedly, Lucy is able to sit upright with support. However, she appears to have difficulty tracking objects visually. Her mother said that she worries about speech development, as Lucy makes only a few vocal sounds, including crying and some vowels.

Family Preferences

Lucy is the youngest of four siblings. She comes from an extended family consisting of her mother and siblings, her grandmother, and an aunt and uncle, who all reside in the same home. Lucy's mother works outside the home, so Lucy is cared for at home by her aunt and older siblings. Lucy's siblings and her aunt are important to include in the assessment process because of their roles as primary caregivers. Each of Lucy's family members has information about her personality, daily communicative behavior, feeding, fussiness, and overall development. Because Lucy has multiple caregivers, the SLP has a unique opportunity to develop teamwork with these key family members through the use of parent/caregiver interview tools with family members.

Developmental Processes

Information provided thus far by Lucy's mother indicated generalized developmental delays in the areas of gross and fine motor, feeding, communication, and visual development. The following questions can be formulated to gather critical information for understanding and planning intervention to support Lucy's progress in developmental and functional skills:

1. What are Lucy's eating patterns, and her likes and dislikes of liquid and solid foods?
2. What are Lucy's general muscle tone and independent mobility skills?
3. What are Lucy's vocalizations, and in what contexts is she most likely to vocalize?
4. What are Lucy's social and gestural communications used with caregivers?
5. In what positions is Lucy most comfortable and observed to vocalize?
6. What degree of physical support is needed to help Lucy maintain sitting?
7. What is Lucy's visual response to her caregivers and objects in her environment?

As discussed, Lucy's extended family plays a critical role in her daily development. Family members may participate to identify Lucy's strengths and needs through a structured interview process, using developmental stages as guidelines for discussion. The Receptive-Expressive Emergent Language Scale (Bzoch & League, 1991) provides an interview guide to determine receptive and expressive milestones, and the results may be scored for normative purposes. Other tools appropriate at this stage of the assessment process include the MacArthur Child Development Inventories for Infants (Fenson et al., 1993), and the Infant/Toddler Checklist for Communication and Language Development (Wetherby & Prizant, 1998).

Individual Differences

Having gathered critical information covering the preceding developmental areas, we can begin to identify the specific characteristics of Lucy's individual prelinguistic communication patterns. We gain the following information through careful observation and parental information:

Results of developmental assessment based on parent report and clinical observations showed that Lucy has low tolerance for solid foods. She can sit upright with support, however, she has yet to walk on "all fours. " She shows interest toward objects presented directly in her line of vision and will reach for those objects. On the other hand, when objects are presented away from Lucy's midline, she is less responsive, probably due to her motor and visual limitations. She demonstrates differentiated cries for hunger, discomfort, and pain. Aside from crying and other reflexive vocalizations (e.g., burping, sneezing), she occasionally laughs, and she is just beginning to make some vocal sounds, including a "grunting" [uh] sound and an "aah" sound. She is particularly vocal when lying on her back during diaper changes. She is also generally more attentive toward familiar family members than to strangers.

This information leads to the hypothesis that Lucy's primary strength is interest in her environment. Her primary weaknesses are in the areas of motor and visual development. These weaknesses may prevent Lucy from gaining everyday experiences in the environment that nondisabled children take for granted. Her present oral motor abilities also suggest that normal speech sound development may be impaired. Additional questions can now be generated for further assessments and focused on Lucy's strengths, as well as further define the range of her motoric and visual limitations.

1. What are Lucy's daily events and what gestural/vocal behaviors does she display?
2. How does Lucy demonstrate her attentiveness toward familiar people?
3. What are the specific food items that Lucy can/cannot tolerate?
4. What are Lucy's imitation skills, both gesturally and vocally?
5. What specific items/events will Lucy attend most/least to?
6. What specific vowel and consonant sounds can Lucy produce?

Assessment instruments that will address these specific questions include the Rossetti Infant-Toddler Language Scale (ITLS) (Rossetti, 1990) and The Early Language Milestone Scale (ELM). The ELM scale uses parent report, incidental observation, and direct testing to evaluate prelinguistic and emerging linguistic skills, including visual response. With respect to Lucy, the assessment of her visual development is particularly important. Coplan and Gleason (1990) have demonstrated that the ELM scale is valid for both normal and at-risk populations. Similar to the ELM scale, the ITLS (Rossetti, 1990) is designed to assess children between the ages of birth and 3 years. The ITLS uses both parent report (and interview) and actual testing of children's social interaction, pragmatics, gestural development, play behavior, language comprehension, and language expression. For Lucy, developmental ages obtained on both the ELM and ITLS measures may not be as critical as the degree of effort and attention she displays on the test items.

Communicative Contexts

Lucy's prelinguistic behavior appears to be tied to three different contexts, her family, daily routines, and response to toys presented at her midline. Lucy is most attentive when interacting with familiar people. Such a context should be stressed as being an important one, with familiar members playing the role as primary interactive partners. Daily routines provide opportunities for Lucy to communicate with her caregivers and for her caregivers to communicate in return, stressing turn taking, vocalization expansion, and vocal and gestural imitation. She responds to items and activities presented at her midline, and this will serve as the foundation for presenting new information to Lucy.

Early Intervention Teams

Events at birth contributing to cerebral palsy seldom bring about only one kind of clinical problem. As already noted, Lucy has difficulties in feeding, motor, and visual impairments, in addition to a delay in communication development. Other problems found to be associated with cerebral palsy include hearing impairment, mental retardation, and seizure activity. Because the problems associated with cerebral palsy are numerous and complex, intervention involves the integrated efforts of many professionals. Rather than schedule separate evaluations for Lucy's family to see these various professionals, the SLP may wish to utilize these persons as consultants while maintaining direct contact with the child and family herself, a transdisciplinary model.

Intervention Strategies

Infants born with special needs and their caregivers require specialized professional support in the early months for optimal communicative interactions. A child with cerebral palsy from birth may have severely limited movement and gestural capabilities, requiring family members to extensively adapt and augment their infant's communicative efforts. The specific areas that need to be strengthened and supported for Lucy's prelinguistic and emerging communication skills with her caregivers include (1) fuller use of gaze patterns to maintain interaction with caregivers, (2) gradual introduction of thicker textures in feeding, and (3) Lucy's discovery that her communicative behaviors have an effect on her family members. The intervention goals, strategies, and suggested models found in Table 4.7 are based on Lucy's develop-

TABLE 4.7	Communication Intervention Strategies for Lucy (Age Seven Months)		
Intervention Goal	**Intervention Strategy**	**Intervention Model**	
Increase chewing of solid foods.	Include small bites of soft foods and thick liquids.	Have OT/PT team member provide feeding program.	
Increase eye gaze and tracking of objects and people.	Introduce colorful, movable objects to visual midline and periphery.		
Develop skills to reach/touch/ activate switches.	Introduce musical/sound making toys (at visual midline) that require switch attention.	Uses language intervention organizational framework (Messick, Anketell, & Chapman, 1987).	
Increase gestural facial expression.	Identify daily routines (e.g., diaper changes) that provide opportunities for face-to-face contact.		
Increase vocalization.	Identify daily routines that elicit frequent vocalization from Lucy and encourage her to vocally imitate.	Milieu teaching and linguistic mapping (Yoder et al., 1994).	
Increase conversational behavior.	Identify daily routines that elicit vocalizations from Lucy and encourage her to "take turns."	Social partnership model (MacDonald & Carroll, 1992).	

mental needs as well as her reported and observed preferences. Her family members all demonstrate active involvement with Lucy; their preferences for certain intervention strategies will determine what priority is placed on the goals outlined.

Example 3: Transitions to Toddlerhood

The conclusion of the infancy period and the beginning of toddlerhood is characterized by the emergence of recognizable language. The following example begins our application of recent findings in studies of emerging language to assessment and intervention planning during the period of toddlerhood.

Josh, age 19 months, was referred for an evaluation of his communication skills, based on his parents' report that he is not yet talking. Josh's mother provided the following information. His birth history is reported to be normal, although he was diagnosed to have Down syndrome at birth. His health history is characterized by a "number of ear infections" that "never seem to clear up." His mother stated that "aside from the infections," his health has been "good." Josh's mother also reported that he cannot yet stand on his own, although he can stand with support. He still drinks fluids from a bottle and is not yet able to tolerate solid foods. Josh communicates with his parents using "only a few sounds," and "lots of gesturing," including gestures for "bye bye" and "eat." When compared to her older child, Josh's mother said, "Josh is not doing much."

Family Preferences

Josh's family consists of his mother, father, and older brother, age 5. His mother coordinates most of the medical and developmental activities with her children, as his father works full time. However, Josh's father is very much involved in the care of his children and keeps well informed about the special needs of his youngest son. Both parents are very much concerned that they do "everything possible to help Josh." His parents' initial comments give an impression that Josh's parents may not perceive his prelinguistic and early linguistic behaviors as strengths. This may alert the SLP that his parents require support and careful guidance to identify every means of communication that Josh exhibits.

Developmental Processes

Having considered the background information, a number of questions can be generated regarding developmental processes present in Josh's communicative behavior. Note that the areas addressed in the preceding description provided by Josh's mother include possible concerns about hearing, motor development, oral motor development, cognitive development, social, and vocal development.

1. Does Josh respond to familiar voices and sounds in his environment?
2. What is Josh's overall muscle tone and body posture in a variety of positions?
3. What are Josh's sucking, swallowing, and chewing patterns?
4. Does Josh demonstrate interest in toys? What types of actions are performed?
5. How does Josh respond or initiate games with family members?
6. What vocal sounds does Josh make? What changes are reported in recent months?
7. What are the types and apparent functions of Josh's communicative gestures?

Based on the areas of concern for Josh, several developmental assessment tools may be appropriate to gather initial information with his parents including the HELP (Furuno et al., 1986), the Sequenced Inventory of Communication Development (SICD) (Hedrick, Prather, & Tobin, 1984), MacArthur Child Development Inventories for Toddlers (Fenson et al., 1993), the Language Development Survey (LDS) (Rescorla, 1989), and the Infant/Toddler Checklist for Communication and Language Development (Wetherby & Prizant, 1998).

At this point in the assessment, general developmental information is needed. Parent report measures such as the CDI for toddlers may be most informative to Josh's parents about developmental skills he demonstrates. Of the other tools listed, the HELP is a nonstandardized developmental scale, and the SICD is a standardized early assessment that also includes several parent report items for children under 20 months of age. There are several advantages to using a tool such as the CDI for initial assessment and intervention planning with Josh's parents. Recall that Josh's mother reported she does not perceive him to be doing much communicating for his age. Through completion of the CDI, with professional support, Josh's parents may be able to identify his specific communication skills and provide the clinician with data for further assessment and initial intervention strategies. Dale (1991) supports the validity of parent report to identify emerging language and communication skills.

The CDI provides two scales, the CDI/Infants and the CDI/Toddlers, to assess preverbal development related to emerging language, including nonverbal gestures, games and routines, actions with objects, imitation of actions, use of early language forms, and the degree of decontextualization present in the young child's language. Dale (1991) reported significant correlations between the CDI/Toddlers and the BSID. Miller, Sedey, and Miolo (1995) recently reported strong predictive correlation between CDI vocabulary scores and MLU. Rescorla (1989) conducted multiple studies of the LDS and reported repeatedly high correlations of the LDS with the BSID, the Preschool Language Scale (PLS) (Zimmerman, Steiner, & Pond, 1992), and the Reynell Expressive and Receptive Language Scales (Reynell, 1985). The LDS was found to be a reliable predictor of language delay with children at 2 years of age. Although each tool is somewhat different in content and in level of communication and language assessed, all have common elements, in particular a focus on current and newly emerging communication and language behaviors.

Individual Differences

With specific developmental information, we will learn more of the developmental bases for Josh's delay in language and begin to identify his individual communication patterns. We gain the following information through careful observation and parental information.

Results of developmental assessment based on parent report and clinical observations showed that Josh responds to many environmental sounds and voices of family members. He appears to understand a number of words that refer to names of family members, to familiar items including his bottle, blanket, teddy bear, and inflated ball with noise makers inside, and to some daily activities including eating, bathtime, and story time. He enjoys sitting in either parent's lap at bedtime to read stories, although he only looks at the pictures fleetingly. Recently, he has begun to pat the pages of the books. Further observation of his body posture showed that Josh pulls to stand on furniture with his back curved and stomach out. He drops to the floor in sitting and generally sits with legs widespread, with his center of balance on his lower back. Feeding patterns were described as "messy" by his mother, with frequent drooling. Observation of chewing skills showed some vertical munching of soft crackers and forward tongue thrusting when attempting to swallow sips of milk from a small plastic tumbler. Interactions with others were generally described as visual and sometimes vocal responses. Josh's parents thought he tended to use gaze patterns to get attention, followed by pointing when he really wants his bottle. Vocal sounds were described primarily as vowels. He was found to use gestures to indicate "up," "bye bye," "eat," and "no."

This information leads to the hypothesis that Josh's strengths lie in his social responsiveness to members of his family and his understanding of familiar events and daily routines. Concerns about motor development and apparently hypotonic patterns (low muscle tone) involve both large and small body movement and control in space as well as feeding skills and preferences. Consultation with other disciplines, including the physical therapist and occupational therapist, is supported by these observations. Additional questions can now be generated for further assessment, as the first steps of supporting parents to become the primary informants about their own child are accomplished.

1. Which environmental sounds are most likely to get a response from Josh?
2. Does Josh respond to particular voices more than others, and if so, how?
3. What differences are found in Josh's responses when his parents name and point to particular toys and familiar objects versus just naming the same items?
4. How does Josh respond to familiar routines, such as bathtime and mealtime?
5. Does Josh attempt to bring favorite toys to family members and to interact?
6. Does Josh enjoy particular pictures and books in his bedtime story routine?
7. In what positions and with what support is Josh most likely to point and reach?
8. To what extent is Josh able to imitate fine motor gestures?

These questions require more specific information about Josh's individual communicative behaviors. Particularly useful at this point are structured parent report measures that help parents catalog more specific understanding of gestural, vocal, and verbal communication and language. Assessment tools that are useful at this point are the Communication and Symbolic Behavior Scales (CSBS) (Wetherby & Prizant, 1993) and Assessing Prelinguistic and Linguistic Behaviors (APLB) (Olswang, Stoel-Gammon, Coggins, & Carpenter, 1987). The CSBS is a normed measure of communicative means, reciprocity, and social and affective signaling that is based on play activities and interactions with objects. Similarly, the APLB is conducted in an observation format to elicit interactions between the child and adults to assess cognitive antecedents to language, communicative intent, production, and comprehension of language. Selection of either tool will yield information that identifies Josh's communicative strengths and needs for intervention.

Communicative Contexts

What are the contexts in which Josh appears to communicate? We know from the work of Bruner (1983) and Snyder et al. (1981) that familiar routines and games are the natural contexts for the expansion and elaboration of early communication forms. We also have learned about the important process of gradual decontextualization in early language. In Josh's case, verbal language has not yet fully emerged, so we might anticipate that his communication behavior is likely to occur in familiar, daily routines with familiar caregivers. Suggested methods to identify communicative contexts include ecological inventories, assessment of play sessions (Kennedy et al., 1991), and direct observations of caregivers and infants.

Early Intervention Teams

Throughout the foregoing discussion of the assessment and initial intervention process for Josh, there are several points of linkage that must made with other professionals. Appropriate team members for the completion of Josh's assessment include the audiologist, pediatrician, nurse practitioner, physical therapist, occupational therapist, social worker, and possibly other professionals. The manner of referral and utilization of other disciplines in the assessment process with Josh and his family can be guided by current understanding of best practice in early intervention and, ultimately, the preferences of Josh's parents.

Intervention Strategies

Although Josh's assessment process has been presented as a linear series of steps leading up to intervention, in actuality the process is not linear. Intervention may begin at any point in the process, whenever a problem has been identified and Josh's parents and the clinician agree to address it. Some of these points in our discussion include reports by Josh's mother of her concern about his use of only a few sounds, frequent ear infections, and general pattern of responding rather than initiating games with his family. Further development of family goals around each of these concerns for Josh will provide opportunities for the clinician to assist the parents. Recommended strategies for each of these concerns are displayed in Table 4.8. General principles to support Josh and his family include enhancing daily routines rather than creating "teaching" situations; expanding play interactions with Josh; identifying functional communication through Josh's use of gestures, vocalizations, and emerging word patterns; and taking a preventative approach to upper respiratory infections.

SUMMARY

The purpose of this chapter was to provide students of speech-language pathology with an overview of typical communication development and potential risks for communication disorders during the infancy and toddlerhood. As part of this overview, biological and environmental factors that contribute to placing the infant at risk for normal communication development were presented. Following a review of typical and at-risk development, approaches to early communication assessment and intervention were discussed with an emphasis on dynamic approaches to determine a child's optimal communication skills with appropriate environmental supports and intervention. An organizational framework developed by the authors, referred to as the CAMI, was provided to assist the SLP to build partnerships with families of young children in the process of assessment and intervention in the context of an early in-

TABLE 4.8	Communication Intervention Strategies for Josh (Age 19 Months)		
Intervention Goal	**Intervention Strategy**	**Intervention Model**	
Monitor general health and ear infections.	Consult with pediatrician on regular basis.	Have Josh undergo periodic audiological testing. Use prevention approach for chronic otitis media (Northern, 1981).	
Increase vocalization repertoire in daily routines and games with family members, especially older brother.	Select favorite routine, such as reading books at night, and pause often to give opportunities for Josh to vocalize before turning pages. Imitate and expand his sounds ("aa . . . ba . . . ," "aa . . . da . . . ," "aa . . . ma . . . ").	Use conversational teaching (MacDonald, 1985; Mahoney & Powell, 1984; MacDonald & Carroll, 1992). Scaffolding structured intervention (Norris & Hoffman, 1990).	
Increase vocal and gestural initiation in games and functional communication.	Before daily activities such as eating, bath time, going in the car, etc. Josh's parents and/or brother should pause and wait for Josh to gesture or vocalize to eat, turn on the bath water, or get picked up to go out to the car.	Enhanced milieu teaching (Kaiser & Hester, 1995). Group intervention (Wilcox, Kouri, & Caswell, 1991).	
Increase Josh's social communication with other children and adults.	Involve Josh in playgroup.		

tervention team. We believe that using a dynamic process that integrates best practice in early intervention including (1) family-centered practices, (2) developmental processes, (3) individual differences, (4) communicative contexts, (5) collaborative teams, and (6) interactive intervention strategies is an appropriate approach to identifying, assessing, and intervening with the youngest and most vulnerable children for the purpose of enhancing communication and language development outcomes for later school and participation in society.

STUDY QUESTIONS

1. Provide a rationale for early identification and intervention with children at risk of communication disorders, based on recent research in developmental neurobiology.
2. Explain the differences between environmental and biological risk factors. Provide examples of each.

3. Describe differences in traditional developmental and naturalistic approaches to assessment with infants and toddlers and identify three types of assessment tools in each category.
4. Identify applications of dynamic assessment for young children at risk of communication disorders.
5. Describe the key components of naturalistic language intervention and describe the rationale for using directives in this context.

REFERENCES

Abel, E., & Sokol, R. (1986). Fetal alcohol syndrome is now the leading cause of mental retardation. *Lancet, 2,* 1222–1224.

Adamson, L. B., & Bakeman, R. (1999). Viewing variations in language development: The communication play protocol. *Augmentative and Alternative Communication, 8,* 2–4.

American Academy of Pediatrics. (1987). Statement of childhood lead poisoning. *Pediatrics, 79,* 458–459.

American Academy of Pediatrics & American College of Obstetricians and Gynecologists. (1993). *Guidelines for perinatal care* (4th ed.). Elk Grove, IL: American Academy of Pediatrics.

American Dietetic Association. (1997). Nutrition management of the infant. Manual of clinical dietetics.

American Speech-Language-Hearing Association. (1989). Issues in determining eligibility for language intervention. *ASHA,* March, 113–118.

American Speech-Language-Hearing Association. (1991). Let's talk: Fetal alcohol syndrome. *ASHA,* August, 53–54.

Bailey, D. B. (1988) Considerations in developing family goals. In D. Bailey & R. Simeonsson (Eds.), *Family assessment in early intervention.* Columbus, OH: Merrill/Macmillan.

Bates, E. (1999). Language and the infant brain. *Journal of Communication Disorders, 32,* 195–205.

Bates, E., Benigni, L., Bretherton, I., Camaioni, L., & Volterra, V. (1979). *The emergence of symbols: Cognition and communication in infancy.* New York: Academic Press.

Bates, E., Bretherton, I., & Snyder, L. (1988). *From first words to grammar: Individual differences and dissociable mechanisms.* New York: Cambridge University Press.

Bates, E., Bretherton, I., Snyder, L., Shore, C., & Volterra, V. (1980). Vocal and gestural symbols at 13 months. *Merrill-Palmer Quarterly, 26,* 408–423.

Bates, E., Thal, D., Whitesall, K., Fenson, L., & Oakes, L. (1989). Integrating language and gesture in infancy. *Developmental Psychology, 25,* 197–206.

Bayley, N. (1993). *Bayley scales of infant development.* San Antonio, TX: The Psychological Corporation.

Billeaud, F. P. (1998). Communication disorders in infants and toddlers: Assessment and intervention (2d ed.). Boston: Butterworth-Heinemann.

Bliele, K. (1997). Where words come from: The origins of expressive language. In R. Paul (Ed.), *Exploring the speech-langauge connection* (pp. 119–139). Baltimore: Paul H. Brookes.

Bluestone, C. (1990). *Update on otitis media: 1990.* Unpublished manuscript, University of Pittsburgh School of Medicine, Pittsburgh.

Brainerd, C. (1978). The stage question in cognitive developmental theory. *Behavioral and Brain Sciences, 1,* 173–182.

Brazelton, T. (1984). Neonatal behavioral assessment scale (2d ed.). White Plains, NY: March of Dimes Materials and Supplies Division.

Brazelton, T. B., & Als, H. (1979). Four early states in the development of mother-infant interaction. *Psychoanalytic Study of the Child, 34,* 349–369.

Brazelton, T. B., Koslowski, B., & Main, M. (1974). The origins of reciprocity: The early mother–infant interaction. In M. Lewis & L. A. Rosenblum (Eds.), *The effect of an infant upon its caregiver* (pp. 49–76). New York: Wiley.

Bricker, D. (1993). Assessment, evaluation and programming system for infants and children, Volume I: AEPS measurement of birth to three years. Baltimore: Paul H. Brookes.

Briggs, M. H. (1993). Team talk: Communication skills for early intervention teams. *Journal of Childhood Communication Disorders, 15,* 33–40.

Briggs, M. H. (1997). A systems model for early intervention teams. *Infants and Young Children, 9,* 66–77.

Bruner, J. (1983). *Child's talk: Learning to use language.* New York: Norton.

Bryant, D., & Ramey, C. (1987). An analysis of the effectiveness of early intervention programs for environmentally at-risk children. In M. Guralnick & F. Bennett (Eds.), *The effectiveness of early intervention for at-risk and handicapped children.* New York: Academic Press.

Butler, K. (1997). Dynamic assessment at the millennium: A transient tutorial for today! *Journal of Children's Communication Development, 19,* 43–54.

Bzoch, K., & League, R. (1991). Receptive-expressive emergent-language test (REEL-2). Austin, TX: Pro-Ed.

Campbell, R. (1987). The integrated programming team: An approach for coordinating professionals of various disciplines in programs for students with severe handicaps. *Journal of the Association for Persons with Severe Handicaps, 12,* 107–116.

Capute, A., & Accardo, P. J. (1978) Clinical linguistic and auditory milestones scale. *Clinical Pediatrics, 17,* 847.

Catlett, C. (1991). ASHAs early intervention projects. *ASHA,* April, 50–51.

Centers for Disease Control and Prevention (2000). *HIV/AIDS surveillance report.* Vol. 11(2).

Chasnoff, I. (1987). Parental effects of cocaine. *Contemporary Ob/Gyn, 26,* 1–8.

Chiocca, E. M. (1998). Language development in bilingual children. *Pediatric Nursing, 24,* 43–47.

Chomsky, N. (1965). *Aspects of the theory of syntax.* Cambridge, MA: MIT Press.

Cochrane, C. G., Farley, B. G., & Wilhelm, L. J. (1990). Preparation of physical therapists to work with handicapped infants and their families: Current status. *Physical Therapy, 70,* 372–380.

Cohen, H. (1990). Case management and care coordination for children with HIV infection. In R. Kozlowski, D. Snider, R. Vietze, & H. Wisniewski (Eds.), *Brain in pediatric AIDS.* Basel, Switzerland: Karger.

Cole, J. G. (1996). Intervention strategies for infants with prenatal drug exposure. *Infants and Young Children, 8,* 35–39.

Comfort, M., & Farran, D. C. (1994). Parent–child interaction assessment in family-centered intervention. *Infants and Young Children, 6,* 33–45.

Coplan, J. (1993). *Early language milestone scale* (2d ed.). Austin, TX: Pro-Ed.

Coplan, J., Contello, K. A., Cunningham, C. K., Weiner, L. B., Dye, T. D., Roberge, L., Wojtowycz, M. A., & Kirkwook, K. (1998). Early langauge development in children exposed to or infected with human immunodeficiency virus. *Pediatrics, 102,* 8.

Coplan, J., & Gleason, J. (1990). Quantifying language development from birth to 3 years using the Early Language Milestone Scale. *Pediatrics, 86,* 963–971.

Crais, E. (1995). Expanding the repertoire of tools and techniques for assessing the communication skills of infants and toddlers. *American Journal of Speech-Language Pathology, 4,* 47–59.

Crawley, S., & Spiker, D. (1983). Mother–child interactions involving two-year-olds with Down syndrome: A look at individual differences. *Child Development, 54,* 1312–1323.

Crees, C. J. (1999) Transitions from spontaneous to intentional behaviors. *Augmentative and Alternative Communication, 8,* 4–7.

Dale, P. (1995). The value of good distinction. *Journal of Early Intervention, 19,* 102–103.

Dale, R. S. (1991). The validity of a parent report measures of vocabulary and syntax at 24 months. *Journal of Speech and Hearing Research, 34,* 565–571.

D'Apolito, K. (1998). Substance abuse: Infant and childhood outcomes. *Journal of Pediatric Nursing, 13,* 307–316.

Dattel, B. (1990). Substance abuse in pregnancy. *Summaries in Perinatology, 14,* 179–187.

DeWeerth, C., van Geert P., Hoijtink, H. (1999). Intraindividual variability in infant behavior. *Developmental Psychology, 35,* 1102–1112.

Donahue, M. L., & Pearl, R. (1995) Conversational interactions of mothers and their preschool children who have been preterm. *Journal of Speech and Hearing Research, 38,* 1117–1125.

Drash, R. W., & Tudor, R. M. (1990). Language and cognitive development: A systematic behavioral program and technology for increasing the language and cognitive skills of developmentally disabled and at-risk preschool children. *Programs in Behavior Modification, 26,* 173–220.

Dunst, C., & Rheingrover, R. (1982). Discontinuity and instability in early development: implications for assessment. In J. Neisworth (Ed.), *Assessment in special education.* Rockville, MD: Aspen.

Ensher, G. (1989). Newborns at risk. *Topics in Language Disorders, 10,* 80–90.

Fenson, L., Dale, R., Reznick, S., Thal, D., Bates, E., Hartung, J., Pethick, S., & Reilly, J. (1993). *MacArthur communicative development inventories.* San Diego: Singular.

Fergusson, D., Woodward, L., & Horwood, L. (1998). Maternal smoking during pregnancy and psychiatric adjustment in late adolescence. *Archives of General Psychiatry, 55,* 721–727.

Fried, R, & Watkinson, B. (1990). 36- and 48-Month neurobehavioral follow-up of children prenatally exposed to marijuana, cigarettes, and alcohol. *Developmental and Behavioral Pediatrics, 11,* 49–58.

Furuno, S., O'Reilly, K., Inatsuka, T., Hosaka, C., Allman, T., & Zeisloft-Falboy, B. (1987). *Hawaii early learning profile.* Palo Alto, CA: Vort.

Gerber, S. (1990). Prevention: *The etiology of communicative disorders in children.* Englewood Cliffs, NJ: Prentice Hall.

Girolametto, L. (1995). Reflections on the origins of directiveness: Implications for intervention. *Journal of Early Intervention, 19,* 104–106.

Glascoe, F. P., & Byrne, K. E. (1993). The usefulness of the Developmental Profile-II in developmental screening. *Clinical Pediatrics, 32,* 203–208.

Gonzalez-Cossio, T., Peterson K. E., Sanin, L., Fishbein S. E., Palazuelos, E., Aro, A., Hernandez-Avila, M., and Hu, H. (1997). Decrease in birth weight in relation to maternal bone lead burden. *Pediatrics, 100,* 856–862.

Gradel, K., Thompson, M. S., & Sheehan, R. (1981). Parental and professional agreement in early childhood assessment. *Topics in Early Childhood Special Education, 1,* 31–39.

Gravel, J., & Wallace, I. (2000). Effects of otitis media with effusion on hearing in the first 3 years of life. *Journal of Speech, Language, and Hearing Research, 43,* 631–644.

Halle, J. W., Baer, D., & Spradlin, J. E. (1981). Teacher's generalized use of delay as a stimulus control procedure to increase language use in handicapped children. *Journal of Applied Behavior Analysis, 14,* 389–411.

Hanson, M. J., & Krentz, M. S. (1986). *Supporting parent–child interactions: A guide for early intervention program personnel.* San Francisco: San Francisco State University, Integrated Special Infant Services Program, Department of Special Education.

Hanson, M. J., Lynch, E. W., & Wayman, K. (1990). Honoring the cultural diversity of the family when gathering data. *Topics in Early Childhood Special Education, 10,* 112–131.

Harding, C., & Golinkoff, R. (1979). *The origins of intentional vocalizations in prelinguistic infants. Precursors of early speech.* New York: Stockton.

Hart, B., & Risely, T. (1975). Incidental teaching of language in the preschool. *Journal of Applied Behavioral Analysis, 8,* 411–420.

Hart, B., & Risely, T. (1995). *Meaningful differences in the everyday experiences of young American children.* Baltimore: Paul H. Brookes.

Hatch, E., & Bracken, M. B. (1993). Caffeine use during pregnancy: How much is safe? *Journal of the American Medical Association, 270,* 46–47.

Hedrick, D., Prather, E., & Tobin, A. (1984). *Sequenced inventory of communication development (revised).* Los Angeles: Western Psychological Services.

Holmgren, K., Lindblom, B., Aurelius, G., Jaling, B., & Zetterstrom, R. (1980). On the phonetics of infant vocalization. In B. Lindblom & R. Zetterstrom (Eds.), *Precursors of early speech.* New York: Stockton.

Hopkins, K., Grosz, J., & Lieberman, A. (1990). Working with families and caregivers of children with HIV infection and developmental disability. Technical report on developmental disabilities and HIV infection. American Association of University Affiliated Programs.

Howard, C., & Lawrence, R. (1998). Breastfeeding and drug exposure. *Obstetric & Gynecological Clinics of North America, 25,* 195–217.

Iacono, T. A. (1999). Language intervention in early childhood. *International Journal of Disability, Development and Education, 46,* 383–420.

Ireton, H., & Thwing, E. (1974). *Manual for the Minnesota Child Development Inventory.* Minneapolis: Behavior Science Systems.

Jones, K., & Smith, D. (1974). Outcomes in offspring of chronic alcoholic women. *Lancet, 3,* 1076–1078.

Jones, H., & Warren, S. (1991). Enhancing engagement in early language teaching. *Teaching Exceptional Children, 23,* 48–50.

Kaiser, A. B., & Hester, R. R. (1995). Generalized effects of enhanced milieu teaching. *Journal of Speech and Hearing Research, 37,* 1320–1340.

Kennedy, M. D., Sheridan, M. K., Radlinshi, S. H., & Beeghly, M. (1991). Play-language relationships in young children with developmental delays: Implications for assessment. *Journal of Speech and Hearing Research, 34,* 112–122.

Kent, R., & Hodge, M. (1991). The biogenesis of speech: Continuity and process in early speech and language development. In J. Miller (Ed.), *Research on child language disorders.* Austin, TX: Pro-Ed.

Klein, M. D., & Briggs, M. H. (1987). *Observation of communicative interaction.* Los Angeles: Mother-Child Communication Project, University of California, Los Angeles.

Kopp, C. (1990). Risk in infancy: Appraising the research. *Merrill-Palmer Quarterly 36,* 117–139.

Linder, T. (1993). *Transdisciplinary play-based assessment.* Baltimore: Paul H. Brookes.

Locke, J. (1994). Gradual emergence of developmental language disorders. *Journal of Speech and Hearing Research, 37,* 608–616.

Lyons-Ruth, K., Connell, D., & Grunebaum, H. (1990). Infants at social risk: Maternal depression and family support services as mediators of infant development and security of attachment. *Child Development, 61,* 85–98.

MacDonald, J. (1985) Language through conversation. In S. Warren and A. Rogers-Warren (Eds.), *Teaching functional language.* Austin, TX: Pro-Ed.

MacDonald, J., & Carroll, J. Y. (1992) A social partnership model for assessing early communication development: An intervention model for preconversational children. *Language, Speech and Hearing Services in Schools, 23,* 113–124.

MacDonald, J., & Gillette, Y. (1985). *Social play: A program for developing a social play habit for communication development.* Columbus, OH: O.S.U. Research Foundation.

Mahoney, G., & Powell, A. (1984). The transactional intervention program, preliminary teachers' guide. Unpublished manuscript. School of Education, University of Michigan, Ann Arbor.

Mays, R. M., & Gillon, J. E. (1993). Autism in young children: An update. *Journal of Pediatric Health Care, 7,* 17–23.

McCathren, R. B., Yoder, P. J., & Warren, S. F. (1995). The role of directives in early language intervention. *Journal of Early Intervention, 19,* 91–101.

McCathren, R. B., Yoder, P. J., & Warren, S. F. (1999). The relationship between prelinguistic vocalization and later expressive vocabulary in young children with developmental delay. *Journal of Speech, Language, and Hearing Research, 42,* 4, 915–924.

McCollum, J. A., & Yates, T. J. (1994). Dyad as focus triad as means: A family-centered approach to supporting parent–child interactions. *Infants and Young Children, 6,* 54–63.

McCormick, L., & Goldman, R. (1978). The transdisciplinary model: Implications for service delivery and personnel preparation for the severely and profoundly handicapped. *AAESPH Review, 4,* 152–161.

McCormick, L., Loeb, D., & Schiefelbusch, R. (1997). *Supporting children with communication difficulties in inclusive settings: School-based intervention.* Boston: Allyn & Bacon.

McElhatton, P., Bateman, D., Evans, C., Pughe, K., & Thomas, S. (1999). Congenital anomalies after prenatal ecstasy exposure. *Lancet, 354,* 1441–1442.

McGonigel, M., Kaufmann, R., & Johnson, B. (1991). Guidelines and recommended practices for the individualized family service plan. Bethesda: Association for the Care of Children's Health.

McKinney, E., Ashwill, J., Murray, S., James, S., Gorrie, T., & Droske, S. (2000). *Maternal–child nursing.* New York: Saunders.

Messick, C., Anketell, M., & Chapman, K. (1987). Language intervention with 0–5 population: An organization framework. Paper presented at the American Speech-Language-Hearing Association Convention.

Miller, J. P., Sedey, A. L., & Miolo, G. (1995). Validity of parent report measures of vocabulary development for children with Down syndrome. *Journal of Speech and Hearing Research, 38,* 1037–1044.

Mitchell, R., & Kent, R. (1990). Phonetic variation in multisyllabic babbling. *Journal of Child Language, 17,* 247–266.

Montgomery, J. K., Valdez, F., & Herer, G. R. (1997). Best practice in school speech language assessment: Using early intervention results. *Journal of Children's Communication Development, 19,* 3–11.

Moore, M. K., & Meltzhoff, A. N. (1978). Object permanence, imitation, and language development: Toward a neo-Piagetian perspective. In R. D. Minifie and L. L. Lloyd. (Eds.), *Communicative and cognitive abilities—Early behavioral assessment.* Baltimore: University Park Press.

Narod, S., Sanjose, S., & Victora, C. (1991). Coffee during pregnancy: A reproductive hazard? *American Journal of Obstetrics and Gynecology, 164,* 1109–1114.

National Institute on Alcohol Abuse and Alcoholism. (1997). Ninth special report to the U.S. Congress on alcohol and health. NIAA/National Institutes of Health Pub. No. 97-4017.

National Institute on Drug Abuse. (1995). Biological mechanisms and perinatal exposure to drugs. *NIDA Research Monograph Number 158.*

Newborg, J., Stock, J., & Wnek, I. (1984). *Batelle developmental inventory.* Allen, TX: DLM/Teaching Resources.

Norris, J. A., & Hoffman, R. (1990). Language intervention within naturalistic environments. *Language, Speech, and Hearing Services in the Schools, 21,* 72–84.

Oller, D. K. (1980). The emergence of the sounds of speech in infancy. In G. Yeni-Komshian, J. Kavanagh, & C. Ferguson (Eds.), *Child phonology* (Vol. 1) (pp. 93–112). New York: Academic.

Oller, D. K., Eilers, R., Neal, A. R., & Schwartz, H. K. (1999). Precursors to speech in infancy: The prediction of speech and language disorders. *Journal of Communication Disorders, 32,* 223–245.

Olswang, L., Stoel-Gammon, C., Coggins, T., & Carpenter, R. (1987). *Assessing prelinguistic and linguistic behavior.* Seattle: University of Washington Press.

Owens, R. (1992). *Language development: An introduction* (3d ed.). Columbus, OH: Merrill/Macmillan.

Paradise, J., Rockette, H., Colborn, K., Bernard, B., Smith, C., Kurs-Lasky, M., & Janosky, J. (1997). Otitis media in 2,253 Pittsburgh-area infants: Prevalence and risk factors during the first two years of life. *Pediatrics, 99,* 318–333.

Paul, R. (1999). Discussion: Early speech perception and production. *Journal of Communication Disorders, 32,* 247–250.

Pine (1992). Maternal style at the early one-word stage: Re-evaluating the stereotype of the directive mother. *First Language, 12,* 169–186.

Proctor. A. (1989). Stages of normal vocal development in infancy: A protocol for assessment. *Topics in Language Disorders, 10,* 26–42.

Public Law 205-17. *Amendments to the Individuals with Disabilities Education Act of 1997.*

Reinharten, D. B., Edmondson, R., & Crais, E. R. (1997). Developing assistive technology strategies for infants and toddlers with communication difficulties. *Seminars in Speech and Language, 18,* 283–301.

Rescorla, L. (1989). The Language Development Survey. *Journal of Speech and Hearing Disorders, 54,* 587–599.

Reynell, J. (1985). *Reynell Developmental Language Scales.* Los Angeles: Webster Psychological Corp.

Rice, M., Buhr, J., & Nemeth, M. (1990). Fast-mapping word-learning abilities of language-delayed preschoolers. *Journal of Speech and Hearing Research, 55,* 33–42.

Robinson, N., & Robb, M. (1997). Early communication assessment and intervention: An interactive process. In D. Bernstein & E. Tiegerman (Eds), *Language and Communication Disorders in Children* (4th ed.) (pp. 155–196). Boston: Allyn & Bacon.

Robb, M., Bauer, H., & Tyler, A. (1994). A quantitative analysis of the single-word stage. *First Language, 14,* 37–48.

Robb, M., Psak, J., & Pang-Ching, G. (1993). Chronic otitis media and early speech development: A case study. *International Journal of Pediatric Otorhinolaryngology 26,* 117–127.

Roberts, J., Wallace, I., & Henderson, F. (1997). Otitis media in young children: Medical, developmental, and educational considerations. Baltimore: Paul H. Brookes.

Robertson, S. B., & Weismer, S. E. (1999). Effects of treatment on linguistic and social skills in toddlers with delayed language development. *Journal of Speech, Language and Hearing Research, 42,* 1234–1248.

Romski, M. A., & Sevcik, R. A. (1999). Speech comprehension and early augmented language intervention: Concepts, measurement, and clinical considerations. *Augmentative and Alternative Communication, 8,* 7–10.

Rossetti, L. (1990). The Rossetti Infant–Toddler Language Scale. Moline, IL: Lingua Systems.

Rutter. M. (1979). Protective factors in children's response to stress and disadvantage. In M. Kent and T. Rolf (Eds.*), Social competence in children.* Hanover, NH: University Press of New England.

Sawyer, D., & Butler, K. (1991). Early language intervention: A deterrent to reading disability. *Annals of Dyslexia, 41,* 55–79.

Sevcik, R. A. (1999). Research with young children at risk of speech/language development disorders. *Augmentative and Alternative Communication, 8,* 1–2.

Shatz, M. (1983). On transition, continuity, and coupling: An alternative approach to communicative development. In R. Golinkoff (Ed.), *The transition from prelinguistic to linguistic communication.* Hillsdale, NJ: Erlbaum.

Shaw, D., & Bell, R. (1993). Developmental theories of parental contributors to antisocial behavior. *Journal of Abnormal Child Psychology, 21,* 25–49.

Shprintzen, R. (1997). *Genetics, syndromes, and communication disorders.* San Diego, CA: Singular.

Shriberg, L., Friel-Patti, S., Flapsen, P., & Brown, R. (2000). Otits media, fluctuant hearing loss, and speech-language outcomes: A preliminary structural equation model. *Journal of Speech, Language, and Hearing Research, 43,* 100–120.

Smith, B., Brown-Sweeney. S., & Stoel-Gammon, C. (1989). A quantitative analysis of reduplicated and variegated babbling. *First Language, 9,* 175–190.

Snow, C. (1979). The role of social interaction and the development of communicative ability. In A. Collins (Ed.), *Children's language and communication.* Hillsdale, NJ: Erlbaum.

Snyder, L., Bates, E., & Bretherton, I. (1981). Content and context in early lexical development. *Journal of Child Language, 8,* 565–582.

Sparks, S. (1989). Assessment and intervention with at-risk infants and toddlers: Guidelines for the speech-language pathologist. *Topics in Language Disorders, 10,* 43–56.

Stark, R. (1980). Stages of speech development in the first year of life. In G. Komishan, J. Kavanagh, & C. Ferguson (Eds.), *Child phonology (Vol. 1).* New York: Academic.

Stoel-Gammon, C., & Cooper, J. (1984). Patterns of early lexical and phonological development. *Journal of Child Language, 11,* 247–271.

Teele, D., Klein, J., Chase, C., Menyuk, R., & Rosner, B. (1990). Otitis media in infancy and intellectual ability, school achievement, speech and language at age 7 years. *Journal of Infectious Diseases, 162,* 685–694.

Tomblin, J. B., Shonrock, C. M., & Hardy, J. C. (1989). The concurrent validity of the Minnesota Child Development Inventory as a measure of young children's language development. *Journal of Speech and Hearing Disorders, 54,* 101–105.

Turnbull, A., & Turnbull, H. (1990). *Families, professionals, and exceptionality: A special partnership* (2d ed.). Columbus, OH: Merrill/Macmillan.

UNICEF (1998). *The state of the world's children.* Oxford, UK: Oxford University Press.

Vihman, M., & Greenlee, M. (1987). Individual differences in phonological development: Ages one and three years. *Journal of Speech and Hearing Research, 30,* 503–521.

Ward, S. (1999). An investigation into the effectiveness of an early intervention method for delayed language development in young children. *International Journal of Language and Communication Disorders, 34,* 243–264.

Warren, S. R., & Gazdag, G. (1990). Facilitating early language development with milieu intervention procedures. *Journal of Early Intervention, 14,* 62.

Warren, S., & Kaiser, A. (1986). Incidental language teaching: A critical review. *Journal of Speech and Hearing Disorders, 51,* 291–299.

Wetherby, A., & Prizant, B. (1992). Profiling young children's communicative competence. In S. Warren & J. Reichle (Eds.), Causes and effects in communication and language intervention (pp. 217–253). Baltimore: Brookes.

Wetherby, A., & Prizant, B. (1998). Communication and symbolic behavior scales. Chicago: Riverside.

Wetherby, A., Prizant, B., & Hutchinson, T. (1998). Communication, social/affective, and symbolic profiles of young children with autism and pervasive developmental disorders. *American Journal of Speech-Language Pathology, 7,* 79–91.

Wilcox, M. J., Kouri, T. A., & Caswell, S. B. (1991). Early language intervention: A comparison of classroom and individual treatment. *American Journal of Speech-Language Pathology, 1,* 49–61.

Wing, C. (1990). Defective infant formulas and expressive language delay: A case study. *Language, Speech and Hearing Services in Schools, 21,* 22–27.

Wyly, M., Allen, J., Pfalzer, S. M., & Wilson, J. R. (1996). Providing a seamless service system from hospital to home: The NICU Training Project. *Infants and Young Children, 8,* 77–84.

Yoder, P., & Warren, S. (1999). Prelinguistic communication intervention may be one way to help children with developmental delays learn to talk. *Augmentative and Alternative Communication, 8,* 11–12.

Yoder, P., Warren, S., Kyoungram, K., & Gazdag, G. E. (1994). Facilitating prelinguistic communication skills in young children with developmental delay II: Systematic replication and extension. *Journal of Speech and Hearing Research, 37,* 841–851.

Zimmerman, I., Steiner, V., & Pond, R. (1992). Preschool Language Scale—3. San Antonio, TX: Psychological Corporation.

Zuniga, J. (1999). Communication disorders and HIV disease. *Journal of the International Association of Physicians in AIDS Care, 2*(4).

CHAPTER 5

Elaine R. Silliman
University of South Florida

Sylvia F. Diehl
University of South Florida

Assessing Children with Language Learning Disabilities

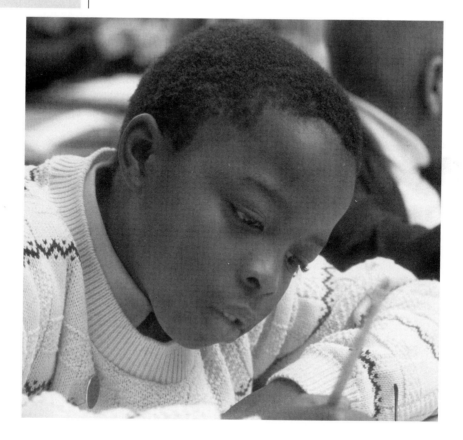

- Understand the influence of the model selected for assessment on the purposes of assessment
- Articulate the synergistic relationship between the purposes of assessment and intervention especially in light of the interpretation of the Least Restricted Environment (LEA) under IDEA
- Apply a decision making framework to ask assessment questions that consider educational standards, grade level expectations, and person-centered planning
- Determine the focus of assessment based on current scientific evidence about relationships between aspects of spoken language knowledge and learning to read, write, and spell
- Select norm reference or alternate assessments that are consistent with the purposes and focuses of assessment and reflect technical knowledge of reliability, validity, and diagnostic accuracy
- Evaluate system patterns for individual children and interpret their possible meanings as these patterns of performance relate to classroom and community challenges
- Utilize the assessment process as a starting point to address new questions and outcomes on an ongoing basis

The 1997 reauthorization by the U.S. Congress of the Individuals with Disabilities Education act (IDEA) and the 1999 regulations for Part B of that act have changed the role of school-based speech-language pathologists. New provisions require a process of educational planning that is premised on collaboration among professionals responsible for children with special needs. Children must now have access to the general education curriculum. The individualized educational plan (IEP) must combine content-area learning with functional curriculum-based assessments and specify "measurable annual goals that support the child's progress in the general curriculum . . . (as well as) nonacademic, and extracurricular programs" (Whitmire, 2000a, p. 194).

As speech-language pathologists, we are responsible for identifying school-age children with language learning disabilities and for designing and implementing effective intervention programs for them in a variety of settings but, most critically, the classroom setting (Bashir, Conte, & Heerde, 1998). Meeting the new mandates of IDEA requires the understanding that successful literacy learning is interconnected with spoken language abilities. For example, we must (1) recognize that the language basis of learning is essential for children's academic success, (2) view both language and literacy learning as central components of assessment, (3) take into account the general education curriculum as a guide for the development of more authentic assessment approaches, and (4) develop skill as a collaborative partner in the educational process. Thus, assessing children's language and communication behaviors, as well as how their language-related abilities support literacy learning, is significant for fulfilling professional responsibilities as a speech-language pathologist.

The task of assessing children's language abilities would be relatively simple if language were easily quantified, like height or weight. However, language is not a single dimension that can be easily measured with a yardstick or scales, like height and weight. Instead, language is a multidimensional, complex, and dynamic system; it involves many interrelated processes and abilities; and it changes from situation to situation depending on why we are talking, where we are talking, whom we are talking with, and what we are talking about. As Miller (1981) pointed out over two decades ago, the elusive nature of language makes it very difficult to measure and quantify. The task is complicated further in the range and variety of behaviors exhibited by individual children with language disorders. Every child evaluated will have a unique pattern of language abilities and a unique profile of problems in understanding and using language. In fact, individual differences will be the rule, not the exception. For example, one child may appear to have an adequate vocabulary and good social communication skills but have significant difficulties with formulating age-appropriate syntax in classroom situations. Another child may appear able to produce a variety of grammatically acceptable utterances for everyday speaking but may use many nonspecific terms such as *that one, it,* and *the thing,* because she has trouble rapidly retrieving the appropriate words for objects, people, and events in particular social situations. Still another child may appear to have acquired a spoken language system consistent with expectations for the preschool years, but is experiencing severe problems in mastering relationships between phonemes and letters, which also affects reading comprehension. One of the challenges in language assessment is to reveal and describe the distinctive pattern of language behaviors for each child with a suspected or known language learning disability.

Another complicating variable in assessment is that, today, an increasingly diverse school population reflects a rich fabric of cultural and linguistic differences. However, the ability to differentiate sociocultural variability in language use from language patterns that result from an impaired system requires comprehensive knowledge of two domains. These are the values and beliefs of the child's culture and the patterns of language and communication that may be characteristic of that culture. An important issue is how these cultural and sociolinguistic factors may positively or negatively influence the expectations of teachers and others for the academic achievement of individual children (Silliman, Bahr, Turner, & Wilkinson, in press; Washington & Craig, 2001). In the case of children who are learning English as a second language, understanding critical linguistic distinctions between the first language and English is also necessary for conducting valid assessment in both languages (Gutiérrez-Clellen, Restrepo, Bedore, Peña, & Anderson, 2000; see also Chapter 8). Approximately 14 percent of school-age children have limited English proficiency; about three-quarters of these are from Spanish-speaking families and "attend high-poverty schools" (Hakuta & Beatty, 2000, p. 12).

The many challenges of the assessment task can be met if four points are kept in mind. First, keep an open and curious mind. Second, develop keen observational skills. Third, maintain a current disciplinary and interdisciplinary knowledge base about language theory and research. Finally, understand how different conceptual frameworks about language and literacy learning lead to different questions and focuses for both assessment and intervention (Apel, 1999; Hewitt, 2000).

This chapter is designed to introduce you to the nature and scope of language assessment in school-age children rather than to provide all of the information necessary for carrying out an in-depth language assessment. As part of this discussion, different types of assessment are described, contrasted, and illustrated with case examples. Five major questions are explored:

1. *Model of assessment:* What conceptual framework about language learning guides the approach to assessment?
2. *Purposes of assessment:* Why are the child's language and communication abilities being assessed?
3. *Focuses of assessment:* What aspects of the child's functioning should be assessed?
4. *Methods of assessment:* How will those aspects be assessed?
5. *Outcomes of assessment:* How will the results of the assessment be interpreted and used?

Although this chapter focuses on assessing children's language and communicative behaviors, other aspects of development also need to be considered in evaluating any child. It is crucial to remember that children's communicative functioning involves not only language knowledge and skills but also cognitive and social knowledge and, when appropriate, physical status and motor abilities. The development of early cognitive and social-communicative behaviors is discussed in Chapter 2. In addition, Chapter 4 discusses the principles of assessing these behaviors in infants and toddlers.

There is also increasing evidence that we should be concerned with children's socioemotional development. Being a competent communicator is intertwined with self-esteem; thus, children's abilities as communicators affect the development of their personal identity and, in turn, significantly influence how others judge their competence (Brinton, Fujiki, & McKee, 1998; Brinton, Fujiki, Montague, & Hanton, 2000; Fujiki, Brinton, Hart, & Fitzgerald, 1999; Redmond & Rice, 1998). As these studies on socioemotional development suggest, we need to be concerned with those situations in which the child spends a good deal of time, such as the classroom, interacting with peers inside and outside of school, and with family at home. Although it may not be possible to obtain information in all of the situations just mentioned, it is important to remember that the assessment of children's language and communicative skills can never be separated from the larger familial and cultural-linguistic contexts of communication (McCauley, 2001). Also, the choice of particular assessment methods should always depend on the purposes for assessing a particular child in relation to the clinical or educational questions being asked.

MODELS AND PURPOSES OF ASSESSMENT

Models of Assessment

Assessment is a problem-solving process. An assessment model can be thought of as the blueprint or a set of assumptions about the process of language learning that guides (1) the clinical questions asked about the functioning of a child's communication system, (2) how this functioning will be interpreted, and (3) the extent to which interpretation can appropriately address the specific set of questions. Models tend to derive from different conceptual frameworks of what language learning is and how it works. Different models are not necessarily always compatible with each other (Chapman, 1991).

Deficit Models and the Discrepancy Concept

Lund and Duchan (1993) illustrate this point about the incompatibility of assessment models. When we ask a deficit question such as, "What is the language deficit and how severe is it?," we are asking a question typically associated with normative/deviance models of assessment. These models tend to define normal versus atypical in terms of the degree of deviance from a statistical mean (Peterson & Marquardt, 1994). This type of statistical definition derives from the average performance of large groups of individuals, called a **norming sample,** and is associated with one general kind of assessment tool: standardized measures of language performance. Another term for a standardized measure is **norm-referenced measure.** All norm-referenced measures have a common standard of comparison. The individual's performance is interpreted in relation to the average performance of a peer group, or those "who are presumably like that person in other respects" (Salvia & Ysseldyke, 2001, p. 30).

Deficit models often have a **discrete-point perspective** on language assessment (Damico, 1991; Shulman, Katz, & Sherman, 1995). In this perspective, language proficiency is viewed as its own system relatively uninfluenced by other systems, such as cognition, memory, or socioemotional factors. Moreover, as mentioned earlier, the language system itself is considered as consisting of separate, or unitary, components, such as sound structure, syntax, or meaning, which implies that each can be assessed independently (Damico, 1991). The purpose of assessment, therefore, is directed to identifying the specific components of the language system that are missing or incomplete—for example, the vocabulary or syntactic structures that the child either does not understand or produce. Often the information obtained is not useful for intervention purposes because it is unrelated to the child's specific needs. Examples of deficit models include auditory (temporal) processing models, in which it is speculated that children have difficulties in attending to rapidly changing aspects of the acoustic signal containing speech stimuli (see, e.g., Tallal, Miller, Jenkins, & Merzenich, 1997), and the specific disabilities model. In the specific disabilities model, the assumption is that breakdowns occur in particular processes, such as auditory perception, auditory memory, or verbal expression, which then lead to weaknesses (deficits) in these areas (Paul, 1995). [For critiques of auditory processing models, see Friel-Patti (1999a, 1999b); Lahey (1988) and Paul (1995) provide similar assessments of specific disabilities models.]

However, information on deficit areas, as gained from norm-referenced measures representing these models, is most commonly used for determining eligibility for speech and language services in the school setting (Casby, 1992; Whitmire, 2000b). Eligibility means deciding (1) whether a language impairment exists and (2) whether the level of severity meets eligibility requirements in accord with the standards of state education departments and local school systems. A long-standing controversy about the use of norm-referenced measures for determining eligibility involves the use of *discrepancy criteria.* The IDEA specifies that, for the identification of a learning disability, a severe discrepancy must be present between intellectual ability and achievement, which can include such areas as oral expression, listening comprehension, basic reading skill, and reading comprehension (Nelson, 1998, p. 97). Thus, the two components of a discrepancy are cognitive ability, as defined by IQ, and language-related abilities that are presumed to support academic achievement. However, in the identification of a language learning disability, the IDEA does not specify that the discrepancy concept must be applied (Whitmire, 2000b). Despite the absence of this requirement in federal law, it appears that the application of the discrepancy concept continues to be common practice in the assessment of children with a possible language learning disability (Casby, 1992; Nelson, 2000; Whitmire, 2000b). For a discrepancy to be present there must be a gap in performance between children's intellectual abilities and their language abilities, which may be converted to a language age. In other words, language abilities must be assessed as being less than expected for the child's intellectual level. Thus, in the assessment of both a learning and a language disability, the IQ score becomes "the benchmark" (Stanovich, 2000, p. 348) from which a discrepancy is measured.

To illustrate, Mary and Johnny are both in grade 2 and have been referred to the school psychologist and speech-language pathologist for assessment. Mary is struggling academically and seems to have significant problems with understanding classroom instructions, but she has formed peer friendships. Upon completion of the assessments, it is found that Mary has at least a 15-point difference between her language age and IQ level, which will likely qualify her for services. Johnny, however, whose IQ and language age are not discrepant, fails to qualify for services even though he has similar language comprehension problems, cannot read, write, or spell, and is socially isolated.

At least four criticisms have been leveled against the discrepancy concept as the basis for determining eligibility for language services.

1. *The theoretical premises of the discrepancy concept are false.* The underlying conceptual assumption for the discrepancy notion is that cognitive development leads language development or, in a somewhat weaker version, that language abilities are always dependent on cognitive abilities (Casby, 1992). The existing scientific evidence does not support this assumption of a unidirectional causal relationship. Although various aspects of cognition and language may be correlated with each other at different developmental points in time, correlation is not identical with causation.

2. *IQ is not predictive of who has a language learning disability or who will respond to intervention.* Nonverbal cognitive measures are typically used to assess the intellectual ability of children with a suspected language disorder, because it is reasoned that they will not do well on verbal measures. The lower boundary of "normal intelligence" is generally defined as a nonverbal IQ of 85. However, the limited evidence to date again shows that nonverbal IQ is not a valid predictor of who will benefit from language intervention (Cole & Fey, 1996). Moreover, other studies show that nonverbal abilities are also affected in many children with a language learning disability (Kamhi, 1996; Parnell, 1995). For example, as a group, children with atypical language learning have problems in so-called nonlanguage areas, such as the complexity of their symbolic play, manipulating visual imagery, and the efficiency of their problem solving. This finding leads Johnston (1994) to speculate

that, "A portion of this disability must reflect the role of language in higher level problem solving. Another portion of the cognitive disability is nonverbal and can be presumed to be responsible for inefficient learning in many domains, including language" (p. 114).

An additional source of evidence that challenges the concept of IQ as a determiner of impairment comes from the field of reading disabilities. Here, a discrepancy is usually defined as a gap between aptitude (IQ) and achievement (either basic reading ability or reading comprehension). However, there is an absence of scientific evidence for the valid application of the discrepancy concept either for the identification of a reading disability or the prediction of instructional outcomes for individual children (Stanovich, 1999, 2000).

3. *Children's performance varies according to the assessment measure and cutoff point.* The particular norm-referenced measures selected for assessing the existence of discrepancy influence the magnitude of the discrepancy (Lubker & Tomblin, 1998). This means that children's performance cannot easily be separated from the content of the assessment measure and how a cutoff score is assigned for atypical performance. A cutoff score is the score that serves as a "decision boundary" (McCauley, 2001, p. 243). Scores above that boundary are considered as normal, while scores below the boundary are viewed as indicating a possible difference from normal variation.

Since every norm-referenced measure has different content and varying cutoff boundaries, the extent to which a discrepancy is evident can result from the combination of measures that are administered rather than reflect a real difference between children's cognitive and language abilities. One serious consequence may be diagnostic inaccuracy in which unacceptable numbers of children who do not have a language learning disability are erroneously classified as having one. This inappropriate interpretation of results from norm-referenced assessment is discussed further in the section on methods of assessment.

4. *Language needs of individual children are ignored.* A final criticism is that the concept of discrepancy, which stems from the notion of deficit areas, does not address what individual children require in terms of language intervention services. In Nelson's (2000) analysis, the appropriate question to ask is, " 'What does this child need?' rather than 'What does the child qualify for?' " (p. 10). However, a long-standing practical obstacle has prevented the adoption of the need-based model. Professional consensus does not exist among school administrators and educational staff on alternative assessment models and alternative eligibility criteria. The perception is that shifting to need-based models will increase caseloads of speech-language pathologists in the public schools, which will then further strain the financial resources necessary to support their services (Ehren, 2000).

Categorical Models

On the other hand, an assessment question, such as "What is causing the language problem?," asks an etiological, or causal, question. Categorical models are common to medically based assessment approaches, in which the task is to differentiate one set of symptom clusters from another in order to arrive at a *category of diagnosis.*

The implication is that the diagnostic category provides some causal account of the disorder—for example, that a child's set of "symptoms" is more consistent with a specific language impairment (or a language learning disability) than with mental retardation or autism. Categorical models may also be concerned with factors that contribute to a profile of severity in certain situations (Nation & Aram, 1991). For example, in the example cited in the previous section, it may be that Johnny has undiagnosed and intermittent otitis media that contributes to a continuous cycle of failure.

The disability categories in the IDEA are based on the categorical model and serve as the vehicle for qualifying children for special education and related services, most typically by determining deficit areas (see the previous section). Additionally, educational funding at federal, state, and local levels for special education services is dedicated to the category (i.e., speech-language impaired, learning disabilities, hard of hearing/deaf, mental retardation, etc). One advantage of this model, according to Paul (1995), is that the categories of disability are an efficient way to convey to different audiences how the problems of one group of children differ from those of another group. A second advantage is that, if contributing causal factors can be identified (Nation & Aram, 1991), then these become important for preventing further increases in severity and for designing more functional language intervention goals and procedures.

However, three major problems, some of which are discussed in Chapter 1 and all of which are related to one another, arise when applying a categorical model derived from medical concepts of "disease" and "disorder" to the behavioral realm. These are reviewed briefly.

1. *The absence of known causes is the rule.* Apparent developmental difficulties exist in language and communication despite the current absence of documented evidence for a known neurobiological etiology or etiologies, which is most often the case (Leonard, 1998). There is some correlational evidence, based on family studies, that certain patterns of language impairment may be inherited (Crago & Gopnik, 1994; Gilger, 1995; Lahey & Edwards, 1995; Rice, 1999; Rice & Wexler, 1996; Tomblin, 1989). From the perspective of genetic analysis, inheritability may at least contribute to individual differences in children's language patterns (Tomblin & Zhang, 1999). Greater specificity about neurobiological and genetic causes of a language learning disability may emerge as rapid advances in the neurosciences, including genetic analysis, continue. In addition, more longitudinal studies that follow children with a language learning impairment into adulthood are necessary in order to understand individual changes over time.

2. *Category overlap is the rule.* A second problem with categorical models is the reliability of the etiological groupings. A presumption is that categories are homogeneous with respect to the behaviors that characterize each. In practice, as Lahey (1988) points out, causal or precipitating factors typically coexist with one another. For example, a child with autism spectrum disorder invariably has language learning problems. Also, current evidence suggests that a language disability and a "learning disability" are not two separate categories, but interrelated in a majority of children studied longitudinally (Catts, Fey, Zhang, & Tomblin, 1999). Moreover, marked in-

dividual differences exist in child-rearing practices that produce different portraits of language and socioemotional development in children with language learning disabilities. Thus, separating causes of a disability from the effects of differences in socialization experiences is almost an impossible task (Lahey, 1988).

3. *Marked variations in individual language profiles is the rule.* Finally, the difference between a language delay and a language disorder is unclear (Kahmi, 1996) and probably not a useful distinction because of the marked heterogeneity in language profiles. One profile is the "catch-up" pattern, whereby children with spoken language problems during their preschool years appear to be within the normal range of variation by school entry; however, this apparent recovery is illusory (Leonard, 1998). The new cognitive and sociolinguistic demands created by schooling stress children's language systems, with the result that they begin to fail academically.

Locke (1994) proposes a second pattern that is not incompatible with the catch-up profile. Initial language development may not be slow or delayed, but protracted. In other words, a late start means that normal "windows of opportunity" for language learning may be less available unless young children are challenged to use their existing linguistic and communicative resources, for example, through early language intervention. However, a recent research review by the National Academy of Sciences (Shonkoff & Phillips, 2000) on the developing brain suggests caution in assuming that critical, or sensitive, periods of development cap the potential for development. Instead, existing evidence points to the finding that critical periods are the exception, and not the rule, in child development. In effect, "the brain remains open to experiences across broad (pathways) of development" (Shonkoff & Phillips, 2000, p. 216). This means that the developing brain maintains more neural plasticity across childhood and adolescence than previously thought and that the nature and quality of experience continuously affect brain development.

With respect to the effects of neural plasticity on a range of outcomes in language development, studies of children with early unilateral (left hemisphere) lesions due to stroke provide natural evidence for a middle-ground perspective and also challenge the Locke (1994) hypothesis on critical periods (Bates, Vicari, & Trauner, 1999). Depending on such factors as the age of lesion onset and lesion location, many of these children proceed to acquire language functions within the normal range of variation. This suggests that variations exist in the amount of neural plasticity in different brain regions and this degree of plasticity plays a crucial role in how the neural mediation of language changes with development and experience (Bates et al., 1999). A puzzling question is why children with a known etiology—unilateral focal lesions—progress better than children without known cortical etiologies, as is the case with a language learning disability. Two possibilities have been proposed (Elman et al., 1996). One is that diffuse cortical abnormalities are present in the cellular architecture, which would not be detectable by neuroimaging techniques that examine brain structure. A second speculation is that abnormalities exist in subcortical structures, which then block a healthy cortex from playing its normal role in language and cognitive development. In either account the neural organization of children with language learning disabilities may differ from the neural organization of children with unilateral focal lesions.

Systems Models

A third kind of assessment question addresses more directly the connection between assessment and intervention (Lund & Duchan, 1993): "What language intervention plan should we design to help this child?" Systems models most often see this question as the important purpose of assessment.

Because of this concern, systems models of assessment tend to share in common a *multidimensional* or *synergistic* perspective on language and communication (Damico, 1991). That is, "Language exists only as an integrated whole and that communication is *highly* influenced by context, cognitive ability, experience, and learning potential" (Shulman et al., 1995, pp. 53–54). In this view, language components are seen as an integrated system whose components interact with each other and with other cognitive and socioemotional systems, such as attention, memory, and inferencing. With regard to inferencing, focuses may include the social presuppositions underlying reasoning about the motivations and intents of communicative interactions as well as the logical reasoning that characterizes sentence and discourse comprehension.

As a result of this multidimensional view, systems models are oriented to discovering and describing patterns of regularity in an individual child's language performance, using normal aspects of development as a reference. Knowing what a child cannot do (a "deficit" view) must be balanced with learning about a child's potential (an "ability" view), what the child is capable of doing more proficiently in particular situations, including the circumstances that might promote a higher level of competence. Systems models may draw from social interactional theories of language development or from information processing theories, which are often concerned with questions about phonological, lexical, and syntactic processing [for further discussion of these theories and their applications to language disability and language intervention, see Hewitt (2000) and Leonard (1998)].

Systems models do not reject the appropriate use of categorical models of assessment, although deficit models would be considered as more incompatible. The major issue concerns the extent to which causal information illuminates how best to meet individual children's needs. For example, even if it is known that a child's language learning disability may be related to maternal drug use during pregnancy, that information alone provides little guidance for developing an individualized IEP that will be implemented through language intervention.

Summary

The model(s) selected for understanding language and communicative behaviors and their disruption should represent a valid conceptual framework about the process of language development. These same models influence clinical and educational practices. Approaches based on discrete point models, such as the deficit model with its associated discrepancy criteria for identification, as well as certain categorical models, often emphasize the language system as consisting of splinter skills. The outcomes of a splinter skill perspective often translate into learning experiences disconnected from functional communication.

In contrast, approaches grounded to more synergistic and multidimensional perspectives value integrating the real communicative processes of listening, speaking, reading, and writing across the curriculum as strategies for "learning how to learn."

Again, these significant differences in assessment and intervention models mean that speech-language pathologists must continuously assess and reassess their clinical practices in light of changing scientific knowledge about children with a language learning disability. They must also continuously reevaluate how children's complex needs can be best met to achieve a range of goals in the academic, nonacademic, communicative, and social arenas.

Purposes of Assessment

The purposes for assessment influence the nature of the information to be obtained, the methods used to obtain the information, and how that information will be interpreted. There are typically four purposes associated with the assessment of children's language and communicative behaviors.

1. *Identification*—Screen children who may be at risk for or suspected of having a language learning disability.
2. *Evaluation*—Determine through a comprehensive assessment whether a language learning disability is present, the nature of strengths and needs, and if the level of severity meets local eligibility requirements.
3. *Intervention*—Design an appropriate language intervention program that addresses needs recognized through the evaluation.
4. *Functional outcomes*—Systematically document ongoing process resulting from intervention goals and procedures, including the extent to which new learning is functionally related to everyday language, communication, academic, and social goals.

This section focuses on the first three purposes. However, as readers contemplate these four purposes, it is important to keep in mind two points. First, as noted in Chapters 1, 4, and 6, assessment and intervention are not two distinct activities. The authenticity of assessment depends on the degree to which it is linked to learning about what the child is capable of in real communicative contexts, given the support to be successful. All good intervention involves ongoing assessment. Second, regarding the functional outcomes purpose, the IDEA amendments require ongoing monitoring and yearly review of children's progress in the general education curriculum. The information obtained from this process is used to determine whether children in placements other than the general education classroom are ready to begin transitioning into that setting on a full-time basis (Maskel, 1999).

Identification

Under the IDEA, federal law does not specify how identification of children with a possible language learning disability must occur. Moreover, parental consent is not required for screening purposes (McCarthy, Cambron-McCabe, & Thomas, 1998). In general, the purpose of screening is to identify whether a child's spoken language learning, including his or her readiness to learn to read, may be sufficiently different to warrant a comprehensive assessment. Those children who perform below a given acceptable level for their age or grade level are recommended for more comprehensive evaluations.

In many school districts, speech-language pathologists are responsible for conducting these brief evaluations of the spoken language abilities of all kindergarten children served by that district. Screening measures can vary, from formal (norm-referenced) measures to clinician-developed measures to parental and teacher questionnaires (for a review, see McCauley, 2001). At the preschool/kindergarten level, McCauley (2001) reports that referral rates resulting from screening may be unnecessarily high or low depending on the screening procedure being used and the cutoff score applied. A related point is that young children enter kindergarten with wide variations in the scope and depth of their conceptual knowledge, including vocabulary knowledge, their familiarity with the alphabet and its relationship to English sounds, and their planning and organizational skills (Shonkoff & Phillips, 2000; Snow, Burns, & Griffin, 1998). Thus, the sensitivity of screening instruments to these individual differences, regardless of whether the instruments are norm referenced or informal methods, as well as their overall reliability and validity, are important considerations in the selection process (McCauley, 2001; Paul, 1995).

Also, parents or teachers may refer some older school-age children for screening because they begin to encounter obvious difficulties, particularly by grade 3, when language must now be used as a primary way to learn. Furthermore, because language disabilities change over time and may look differently depending on the nature of cognitive, linguistic, social, and academic participation requirements, some students may not experience serious academic problems until they enter middle school or even high school (Bashir & Strominger, 1996; Ehren, 1994; Singer & Bashir, 1999). The following description by George, age 16, captures the organizational and formulation difficulties that emerge when students enter high school.

> With writing and talking, too much information floods my mind at once. I don't know how to present it in a clear way. I especially have a hard time when I lose focus of what I want to say or when I lose my organization. . . . I often only "half bake" an argument (Singer & Bashir, 1999, p. 265).

At this level, the curriculum demands the application of more complex cognitive and linguistic strategies for planning, organizing, and comprehending a wide variety of curricular contents in the spoken and print domains. The expectation is that students are also capable of effectively expressing what they think and know in both the spoken and print arenas.

Evaluation

Regardless of how or when a child or adolescent with a potential language problem is located, the second purpose is to determine whether a language learning disability is present. The IDEA specifies six important requirements in regard to the evaluation process (McCarthy et al., 1998; Osborne, in press).

1. States, and subsequently, local school districts, must establish procedures to make certain that all students with disabilities, including language learning disabilities, are appropriately evaluated.
2. These procedures, including any assessment instruments, must not be culturally, racially, or linguistically biased.

3. Personnel who have been properly trained must administer and interpret assessment instruments.
4. No single criterion or procedure can be used to determine a child's educational placement, which means that multiple sources of information must comprise the process of evaluation.
5. Parents must give consent and participate in all decisions concerning their child's evaluation or educational placement.
6. If the parents disagree with the school district's evaluation, the IDEA provides them with the right to an independent evaluation. However, unless the parents can demonstrate that the school district's evaluation was inappropriate, a school district is not required to pay for an independent assessment. According to court rulings, a school district is obligated to consider recommendations from an independent evaluation, but they do not have to adopt any of these recommendations (Osborne, in press).

The purpose of a comprehensive evaluation should lead to the formulation of specific clinical questions that then guide how the language and communication system will be assessed. Because it is not possible to sample a child's understanding and use of all components of language—its phonology, semantics, syntax, and discourse—and the interactions of these components across multiple situations, the importance of *asking specific and answerable questions* cannot be overestimated. Questions such as "What are the child's comprehension abilities?" or "What is the child's vocabulary knowledge?" are not answerable because they are global questions. On the other hand, questions, such as "What inferencing strategies does the child use to understand familiar versus less familiar stories?" and "What lexical diversity does the child demonstrate in producing spoken versus written narratives?" are answerable. The depth to which these questions can be answered will depend on the requisite knowledge of the speech-language pathologist about how to elicit valid information on inferencing and vocabulary diversity in particular situations and then how to interpret the results.

Based on the chain of evidence gathered during the assessment, the next step is to address two questions. Does the evidence support the conclusion that this child will continue to develop normally in either basic language learning or the use of language to learn? Or does the evidence lead to the conclusion that intervention is required in order to maximize opportunities for further language and academic development? If intervention is indicated, then, under current federal law as well as most state laws, for financial reimbursement purposes the child must qualify for special education services, such as speech-language pathology services, which may or may not be a related service, depending on the particular state. For example, instead of a related service where children are typically "pulled out" of the classroom and seen in small groups, some states define speech-language pathology as a special education area. In this definition, speech-language pathologists can serve as special education teachers in classrooms for children with language learning disabilities. As Osborne (in press) notes, regardless of how services are delivered, their scope, intensity, and duration can be critical for determining whether or not a child receives a free and appropriate education from an Individualized Educational Plan

(IEP). Furthermore, courts have also ruled that, if evaluation procedures are not in compliance with federal or state requirements, then the IEP can be invalidated (Osborne, in press).

If it is determined that a child has a language learning disability even in the absence of a known etiology, it becomes important to assist teachers, parents, and others to understand that this condition is persistent and chronic (Elman et al., 1996; Leonard, 1998). Children do not "catch up" in the sense of being in phase with children of their own age or grade level. In fact, data are now emerging at the postsecondary level, based on two decades of experience with the IDEA and its predecessor, The Education of the Handicapped Act of 1975, on the persistent, although often residual, nature of a language and learning disability (Bashir, Goldhammer, & Bigaj, 2000; Battle, in press).

However, as mentioned earlier, individual profiles change qualitatively over time. The process of change is propelled by interactions between neurobiological and social factors. Neurobiological factors regulate developmental advances in the complexity of neural organization. Social factors concern the interpersonal contexts that constitute experiences in the home, school, and community. The extent to which these interpersonal contexts support the development of resilience and self-esteem then interacts with how the individual manages psychologically the challenges that novel experiences present. For example, if children are continuously faced with failure as competent learners and communicators, to cope with feelings of incompetence, they may learn to "keep a low profile" (the so-called quiet or withdrawn child) (Brinton et al., 2000; Donahue, Symanski, & Flores, 1999; Fujiki et al., 1999). Others may present an aggressive "acting-out" profile when interacting with teachers or peers (Donahue, 1994). In either case the end result may be the Matthew effect (Stanovich, 2000), in which the rich get richer and the poor get poorer. Those with a negative Matthew effect are children with "inadequate vocabularies—who read slowly and without enjoyment—read less and as a result have slower development" (Stanovich, 2000, p. 184), and a reduced motivation to learn that then leads to further cycles of failure. An outcome for many, which can begin as early as grade 4, is emotional disengagement from school and formal dropping out in high school (National Research Council, 1999). Conversely, those who display positive Matthew effects demonstrate achievement early in their school careers, which then allows them to capitalize on their educational experiences because success promotes engagement and the motivation to learn.

Intervention

Once a child is identified as demonstrating a language learning disability, the third purpose of language assessment takes precedence: designing an appropriate language program. Under the 1997 reauthorization of the IDEA and the implementation of the 1999 Part B regulations, educational planning for intervention must extend beyond spoken language needs. Individualized educational planning must continue to consider the most appropriate educational placement, a decision that is intertwined with the least restrictive environment (LRE). However, since 1999, an additional component must be included: the development of an IEP that promotes access to the general education curriculum and incorporates subject-area content.

Because of the emphasis on the general education curriculum, speech-language pathologists now have two new intervention purposes. One involves the integration of content-area learning as a key element of intervention programs (Whitmire, 2000a). The other pertains to the development of collaborative partnerships with general education teachers so that intervention goals are integrated with curriculum goals in the classroom in combination with any necessary modifications that will meet a child's unique needs.

Appropriate Placement and the LRE.   The 1997 reauthorization of the IDEA did not change an important cornerstone of service delivery. The appropriate education and related services necessary for that child to achieve satisfactorily must be ascertained. An issue is that neither the IDEA nor the 1999 federal regulations that implement its provisions provide any further guidance on the meaning of "appropriate." Because programs are supposed to be individualized, an intervention program appropriate for one student may not be appropriate for another student. As reviewed by Osborne (in press), various court decisions have provided the rule of thumb that an educational program must provide the student with a meaningful educational benefit. This is interpreted to mean that a particular placement must reasonably be expected to result in measurable progress toward the goals and objectives specified in the student's IEP.

The IDEA continues to require that every effort be made to keep a child in the least restrictive environment (LRE), which is often interpreted as the general education classroom. In fact, all efforts must be directed initially, including all aids and supports for the teacher and child, toward keeping the child in the general education classroom. It is important to remember that the IDEA prohibits decision making about the LRE based on a student's category of disability (Bateman, 1995). Instead, decision making must proceed on a case-by-case basis. In other words, a child's individual needs should determine the appropriate placement. To illustrate, the fact that a child has a language disability does not mean that the child must be placed in a classroom for children with language disability. Because a classroom for children with language disabilities is more restrictive than a general education classroom, in that situation the overarching priority should be to support the child's eventual inclusion and success in the general education classroom.

Inclusion.   It is now well accepted that the context of instruction exerts strong influences over what a child learns and how learning occurs. In the last fifteen years, the education of children with disabilities has become a focal point of controversy in special education (Kavale & Forness, 2000). Initially, children with disabilities attended separate classes. If a child was deemed "ready," *integration* into a general education elementary or secondary classroom was then attempted for half the school day, with the remainder spent in special services such as a resource room. The term *mainstreaming* was used to describe access into general education classes (Kavale & Forness, 2000; Westling and Fox, 2000), most typically, physical education, art, or music. Often, mainstreaming involved a "sink-or-swim" approach in that additional support or modifications were not necessarily provided to assist mainstreamed children in being successful. Philosophically, the integration/mainstreaming views of education considered the child with disabilities as someone who had to fit into existing instructional practices. If the child had adequate skills to keep up with the rest of the class, then the placement was deemed appropriate. In other words, the child needed to know how to swim before taking swimming lessons.

Recently, the philosophy of *inclusion* has taken center stage. Unlike either integration or mainstreaming, inclusion focuses on the restructuring of schools to accept and provide for the needs of all students. Inclusion emerged from concerns that special education was a segregated education. In a democratic society, specialized instruction and support should be provided to any student who needs assistance, not just those who have special education needs. Although in theory the inclusion philosophy reflected the needs-based model discussed earlier in this chapter, unfortunately, it poses some of the same fiscal challenges for service delivery cited previously. In addition, real inclusion requires significant reform of educational philosophy and school organization, neither of which has proceeded at even a moderate rate of change. It should be noted that the IDEA does not specify inclusion as a placement. Instead, the IDEA specifies that a continuum of services must be provided in accord with a child's needs. Inclusion is one option in the LRE continuum.

Summary

Currently, there is great variability in the interpretation of the LRE and the continuum of services. Educational programs extend from totally self-contained center schools to the full inclusion of all children with disabilities in the general education setting. However, under the IDEA, the decision-making process about the LRE excludes preconceived notions about the disability category serving as the determinant of educational placement. Rather, in utilizing a needs-based model, the assessment purposes for identification, evaluation, and intervention purposes ultimately should be directed to answering two interrelated questions: "What kind of accommodations, adaptations, and strategies are needed to make instruction effective for this child?" and "What situation can best maximize achievement of the child's unique needs?"

In conclusion, simple access to general education classroom experiences, such as offered through mainstreaming, or even the equal opportunity afforded through inclusion, by themselves are insufficient to meet every child's language, literacy, and socioemotional learning needs. The pathway to success for many children with language learning disabilities should be paved with high-quality classroom instruction that offers appropriate supports, including peer support, combined with high expectations for achievement (Allington & Baker, 1999). Collaborative partnerships are a cornerstone of a high-quality inclusive education (Giangreco, 2000). Forging collaborative partnerships where assessment and intervention goals are embedded in high-quality instruction means that prospective speech-language pathologists need to become knowledgeable about and have practical experiences with successful models of collaborative service delivery (Giangreco, 2000; see also Chapter 9). They must also develop knowledge about effective instructional practices for whole-group and small-group learning in the general education classroom (Silliman, Ford, Beasman, & Evans, 1999).

FOCUSES OF ASSESSMENT

Once the major purpose for the language assessment is decided on, the next problem to solve is choosing the language behaviors that will serve as the focus of assessment. Language and communication assessment with school-age children should concentrate on a child's knowledge and uses of language in relation to developmental and educational expectations. Therefore, a starting point for decision making about the focuses of assessment is to consider the educational standards, benchmarks, and academic expectations in place for particular grade levels. Figure 5.1 outlines a decision plan for selecting language-related literacy behaviors to target in assessment. This plan is consistent with the implementation of educational standards and benchmarks that many school systems in the United States have adopted. An important point to reflect on in thinking about standards and benchmarks is that literacy is more than learning to read and write. The twenty-first century is a digital world that thrives on the explosion of information; therefore, it is no longer adequate to think of literacy as just a unitary concept premised on mastering the alphabet. Instead, multiple literacies, such as information literacy, computer literacy, technology literacy, cultural literacy, and media literacy, among others, are challenging traditional concepts of what it means to be literate (Tyner, 1998). All are considered as new expressions of communicative knowledge (Tyner, 1998). Because these multiple literacies are tools for enriching our understanding, and not ends in themselves, the extent to which they will meaningfully enhance what we know and are able to do in this age of information remain speculative (Gardner, 2000).

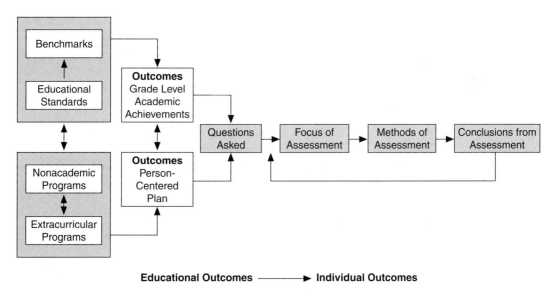

FIGURE 5.1

A Decision Plan for Determining the Focuses of Assessment

A DECISION PLAN FOR DETERMINING THE FOCUSES OF ASSESSMENT

Educational Outcomes

Standards, Benchmarks, and Grade-Level Academic Achievements

Standards-based education is oriented to specific outcomes for all students, including those with disabilities. The 1997 IDEA amendments require that all states include students with disabilities in statewide measures of educational outcomes; however, if students cannot be included in these assessments, with or without appropriate accommodations, then they must be given alternate assessments (Thurlow, House, Scott, & Ysseldyke, 2000; Westling & Fox, 2000). However, considerable inconsistency exists among states about what are acceptable accommodations (Thurlow et al., 2000).

The concept of standards-based education is rooted to a basic belief: "Society must make clear what it expects from schools by setting standards that describe what students should know and be able to do; and schools and school systems must be held accountable for making sure students meet these standards" (Elmore, 1999–2000, p. 6). As of 1999, forty-nine of fifty states employ statewide assessments (Thurlow et al., 2000). As shown in Figure 5.1, states establish **educational standards.** In turn, these content or performance standards become the basis for developing benchmarks. A **benchmark** is a key skill expected to be learned in a particular grade (Westling & Fox, 2000), which is then translated into expected academic achievements. Standards and benchmarks are the components that a state uses to evaluate the *instructional practices* that their schools employ at various grade levels to achieve the anticipated *educational outcomes.*

Tables 5.1 through 5.4 provide illustrations of the Sunshine State Standards developed by the Florida Department of Education (1996). They show how the same language arts standard for the reading process is translated into more complex benchmarks and expectations for achievement at each grade level, from kindergarten through high school. Other language arts standards can be found across grade levels for writing, spoken language comprehension and expression, the forms and functions of language, and knowledge of discourse genres, from narratives to poetry and drama. In addition to the language arts, there are also standards for mathematics, science, social studies, the arts, health, and physical education (Florida Department of Education, 1996). The benchmarks and grade-level expectations for the language arts are also generally consistent with large-scale research evaluations by various National Research Council of the National Academy of Sciences and federally created review panels (Burns, Griffen, & Snow, 1999; National Reading Panel, 2000; National Research Council, 1999; Snow et al., 1998). The evaluations of these groups present a strong consensus on the language and literacy experiences and educational practices that facilitate success in reading, writing, and spelling.

While the language arts examples in Tables 5.1 through 5.4 are based on one state, many states have comparable standards. Because speech-language pathologists must be concerned with children's ability to manage the content areas of the general education curriculum, they should become familiar with the standards, benchmarks,

TABLE 5.1	**Examples of an Educational Standard, Benchmarks, and Grade-Level Expectations in Language Arts—Kindergarten to Grade 2 (Florida Sunshine State Standards)**

Educational Standard: The student uses the reading process efficiently

Benchmark	Kindergarten Expectations	Grade 1 Expectations	Grade 2 Expectations
1. Predicts topic of a passage based on its title and illustrations	• Uses titles and illustrations to make oral predictions	• Uses prior knowledge, illustrations, and text to make predictions	• Uses prior knowledge, illustrations, and text to make and confirm predictions
2. Identifies words and constructs meaning from text, illustrations, graphics, and charts using strategies such as phonological, word structure, and context strategies	• Understands organization of print (locating print on page, identifying parts of a book, etc.); knows letter names (upper and lower case), sounds of letters, rhyming words; identifies words having same initial and final sounds; understands print conveys meaning	• Applies basic elements of phonemic analysis (e.g., segments, blends, substitutes sounds in words); uses sound/symbol relationships and structural cues to decode words (e.g., word order, sentence boundaries); uses context cues to construct meaning (e.g., illustrations, knowledge of story and topic)	• Blends sound components into words; applies knowledge of beginning letters (onset) and spelling patterns (rimes) in single and multisyllabic words as decoding cues; uses variety of structural cues to decode unfamiliar words (e.g., word order, prefixes, suffixes, verb endings); uses variety of context cues to construct meaning (diagrams, titles, headings, etc.)
3. Uses knowledge of appropriate grade, age, and developmental level vocabulary in reading	• Identifies high-frequency words, words that name persons, place, things, and action; identifies and sorts common words from within basic categories (e.g., colors, shapes, foods); uses variety of sources to build vocabulary (e.g., word walls, other people, life experiences); develops vocabulary by discussing characters and events from a story	• Identifies and classifies common words from within basic categories; uses knowledge of individual words in unknown compound words to predict their meaning; uses resources and references to build upon word meanings (e.g., illustrations, knowledge of story and topic, beginning dictionaries, and available technology)	• Identifies simple, multiple-meaning words; uses knowledge of contractions, base words, and compound words to determine word meanings; uses knowledge of prefixes (e.g., *un-, re-, pre-, mis-*) and suffixes (*-er, est-, -ful*) to determine word meaning; develops vocabulary by reading independently, and discussing familiar and conceptually challenging selections

TABLE 5.2   Examples of an Educational Standard, Benchmarks, and Grade-Level Expectations in Language Arts—Grades 3 to 5 (Florida Sunshine State Standards)

Educational Standard: The student uses the reading process efficiently

Benchmark	Grade 3 Expectations	Grade 4 Expectations	Grade 5 Expectations
1. Uses table of contents, index, headings, captions, illustrations, and major words to anticipate or predict content and purpose of a reading selection	• Uses text features to predict content and monitor comprehension (e.g., table of contents, indexes, captions, illustrations, key words, previewing of text); applies knowledge of formats, ideas, plots, and elements from previous reading to generate questions and make predictions about text content	• Uses text features to predict content and monitor comprehension (e.g., glossary, headings, side headings, paragraphs, and print variations, such as italics, boldface, and underline); integrates prior knowledge with text features to generate questions and make predictions about text content	• Extends previously learned prereading knowledge and skills from grade 4 to increasingly complex reading of texts, assignments, and tasks
2. Selects from a variety of simple strategies to identify words and construct meaning from various texts, illustrations, and graphics. Strategies include phonological, word structure, contextual, self-questioning, confirming of predictions, retelling and visual cue strategies	• Uses decoding strategies to clarify pronunciations (e.g., less common vowel patterns, homophones); applies context clues (e.g., known words, phrases, and structures) to infer meaning of new/unfamiliar words, including synonyms, antonyms, and homophones; uses a variety of word structures to construct meaning (e.g., affixes, roots, homonyms, antonyms, synonyms, and word analogies); establishes purpose for reading (e.g., entertainment, skimming for facts, answering a specific question)	• Extends previously learned knowledge and skills from grade 3 to increasingly complex reading selections, assignments, and tasks (e.g., decoding, context clues, prediction, variety of word structures, constructing meaning, reading purposes)	• Extends previously learned knowledge and skills from grade 4 to increasingly complex reading selections, assignments, and tasks (e.g., decoding, context clues, prediction, variety of word structures, constructing meaning, reading purposes)

TABLE 5.3 Examples of an Educational Standard, Benchmarks, and Grade-Level Expectations in Language Arts—Grades 6 to 8 (Florida Sunshine State Standards)

Educational Standard: The student uses the reading process efficiently

Benchmark	Grade 6 Expectations	Grade 7 Expectations	Grade 8 Expectations
1. Applies background knowledge of the subject and text structure to make complex predictions of content, purpose, and organization of the reading selection	• Predicts ideas or events that may take place in the text, gives rationale for predictions, and confirms and discusses predictions as the story progresses; uses prereading strategies before reading (e.g., asks "what do I know" questions or skims text headings, bold type, and other text features); makes predictions about purpose and organization using background knowledge and text structure knowledge; reads and predicts from graphic representations (e.g., illustrations, diagrams, graphs, and maps)	• Extends and applies previously learned prereading knowledge and skills from grade 6 with increasingly complex reading selections, assignments, and tasks	• Extends and applies previously learned prereading knowledge and skills from grade 7 with increasingly complex reading selections, assignments, and tasks
2. Demonstrates consistent and effective use of interpersonal and academic vocabularies in reading, writing, listening, and speaking	• Identifies word parts, such as prefixes, suffixes, and root words; uses word origins as a strategy to understand historical influences in word meaning; analyzes word relationships, such as analogies; distinguishes denotative and connotative word meanings; learns new words in a consistent manner (e.g., through reading and writing activities)	• Extends the vocabulary-building expectations of grade 6 using grade 7 or higher-level vocabulary	• Extends the vocabulary-building expectations of grade 7 using grade 8 or higher-level vocabulary

and grade-level expectations that have been implemented in their own states. This information can serve as a framework for developing specific assessment questions about individual children and the selection of language and literacy behaviors that will serve as the focus of assessment. The rationale for this recommendation is that a review of the grade-level expectations in the four tables makes obvious that language and communication are the basic foundation of all school-based learning because they mediate instructional practices. As Bashir et al. (1998) observe, ". . . if

TABLE 5.4	**Examples of an Educational Standard and Four Benchmarks in Language Arts—Grades 9 to 12 (Florida Sunshine State Standards)**

Educational Standard: The student uses the reading process effectively

Benchmark

1. Selects and uses prereading strategies appropriate to the text, such as discussion, making predictions, brainstorming, generating questions and previewing, to anticipate content, purpose, and organization of a reading selection.

2. Selects and uses strategies to understand words and texts and to make and confirm inferences from what is read, including interpreting diagrams, graphs, and statistical illustrations.

3. Refines vocabulary for interpersonal, academic, and workplace situations, including figurative, idiomatic, and technical meanings.

4. Applies a variety of response strategies, including rereading, note taking, summarizing, outlining, writing a formal report, and relating what is read to his or her own experiences and feelings.

Note: Grade-level expectations in language arts have not yet been developed for grades 9–12.

educational teams are to appreciate the factors that influence the academic success of children with LLDs [language learning disabilities], they need to understand the roles that language and communication serve in the educational process and specifically in classroom contexts" (p. 5).

Person-Centered Planning

Person-Centered Plan.   Figure 5.1 also features the importance of considering communication and language contexts other than the classroom in outcome planning. Children with language learning disabilities often have significant difficulty in appropriately inferring peers' social intent and using language effectively for a wide variety of social interactional purposes, including how to participate in cooperative learning activities (e.g., Brinton et al., 2000; Donahue, in press; Donahue et al., 1999). Without addressing both academic and nonacademic communication demands, children with a language learning disability are often primed for failure when interacting with peers, both at school and later in vocational settings. Lack of acceptance often translates into less than positive roles in community life. [For further detail on assessment procedures in the socioemotional domain, see Prelock (in press).]

Person-centered planning shifts the focus of setting outcomes to include the person with disabilities, his or her family, community, and friends. Although person-centered approaches were developed for children with severe disabilities, the tenets of the planning process can also significantly enhance the quality of planning for children with language learning disabilities. There are many widely used person-center planning tools that can serve as companion tools for academic planning, such as Personal Futures Planning (Mount & Zwernik, 1988), McGill Action Plans (MAPS) (Forest & Lusthaus, 1990), and Planning Alternative Tomorrows with Hope (PATH) (Pearpoint, O'Brien, & Forest, 1993). Person-centered planning becomes especially important as the child reaches mid-adolescence. IDEA 97 requires that an individual transition plan (ITP) be written as part of the IEP by the time a child is 14 years old (Snell & Brown, 2000). The ITP is intended to help transition the student from school to adult life. The role of the speech-language pathologist in this process is often vital to success in both the academic and community settings.

A Case Study.   Consider Brian, an eleventh-grade student, who was recently enrolled in the local high school in the LLD program. At sixteen, Brian had met the academic reading and spelling benchmarks for the fifth grade; the writing benchmarks for third grade; and the math benchmarks for seventh grade. It was anticipated by the school that Brian would not receive a regular high school diploma but would receive a certificate of attendance. Given his multiple language and communication needs and his age, setting priorities for his language intervention was crucial. Personal futures planning became an important part in this prioritizing process. The three main steps involved in the personal futures planning process are as follows.

1. Develop a personal profile that involves gathering key information about the student and his or her capacities. This profile does not typically involve formal assessment but, instead, relies on information about the person's background (health history, experiences, critical events, current situation, family issues, and relationship to the community), quality of life (accomplishments, routines, lifestyle patterns, choices), and activities that are enjoyed and not enjoyed. The person with disabilities is a key part in the whole process and participates as actively as possible in each step.
2. Based on this information, design an action plan for the person that involves identifying desirable images of the future, identifying obstacles and opportunities, and identifying problem-solving strategies that might resolve obstacles and, subsequently, maximize the realization of opportunities.
3. Form a network of support people who commit to ensure the success of the plan (Westling & Fox, 2000).

For Brian, this process revealed a young man who, according to his parents, had received inconsistent reading instruction. They reported that approaches to Brian's reading instruction seemed to change from year to year and from teacher to teacher. Furthermore, they stated that he often seemed to be presented with skills that had previously been learned. His parents added that making and keeping friends was a challenge for him, which they believed was due largely to his language and communication problems. For example, Brian interrupted conversational partners frequently, seldom initiated or sustained eye gaze (a way of conveying interest in one's conversational partner and monitoring their understanding), and often dominated the conversational topics. On the other hand, they saw Brian as a motivated learner who never missed a day of school, always completed his homework, as well as chores at home, such as yard work. Brian stated that his main interests were football, animals, and agriculture. When asked, Brian said he had not made any friends at school but that he wanted to have a close friend. Finally, Brian and his family articulated images of his future that included passing the driver's license test, forming at least one close friendship, and obtaining some work-related experience.

The speech-language pathologist took this information and adjusted her assessment plan to incorporate two focuses: (1) the spoken language and discourse skills that would help Brian cultivate friendships and interview for jobs and (2) the literacy-related skills that would support passing the driver's test and filling out job applications. Brian's teachers similarly incorporated academic achievement outcomes that would support Brian and his family in their future planning. The guidance counselor and the driver's education teacher were enlisted to join the planning team for future meetings.

Summary

Diagnostic planning can no longer be rooted solely in the individual. The speech-language pathologist must now incorporate knowledge about educational benchmarks and the general curriculum, as well as person-centered knowledge, before the actual diagnostic process can begin. As Figure 5.1 outlines, articulation of the diagnostic process with the standards set in the general education environment is essential for the success of individual children in that context. In addition, comprehensive planning must include communicative contexts and abilities outside the classroom. It is often these social communication challenges that reduce the vocational and social opportunities available to individual children as they transition from school to adult life. Thus, an assessment framework should incorporate educational and noneducational outcomes. This type of assessment plan will better ensure that the diagnostic questions asked, the focus of assessment, and the methods of language assessment will be consistent with intervention and instructional practices that mesh educational and community goals.

Individual Outcomes

As shown in Figure 5.1, once the educational milieu is understood, including the expectations for achievement at various grade levels, then specific decisions can be made about the areas of spoken language that should be assessed. These decisions should be made in the context of what is known about the prerequisite language-related abilities that are correlated with successful literacy learning at various ages. One limitation for making these decisions is that more research-based information is available about language–literacy connections for school-age children in kindergarten through grade 3 than for the upper elementary grades, middle school, or high school.

A second constraint for decision making is an imbalance in the areas that have been studied. For example, over the past 15 years, more research resources have been allocated to understanding the process of learning to read, specifically relationships among children's development of phonological sensitivity, mastering the alphabetic principle, and print word recognition (decoding), than to other language domains.

One reason for this imbalance is that the specific spoken language abilities required for learning to read are easier to define than are other abilities, such as those required for reading comprehension (Kamhi & Catts, 1999a, in press).

A third reason previously alluded to also qualifies decision making about the focuses of assessment. Little is known on how variations in instructional practices at the classroom level affect the individual language and learning profiles that children present. For example, the reading instruction provided to poor readers, like the case of Brian in the last section, may be less than optimal, which then creates another kind of Matthew effect. Less skilled learners often receive less meaningful and challenging instructional experiences and, as a consequence, learning to read is further inhibited (National Reading Panel, 2000; Stanovich, 2000). Another consequence of inadequate instruction may be that more advanced language learning is suppressed. If reading and writing are not accessible skills, then the acquisition of new language knowledge is also markedly suppressed.

Focus of Assessment

Three components of the spoken language system should be considered as focuses for assessment because of their association with learning to read, write, and spell. These are (1) phonological sensitivity, (2) lexical diversity, which is related to morphological sensitivity, and (3) syntactic diversity, including morphosyntactic sensitivity. The term "association" as used here means that statistical correlations from a variety of studies predict possible relationships, which may range from strong to weak, but that these relationship should not yet be interpreted as causal. The reason for caution in interpretation is due to three factors. First, different studies are conducted with different populations and different methods. A few studies may be longitudinal; most investigate children's knowledge at one point in time rather than over time. Thus, results across studies cannot always be easily compared. Second, predictor abilities change. Based on longitudinal studies, different sets of language-related variables predict reading outcomes at different ages (Scarborough, in press). Third, once children enter school, the nature of their instruction in reading, writing, and spelling influences their language-related knowledge, which, in turn, affects what they know about these literacy processes. If children with language learning disabilities do not have sufficient experiences and instruction with reading, writing, and spelling in meaningful literacy activities, then they will not advance their language skills (Scott, in press). Therefore, "causality" is not a unidirectional phenomenon by which the language disability causes the problems with literacy learning as a consequence. Instead, consistent with negative and positive Matthew effects, the relationship is a reciprocal, or bi-directional, one for which it is difficult to disentangle causes from consequences (Catts & Kamhi, 1999).

Phonological Sensitivity

Overview.   The basic phonological system is predicated on the existence of a phonological code that allows speech to be produced. This basic system is first used in a primarily automatic way to formulate and execute speech. Phonemes are the smallest relevant sound units in any language, because they signal meaning differences among words. A change in a phoneme creates a different word. For example, the words *bat, fat, cat, mat,* and *sat* differ only in the first sound, and yet they all mean something different because /b/, /f/, /k/, /m/, and /s/ are different phonemes in English. Most children achieve adult speech production no later than age 7 years (Hodson, 1994).

There is a difference, however, between holistic use of phonemic structure to produce intelligible speech and the ability to analyze more consciously segments of that structure for a new purpose, to recognize and spell printed words. This requires that the child shift from a holistic orientation to an analytical orientation toward sound segments, a development that it is not all or none, but gradual, beginning in very early childhood. The task confronting the child is made all the more difficult because nothing exists in alphabetic information that signals to the child the specific linguistic units that print symbolizes (Blachman, 1994). Because phonemes are abstract categories (unlike syllables, phonemes have no acoustic correlates in the speech stream), correspondences must be inferred between phonemic structure and their alphabetic counterparts.

Phonological sensitivity refers to the more formal conscious, or "metalinguistic," awareness that the sound structure of spoken language can be manipulated (Lonigan, Burgess, & Anthony, 2000). This sensitivity is an important aspect of emerging literacy because "Getting started in alphabetic reading depends critically on mapping the letters and spellings of words into the speech units that they represent; failure to master word recognition can impede text comprehension" (Snow et al., 1998, p. 6). Word recognition, decoding, and word identification are often interchangeable terms.

Asking Relevant Questions about Ryan's Phonological Sensitivity.   When basic alphabetic reading and spelling skill has not been attained, the consequences can be devastating. Figure 5.2 depicts Ryan's descriptive narrative writing (and spelling) sample on "My Favorite Hobby." Ryan is a 14-year-old male who has been in a self-contained class for specific learning disabilities for six years. He also has received

FIGURE 5.2

Ryan, Age 14—"My Favorite Hobby"

*Note: All spellings, punctuation, and spacing are preserved.

> My favoritehobb is a
> bisigll it is red nad god nad ithos
> a lit unrbu bisill it has rims it has
> hibrollix I like my bisigll I
> ribib   breba it is fun ribib my bisigll I klintt
>   ureba
> wen I my it hom. I go
> to the mobes I lak my
> bisigll up I bo trix wit my bisix

speech-language services as a resource service for six years. Given the problems evident in his written narrative, a strong case can be made that neither Ryan's language nor literacy needs have been appropriately identified. There are three overlapping components of phonological sensitivity, all of which are applicable to Ryan either singly, or most likely, in combination.

1. *Phonological awareness.* Phonological awareness is a concept that indexes phonological sensitivity about the segmental (phonemic) properties of words (Gottardo, Stanovich, & Siegel, 1996). Five findings are pertinent.

   (a) This type of phonological sensitivity originates as a spoken language skill that, eventually, is transformed in a manner that allows children to analyze and manipulate the phonemic structure of words more consciously (Torgesen & Wagner, 1998), for example, by segmenting words into phonemes or blending phonemes to produce real words. Ryan has never been assessed for his segmental understanding of phoneme structure. A specific question to ask would be whether he has achieved this basic understanding, as well as the degree of his letter-recognition ability.

   (b) As strategies, phoneme segmentation assists students to generate more complex spellings, while blending supports the decoding of words (National Reading Panel, 2000). Ryan cannot yet decode or spell high-frequency words easily, effortlessly, or automatically; instead, as he has been taught, he relies on context clues, which is not a helpful strategy given his conceptual struggles with phoneme–grapheme correspondences.

   (c) A large number of studies have consistently found that children's level of phonological awareness at kindergarten is highly predictive of who will be a good reader and who will be a poor reader at grade 3 (for reviews, see Catts & Kamhi, 1999; Kamhi & Catts, in press; Keogh, in press; Snow et al., 1998). Information on Ryan's abilities in the lower elementary grades is unavailable; however, at age 14 years, he has yet to achieve grade 1 expectations for reading achievement, much less middle school expectations (see Tables 5.1 and 5.3).

   (d) Reading and spelling are both language-based skills (Kamhi & Catts, in press; Kamhi & Hinton, 2000). Decoding ability depends on phonological and lexical knowledge, whereas spelling ability depends on phonological, orthographic, and morphological knowledge. The contributions of phonological awareness to word recognition are also highly correlated with children's initial abilities to produce accurate spellings (Ehri, 2000; Nunes, Bryant, & Bindman, 1997; Treiman & Bourassa, 2000), a finding that holds for Ryan. Good readers are also good spellers, although the reverse does not always hold true (Kamhi & Hinton, 2000).

   (e) The specific role of phonological awareness as a factor in the spelling problems that are encountered in writing by children with language learning disabilities has not been well studied (Berninger, 2000). One speculation is that the very complexity of the writing process may cause children to attend less to spelling (Windsor, Scott, & Street, 2000). With regard to Ryan, this speculation might be addressed by assessing his ability to spell high-frequency words, such as *and, when,* and *do,* when not also engaged in writing a narrative [see Scott (2000) for assessment procedures].

2. *Phonological memory.* In the print domain, phonological memory refers to the conversion process by which orthographic information (letters and letter patterns) are recoded and temporarily stored in working memory for translation into phonological representations (Tunmer & Chapman, 1998). In other words, the word-recognition processes that are part of phonological memory transform print (orthographic representations) into words (phonological representations) for decoding and in a similar manner convert words into print, for example, for spelling (Ehri, 2000).

   (a) Phonological memory codes also serve as a process for storing linguistic information in long-term memory (Catts & Kamhi, 1999). Impaired phonological memory, or the inability to convert letters and letter patterns rapidly into their corresponding phonological representations, makes it difficult to perform phonemic blending (Torgesen & Wagner, 1998). Whether Ryan can perform blending tasks has not been asked.

   (b) Conversely, when children cannot easily transform phoneme sequences into the letter sequences that comprise spellings, their memory for spellings is compromised (Ehri, 2000). Figure 5.2 suggests that this may be the situation for Ryan. It might be that his many, although inconsistent, letter reversals, such as *nad* for *and, b* for *d* in *hydraulics* ("hibrollix"), *do* ("bo"), and *riding* ("ribib"), originate in orthographic problems involving memory for correct letter sequences. Children who have mastered sound–symbol correspondences should have a richer memory for spellings (Catts & Kamhi, 1999). Ryan's letter reversals may be one more indicator of insufficient phonological awareness being attained.

3. *Phonological retrieval.* Phonological retrieval is the ability to recall easily phonological information that is stored in long-term memory (Catts & Kamhi, 1999).

   (a) This ability is commonly assessed by timed serial naming tasks, either printed letters, digits, colors, objects, or nonwords. The rationale is that "Theoretically, rapid-naming tasks are linked to reading because they are thought to index the speed of processes that are intrinsically related to the cognitive activities involved in word identification" (Torgesen & Wagner, 1998, p. 223). Ryan's ability to retrieve items rapidly has not been assessed; thus the possible contributions of retrieval breakdowns to his present status might be formulated as a specific question to pursue through assessment.

   (b) The reading and spelling problems of some children like Ryan may be related to problems with not rapidly accessing phonological information. It should be noted that the strength of the evidence to support this possibility is less than exists for the influences of phonological awareness and phonological memory (Catts & Kamhi, 1999).

Summary.   The three components of phonological sensitivity reflect the new ways in which the functions of phonological representations must be shifted from everyday listening and speaking to the translation of alphabetic information into meaning if children are to learn to read, write, and spell. The ultimate goal of reading is comprehension. In middle school and high school, problems with reading comprehension explain most of the variation in reading ability (Swank & Catts, 1994). A history of struggle with word recognition, such as Ryan shows, leads to significant problems with reading comprehension. Therefore, the integrity of phonological representations may be a primary factor accounting for why students like Ryan do not develop the phonological sensitivity necessary for rapid and effective uses of phonological recoding, awareness, and retrieval processes, and, thus, continue to have serious problems with reading comprehension. A major controversy, however, is whether this "phonological core deficit hypothesis" is sufficient to explain the reading and spelling problems of students with language learning disabilities like Ryan, or whether other language-related abilities, to be mentioned shortly, must also be considered.

A final point concerns the child who may have a "speech problem." Although the data are conflicting (Hodson, 1994), evidence suggests that, as a group, children whose sole problem is less accurate production of certain phonemes but whose speech is *intelligible* do not encounter problems in learning to read, write, and spell (Catts, 1991, 1993; Catts, Hu, Larrivee, & Swank, 1994). However, severe to profound intelligibility problems, referred to as an *expressive phonological disorder* (Hodson, 1994), may reflect underlying disruptions in the representation and use of the phonological code and affect proficiency in decoding and spelling (Clark-Klein & Hodson, 1995; Larrivee & Catts, 1999). These children should receive as early assessment as possible. On the other hand, many children who have significant problems with the full development of phonological sensitivity do not have any disruptions in their basic phonological system as used for speech production.

Lexical Diversity and Morphological Sensitivity

Overview.   Words are phonological structures; they consist of phonemes: "If we have perceived or produced a word, whether in speech or in reading, we have in fact engaged a phonological structure" (Liberman & Shankweiler, 1991, p. 5). Thus, our mental lexicon, where vocabulary meanings are stored, consists of both lexical and phonological information. The ability to read less familiar words and to employ effective strategies for reading comprehension are both strongly correlated with a rich network of vocabulary meanings (Kamhi & Catts, 1999b; Nagy & Scott, 2000; National Reading Panel, 2000; Stanovich, 2000). The important point is that children who have problems with phonological sensitivity very likely will also have less diverse vocabularies and, as a result, will be poorer readers, writers, and spellers. This interaction among the phonological and lexical components is but one illustration of the synergy that characterizes the linguistic and communicative systems.

Education promotes a *literate lexicon,* the use of words that are more common to the language of instruction and formal writing (Nippold, 1998). Because of the influence of reading, writing, and spelling, the rate of vocabulary growth increases dramatically during the school-age years. It is estimated that from grade 1 to grade 3, vocabulary size on average increases by 9,000 words, and from grades 3 to 5 by

20,000 words (Anglin, 1993). Although reading skill and vocabulary diversity are related, again, specific causal connections have not been demonstrated with regard to how direct instruction in vocabulary improves reading comprehension (National Reading Panel, 2000). Furthermore, estimates of vocabulary diversity depend on what is meant by "knowing a word." At least three types of knowledge affect the diversity of new-word learning (Nagy & Scott, 2000).

1. Knowing a word is a matter of degree, from highly familiar to "have heard it, but aren't really sure what it means."
2. Words often have multiple meanings, and their complexity can increase with figurative language demands (Nippold, 1998; Milosky, 1994). In the classroom, figurative expressions are a common device for making a point (e.g., "Let's not put the cart before the horse").
3. Individual word learning is always interrelated with other word meanings and does not occur in isolation. For example, familiarity with "hot," "cold," and "cool" means that some understanding of "warm" exists even if that word has not been encountered (Nagy & Scott, 2000).

Asking Relevant Questions about Ryan's Morphological Sensitivity in His Lexical Development.   Morphology generally refers to the linguistic process by which words are formed and related to one another. Sensitivity to these morphological relations is believed to further skill in word-level reading and spelling because it supports children's learning of new word meanings (Snow et al., 1998). A review of the benchmarks and grade-level expectations outlined in Table 5.2 for grades 3 to 5 provides practical evidence for the influence of morphological sensitivity in more advanced lexical development. Beginning in grade 3, children are expected to begin applying their knowledge of word-formation processes as linguistic strategies for inferring the meaning of new or less familiar words. By grade 6 (see Table 5.3), they are expected to be "word detectives" who can use their concepts of word parts to derive new meanings in a consistent manner through reading and writing.

Two types of morphology contribute to new word learning: inflectional morphology and derivational morphology. **Inflectional morphology** extends word meaning, for example, through tense and plural inflectional markers, but does not transform it into a new word (Hoff, 2001). For example, inflectional morphemes, such as the plural -*s*, can be added to words after derivational morphemes, but not the reverse; hence people who "zib" for a living are "zib*bers*" and not "zib*ser*" (Hoff, 2001, p. 192), where the suffix -*er* follows the plural -*s*.

However, knowledge of derivational morphology is key for advancing vocabulary knowledge in grades 3 to 5 and beyond, although, as just mentioned, particular causal connections have not been identified. **Derivational morphology** involves prefixes (-*un, bi-, trans-, re-*), suffixes (-*ly, -er, -ful, -ment*), compounded words (*baseball, hotdog, blackberry*), and combining forms, such as *micro-, photo-, -ology,* and -*itis* (Moats, 2000, p. 75). During reading, how might children use their knowledge of derivational morphology to problem-solve an unfamiliar word? Consider whether each of the three sets of words below comes from (are derived from) the same root word (Anglin, 1993):

- *Bash/bashful.* In this set, the words are phonetically similar (they share similarity in the form of their pronunciation), but they are semantically unrelated.
- *Cat/kitten.* This pair is semantically identical, but only phonetically similar.
- *Teach/teacher.* This pair is related phonetically, semantically, and morphologically because of the *-er* derivational form (suffix).

In guessing words from context, younger elementary-age children might use either a semantic similarity strategy (*cat/kitten*), which would lead to a correct judgment, or a phonetic similarity strategy, for example, sounding-out *bashful,* which might not lead to a correct outcome. The ability to apply derivational strategies for new word meanings is gradually acquired throughout the school years (Anglin, 1993; Windsor, 1994). The use of linguistic context for this purpose requires some degree of morphological sensitivity (Nagy & Scott, 2000).

The application of derivational strategies is also essential for being a good speller (Bear, Invernizzi, Templeton, & Johnston, 2000; Snow et al., 1998; Templeton & Morris, 2000). Spelling skill includes the understanding of words that are *semantically transparent* (Nagy & Scott, 2000) or root forms of words that are predictably related in their spelling and meaning but that require comparison of subtle phonetic variations to form a new word. Examples are (Bear et al., 2000, p. 252)

- *Confide/confidence.* Vowel alteration pattern; the vowel in the second syllable of *confide* becomes a schwa (unstressed) in *confidence.*
- *Critic/criticize.* Consonant alteration pattern; pronunciation shifts from /k/ in *critic* to /s/ in *criticize.* Thus, the student who spells *confident* as (confadent) or *criticize* as "critisiz" is capable of thinking about how the orthographic representation remains constant despite alterations in pronunciation (Templeton & Morris, 2000).

To return to Figure 5.2, Ryan's writing sample, readers can discern some information about his basic knowledge of inflectional morphology as applied to writing. He demonstrates appropriate use of relatively simple subject–verb agreement involving the copula verb *is* (My favoritehobb[y] is a bisigll [bicycle]), other auxiliary verbs (ithos[has] a lit[light], it has rims), and, to a lesser extent, plurals (I go to the mobes [movies]), I bo [do] trix [tricks] wit [with] my bisix [bicycle]). There is no evidence of a derivational strategy in this sample, which lacks lexical diversity in general. An important question to ask about Ryan's lexical knowledge base at age 14 years is his level of morphological sensitivity. For example, if given a root word, such as *oppose,* and a linguistic context such as "The New York Yankees always beat their _____," can Ryan readily apply derivational strategies in the spoken realm, as well as in spelling? Is there a gap between his use of spoken language derivational strategies and what he is able to demonstrate in spelling? Asking such questions about what Ryan can do appears important for further understanding his strengths and needs. [For types of morphological assessment tasks, see Carlisle (1987) and Moats (2000).]

Summary.   The various components of phonological sensitivity govern children's ability to transform letter sequences into their phonemic counterparts and constitute the conceptual discovery of the alphabetic principle (Snow et al., 1998). This break-through then opens new doors for lexical acquisition that are afforded through reading, writing, and spelling. The role of morphological sensitivity in advancing word recognition and spelling skills, specifically, the relevance of derivational relationships, has been an overlooked area of instructional practice (Moats, 2000). Students like Ryan, if they are to progress in achieving benchmarks through the development of explicit and systematic approaches to vocabulary learning, require assessment of their level of morphological sensitivity beginning in the lower primary grades.

Syntactic Diversity and Morphosyntactic Sensitivity

Depending on the particular definition, the term "grammar" may actually subsume several levels of language form, its phonology, syntax, and morphology, referred to in the previous section, or may refer only to the syntactic component. The ability to process syntactic relationships easily brings the child beyond decoding to the level of reading comprehension (Scarborough, in press; Westby, in press). For example, the benchmarks in Tables 5.2 and 5.3 for grades 3 to 8 implicate the importance of increasingly sophisticated syntactic strategies for the construction of meaning from text. However, only a small amount of research has directly addressed the role of either syntactic comprehension or production as a primary risk factor in the failure to become a proficient reader or writer. One reason may be the difficulty of separating in real-life use the syntactic level of organization from the morphological, lexical, and discourse levels of organization. A second reason might be due to the fact that different disciplines have been interested in different questions. For example, researchers in the communication sciences and disorders have focused primarily on defining the nature of spoken language impairment, without examining possible connections to reading or writing abilities. In comparison, researchers in reading disabilities have been concerned primarily with refining the contributions of phonological awareness, phonological memory, and phonological retrieval to reading failure and have not attended to other spoken language abilities, such as the lexical and syntactic domains, to the same extent (Scarborough, in press). Because the syntactic area is an important focus area of assessment in both speaking and writing, it is also an area central to any assessment plan.

Overview: Basic and Later-Developing Syntax. As noted in Chapter 2, starting around age 18 to 24 months and continuing throughout the preschool and school-age years, English speaking children acquire a basic knowledge of three interrelated aspects of syntax.

- The first aspect is clause structure. The basic unit of early spoken syntax is the clause. All clauses contain at a minimum a subject and a verb phrase, although the subject may be omitted in imperative sentences (e.g., "See the doggie."). In other words, a main clause always contains a verb or verb phrase, and the type of clause depends on the nature of the verb.
- The second critical area pertains to underlying grammatical representations for tense and agreement in finite and nonfinite clauses. In English, finite clauses are those clauses in which it is *obligatory* for the verb to have inflectional morpho-

logical markers that specify past tense and third-person subject agreement for regular forms. For example, in "The cow jump*ed* over the moon," the *-ed* form may be pronounced as *-t* ["jumped"] or *-d* ["played"]. Nonfinite clauses, in comparison, do not have obligatory requirements for tense and agreement, e.g., "The cow is go*ing* home" or "The cow was go*ing* home." In this last situation, the *-ing* inflectional marker does not index tense, but aspect, which refers to whether an activity is completed or ongoing. Participles, such as *-ing,* denote the progressive aspect, whereas *-n* forms, as in "The cow has gone home," specify the perfect aspect or completion of activity (Radford, Atkinson, Britain, Clahsen, & Spencer, 1999). This aspect of development is often referred to as the *morphosyntactic component,* because of the interface between inflectional morphology and syntax (Rice, Wexler, Marquis, & Hershberger, 2000).

- The third area concerns the emergence and consolidation of basic high-frequency syntactic devices for coordination and subordination, which then allow the formation of interclausal structures. Beginning around age 24 months and continuing through adolescence, children begin to acquire increasingly sophisticated syntactic devices for producing interclausal structures that advance the complexity and flexibility of expression. The diversity of these interclausal structures expand noun-phrase information through coordination and combine and condense clausal information through subordination, as seen in Table 5.5, for example, through the embedding of nominal, adverbial, and relative clauses. Thus, in developing a repertoire of high-frequency interclausal structures, the child can use a syntactic code that is best designed to meet the rapid temporal processing demands of face-to-face communication (Scott, 1995). However, these high-frequency structures tend to be "used with a restricted range of meaning and intention as well as structural flexibility" (Scott, 1988a, p. 50).

Contrasted with the high-frequency structures of spoken language, the syntactic structures of writing, particularly for expository texts, tend to be more low frequency. Low-frequency syntactic constructions are those more characteristic of a literate communication style in both writing and speaking. These advanced "low-frequency" structures contribute to syntactic diversity and slowly emerge during the school-age years. Writing may be a major catalyst for advancing syntactic diversity for at least four reasons.

- First, recall that the basic grammatical unit of speaking is the clause, not the sentence. The grammatical concept of "sentence" may actually develop through the nature and scope of writing experiences in the lower elementary grades, which then influences the development of syntactic diversity (Scott, 1995, 1999). In other words, spoken language experiences may be a less effective approach for teaching students with a language learning disability, like Brian and Ryan, about syntactic units because the primary unit of spoken language are clause units linked together via coordinates and simple subordinates.
- Second, when children start to master the notion of sentence, their writing productivity increases as assessed through sentence length at the level of noun and verb phrases (Scott & Windsor, 2000). For example, children formulate (1) more

TABLE 5.5	Spoken Interclausal Structures: High-Frequency Syntactic Devices for Coordination and Subordination	
Clause Type	**Example**	**Emerging Complexity**
Coordination		
1. Additive (simultaneous) and temporal (sequential) conjoining of events (Lahey, 1988)		Well-developed by age 2½ years; most common coordinate across childhood particularly in narrative discourse and with the subject repeated (Scott, 1988a; Lahey, 1988)
(a) Sentential *and* with same verb in both clauses	He drinks milk *and* he drinks it with a straw (simultaneous event order)	
(b) Sentential *and* with different verbs in both clauses	He drinks milk *and then* he eats the cupcake (sequential event order)	
(c) Phrasal (co-referential) *and*; subject of second clause deleted	He drinks milk *and then* eats the cupcake (sequential event order)	
2. Causal, adversative, comparative (see also adverbial clauses)	I'm gonna wet my hair *and* get it tangled up (causal) My hair got tangled up *because* I wet it (causal) I wanted to wet my hair *so* it would get tangled (causal), *but* I didn't do it (adversative) I wanted to get my hair wet *like* mommy (comparative)	Because, *so, but, like* uncommon before late preschool years (Lahey, 1988); occur less frequently than *and* in oral narrative through adolescence (Scott, 1988a)

complex and elaborated noun phrase constructions ("*The flaming red sun* sank into *the brilliantly illuminated horizon*"), (2) series constructions ("*The Internet offers many opportunities for shopping, such as computers, clothes, jewelry.* . . . "), and (3) verb-phrase expansions that include auxiliaries and modals (e.g., "Benton High School *had received* many new books for their library; He wished that he *could have* been smarter.") (Scott, 1995).

- Third, discovery of the grammatical concept of sentence allows children to employ more sophisticated coordinates to link independent clauses ("He lost his

Clause Type	Example	Emerging Complexity
Subordination		
1. Nominal clauses (typically, infinitive as complement in object position)	He's trying *to make a sandwich* Mary didn't want *to cry*.	Earliest subordinated form to emerge (27 to 30 months) (Tyack & Gottsleben, 1986; Wells, 1985). Object position frequent complement position because is easiest to mark new information in what is last said (Scott, 1988b)
2. Adverbial clauses (time and reason as complements in object position)	You can go *when* I do. (time) They went home *because* they were mad. (reason)	*Because* and *when* most frequent adverbial clauses in object position in the everyday and narrative discourse of preschool children (Scott, 1988a)
3. Relative clauses (as complements in object position; includes *what, who, which,* and *that* as relative pronouns in *wh-* and *that* clauses)	Do you know *what* I know? The boy didn't know *who* owned the dog. Harry could always figure out *which* answer was correct.	*Wh-* clauses emerge about age 4 years (Hoff, 2001; Wells, 1985), but *that* clauses not frequent in preschool years (Tager-Flusberg, 2001; Tyack & Gottsleben, 1986); both *wh-* and *that* clauses appear more often at ages 8 to 10 years in narratives (Strong, 1998), but marked or unmarked *that* still preferred over *wh-* at ages 6 to 10 years.
	And the end of the story is [*that*] My-My and Rosie went west (unmarked for *that*, but is co-referential with the main clause *And the end is*) (Romaine, 1984, p. 85) There's lot's of people *that* got hurt (*that* preferred to *who* to mark interclausal relations) Do you think *that* I can go? (marked)	

wallet and, *therefore,* could not buy dinner.") and subordinating coordinates to connect dependent clauses ("*Although* he lost his wallet, he still managed to buy dinner.") (Westby & Clauser, 1999).

- Finally, around age 10 years, with sufficient experience, writing tends to become increasingly differentiated from speaking and, at the same time, becomes progressively more subordinated than spoken language (Scott, 1988b, 1999), as assessed by the terminable unit (T-unit) or communication unit (C-unit), which are measures for assessing clausal density. For example, children's syntactic repertoire becomes more diverse when they can increase clausal density through utilizing such devices as (1) adverbial clauses of condition (*"When the ghost knows about you,* he will haunt you."); (2) center-embedded relative clauses ("The other frog *[that] he had* was older.") (Strong, 1998, p. 47); (3) adverbial clauses with nonfinite verbs (*"Having seen the house,* she decided not to buy it."); and (4) nominal clauses shifted from object to subject position (*"What bothered President Lincoln* was the long duration of the war.") (Scott, 1988b; Scott & Stokes, 1995).

Asking Relevant Questions about Jay's Basic Syntactic Ability.   As the benchmarks and grade-level expectations for grade 1 and beyond document (see Tables 5.1 to 5.4), proficient reading requires morphosyntactic sensitivity or awareness. This involves "Being able to talk about language, pull its units apart and put them back together, compare and contrast words, [and] reorganize paragraphs and topic sentences" (Wallach & Butler, 1994, p. 8). To meet literacy expectations, children must be able to think and talk about grammatical units, such as words, clauses, and sentences, in explicit ways. Children who have not yet mastered critical aspects of inflectional morphology, therefore, may be at significant risk in learning to read, write, and spell (Scarborough, 1998).

Consider the following description of Jay, now 5 years old and enrolled in a longitudinal study of children with language impairment (Jay has been receiving language intervention since age 3 years) (Rice, 1999):

> The initial round of testing determined that Jay's [inflectional] morphological development showed a profile that proved to be characteristic of other children in the affected [language impairment] group. Some grammatical rules were evident, whereas others were not. On the unaffected side were rules governing plurals, the verbal inflection, *-ing* (author's italics), and prepositions. Jay said these sentences clearly: (1) Those guys got sore legs"; (2) "That baby's taking a nap"; and (3) "The babies sleep in this bed." . . . In these ways, Jay's grammar was very similar to that of unaffected, typically developing children. In other ways, Jay's grammar was very different from that of his age peers. This was evident in utterances involving grammatical tense marking, [for example], (4) "This thing drop"; (5) "Dad sleep here"; (6) Her fine"; and (7) "He going to fall". . . . His reading readiness skills are limited, and he subsequently encounters difficulty with the transition to reading (pp. 331–332).

Is Jay's variability in the use of grammar due to the fact that he does not understand tense? Recent evidence suggests otherwise. By drawing on recent research in spoken syntactic development, the speech-language pathologist may ask the answerable question of whether Jay's profile is consistent with a distinctive clinical marker of spoken language impairment. This diagnostic marker involves verb morphology, specifically, a selective impairment in the syntactic contexts in which finiteness marking of verb tense is mandatory (Leonard, 1998; Rice, 1999). *Mandatory* means that the inclusion of the inflections for tense and agreement is obligatory in Standard American English finite clauses in order for an utterance to be grammatically acceptable.

One explanation of the variability in Jay's production of the inflectional morphemes that index tense and agreement is *morphosyntactic* (Rice, 1999; Rice, Cleave, & Oetting, 2000). Finite morphosyntactic clausal contexts include:

- *-s* with third-person singular present-tense subjects ("Michael walk*s*")
- *-ed* to specify past tense regardless of subject–verb agreement ("Michael and Paul walk*ed* home")
- *Be* forms as auxiliary verbs (*is, am, were, was, were,*) where tense and subject–verb agreement are necessary ("Michael *is* walking home"; "Michael and Paul *were* walking home")
- *Do* forms (do, does, did), where tense and agreement are also obligatory ("Michael *does* often walk home"; "Michael and Paul *did* often walk home").

Longitudinal data (Rice et al., 2000) show that error patterns with basic past-tense marking of regular finite verbs (e.g., *brush, kick, pick, play*) continue through age eight for many children. This suggests an incompleteness of underlying syntactic representations for children like Jay.

An alternative explanation of Jay's grammatical problems is attributed to *morphophonological* representations (Leonard, 1998). Morphophonology is the interface between phonology and morphology. The morphophonological account would attribute Jay's "bare stem marking" (zero marking) of finite verb relations as due to the lower phonetic prominence (less duration and stress) of the *-ed/-s* affixes, including the *-t* and *-d* allophonic variations of *-ed*, in spoken language processing. This surface phonology explanation suggests that weaker representations exist for this class of inflectional morphemes due to a history of "incomplete processing" (Leonard, 1998, p. 252), particularly when spoken language processing demands increase. A result is protracted acquisition of morphophonological patterns for tense and agreement in finite clauses. According to Rice et al. (2000), most research in this area has adopted the morphophonological perspective, e.g., "How do children learn the phonological properties of past tense?" (p. 1130). The morphosyntactic account, on the other hand, argues that the marking of finiteness is an obligatory syntactic principle that applies in spite of variations in the surface phonology (Rice, 1999; Rice et al., 2000).

Regardless of whether the morphosyntactic or morphophonological account is ultimately validated, it seems safe to assume that chronic problems with finite morphosyntactic contexts and related semantic/syntactic cues interact to affect new spoken word learning (Rice et al., 2000). These same problems may also influence the lexical learning of students like Jay, whose problems with morphosyntactic sensitivity become obvious when they must depend on more advanced derivational morphology strategies for learning to read and spell.

Asking Relevant Questions about the Syntactic Diversity of Ryan's Writing.   Most state assessments include the evaluation of children's ability to write. For example, by grade 4 it is expected that students are capable of writing, "for public and private purposes in a variety of literary forms, including poems, stories, reports, and personal narratives. They write to persuade, using order of importance and classifying . . . advantages and disadvantages. They use writing according to purpose and intended audiences" (Center for Research on Evaluation, Standards, and Student Testing, 1998, p. 31). The sample of Ryan's writing about his favorite hobby (see Figure 5.2) serves as a metaphor for many students who, at age 14, still cannot write in a manner that would even begin to meet grade 4 standards. The important question to ask is what sources of difficulty might account for this outcome.

A starting point to address this question as a focus of assessment is to under-stand writing as a process that integrates the metacognitive and metalinguistic spheres. Much of everyday speaking is less planned. From a metacognitive per-spective, writing requires more advance planning and self-regulation than everyday speaking (Graham, Harris, & Troia, 2000; Westby & Clauser, 1999). The need to plan ahead more explicitly in order to manage composing strategies may push chil-dren to attend to such syntactic units as the sentence because written language is more consistent, with a complex linguistic code (Scott, 1995). The issue is that many chil-dren with a language learning disability continue to "write like talk" rather than "write like books" (Silliman & Wallach, 1991, in Wallach & Butler, 1994, p. 9), even as adolescents, regardless of whether this more oral style is appropriate for the in-tended communicative purpose and audience. For example, Ryan's written descrip-tion of his favorite hobby has this "write like talk" quality, most likely because he does not have available effective strategies for self-regulation, planning, and com-posing that would support his learning to write in a more literate way (Graham & Harris, 1999).

A second question to be answered relates to the metalinguistic domain. Until re-cently, there has been little formal study of the writing approaches of children with language learning disabilities. One promising avenue is to compare the genre of pro-duction (narrative versus expository) and the modality of production (speaking ver-sus writing) in the same children, assuming that they have developed some level of writing skill. Recent studies have begun to investigate the spoken/written syntactic complexity of narrative and expository summaries in 9 to 12 year-old children with language learning disability. Two consistent sets of findings emerge; both are perti-nent for understanding the writing struggles, which students like Ryan constantly face. First, in terms of morphosyntactic sensitivity, in contrast to chronological-age peers and language-age peers, children with language learning disability failed to mark verb finiteness in writing, specifically, the past tense *-ed*, as well as the irregular past tense (Windsor et al., 2000). This pattern is found well past the age when these forms are mastered in writing development (e.g., Nunes et al., 1997) and may reflect per-sisting problems in developing the level of morphosyntactic awareness required for the spellings that support writing expression. A reexamination of Ryan's narrative provides suggestive evidence that, although he uses verb finiteness in obligatory con-texts, he is selecting bare-stem forms. In other words, past tense is unmarked for any regular verb form (*like, lock*), irregular form (*has, ride, go*), or *be/do* forms (*is, do*) (spellings have been translated into conventional words; punctuation is retained from the original):

My favorite hobby is a bicycle...it is red and gold and it has a light...under bicycle it has rims...it has hydraulics.... I like my bicycle.... I riding [unknown word]...it is fun riding my bicycle. . . . I can't [unknown word] when I my it home. I go to the movies. . . . I lock my bicycle up. . . . I do tricks with my bicycle

Obviously, longer writing samples need to be collected for any meaningful conclusions; however, it would be equally important to obtain narrative and expository samples of Ryan's spoken language use to compare and contrast morphosyntactic patterns in the marking of finite verb clauses.

The second pattern emerging from research on spoken–written contrasts concerns syntactic productivity and complexity. Regardless of discourse genre (narrative or expository), children with a language learning disability were less productive in the amount of writing generated (they produced fewer total words) (Scott & Windsor, 2000). They also produced on average fewer words per T-unit in the narratives, which suggested differences in the degree to which complexity was present in the formulation of noun and verb phrases. Note that Ryan's descriptive narrative contains minimal "nonclausal" complexity. Both noun and verb phrases are relatively brief and redundant in the information offered. This type of productivity pattern is also consistent with the minimalist, or "retrieve and write" (Graham & Harris, 1999, p. 256), approach that indicates the absence of preplanning and self-regulation of the writing process (e.g., missing words in the sample), as well as a general absence of attention to audience needs. A final relevant point pertains to Ryan's primitive concepts about word boundaries and punctuation, which may be an outcome of his not yet understanding the notion of sentence. Scott (1999) makes the case that punctuation patterns provide explicit insight into children's theories about grammar and text, for example, the knowledge that punctuation is a convention governed by phrase or clause boundaries.

Some Conclusions about the Focuses of Assessment

The case has been made that decisions about the focuses of assessment should be motivated by two intersecting factors. One factor involves general knowledge of: (1) the educational standards, benchmarks, and grade-level expectations that comprise the general education curriculum in a particular state and (2) how these standards and expectations are implemented in the school system that the child of interest attends. The second factor is derived from professional knowledge. Potential assessment areas should reflect evidence-based findings on the spoken language components that, developmentally, are associated with the prediction of success in reading, writing, and spelling at various ages. A functional assessment plan should then combine knowledge of educational standards and expected outcomes with clinical knowledge of the language components that appear critical for the individual child being able to achieve successful outcomes. A functional assessment has to involve careful description of what children can do, the difficulties they encounter, and the instructional and peer situations that facilitate or hinder effective communication.

As discussed in this section, children and adolescents with language learning disabilities, like Ryan and Jay, can demonstrate various patterns that are not mutually exclusive and that also represent the challenges they must confront every day in the spoken and written modalities. Furthermore, the nature of the problems that result from meeting new or different challenges will change over time as communicative and educational expectations are increased. They may struggle with the phonological sensitivity correlated with effective decoding ability, the morphological sensitivity related to attaining a rich storehouse of literate vocabulary meanings, and the morphosyntactic sensitivity that plays a critical role in advancing their understanding and use of grammatical complexity. At the discourse level, they also have difficulty with easily or efficiently planning and organizing information, which may be made the most visible when they attempt to write. At the metacognitive level, they may manifest problems in being able to manage their own learning, which also can seriously affect strategies for reading comprehension (National Reading Panel, 2000). Because the linguistic/discourse system is an integrated system that continuously interacts, breakdowns in any single component, for example, problems in the marking of finite verb relations, can affect the integrity of functioning of the other components, such as the productivity and complexity of spoken and written narratives. To the greatest extent possible, the focuses of assessment should aim to examine these dynamic system interactions (Silliman, Jimerson, & Wilkinson, 2000) through the methods selected for assessment.

METHODS AND OUTCOMES OF ASSESSMENT

As outlined in Figure 5.1, after determining the purposes and focuses of assessment, the next step concerns "how" to obtain the information to answer the questions being asked. This aspect of the assessment plan has two subcomponents: selection of assessment methods, and the analysis and interpretation of the information gathered; thus, the methods selected are a critical decision because they link the questions asked with the conclusions reached.

Assessment procedures should be chosen that provide the relevant information in accord with educational standards, developmental level, and grade-level expectations. Procedures should always be appropriate for the child's current level of knowledge and abilities. Flexibility in planning is also required, because particular assessment procedures may not turn out to be suitable; therefore, alternative procedures should be part of planning. The specific interpretation of results and subsequent recommendations for whether intervention is warranted will depend, to a large extent, on the questions driving assessment. A critical issue is that assessment procedures should yield clear directions for an intervention plan that is linked to the general education curriculum, if such a plan is recommended as the outcome.

This section addresses traditional and alternative assessment methods and includes a minicase example as a means for applying methods to the interpretation of outcomes. It is recognized that detailed information should also be obtained from a variety of sources about children's physical and medical status that may be contributing factors, as well as their language, communicative, socioemotional, and academic abilities. These sources on past and current functioning include parents (or primary caregivers), other family members, physicians, psychologists, teachers, and the child of interest, who should be an active participant in any evaluation. For example, a child interview can help to validate how the child interprets the world of classroom discourse by using an interview format designed for this specific purpose (e.g., Morine-Dershimer, 1985). Because of space considerations, only diagnostic tools are emphasized within the contexts of traditional and alternative approaches to assessment.

Traditional Methods of Assessment

Traditional assessment methods generally refer to norm-referenced, or standardized, tests and criterion-referenced measures. With norm-referenced procedures, the interpretation of an individual child's performance is based on comparison to a group standard of performance. In this situation, the standard of comparison is the child's *relative standing* in relation to the larger group norms, such as a percentile ranking or the degree of the standard deviation from the mean group score. In criterion referencing, the child's performance is interpreted according to a predetermined standard, such as "When given ten spelling words, how many does Mary spell correctly?" or "Does Mary mark verb finite clauses in an oral narrative with 100% accuracy?" The standard for comparison is an *absolute standard,* because the performance criteria are determined in advance (Salvia & Ysseldyke, 2001).

In general, normative interpretations are often applied to the identification of a language learning disability for a practical reason. Standardized measures are less time consuming to administer than is the planning, analysis, and interpretations often associated with descriptive measures (McCauley, 2001). Descriptive measures can include, but are not limited to: (1) language or discourse samples collected from a variety of communicative activities, (2) direct observations of child interactions in the classroom, (3) elicitation procedures employed to obtain specific information on children's comprehension or production of various aspects of the linguistic/discourse system, and (4) tasks designed specifically to explore a child's learning potential. The examination of learning potential is also called *dynamic assessment,* because assessment and an intervention are integrated to investigate how much support a child needs to be successful with a particular task. Criterion-referenced interpretations are preferred when the purpose is to plan or evaluate the outcomes of instructional or intervention practices that have been implemented with individual children (McCauley, 1996; Salvia & Ysseldyke, 2001). Because criterion-referenced measures are commonly found in alternative assessments, they will be expanded on when alternative assessments are described.

Norm-Referenced Measures

Table 5.6 lists twenty-four tests that can be selected to assess the comprehension or production of spoken language functioning in school-age children and adolescents. Even a brief skimming of this table shows that most measures are heavily weighted toward the lexical/semantic and syntactic domains. In addition, none of these measures includes literacy-related components. Table 5.7 outlines fourteen literacy-related tests that sample the domains of phonological sensitivity, reading comprehension,

TABLE 5.6   Selected Language Tests by Type of Score, Components Assessed, and Age Range

Test Authors	Type of Score			Comprehension				Production				Ages
	SS	AE	%	SYN	SEM	PRG	DIS	SYN	SEM	PRG	DIS	
ASSET: Assessing Semantic Skills through Everyday Language (Barret, Bowers, & Huisingh, 1988), Linguisystems)	X	X	X		X				X			3–9:11
CASL: Comprehensive Assessment of Spoken Language (Carrow-Woolfolk, 1999, American Guidance Service)	X	X	X	X	X	X		X	X	X		3–21
Clinical Evaluation of Language Fundamentals (CELF)—3 (Semel, Wiig, & Secord, 1995, Psychological Corp.)	X	X	X	X	X			X	X			6–21
Comprehensive Receptive and Expressive Vocabulary Test (CREVT) (Wallace & Hammill, 1994, Pro-Ed)	X	X	X		X				X			4–17:11
Expressive One-Word Vocabulary Test (EOWVT), 2000 Edition (Gardner, 2000, Linguisystems)	X	X	X						X			2–18:11
OWLS Listening Comprehension and Oral Expression Scales (Carrow-Woolfolk, 1995, American Guidance Service)	X	X	X	X	X			X	X			3–21
Peabody Picture Vocabulary Test (PPVT)—III (Dunn & Dunn, 1997, American Guidance Service)	X	X	X		X							2:6–90:11
Preschool Language Scale (PLS)—3 (Zimmerman, Steiner, & Pond, 1992, Psychological Corp.)	X	X	X	X	X			X	X			Birth–6
Receptive One-Word Vocabulary Test (ROWVT), 2000 Edition (Gardner, 2000, Linguisystems)	X	X	X		X							2–18:11

Test Authors	Type of Score			Comprehension				Production				Ages
	SS	AE	%	SYN	SEM	PRG	DIS	SYN	SEM	PRG	DIS	
Test for Auditory Comprehension of Language (TACL)—3 (Carrow-Woolfolk, 1999, Psychological Corp.)	X	X	X	X	X							3–9:11
Test of Adolescent/Adult Word Finding (German, 1989, American Guidance Service)	X		X						X			12–80
Test of Adolescent and Adult Language (TOAL)—3 (Hammill et al., 1994, American Guidance Service)	X		X	X	X			X	X			12–24:11
Test of Early Language Development (TELD)—3 (Hresko, Reid, & Hammill, 1999, American Guidance Service)	X	X	X	X	X			X	X			2–7:11
Test of Language Competence—Expanded Edition (Wiig & Secord, 1989, Psychological Corp.)	X	X	X	X	X			X	X			5–18
Test of Language Development (TLD)—3 Primary/Intermediate (Hammill & Newcomer, 1997, Psychological Corp.)	X	X	X	X	X			X	X			P 4:8–8 I 8–12:11
Test of Pragmatic Language (TOPL) (Phelps-Terasaki & Phelps-Gunn, 1992, Pro-Ed)		X	X							X		3–15:6
Test of Word Finding (TWF)—2 (German, 2000, Pro-Ed)	X		X						X			4–12:11
Test of Word Finding in Discourse (TWFD) (German, 1991, DLM)	X		X		X				X			6:6–12:11
Test of Word Knowledge (TOWK) (Wiig & Secord, 1992, Psychological Corp.)	X	X	X		X				X			5–18

(continued)

TABLE 5.6 *(continued)*

Test Authors	Type of Score			Comprehension				Production				Ages
	SS	AE	%	SYN	SEM	PRG	DIS	SYN	SEM	PRG	DIS	
Utah Test of Language Development (UTLD)—3 (Mecham, 1989, Pro-Ed)	X	X	X	X	X			X	X			3–9:11
Wiig Criterion Referenced Inventory of Language (Wiig, 1990, Psychological Corp.)								X	X	X		4–13
Woodcock Language Proficiency Battery (WLPB) (Woodcock, 1991, Psychological Corp.)	X	X	X	X	X			X	X			2–90+
The WORD Test—Revised (Elementary) (Huisingh et al., 1989, Linguisystems)	X	X	X						X			7–11
The WORD Test—Adolescents (Zackman et al., 1989, Linguisystems)	X	X	X						X			12–17

Note: SS = Standard score; AE = Age equivalent; % = Percentile; SYN = Syntactic focus; SEM = Lexical/semantic focus; PRG = Pragmatic focus; DIS = Discourse focus.

oral reading accuracy and fluency, spelling, and writing. The norm-referenced tests in these two tables do not represent an exhaustive listing; rather, the two tables show some of the more recent and commonly used measures.

An important skill for speech-language pathologists to acquire is how to review critically the examiner or technical manual that should accompany any norm-referenced measure. Because speech-language pathologists are test consumers and tests are commercially prepared to be sold, the wise professional consumer should adopt a "show me" attitude (Salvia & Ysseldyke, 2001, p. 664). A basic understanding of standards for psychometric adequacy in test construction and standardization is essential to attain in order for the process of decision making in test selection to be an informed one.

The Selection of Norm-Referenced Measures for Language and Literacy Assessments

Standardized language and literacy tests, including screening measures, are psychometric creations rooted in concepts of statistical probability (see the earlier discussions of deficit models and discrepancy criteria). These norm-referenced measures provide a uniform set of instructions and content to elicit particular behaviors and a specific way to score and interpret these behaviors. They may also consist of

TABLE 5.7 Selected Literacy Related Tests by Type of Score, Components Assessed, and Age Range

Test (Authors)	Type of Score			General Content Area					Ages
	SS	AE/GE	%	Phon. Sensit.	Read. Comp.	Oral Read.	Spelling	Writing	
Comprehensive Test of Phonological Processing (CTTOP) (Wagner, Torgesen, & Rashotte, 1999, Pro-Ed)	X	X	X	X					5–24:11
Gray Oral Reading Test (GORT)—3 (Wiederholt & Bryant, 1992, Pro-Ed)	X	X	X		X	X			7–18:11
OWLS: Written Expression Test (Carrow-Woolfolk, 1996, American Guidance Service)	X	X	X				X	X	5–21
Phonological Awareness Test (PAT) (Robertson & Salter, 1997, Linguisystems)			X	X					5–7
Test of Early Reading Ability (TERA)—2 (Reid, Hresko, & Hammill, 1989, American Guidance Service)	X		X	X					3–9:11
Test of Phonological Awareness (TOPA) (Torgesen & Bryant, 1994, Psychological Corp.)	X		X	X					5–8
Test of Early Written Language (TEWL) (Hresko, Herron, & Peak, 1996, Psychological Corp.)	X	X	X					X	4–10:11
Test of Reading Comprehension (TORC) (Brown, Hammill, & Wiederhot, 1995, American Guidance Service)	X		X		X				7–17
Test of Written Language (TOWL) 3d Edition (Hammill & Larsen, 1996, Pro-Ed)	X	X	X				X	X	7:6–17:11

(continued)

TABLE 5.7 *(continued)*

Test (Authors)	SS	AE/GE	%	Phon. Sensit.	Read. Comp.	Oral Read.	Spelling	Writing	Ages
Test of Word Reading Efficiency (TOWRE) (Torgesen, Wagner, & Rashotte, 1999, Pro-Ed)	X	X	X			X			6–24:11
Test of Written Expression (TOWE) (McGee, Bryant, Larsen, & Rivera, 1995, Pro-Ed)	X		X					X	6:6–14:11
Test of Written Spelling (TWS) (Larsen, Hammill, & Moats, 1999, Pro-Ed)	X	X	X				X		6–17:6
Woodcock Language Proficiency Battery (WLPB) (Woodcock, 1991, Psychological Corp.)	X	X	X		X	X	X	X	2–90+
Woodcock Reading Mastery Test (Woodcock, 1998, American Guidance Service)	X	X	X		X	X			5–75+

Header spanning: "Type of Score" spans SS, AE/GE, %; "General Content Area" spans Phon. Sensit., Read. Comp., Oral Read., Spelling, Writing.

Notes: SS = Standard score; AE/GE = Age equivalent/grade equivalent; Phono. Sensit. = Phonological sensitivity focus; Read Comp. = Reading comprehension focus; Oral Read. = Oral reading focus.

contrived tasks whose correspondence to real-life communication, whether defined as listening, speaking, reading, or writing, is often questionable. A major assumption underlying the construction of all norm-referenced measures is the homogeneity of children's performance; that is, regardless of individual differences, similar patterns of performance can be expected from all children.

As summarized in Table 5.8, norm-referenced measures vary along eight dimensions. There is no perfect test, just as there is no perfect method of assessment regardless of which approach to assessment is selected. The goal of reviewing an examiner or technical manual is the degree to which a particular measure deviates from reasonable standards of psychometric (measurement) adequacy for each of the dimensions. The extent of variation within and across these eight dimensions significantly affects the reliability and validity of the measure.

Reliability.   Reliability, a subcomponent of validity, concerns the consistency of measurement. A test can never meet validity standards if it is not reliable; however, reliability does not guarantee validity (see Table 5.8). The overall reliability of any test

TABLE 5.8	Eight Dimensions of Variation in Norm-Referenced Measures and Effects on Psychometric Adequacy for Diagnostic Purposes	
Dimension	**Key Features**	**Outcome**
1. Conceptual model and purposes	• Conceptual model reflects era in which test developed • Models of assessment often describe similar language learning problems differently • Test purposes should clearly derive from conceptual model (Lund & Duchan, 1993)	• Affects construct validity—internal validity or adequacy of test's theoretical premises in relation to its purpose
2. Focus targeted	• Global test titles often mislead as to the actual focus • Real focus can only be determined from careful analysis of the kinds of behaviors included	• Affects content validity—degree to which (a) clear rationale given for selection of test items, (b) test items reflect specific behaviors being measured, and (c) test items are consistent with the constructs being used to measure the behaviors
3. Range of difficulty	• Must demonstrate that range of item selection and difficulty are related to purpose and focus	• Affects content validity
4. Depth of assessment	• More global the focus or wider the age ranges covered, the less are opportunities for in depth assessment at any age	• Affects construct and content validity

5. Methods for quantifying performance	• Different kinds of scores are based on different scales of measurement
	• Most common scores
	  (a) Age-equivalent/grade-equivalents scores
	  (b) Percentile ranks
	  (c) Standard scores
	
	• Regardless of scoring method, every test score has measurement error
	
	• Cutoff score for diagnostic decision making varies from test to test
		
		• Affects reliability—consistency or generalizability of measurement across similar testing situations
		• Affects overall validity

6. Nature of standardization sample for obtaining norms	• Sufficiency of norms depends on
	  (a) Adequacy of sampling plan
	  (b) Representativeness of sample for intended assessment purposes
	  (c) Total number included and distributions of subtotals within age levels or diagnostic categories in accord with intended assessment purposes
	  (d) Age of norms
	  (e) Relevance of norms for assessment purposes
		• Affects reliability (stability of norms) and overall validity

(continued)

TABLE 5.8 *(continued)*

Dimension	Key Features	Outcome
7. Nature of reliability data	• Consistency and stability of scores always affected by some degree of random measurement error (a) Degree to which test/subtest items are measuring the same behaviors (internal consistency) (b) Consistency of scoring across different administrators or examiners (interexaminer reliability) (c) Stability of scores over time (test–retest reliability) (d) Magnitude of error in estimating that an individual's obtained score and true score would be similar if the test was taken repeatedly	• Affects overall validity of assessment • Greater the reliability, the less is standard error of measurement (SEM)
8. Nature of validity data	• Extent to which "testing process leads to correct inferences about a specific person in a specific situation for a specific purpose" (Salvia & Ysseldyke, 2001, p. 145) • Sources of external evidence (a) Content validation 　(1) Appropriateness and relevance of items 　(2) Scope and completeness of items 　(3) How items assess content, e.g., response format (b) Criterion-related validation 　(1) Concurrent validation— degree to which content of target measure and an existing measure are related 　(2) Predictive validity—degree to which target measure predicts future performance in same or related content area (c) Diagnostic validation—extent to which an empirically validated cutoff point clearly discriminates disability "membership" from typically developing "membership"	• Validation evidence may result in legitimate inferences about a group's performance, but not produce valid inferences about an individual's performance • Construct validation of a measure depends on how accrual of external validity evidence supports underlying model or inferences drawn from model in predictable ways

Sources: Hutchinson, 1996; McCauley, 2001; Salvia & Ysseldyke, 2001.

is related to its possible sources of error (Hutchinson, 1996; McCauley, 2001; Salvia & Ysseldyke, 2001). These sources include (1) the size and characteristics of the standardization sample, (2) the extent to which items in a test or subtest are measuring the same behaviors (item or internal consistency), (3) variability in examiner scoring (interexaminer reliability), (4) too short or too long test–retest intervals (test–retest reliability), and (5) situational variations in testing conditions (the testing room is noisy, children become bored or do not understand instructions or even the purpose of test participation, etc.). The general guideline is that diagnostic measures should have reliability coefficients of at least .90, while screening measures should have reliability coefficients of at least .80 (Salvia & Ysseldyke, 2001).

Measurement error is also a significant factor affecting the confidence that test consumers can have in the accuracy of an individual child's obtained score. This type of measurement error should be reported as the "margin of error," or a confidence interval, for each test score as derived from the standard error of measurement (Hutchinson, 1996). Also, confidence intervals should always be included in clinical or educational reports of a child's test performances. The error margin around an obtained score should be considered in decision making.

Validity. In the broadest sense, the validity of a measure does not reside in the test itself. Unlike reliability, which is related to sources of error, validity is a property of the evidence gathered over time and the inferences drawn from that evidence that the measure's results are consistent with its purposes (Hutchinson, 1996; Salvia & Ysseldyke, 2001) (see Table 5.8). For this reason, it is important that the test purposes are stated explicitly in an accompanying manual, because it is this statement of purpose that "helps to define the boundaries the test maker has placed around the *construct* [author's italics] of the test" (Hutchinson, 1996, p. 110). The underlying construct can be a conceptual framework or model or a set of skills presumed related to particular achievements. For example, many commonly used vocabulary measures are "atheoretical." They are not grounded to developmental models of how children acquire a lexicon over time; instead, they are collections of single word meanings, and children's skills in either the comprehension or production of these meanings are predicted to increase with age. This underlying construct then serves as the basis for the selection of content (vocabulary items) that represent the behaviors to be evaluated. The process for content selection should also be stated clearly (Hutchinson, 1996; McCauley, 2001).

As Table 5.8 suggests, the process for validating the underlying premises of a norm-referenced measure is complex. Validation is best considered as the external evidence presented about the degree to which a measure's content (the language domain being assessed) is related to its intended purposes; therefore, a technical manual should present more than superficial evidence of external or "face" validity in regard to content, criterion-related, and diagnostic validity (McCauley, 2001). This standard is particularly important in the case of measures that have a diagnostic purpose. Any measures intended for identification (or screening) purposes should provide strong experimental evidence that it has both *test sensitivity* and *test specificity*. In other words, the measure's content has discriminative power. It can classify with a high standard of accuracy true positives (positive results that demonstrate sensitivity to children who have a language learning disability) and exclude true negatives (negative results that demonstrate specificity about children who do *not* have a language learning disability). A measure that has discriminative power in its diagnostic accuracy as a classification tool should not produce unacceptable proportions of false positives or false negatives. Plante and Vance (1994) recommend that a diagnostic accuracy of 90% could be evaluated as good, a diagnostic accuracy of 80% to 89% should be considered as only fair, and a diagnostic accuracy of less than 80% is unacceptable.

Diagnostic accuracy, however, is always a product of either the standard deviation point or the percentile rank that serves as the boundary for a classification decision. This lower boundary is referred to as the *cutoff point*. Children who perform below the cutoff point, for example, below 2 standard deviations from the mean or below the 10th percentile on language measures, may be candidates for language intervention, depending on the criterion that a particular school system (or clinical setting) employs. However, different cutoff points produce different trade-offs between the test sensitivity and test specificity components of diagnostic accuracy.

Test Validity and Diagnostic Accuracy.   Technical manuals still do not routinely contain data on diagnostic accuracy, perhaps due to the concern of test makers that less than acceptable accuracy levels will hinder the sale of their product. As a consequence, speech-language pathologists and others concerned with identification decisions must search out independent studies peer reviewed in journals for this essential information.

An illustration of the clinical requirement for norm-referenced language and literacy measures to demonstrate diagnostic accuracy comes from the work of Gray, Plante, Vance, and Henrichsen (1999). These authors studied four single-word vocabulary measures that speech-language pathologists commonly use in diagnostic decision making. Among the questions asked were whether these vocabulary tests discriminated "between children with normal and impaired language with acceptable levels of sensitivity and specificity" (Gray et al., 1999, p. 198). This question is a critical one, because language assessment is concerned with individual differences, not group differences. None of the measures evidenced discriminative power for either sensitivity or specificity; diagnostic accuracy ranged from a low of 68% to a high of only 77%. It was also found that if a cutoff point was selected that did maximize classification accuracy, the majority of children with a language learning impairment obtained scores within 1 standard deviation of the mean or the normal range of variation. Thus, even if a cutoff point of 1.5 standard deviations had been established, many of the children with a language learning impairment would not have been identified by any of these four measures.

Gray et al. concluded that although these particular vocabulary measures had basic construct validity (they did assess vocabulary skill), construct validity by itself was insufficient to support a diagnostic purpose. These vocabulary measures did not accurately identify children with or without a language learning disability at acceptable levels. Approximately 23% of children in both groups were either overidentified (falsely identified as positive) or underidentified (falsely identified as problem free). The issue of the diagnostic accuracy of norm-referenced measures is reflected in the case study of Jack, which is presented next.

Jack's Profile on Norm-Referenced Assessment

Jack is 8 years old and in a grade 2 classroom. He has struggled academically since beginning kindergarten but has not been identified as needing additional educational services. Although he has not yet repeated a grade, he still has not met grade 1 expectations in reading. For example, Jack is still struggling with sound--letter correspondences. His teacher believes that an underlying language problem may be responsible for his academic problems and has referred Jack for a language evaluation to the school diagnostic team, which includes a speech-language pathologist. As part of the information-gathering phase of the assessment, the speech-language pathologist learns from Jack's parents that Jack never liked to be read to when he was a preschooler and withdrew into silence when asked questions about events occurring in story books. As a result, Jack's mother reported that she stopped book reading with him when he was four years old because he disliked it so much. When Jack began school, the parents reinitiated book reading and found that he would only respond to short stories that had many pictures. The parents did not state any concerns about Jack's language development, but described him as a child who did not like to talk much, in contrast to his two older brothers.

Jack has been selected to highlight the purposes, methods, and outcomes of norm-referenced assessment for three reasons. First, he is typical of many children whose language problems may not emerge in a visible way until they enter school. Second, he also demonstrates how the subtle nature of problems in more advanced language learning may function as barriers in learning to read. Finally, Jack represents those children for whom no discrepancy exists between their scores on language and literacy tests and their nonverbal intelligence scores, yet who are seriously struggling in communicative and academic domains.

Measures Selected.   In this situation, the broader question asked about Jack was a diagnostic question: Did he have a language learning disability? A related question, narrower in scope, and thus more directly answerable, concerned whether Jack's level of phonological sensitivity was sufficient for the current instructional demands of learning to decode. The speech-language pathologist decided to administer two measures. The first was the Clinical Evaluation of Language Fundamentals (CELF)—3 (Semel, Wiig, & Secord, 1995), a norm-referenced measure of spoken language that focuses primarily on the semantic and syntactic domains in assessing comprehension and production. The CELF—3 has a clear diagnostic purpose stated in the examiner's manual, which also outlines a conceptual model of fundamental language functioning adapted from Lahey (1988). This model stresses interactions between semantics (content) and syntax (form).

The second measure that the speech-language pathologist selected was the Comprehensive Test of Phonological Processing (CTOPP) (Wagner, Torgesen, & Rashotte, 1999). The CTOPP is also a norm-referenced measure, but one premised on the extensive research that has examined phonological processing abilities as a predictor of learning to read. Among its four purposes are two diagnostic aims: "to identify individuals who are significantly below their peers in important phonological abilities [and] to determine strengths and weaknesses among developed phonological processes" (Wagner et al., 1999, p. 13). Phonological processing (or phonological sensitivity) is examined in three areas that research has found to be correlated: phonological awareness, phonological memory, and rapid naming of digits and letters.

Interpretation and Outcomes.   Jack's performances on the CELF—3 and the CTOPP are presented in Table 5.9.

1. *Standard score interpretations.* The CELF—3 and CTOPP quantify performance with standard scores (SS), which are derived scores. This means that raw scores have been converted into an equal-interval scale of measurement so that a standard distribution is produced in relation to the normal curve and different subtests (or even different tests) can be compared with one another. This standard distribution always has a specific mean and the same interval between each standard deviation (SD) (for further discussion on the benefits of standard scores and why age/grade-equivalent scores should not be used, see McCauley, 2001; Salvia & Ysseldyke, 2001; also see the CTOPP examiner's manual [Wagner et al., 1999, p. 43]).

TABLE 5.9   **Jack's Scores on the Clinical Evaluation of Language Fundamentals—3 (CELF—3) and the Comprehensive Test of Phonological Processing (CTOPP)**

Celf—3 Subtest	Standard Score (SS)	Confidence Interval (68% Level)	Percentile Rank	Confidence Interval (68% Level)
1. Sentence Structure	12	10–14	63	50–91
2. Concepts and Directions	8	7–9	25	16–37
3. Word Classes	6	5–7	9	5–16
Receptive Language Score	90	85–95	30	16–37
4. Word Structure	12	11–13	75	63–84
5. Formulated Sentences	10	9–11	50	16–84
6. Recalling Sentences	6	5–7	9	5–16
Expressive Language Score	96	92–100	39	30–50

CTOPP Subtest	Standard Score (SS)	Description	Confidence Interval (90% Level)	Description
1. Elision	6	Below average		
2. Blending Words	9	Average		
3. Blending Nonwords	9	Average		
Phonological Awareness Composite	87	*Below average*	77–97	*Poor to average*
4. Memory for Digits	6	Below average		
5. Nonword Repetition	6	Below average		
Phonological Memory Composite	76	*Poor*	66–86	*Very poor to below average*
6. Rapid Digit Naming	8	Average		
7. Rapid Letter Naming	7	Below average		
Rapid Naming Composite	85	*Below average*	75–95	*Poor to average*

Notes: CELF—3, Mean SS Subtests = 10, SD = 3; CELF—3, Mean Receptive/Expressive SS = 100, SD = 15; CTOPP, Mean SS Subtests = 10, SD = 3; CTOPP Composite SS = 100, SD = 15.

Note that on two of the CELF—3 subtests shown in Table 5.9, Word Classes and Recalling Sentences, Jack scored below 1 SD (mean = 10 ± 3, or 7 to 13), receiving an SS of 6. However, both of Jack's composite scores were within 1 SD of the mean (100 ± 15, or 85 to 115) despite his lower obtained scores on these two subtests. His performance on the CTOPP differed somewhat in comparison to the CELF—3. He scored below 1 SD on three subtests (mean = 10 ± 3, or 7 to 13): Elision ("Say *mat* without saying the /m/"), Memory for Digits (repeat a series of numbers in the same order in which they are heard), and Nonword Repetition (repeating nonwords, such as *"meb," "zid,"* and *"wudoip"*). The test authors report that SS are more reliable for the composite scores than for the individual subtest scores. Thus, as Table 5.9 shows, Jack scored within 1 SD on the two of the three phonological processing composites (mean = 100; SD = 15, or 85 to 115), Phonological Awareness and Rapid Naming, but below 1 SD on the third composite, Phonological Memory.

2. *Percentile ranking interpretation.* Another score of relative standing for quantifying performance is the percentile ranking. On the two CELF—3 composites, Jack's obtained ranks are the 30th percentile and the 39th percentile, respectively (percentile ranks for the CTOPP have not been included, but are available in the examiner's manual). Often, percentile ranks are not standard scores (although they may be), because they are based on another scale of measurement, an ordinal scale in which the ranks between intervals are unequal. However, they are derived scores because they have been transformed from raw scores to indicate the percentage of individuals whose scores fall at or below a specific raw score (see Salvia & Ysseldyke, 2001, for further discussion). Unlike standard scores, percentile ranks cannot be averaged or combined into a composite (McCauley, 2001). A major advantage of percentile ranks is that they report relative standing in a group in a way that parents and professionals can easily understand. In terms of the normal-curve distribution, Jack's percentile rankings on the two language scores, as would be expected from the SS composites, correspond to the normal range of variation (within 1 standard deviation).

3. *Confidence interval interpretations.* A confidence interval represents the standard error margin of Jack's obtained standard scores and percentile rankings. In other words, if Jack was repeatedly administered the CELF—3 or the CTOPP, what might be his true score?

Let's first examine the CELF—3. From the examiner's manual (Semel et al., 1995), we can find the confidence intervals for his two language composite scores, which account for a standard error of measurement around the obtained score. These confidence intervals indicate that, at the 68% level of confidence, Jack could obtain (1) a score as low as 85 and as high as 95 on the receptive subtests and (2) a score as low as 92 and as high as 100 on the expressive subtests if he took these subtests more than once. For either the receptive or expressive content area, the probability is that 68 of 100 times Jack's true scores would fall with these confidence intervals, both of which are within the normal range of variation. However, the chances remain that, 32 of 100 times, his true score might be lower than 85 and 92 or higher than 95 and 100 (on the CELF—3, the margin of error can also be increased to the 90% level of confidence). The confidence intervals for the percentile rankings would be interpreted similarly.

Turning to the confidence intervals for the CTOPP SS (recall that the composite SS is more reliable than the individual SS for the subtests), this time the probability for the margin of error around the obtained scores has been increased to the 90% confidence level, which is a more stringent estimate. In this situation, if Jack took the CTOPP repeatedly, 90 of 100 times his composite score, for example, for the Phonological Awareness Composite, could be as low as 77 and as high as 97. However, 10 of 100 times the likelihood is that this composite "true" score could be lower than 77 or higher than 97. With this more stringent estimate of the intervals for Jack's true score, note that all three composites become more worrisome relative to their lower boundaries. For example, a lower boundary SS of 66 for Phonological Memory would be more than 2 standard deviations below the mean of 100.

4. *Some factors affecting the reliability and validity of interpretations.* Both measures have strengths and weaknesses in relation to the eight dimensions that affect psychometric adequacy. By carefully reviewing the examiner or technical manuals for both measures, the speech-language pathologist should become knowledgeable about the dimensions that might have the most effect on reliability and validity and, as a consequence, influence how results are interpreted. Independent evaluations of a measure should also be sought in journal articles or in textbooks that deal with assessment or tests and measurement.

An important decision is to consider the overall validity of any measure that is intended for diagnostic purposes. The CELF—3 is a tool for the diagnosis of a language learning disability; however, its diagnostic accuracy as reported in the technical manual (Semel et al., 1995, p. 64) is only 71%, an accuracy level that Plante and Vance (1994) consider unacceptable. Thus, the diagnostic purpose of such an instrument would be compromised due to the absence of diagnostic validity.

Although the CTOPP appears to have construct validity relative to its conceptual framework (Salvia & Ysseldyke, 2001), it does not provide data on classification accuracy, which may be a drawback to its diagnostic use. Instead, the test authors offer a discrepancy analysis as a method to determine whether the differences between two test scores, such as two composite scores or two subtest scores, are sufficiently different to be clinically meaningful. A discrepancy analysis concerns the reliability of measurement, specifically, whether the magnitude of a difference in two test scores is sufficiently different to be practically significant. As Salvia and Ysseldyke (2001) point out, that a difference is real does not mean that it is "rare" (p. 140). For example, Jack had an 11-point "real" difference between his Phonological Awareness Composite score (SS = 87) and his Phonological Memory Composite score (SS = 76). On the surface, this gap appears to be important. The issue is whether the size of this discrepancy is one that occurs so infrequently that it can be interpreted as having practical clinical or educational significance for the individual child. According to the examiner's manual (Wagner et al., 1999, p. 52), for a discrepancy between these two composite scores to be a clinically meaningful one, the difference score must be at least 15 points. Jack's difference does not reach that critical value. The concepts of critical values and clinically meaningful differences are equally pertinent for the overall use of discrepancy criteria in the classification of a language or learning disability, because uncommon differences in two scores and their meaningfulness are always a function of the reliability of the tests themselves. For example, the reliability coefficients of the CTOPP do not consistently meet the .90 minimum standard for decision making about individual children older than age 6 years. This limitation is attributed to problems with sample representativeness (Salvia & Ysseldyke, 2001); thus, the internal consistency of this measure may be suspect for children who are age 7 or older.

Answering the Evaluation Questions.   Given some of the issues raised with the reliability and validity of these two measures, how should Jack's overall performance on these two measures be interpreted? Does the evidence support the conclusion that Jack (1) presents with a language learning disability (the eligibility question) and (2) requires intervention that will support his language and academic development (the need question)? Answering these questions in a competent manner requires that speech-language pathologists go beyond test scores and apply their professional judgment to the interpretation of performance patterns.

The eligibility answer for Jack is not clear-cut. Although he encountered some difficulty with two subtests, Word Classes and Recalling Sentences, on the CELF—3, the major spoken language measure, he otherwise performed within the normal range of variation. The meaning of the difference in these subtest scores in contrast to other subtest scores may not be practically important, because the CELF—3 does not provide critical reliability values on how big the magnitude of a difference must be to be significant. The Word Classes subtest is a semantic memory task. It requires that a child of Jack's age listens to a series of three words, such as *button, shirt,* and *chair,* and determine which two words represent a larger superordinate category. The Recalling Sentences subtest is a verbatim repetition task. The child must repeat exactly the sentences (syntactic elements) presented, which increase in length and in the inclusion of literate word meanings, e.g., "The rabbit was not put in the cage," and "Was the van preceded by the ambulance?" Successful performance involves the application and coordination of metacognitive strategies to hold information actively in short-term memory, while engaging in some level of metalinguistic analysis to separate structure from meaning (Ricciardelli, 1993; Semel et al., 1995). The need to attend to multiple strategies may have taxed Jack's attentional resources for language processing at this point in time. Most important, the extents to which these processing requirements are reflected in Jack's real-life decoding problems are unclear, although they may contribute indirectly to his predicted struggles with comprehension in both spoken and written language. But the nature of the connections remains blurred, as do implications for a language intervention plan integrated with benchmarks and grade-level curriculum expectations. Therefore, answering the question from the norm-referenced information about whether Jack has a language learning disability remains clinically ambiguous.

On the other hand, Jack clearly has real-life educational needs, as documented by his struggles in learning to read. Taking into account the 90% confidence intervals for his obtained score, his struggles are reflected in the borderline performance on the CTOPP for two of the three components of phonological processing and below expectations for the phonological memory component. The diagnostic implications of his performance patterns can be addressed more specifically in contrast to the CELF—3 performance patterns. Jack's degree of phonological sensitivity is inconsistent with developmental expectations. He still appears to be struggling with the segmental (phonemic) properties of words (phonological awareness), encountering difficulties with easily translating print into words in order to access their meanings readily (phonological memory), and, in addition, may be having related problems in easily recalling phonological information from long-term memory (phonological retrieval). The evidence points to the conclusion that Jack is experiencing problems, at a minimum, with the language-related processes strongly associated with the development of alphabetic reading and the prediction of reading success at grade 3 (Catts et al., 1999; Snow et al., 1998). Assisting Jack's potential to benefit from instruction or intervention in alphabetic reading should now be addressed collaboratively with his classroom teacher and other educational staff. This task is best approached through alternative assessments.

Alternative Assessments

Alternative assessments are typically directed to the process of learning in contrast to the focus of traditional assessments on the "products" of learning. In other words, traditional assessments, such as norm-referenced assessments, examine what has or has not been learned according to the individual's child's relative ranking in a normative group. Because of this focus, traditional methods of assessment often lack the flexibility to foster meaningful intervention in real-life activities and situations or to track the effectiveness of particular intervention procedures. This inflexibility does not allow the consideration of four important factors that influence individual children's engagement in learning. These factors are (1) the context of learning (Villa & Thousand, 1995), (2) information about children's understanding of and quality of thinking in problem solving (McMillan, 2001), (3) the influences of motivation, personality, social, and multicultural factors on learning (Meltzer & Reid, 1994), and (4) the complex interactions between development and curriculum. For these reasons, the concept of authenticity has become an important element in assessment (McMillan, 2001).

Authenticity is defined practically as how closely the content selected for assessment relates to real communicative contexts within the curriculum and the community. Authenticity can be viewed through three dimensions (Elliot, 1994): (1) response type, (2) nature of the task, and (3) relevance to instruction. Response type is the amount of interaction expected on the part of the student. Low interaction expectations would involve such responses as circling an item or pointing to a picture. High interaction expectations might feature writing a book report or participating in a debate. The nature of the task pertains to whether the diagnostic task involves a more contrived task, such as repeating nonsense words, or a task based more on functional activities, such as reading a letter from a friend. Relevance to instruction addresses the alignment of the alternative assessment with the classroom curriculum and expected academic outcomes (Witt, Elliott, Daly, Gresham, & Kramer, 1998). Alternative assessment methods are diverse in choice.

Two complementary possibilities for more authentic assessment of language and literacy abilities are briefly described here in order to sketch the different information that may be obtained with elementary-age students like Jack, as well as older students. These possible methods are curriculum-based assessment and portfolio assessment. As with norm-referenced methods, each has strengths and limitations. For example, it is also critically important to establish the reliability and validity of these methods. However, it is essential to note that these alternatives to traditional assessment are not synonymous with informal or unstructured observations. They are descriptive, grounded in conceptual frameworks and related research about language and communication development and its disruption, and require planning and organization to implement and interpret appropriately.

Curriculum-Based Assessments

Curriculum-based assessment uses tasks that often are teacher constructed and whose content examines directly the skills expected to be attained at a particular grade level (Salvia & Ysseldyke, 2001). There are multiple purposes for the use of curriculum-based assessment measures, such as appraising children's current levels of ability, determining their capacity to benefit from instruction, deriving instructional goals, and tracking of individual progress along a continuum of curricular objectives (Westling & Fox, 2000). In considering methods consistent with curriculum-based assessment, several points are relevant.

What Is Curriculum-Based Language Assessment?   First, Nelson's (1998) distinction between curriculum-based assessment and curriculum-based language assessment should be understood. In curriculum-based language assessment, the primary role of the speech-language pathologist is not to construct tests to determine how well a component of the curriculum has been learned. Instead, the goal is to "use samples of the real curriculum . . . to analyze the student's curriculum-based language processing abilities' (Nelson, 1998, p. 402) in order to answer a specific question (see Chapter 9). Answerable questions might include the effectiveness of instruction in phonological sensitivity or whether instructional modifications are indicated, and if so, what they should be (Jones, Southern, & Brigham, 1998; Kratcoski, 1998).

The process of evaluating a child's ability to benefit from instructional assistance should incorporate a clear focus of assessment in the selection of specific language and literacy behaviors, often referred to as target behaviors. The focus of assessment should then lead to a decision about the appropriate methods to collect data, such as systematic observation of the target behaviors the child uses in teacher-directed versus peer-directed learning activities (Silliman & Wilkinson, 1991). Other methods may center on the analysis of children's various written products to assess their application of the target behaviors, such as planning and text organization strategies, the use of derivational morphology strategies, or the level and type of syntactic complexity produced (Silliman et al., 2000). This form of curriculum-based language assessment is consistent with the integration of assessment and instruction (or intervention) where actual language learning processes in the classroom serve to inform diagnostic decision making.

How Does Curriculum-Based Assessment Differ from Performance-Based Assessment?   A second point to consider is that curriculum-based language assessment differs from performance-based assessment by not being tied to one specific performance or product, for example, preparing, writing, and orally presenting a report on the habitats of reptiles. This activity may represent the content and strategies that a child has learned to overcome a given challenge (e.g., problems in organizing, writing, and presenting a report orally). Performance-based assessment centers on the direct observation of the individual performing a skill or competency, such as the quality of the report and its presentation, and then applies a scoring rubric for evaluation of the outcome (Coutinho & Malouf, 1992; McMillan, 2001). A **scoring rubric** is a guide that uses specific criteria to distinguish between levels of student proficiency, usually with a rating scale (McMillan, 2001) (state-wide assessments of student achievements are often based on scoring rubrics). Performance-based assessments can be incorporated as part of curriculum-based language assessment.

The Role of Criterion-Referenced Measures in Curriculum-Based Assessment.   The third relevant point to consider in adopting curriculum-based assessment and its modifications for language assessment is that, unlike the qualitative scoring rubrics of performance-based assessment, evaluation of outcomes is frequently connected to criterion-referenced measures. As mentioned earlier, criterion-referenced measures interpret individual performance in relation to a predetermined behavioral criterion (McCauley, 1996). Today, commercial test makers are developing more criterion-referenced, or standards-referenced, tests for state and district assessments (McMillan, 2001).

As contrasted with the relatively broad domains of norm-referenced measures, criterion-referenced measures examine more narrow content domains in a comprehensive manner, such as the progressive results of a particular set of intervention procedures for the skill acquisition of individual children (McCauley, 2001). They also are more discriminating than norm-referenced measures in terms of identifying curricular achievements and the sequence of achievements, because content is tied to what is being learned. As such, criterion-referenced measures, like scoring rubrics, are designed to differentiate specific levels of performance. Unlike the recommended standard scores derived from raw scores on norm-referenced measures, performance on criterion-referenced measures is often summarized with raw scores (how many responses to questions were answered appropriately, the number of times particular story elements were recalled, whether less familiar words can be identified with 90% accuracy, etc.) (McCauley, 2001). Similar issues pertain to the item construction and interpretation of criterion-referenced measures as affect norm-referenced measures. Formats must be standardized, a representative sample of content must be selected, appropriate response formats must be chosen, and psychometrically derived cutoff points should be established (McCauley, 2001; Salvia & Ysseldyke, 2001).

Curriculum-Based Language Assessment for Jack.   In assessing how Jack decodes and how he attempts to gain meaning from what he is reading, the speech-language pathologist must first be familiar with the particular reading program being used in the classroom. A child's problems in reading are not separate from the instructional practices employed to teach alphabetic reading and the construction of meaning. The chief point to remember from scientific evaluations of reading programs (National Reading Panel, 2000) is that no one "right" program or approach exists; rather it is the components comprising instructional practices that matter. Moreover, instruction should be verbally explicit for children about the connection between phonological awareness activities and the resulting benefits for learning to read.

In teaching children to acquire phonemic awareness, the evidence supports that four features should be incorporated into meaningful reading activities (National Reading Panel, 2000; Torgesen et al., 2001). These features are: (1) engage and motivate children, (2) focus on one or two phoneme manipulation skills, such as blending and segmenting phonemes, (3) include letters for phoneme manipulation across materials and activities, and (4) provide intensive instruction over time, but sequence activities so that they are not more than 30 to 50 minutes long for any single session. How long "it takes" for an individual child to learn the necessary skills for word recognition will vary depending on instructor/clinician qualifications, the goals of instruction, how many skills are being taught, and the nature of difficulties that the child is encountering, which may require further modifications to the components of instruction (National Reading Panel, 2000; Torgesen et al., 2001).

The classroom teacher and the speech-language pathologist collaboratively implemented in the classroom a plan for Jack and two other children encountering similar decoding difficulties (for classroom-based collaborative strategies, see DiMeo, Merritt, & Culatta, 1998; Silliman et al., 1999). This plan was a modification of the phonological awareness program developed and validated on a preliminary basis by Gillon (2000) for children with spoken language impairment. Specifically, Jack and his two peers engaged in a range of explicit phonological awareness activities for thirty minutes a day, five days a week, for three months. The components of the plan systematically emphasized blending and segmentation and the linking of monosyllabic spelling patterns to phoneme patterns (e.g., *-at, -ake, -ing*). The classroom teacher and the teacher assistant assisted Jack in continually applying his new learning through reading experiences with specially created minibooks and the use of word sorts for spelling (Bear et al., 2000). Through writing, including computer-assisted instruction, Jack then created his own minibooks that included the spelling-phoneme patterns he was learning. Once Jack could reach 100% accuracy in decoding particular spelling-phoneme patterns, a new set of patterns was introduced.

At the beginning of the intervention, Jack was only able to decode basic word patterns 35% of the time when reading aloud during reading group. Over the course of the three-month curriculum-based language assessment, Jack's progress in recognizing increasingly less familiar spelling-phoneme patterns was graphed (progress was not always consistent, but Jack did consistently show that he was responsive to this approach). At the end of the three-month period, he had acquired a substantially larger sight-word vocabulary that could be applied to more challenging reading materials. He now could decode twenty word patterns and spell them accurately in writing his ministories at 90% to 100% levels of accuracy. Thus, the curriculum-based language assessment determined that, although Jack was still below grade-level expectations, with explicit and systematic instruction in the components of phonological sensitivity, he was responsive to instruction, could benefit from it, and evidenced authentic progress in shifting to a more analytical approach to alphabetic reading. In a real sense, the plan used with Jack was dynamic in that it allowed the ongoing assessment of Jack's responsiveness to classroom intervention that was sufficiently challenging, but not overwhelming, for him and permitted any necessary modifications to be made as he showed the need for adjustments. At the same time, the intervention plan helped to reduce negative Matthew effects (Stanovich, 2000), because Jack began to see himself as capable of successful learning.

Portfolio Assessment

Portfolio assessment is a systematic, purposeful collection of student work that tells the story of students' efforts, progress, or achievement in certain curriculum areas (Kratcoski, 1998; Mabry, 1999). A portfolio should not be an exhaustive conglomeration of children's work but rather carefully chosen products that represent the learning process. It may or may not be authentic, depending on the context of the products collected, and may include many forms of assessment. Student participation in the selection of portfolio content and in self-reflection, as well as clear reasons for the inclusion of certain works, is vitally important (Salvia & Ysseldyke, 2001).

When planning and evaluating a child's portfolio, the speech-language pathologist should answer the following questions (Kratcoski, 1998; Mabry, 1999; Taylor, 2000):

- What conceptual content and physical format will guide the portfolio?
- What types of products should be included?
- What are the scoring and evaluation criteria?
- What information does the portfolio yield about the child's current development?
- What patterns of performance are evident?
- Where should instruction go next?
- What supports are needed for the next step?

Portfolios can provide information not readily available from other types of assessment. Depending on the assessment focus, portfolio products could include language samples, observations, work samples (e.g., Jack's minibooks), child interest inventories, teacher interviews, peer interviews, student interviews, checklists, and criterion-referenced data. Since multiple products are collected that represent the entire learning process, portfolio assessment allows for a more complete view of the learner. Additionally, portfolio assessment is attractive to parents, since identifying and communicating about specific patterns and processes is more visible due to the direct application to their child's current work (Kratcoski, 1998; Westling & Fox, 2000). For example, changes in Jack's ability to decode more easily were reflected in the increasing difficulty of the minibooks that he could read and that he created. Sharing this aspect of his portfolio with his parents conveyed a real indicator of his continual progress.

Reliability and Validity of Alternative Assessments

As with norm-referenced measures, similar issues surround the reliability and validity of alternative methods of assessment. There is a tendency not to hold alternate assessments to the same standards as traditional assessments, because validity is often difficult to assess when professional judgments are an important basis for evaluation (McMillan, 2001). However difficult it is, it is imperative that the reliability and validity of alternative assessments be considered seriously and every effort made to ensure their technical quality. Table 5.10 outlines the standards for this technical adequacy.

TABLE 5.10	Issues Affecting Reliability and Validity in Alternative Assessments and Strategies to Reduce the Risk of Violations

Category	Issue	Strategies to Reduce Risk
Reliability	• Measurement error • Judgment bias	• Plan multistage assessment • Create scoring criteria carefully • Construct clear and objective scoring rubrics/criteria • Use skilled raters • Use multiple raters
Construct validity	• Theoretical constructs poorly defined; poor definition of instructional process	• Understand personal philosophies of assessment clearly • Define profile of targeted skills clearly (develop table of specifications, rubrics, etc.)
Content validity (Instructional validity—tied to degree of authenticity)	• Unclear definitions of content areas to be assessed	• Plan curriculum-based assessments and portfolio items systematically to make certain a representative sample of both content and process is obtained. • Choose assessment tasks that are highly related to curriculum and the community • Observe systematically in multiple contexts
Criterion-related validity	• Evidence of consistency within a skill and over time needed for prediction	• Obtain multiple examples of same skill (concurrent validity) • Obtain multiple examples of skills over time (predictive validity)

Sources: McMillan, 2001; Salvia & Ysseldyke, 2001.

Reliability.   The reliability, or consistency, of measurement in alternative assessment is highly dependent on the training and skill of the team members involved in the assessment. Because the speech-language pathologist, in concert with other educational team members such as the classroom teacher or reading teacher, will be making joint decisions about the quality of performance, there is room for measurement error similar to norm-referenced measures. Every "examiner" will have different biases and varying levels of skill, which are reflected in their scoring judgments. Well-trained professionals demonstrate more consistency in their judgments than do students-in-training, whose judgments are typically unreliable due to inexperience (Mabry, 1999).

Variability in individual student achievement must also be considered for its effects on measurement error, especially with performance-based measures. For example, the classroom teacher and speech-language pathologist agreed that Lynn, a middle-school student with a language learning disability, needed to work on lexical diversity by expanding on the semantic relationships she expressed in her writing of sentences. Five types of cohesion (semantic ties that relate meaning across sentence boundaries) were identified to be included in an instructional activity, which involved a mini-unit on self-concepts and relationships. The purpose of assessment targeted by the team was to identify improvements in the spontaneous uses of cohesive devices in Lynn's sentence construction. A book report, assigned to culminate the mini-unit, was examined for the type, frequency, and semantically appropriate uses of these cohesive devices. However, the book report could have been written during a week in which Lynn had a bad cold, which influenced her product. Multistage assessment, which is staggered over a longer period of time rather than as a one-time assessment, would strengthen the reliability of judgments. Multistage assessment provides a more comprehensive overview of a student's strengths and needs and facilitates the refinement of more appropriate instructional methods. Using appropriate observational techniques and working collaboratively also serves to diminish sources of measurement error, as well as the judgment bias rooted in either unrealistic or overly flexible beliefs about standards that individual students should meet (McMillan, 2001).

Whether the criterion-referenced interpretations compare individual student performance to predetermined standards or to other students must also be considered in alternative assessments (Herman & Winters, 1994; McMillan, 2001; Shapley & Bush, 1999; Westling & Fox, 2000). Statewide portfolio assessments typically have low reliability and validity mainly because of poorly defined scoring rubrics (Calfee & Perfumo, 1993). When comparing students to others, reliability is heightened by uniform portfolio content, and by raters who are experienced, well trained, and who understand performance criteria (Herman & Winters, 1994; Shapley & Bush, 1999). However, a trade-off is that the need for standardization of portfolio contents may compromise the flexibility necessary to reflect local curriculum and instructional practices.

Validity.   As shown in Table 5.10, construct validity depends largely on a shared frame of reference by all team members about teaching and learning and how these beliefs will be reflected in the overall assessment process and the assessments aims specifically. Agreement is crucial, because the absence of agreement will have significant consequences for both the reliability and validity of any alternative assessment conducted.

Evidence that skills are being measured in a fair and balanced manner that are representative of students' abilities is a necessary prerequisite to support content validity. Content validity in this instance refers to the sample of skills selected to represent achievement and also the context of that selection. In the Lynn example cited under reliability, all cohesive devices being targeted in instruction were being noted. If, however, only one cohesive device was chosen to be representative of her ability, then content validity could be compromised. An additional consideration in this example is that the assessment examined only one genre, a book report, which may not be representative of Lynn's ability to use cohesive devices in other writing genres. For example, certain kinds of cohesion may occur more often in her daily journal writing or in a narrative assignment. Examination of Lynn's use of cohesive devices in a variety of writing genres would establish stronger content validity for the instructional practices that result in skill acquisition.

The instructional validity of alternative assessment is a component of content validity and is related directly to its authenticity, which is a strength of most alternative assessments (Salvia & Ysseldyke, 2000). Tasks used in assessment unrelated to the curriculum or that have no community application may have poor instructional validity, whereas tasks that directly relate to the curriculum have better instructional validity. In Lynn's case, the assessment is related directly to the curriculum and has the potential to demonstrate strong instructional validity. Validity in these instances is not a matter of existence or nonexistence but the degree to which performance on tasks represents instructional goals and outcomes (Mabry, 1999).

Criterion-related validity is the ability to infer a student's performance on a similar skill or to predict performance on this skill in the future. It can be measured through the individual's ability to apply related skills in appropriate situations for appropriate purposes. Support for criterion-related validity depends on the ability to select multiple examples that demonstrate the skill in different situations and the progression of the learning over time (McMillan, 2001). Since no statistical analyses are performed to determine whether a relationship exists between performance and the criterion, evidence must be provided in other ways. Criterion validity is of concern when using performance-based measures, such as a book report. Judgments that are tied to one product often do not allow patterns of performances to emerge. In the Lynn example, the book report genre may have encouraged Lynn to use one form of cohesion more frequently than another. No inference, then, could be made about Lynn's ability to use similar cohesive devices in other forms of writing.

CONCLUSION

In this chapter, we have presented a framework for in-depth language assessment of school-age children, which has three interconnected strands. The first strand embeds assessment within a perspective of language as a multidimensional and dynamic system of human communication that cannot readily be split into independent parts. This holistic view of language should influence the model of assessment that is adopted for answering clinical questions about the language and literacy development of individual children and adolescents, their needs, and how these needs are best addressed through relevant instructional and intervention practices.

The second strand emphasizes the linking of assessment models and methods to two critical elements: the legal requirements of the IDEA and the functional need for a clear bridge between an assessment model and educational standards and grade-level expectations for academic achievement. Across grade levels, these standards and expectations share the attainment of critical literacy through proficiency in using the language tools of reading, writing, and spelling. In the digital world of the twenty-first century, these tools of alphabetic literacy function as gatekeepers for access to other literacies, such as computer and information literacies. Today, multiple literacies are essential for transacting competently as citizens in the global community that now characterizes everyday human communication.

The third strand considers individual outcomes of an assessment model from the perspective of those language-related behaviors that research evidence supports as having a significant relationship to the acquisition of skills in alphabetic literacy. Three domains were identified as focuses of assessment: phonological sensitivity, lexical diversity and its association with morphological sensitivity, and syntactic diversity, which derives its roots from morphosyntactic sensitivity. These areas are not mutually exclusive of each other or of other language domains because of the synergism among the different components of the language system. A key challenge for assessment is to examine these system interactions across the spoken and written modalities. Another assessment challenge is that different clusters of problems may emerge at different points in a child's school career because of the combined effects of developmental changes and social interactional experiences, including instructional experiences. Thus, the methods of assessment selected to describe these system patterns, whether norm-referenced or alternative assessments, should lead to clear directions for interpreting the specific classroom challenges that individual children are facing and potential solutions for assisting them to meet these challenges successfully.

Language is a highly complex human behavior and language assessment is also complex, as well it should be. Unraveling this complexity about an individual child should be approached as an exciting opportunity for problem solving. Effective decision making requires that the well-prepared speech-language pathologist must be armed with considerable professional knowledge about the reciprocity between more advanced language development and literacy learning. The well-prepared speech-language pathologist must also have considerable technical knowledge about the strengths and limitations of any method that will be selected to reveal these complex patterns of performance.

STUDY QUESTIONS

1. How do different models of assessment influence the purposes for assessing children's language? In what ways do the four major purposes for assessment affect decisions made about the focus and methods of assessment?

2. Read this statement carefully: "Literacy is more than learning to read and write." Identify the interactive components of language that guided your recognition of the individual words and understanding of the whole statement. What kinds of content and strategy knowledge did you draw on to interpret the statement's meaning?

3. What are some aspects of phonological sensitivity, lexical diversity, morphophonological sensitivity, and syntactic diversity associated with reading, writing, and spelling? Discuss specific areas that you would include in a comprehensive language evaluation directed to determining a kindergarten-age child's development of necessary skills in emergent literacy.

4. What aspects of phonological sensitivity, lexical diversity, morphophonological sensitivity, and syntactic diversity seem related to the flexible use of reading and writing as tools for learning? Discuss specific areas that you would include in a comprehensive language evaluation of a grade 3 child's abilities to manage critical literacy demands in his or her classroom.

5. Compare differences in the kinds of information obtained from norm-referenced tests versus criterion-referenced tests, including alternative assessment approaches. Then, discuss the reliability and validity concerns of both. Next, focus on how standards for measurement adequacy are similar or different for norm-referenced approaches contrasted with alternative assessment approaches. Finally, justify the situation(s) in which you would recommend using standardized versus non-standardized measures.

6. You are responsible for assessing a 14-year-old female in grade 8 who is suspected of having problems in "semantic and syntactic development" and whose reading skill is the equivalent of grade 2. Using a decision plan that incorporates educational and noneducational outcomes, outline a specific plan of assessment oriented to description of the child's current level of competence. Your goal is to determine whether this child actually has a language impairment. Include in your plan: (a) two answerable question(s) you want to address; (b) the specific areas of linguistic/communicative functioning, to be evaluated; (c) the methods and situations to be selected for assessment; and (d) the procedures to be used. Be sure that the methods you choose, including any standardized tests, are age appropriate and will meet your assessment purposes. Justify the procedures you choose on these bases.

7. Assume that the grade 8 child you assessed in Question 6 is found to be significantly below age/grade expectations in her level of morphophonological sensitivity and syntactic diversity in both oral and written discourse. She is within the normal age range for vocabulary recognition as assessed by a standardized measure, but her teacher reports that, in the classroom, she has a "limited vocabulary" in her writing. Your goal is to maintain this child in the regular classroom setting, thus you are now concerned with determining what supports this child needs to reach her upper level of competence. Outline the additional information you would need to plan an intervention program that meets the child's specific needs and can be integrated with the academic and social requirements of the classroom. What alternative assessment procedures would you use to determine whether the intervention plan is effective over a three-month period of time?

REFERENCES

Allington, R. L., & Baker, K. (1999). Best practices in literacy instruction for children with special needs. In L. B. Gambell, L. M. Morrow, S. B. Neuman, & M. Pressley (Eds.), *Best practices in literacy instruction* (pp. 292–310). New York: Guilford Press.

Anglin, J. M. (1993). Vocabulary development: A morphological analysis. *Monographs of the Society for Research in Child Development, 58* (10, Serial No. 238).

Apel, K. (1999). Checks and balances: Keeping the science in our profession. *Language, Speech, and Hearing Services in Schools, 30,* 98–107.

Bashir, A. S., Conte, B. M., & Heerde, S. M. (1998). Language and school success: Collaborative challenges and choices. In D. M. Meritt & B. Culatta (Eds.), *Language intervention in the classroom* (pp. 1–36). San Diego, CA: Singular.

Bashir, A. S., Goldhammer, R. F., & Bigaj, S. J. (2000). Facilitating self-determination abilities in adults with LLD: Case study of a postsecondary student. *Topics in Language Disorders, 21*(1), 52–67.

Bashir, A. S., & Strominger, A. Z. (1996). Children with developmental language disorders: Outcomes, persistence, and change. In M. D. Smith & J. S. Damico (Eds.), *Childhood language disorders* (pp. 119–140). New York: Thieme.

Bateman, B. D. (1995). Who, how, and where: Special education issues in perpetuity. In J. M. Kaufman & D. P. Hallahan (Eds.), *The illusion of full inclusion: A comprehensive critique of a special education bandwagon* (pp. 75–90). Austin, TX: Pro-Ed.

Bates, E., Vicari, S., & Trauner, D. (1999). Neural mediation of language development: Perspectives from lesion studies of infants and children. In H. Tager-Flusberg (Ed.), *Neurodevelopmental disorders* (pp. 533–581). Cambridge, MA: MIT Press.

Battle, D. E. (in press). Legal issues in serving postsecondary students with disabilities. In K. G. Butler & E. R. Silliman (Eds.), *Speaking, reading, and writing in children with language learning disabilities: New paradigms for research and practice*. Mahwah, NJ: Lawrence Erlbaum.

Bear, D. R., Invernizzi, M., Templeton, S., & Johnston, F. (2000). *Words their way: Word study for phonics, vocabulary, and spelling instruction*. Upper Saddle River, NJ: Merrill.

Berninger, V. W. (2000). Development of language by hand and its connections with language by ear, mouth, and eye. *Topics in Language Disorders, 20*(4), 65–84.

Blachman, B. A. (1994). Early literacy acquisition: The role of phonological awareness. In G. P. Wallach & K. G. Butler (Eds.), *Language learning disabilities in school-age children and adolescents: Some principles and applications* (pp. 253–274). Boston: Allyn & Bacon.

Brinton, B., Fujiki, M., & McKee, L. (1998). The negotiation skills of children with specific language impairment. *Journal of Speech, Language, and Hearing Research, 41,* 927–940.

Brinton, B., Fujiki, M., Montague, E. C., & Hanton, J. L. (2000). Children with language impairment in cooperative work groups: A pilot study. *Language, Speech, and Hearing Services in Schools, 31,* 252–264.

Burns, M., Griffin, P., & Snow, C. E. (1999). *Starting out right: A guide to promoting children's reading success*. Washington, DC: National Academy Press.

Calfee, R. C., & Perfumo, P. (1993). Student portfolios: Opportunities for a revolution in assessment. *Journal of Reading, 36,* 532–537.

Carlisle, J. F. (1987). The use of morphological knowledge in spelling derived forms by learning-disabled and normal students. *Annals of Dyslexia, 9,* 247–266.

Casby, M. W. (1992). The cognitive hypothesis and its influence on speech-language services in schools. *Language, Speech, and Hearing Services in Schools, 23,* 198–202.

Catts, H. W. (1991) Early identification of reading disabilities. *Topics in Language Disorders, 12*(1), 1–16.

Catts, H. W. (1993). The relationship between speech-language impairments and reading disabilities. *Journal of Speech and Hearing Research, 36,* 948–958.

Catts, H. W., Fey, M. E., Zhang, X. & Tomblin, J. B. (1999). Language basis of reading and reading disabilities: Evidence from a longitudinal investigation. *Scientific Studies of Reading, 3,* 331–361.

Catts, H. W., Hu, C.-F., Larrivee, L., & Swank, L. (1994). Early identification of reading disabilities in children with speech-language impairments. In R. V. Watkins & M. L. Rice

(Eds.), *Specific language impairments in children* (pp. 145–160). Baltimore: Paul H. Brookes.

Catts, H. W., & Kamhi, A. G. (1999). Causes of reading disabilities. In H. W. Catts and A. G. Kamhi (Eds.), *Language and reading disabilities* (pp. 95–127). Boston: Allyn & Bacon.

Center for Research on Evaluation, Standards, and Student Testing (CRESST) (1998). *Writing framework and specifications for the 1998 National Assessment of Educational Progress.* Washington, DC: National Assessment Governing Board.

Chapman, R. S. (1991). Models of language disorders. In J. Miller (Ed.), *Research on child language disorders: A decade of progress* (pp. 287–297). Austin, TX: Pro-Ed.

Clark-Klein, S., & Hodson, B. W. (1995). A phonologically based analysis of misspellings by third graders with disordered-phonology histories. *Journal of Speech and Hearing Research, 38,* 839–849.

Cole, K. N., & Fey, M. E. (1996). Cognitive referencing in language assessment. In K. N. Cole, P. S. Dale, & D. J. Thal (Eds.), *Assessment of communication and language* (pp. 143–160). Baltimore: Paul H. Brookes.

Coutinho, M., & Malouf, D. (1992). Performance assessment and children with disabilities: Issues and possibilities. *Teaching Exceptional Children, 25*(4), 62–67.

Crago, M. B., & Gopnik, M. (1994). From families to phentotypes: Theoretical and clinical implications of research into the genetic basis of specific language impairment. In R. V. Watkins & M. L. Rice (Eds.), *Specific language impairment in children* (pp. 35–51). Baltimore: Paul H. Brookes.

Damico, J. S. (1991). Descriptive assessment of communicative ability in limited English proficient students. In E. V. Hamayan & J. S. Damico (Eds.), *Limiting bias in the assessment of bilingual students* (pp. 157–217). Austin, TX: Pro-Ed.

DiMeo, J. H., Merritt, D. D., & Culatta, B. (1998). Collaborative partnerships and decision making. In D. D. Merritt & B. Culatta (Eds.), *Language intervention in the classroom* (pp. 37–97). San Diego, CA: Singular.

Donahue, M. L. (1994). Differences in classroom discourse styles of students with learning disabilities. In D. N. Ripich & N. A. Creaghead (Eds.), *School discourse problems* (2d ed.) (pp. 229–261). San Diego, CA: Singular.

Donahue, M. L. (in press). "Hanging with friends": Making sense of research on peer discourse in children with language and learning disabilities. In K. G. Butler & E. R. Silliman (Eds.), *Speaking, reading, and writing in children with language learning disabilities: New paradigms for research and practice.* Mahwah, NJ: Lawrence Erlbaum.

Donahue, M. L., Szymanski, C. M., & Flores, C. W. (1999). When "Emily Dickinson" met "Steven Spielberg": Assessing social information processing in literacy contexts. *Language, Speech, and Hearing Services in Schools, 30,* 274–284.

Ehren, B. (1994). New directions for meeting the academic needs of adolescents with learning disabilities. In G. P. Wallach & K. G. Butler (Eds.), *Language learning disabilities in school-age children and adolescents: Some principles and applications* (pp. 393–417). Boston: Allyn & Bacon.

Ehren, B. J. (2000). Views of cognitive referencing from the pragmatist's lens. *Newsletter of the Special Interest Division 1, Language Learning and Education, American Speech-Language-Hearing Association, 7*(1), 3–8.

Ehri, L. C. (2000). Learning to read and learning to spell: Two sides of a coin. *Topics in Language Disorders, 20*(3), 19–36.

Elliott, S. N. (1994). *Creating meaningful performance assessments: Fundamental concepts.* Reston, VA: Council for Exceptional Children.

Elman, J. L., Bates, E. A., Johnson, M. H., Karmiloff-Smith, A., Parisi, D., & Plunkett, K. (1996). *Rethinking innateness: A connectionist perspective on development.* Cambridge, MA: MIT Press.

Elmore, R. F. (1999–2000, Winter). Building a new structure for school leadership. *American Educator, 23*(4), 6–13, 42–44.

Florida Department of Education (1996). *Sunshine State Standards.* http://www.firn.edu/doe/curric/prek12/frame2.htm

Forest, M., & Lusthaus, E. (1990). Everyone belongs with the MAPS Action Planning System. *Teaching Exceptional Children, 22*(2), 32–35.

Friel-Patti, S. (1999a). Specific language impairment: Continuing clinical concerns. *Topics in Language Disorders, 20*(1), 1–13.

Friel-Patti, S. (1999b). Clinical decision making in the assessment and intervention of central auditory processing disorders. *Language, Speech, and Hearing Services in Schools, 30,* 345–352.

Fujiki, M., Brinton, B., Hart, C., & Fitzgerald, A. (1999). Peer acceptance and friendship in children with specific language impairment. *Topics in Language Disorders, 19*(2), 34–48.

Gardner, H. (2000). *The disciplined mind: Beyond facts and standardized tests, the K–12 education that every child deserves.* New York: Penguin Books.

Giangreco, M. F. (2000). Related services research for students with low-incidence disabilities: Implications for speech-language pathologists in the classroom. *Language, Speech, and Hearing Services in Schools, 31,* 230–239.

Gilger, J. W. (1995). Behavioral genetics: Concepts for research and practice in language development and disorders. *Journal of Speech and Hearing Research, 38,* 1126–1142.

Gillon, G. T. (2000). The efficacy of phonological awareness intervention for children with spoken language impairment. *Language, Speech, and Hearing Services in Schools, 31,* 126–141.

Gottardo, A., Stanovich, K. E., & Siegel, L. S. (1996). The relationships between phonological sensitivity, syntactic processing, and verbal working memory in the reading performance of third-grade children. *Journal of Experimental Psychology, 63,* 563–582.

Graham, G., & Harris, K. R. (1999). Assessment and intervention in overcoming writing difficulties: An illustration from the self-regulated strategy development model. *Language, Speech, and Hearing Services in Schools, 30,* 255–264.

Graham, S., Harris, K. R., & Troia, G. A. (2000). Self-regulated strategy development revisited: Teaching writing strategies to struggling writers. *Topics in Language Disorders, 20*(4), 1–14.

Gray, S., Plante, E., Vance, R., & Henrichsen, M. (1999). The diagnostic accuracy of four vocabulary tests administered to preschool-age children. *Language, Speech, and Hearing Services in Schools, 30,* 196–206.

Gutiérrez-Clellen, V. F., Restrepo, M. A., Bedore, L., Peña, E. & Anderson, A. (2000). Language sample analysis in Spanish-speaking children: Methodological considerations. *Language, Speech, and Hearing Services in Schools, 31,* 88–98.

Hakuta, K., & Beatty, A. (Eds.) (2000). *Testing English-language learners in U.S. schools: Report and workshop summary.* Washington, DC: National Academy Press.

Herman, J., & Winters, L. (1994). Portfolio research: A slim collection. *Educational Leadership, 52*(2), 48–55.

Hewitt, L. E. (2000). Does it matter what your client thinks? The role of theory in intervention: Response to Kamhi. *Language, Speech, and Hearing Services in Schools, 31,* 186–193.

Hodson, B. W. (1994). Helping individuals become intelligible, literate, and articulate: The role of phonology. *Topics in Language Disorders, 14*(2), 1–16.

Hoff, E. (2001). *Language development* (2d ed.). Belmont, CA: Wadsworth/Thomson Learning.

Hutchinson, T. A. (1996). What to look for in the technical manual: Twenty questions for users. *Language, Speech, and Hearing Services in Schools, 27,* 109–121.

Johnston, J. R. (1994). Cognitive abilities of children with language impairment. In R. V. Watkins & M. L. Rice (Eds.), *Specific language impairments in children* (pp. 107–121). Baltimore: Paul H. Brookes.

Jones, E., Southern, W., & Brigham, F. (1998). Curriculum-based assessment: Testing what is taught and teaching what is tested. *Intervention in School and Clinic, 33,* 239–249.

Kamhi, A. G. (1996). Linguistic and cognitive aspects of specific language impairment. In M. D. Smith & J. S. Damico (Eds.), *Childhood language disorders* (pp. 97–116). New York: Thieme.

Kamhi, A. G., & Catts, H. W. (1999a). Language and reading: Convergence and divergence. In H. W. Catts and A. G. Kamhi (Eds.), *Language and reading disabilities* (pp. 1–24). Boston: Allyn & Bacon.

Kamhi, A. G., & Catts, H. W. (1999b). Reading development. In H. W. Catts and A. G. Kamhi (Eds.), *Language and reading disabilities* (pp. 25–49). Boston: Allyn & Bacon.

Kamhi, A. G., & Catts, H. W. (in press). The language basis of reading: Implications of classification and treatment of children with reading disabilities. In K. G. Butler & E. R. Silliman (Eds.), *Speaking, reading, and writing in children with language learning disabilities: New paradigms for research and practice.* Mahwah, NJ: Lawrence Erlbaum.

Kamhi, A. G., & Hinton, L. N. (2000). Explaining individual differences in spelling ability. *Topics in Language Disorders, 20*(3), 37–49.

Kavale, K. A., & Forness, S. R. (2000). History, rhetoric, and reality: Analysis of the inclusion debate. *Remedial and Special Education, 21,* 279–296.

Keogh, B. (in press). Research on reading and reading problems: Findings, limitations, and future directions. In K. G. Butler & E. R. Silliman (Eds.), *Speaking, reading, and writing in children with language learning disabilities: New paradigms for research and practice.* Mahwah, NJ: Lawrence Erlbaum.

Kratcoski, A. (1998). Guidelines for using portfolios in assessment and evaluation. *Language, Speech, and Hearing Services in Schools, 29,* 3–10.

Lahey, M. (1988). *Language development and language disorders.* New York: Macmillan.

Lahey, M., & Edwards, J. (1995). Specific language impairment: Preliminary investigation of factors associated with family history and with patterns of language performance. *Journal of Speech and Hearing Research, 38,* 643–657.

Larrivee, L. S., & Catts, H. W. (1999). Early reading achievement in children with expressive phonological disorders. *American Journal of Speech-Language Pathology, 8*(2), 118–128.

Leonard, L. B. (1998). *Children with specific language impairment.* Cambridge, MA: MIT Press.

Liberman, I. Y., & Shankweiler, D. (1991). Phonology and beginning reading: A tutorial. In L. Rieben & C. A. Perfetti (Eds.), *Learning to read: Basic research and its implications* (pp. 3–17). Hillsdale, NJ: Lawrence Erlbaum.

Locke, J. L. (1994). Gradual emergence of development language disorder. *Journal of Speech and Hearing Research, 37,* 608–616.

Lonigan, C. J., Burgess, S. R., & Anthony, J. L. (2000). Development of emergent literacy and early reading skills in preschool children: Evidence from a latent-variable longitudinal study. *Developmental Psychology, 36,* 596–613.

Lubker, B. B., & Tomblin, J. B. (1998). Epidemiology: Informing clinical practice and research on language disorders of children. *Topics in Language Disorders, 19*(1), 1–26.

Lund, N. J., & Duchan, J. F. (1993). *Assessing children's language in naturalistic contexts* (3d ed.). Englewood Cliffs, NJ: Prentice-Hall.

Mabry, L. (1999). *Portfolios plus: A critical guide to alternative assessment.* Thousand Oaks, CA: Corwin.

Maskel, S. (1999). Transition to the general classroom and content areas. In J. R. Birsh (Ed.), *Multisensory teaching of basic language skills* (pp. 399–419). Baltimore: Paul H. Brookes.

McCarthy, M. M., Cambron-McCabe, N. H., & Thomas, S. B. (1998). *Public school law: Teachers' and students' rights* (4th ed.). Boston: Allyn & Bacon.

McCauley, R. J. (1996). Familiar strangers: Criterion-referenced measures in communication disorders. *Language, Speech, and Hearing Services in Schools, 27,* 122–131.

McCauley, R. J. (2001). *Assessment of language disorders in children.* Mahwah, NJ: Lawrence Erlbaum.

McMillan, J. (2001). *Classroom assessment: Principles and practice for effective instruction.* Boston: Allyn & Bacon.

Meltzer, L., & Reid, D. K. (1994). New directions in the assessment of students with special needs: The shift towards a constructivist perspective. *Journal of Special Education, 28,* 338–355.

Miller, J. (1981). *Assessing language production in children: Experimental procedures.* Austin, TX: Pro-Ed.

Milosky, L. M. (1994). Nonliteral language abilities: Seeing the forest for the trees. In G. P. Wallach & K. G. Butler (Eds.), *Language learning disabilities in school-age children and adolescents: Some principles and applications* (pp. 275–303). Boston: Allyn & Bacon.

Moats, L. C. (2000). *Speech to print: Language essentials for teachers.* Baltimore: Paul H. Brookes.

Morine-Dershimer, G. (1985). *Talking, listening, and learning in elementary classrooms.* New York: Longman.

Mount, B., & Zwernik, K. (1989). *It's never too early, it's never too late: A booklet about personal futures planning.* St. Paul, MN: Metropolitan Council.

Nagy, W. E., & Scott, J. A. (2000). Vocabulary processes. In M. L. Kamil, P. B. Mosenthal, P. D. Pearson, & R. Barr (Eds.), *Handbook of reading research* (Vol. III) (pp. 269–284). Mahwah, NJ: Lawrence Erlbaum.

Nation, N. E., & Aram, D. M. (1991). *Diagnosis of speech and language disorders* (2d ed.). San Diego, CA: Singular.

National Reading Panel (2000). *Teaching children to read: An evidence-based assessment of the scientific research literature on reading and the implications for reading instruction.* Bethesda, MD: NICHD Clearinghouse.

National Research Council (1999). *Improving student learning: A strategic plan for education research and its utilization.* Washington, DC: National Academy Press.

Nelson, N. W. (1998). *Childhood language disorders in context: Infancy through adolescence* (2d ed.). New York: Merrill-Macmillan.

Nelson, N. W. (2000). Basing eligibility on discrepancy criteria: A bad idea whose time has passed. *Newsletter of the Special Interest Division 1, Language Learning and Education, American Speech-Language-Hearing Association, 7*(1), 8–12.

Nippold, M. A. (1998). *Later language development: The school-age years and adolescent years* (2d ed.). Austin, TX: Pro-Ed.

Nunes, T., Bryant, P., & Bindman, M. (1997). Spelling and grammar—The necsed move. In C. A. Perfetti, L. Rieben, & M. Fayol (Eds.), *Learning to spell: Research, theory, and practice across languages* (pp. 151–170). Mahwah, NJ: Lawrence Erlbaum.

Osborne, A. G., Jr. (in press). Legal, administrative, and policy issues in special education. In K. G. Butler & E. R. Silliman (Eds.), *Speaking, reading, and writing in children with language learning disabilities: New paradigms for research and practice.* Mahwah, NJ: Lawrence Erlbaum.

Parnell, M. M. (1995). Characteristics of language disordered children. In H. Winitz (Ed.), *Human communication and its disorders: A review* (Vol. IV) (pp. 171–275). Timonium, MD: York Press.

Paul, R. (1995). *Language disorders from infancy through adolescence.* St. Louis: Mosby.

Pearpoint, J., O'Brien, J., & Forest, M. (1993). *PATH: Planning alternative tomorrows with hope.* Toronto, Canada: Inclusion Press.

Peterson, H. A., & Marquardt, T. P. (1994). *Appraisal and diagnosis of speech and language disorders* (3d ed.). Englewood Cliffs, NJ: Prentice-Hall.

Plante, E., & Vance, R. (1994). Selection of preschool speech and language tests: A data-based approach. *Language, Speech, and Hearing Services in Schools, 25,* 15–24.

Prelock, P. (in press). Communicating with peers in the classroom context: The next steps. In K. G. Butler & E. R. Silliman (Eds.), *Speaking, reading, and writing in children with language learning disabilities: New paradigms for research and practice.* Mahwah, NJ: Lawrence Erlbaum.

Radford, A., Atkinson, M., Britain, D., Clahsen, H., & Spencer, A. (1999). *Linguistics: An introduction.* Cambridge, UK: Cambridge University Press.

Redmond, S. M., & Rice, M. L. (1998). The socioemotional behaviors of children with SLI: Social adaptation or social deviance? *Journal of Speech, Language, and Hearing Research, 41,* 688–700.

Ricciardelli, L. A. (1993). Two components of metalinguistic awareness: Control of linguistic processing and analysis of linguistic knowledge. *Applied Psycholinguistics, 14,* 349–367.

Rice, M. L. (1999). Specific grammatical limitations in children with specific language impairment. In H. Tager-Flusberg (Ed.), *Neurodevelopmental disorders* (pp. 331–359). Cambridge, MA: MIT Press.

Rice, M. L., Cleave, P. L., & Oetting, J. B. (2000). The use of syntactic cues in lexical acquisition by children with SLI. *Journal of Speech, Language, and Hearing Research, 43,* 582–594.

Rice, M. L., & Wexler, K. (1996). A phenotype of specific language impairment: Extended optional infinitives. In M. L. Rice (Ed.), *Toward a genetics of language* (pp. 215–237). Mahwah, NJ: Lawrence Erlbaum.

Rice, M. L., Wexler, K., Marquis, J., & Hershberger, S. (2000). Acquisition of irregular past tense by children with specific language impairment. *Journal of Speech, Language, and Hearing Research, 43,* 1126–1145.

Salvia, J., & Ysseldyke, J. E. (2001). *Assessment* (8th ed.). Boston: Houghton Mifflin.

Scarborough, H. S. (1998). Early identification of children at risk for reading disabilities: Phonological awareness and some other promising predictors. In B. K. Shapiro, P. J. Accardo, & A. J. Capute (Eds.), *Specific reading disability: A view of the spectrum* (pp. 75–107). Timonium, MD: York Press.

Scarborough, H. S. (in press). Connecting early language and literacy to later reading (dis)abilities: Evidence, theory, and practice. In S. Neuman & D. Dickinson (Eds.), *Handbook for research in early literacy.* New York: Guilford.

Scott, C. M. (1988a). Producing complex sentences. *Topics in Language Disorders, 8*(2), 42–62.

Scott, C. M. (1988b). Spoken and written syntax. In M. Nippold (Ed.), *Later language development: Ages nine through nineteen* (pp. 49–95). Boston: College-Hill.

Scott, C. M. (1995). Syntax for school-age children: A discourse perspective. In M. E. Fey, J. Windsor, & S. F. Warren (Eds.), *Language intervention: Preschool through the elementary years* (pp. 107–143). Baltimore, MD: Paul H. Brookes.

Scott, C. M. (1999). Learning to write. In H. W. Catts & A. G. Kamhi (Eds.), *Language and reading disabilities* (pp. 224–258). Boston: Allyn & Bacon.

Scott, C. M. (2000). Principles and methods of spelling instruction: Applications for poor spellers. *Topics in Language Disorders, 20*(3), 66–82.

Scott, C. M. (in press). A fork in the road less traveled: Writing intervention based on language profile. In K. G. Butler & E. R. Silliman (Eds.), *Speaking, reading, and writing in children with language learning disabilities: New paradigms for research and practice.* Mahwah, NJ: Lawrence Erlbaum.

Scott, C. M., & Stokes, S. L. (1995). Measures of syntax in school-age children and adolescents. *Language, Speech, and Hearing Services in Schools, 26,* 309–319.

Scott, C. M., & Windsor, J. (2000). General language performance measures in spoken and written narrative and expository discourse of school-age children with language learning disabilities. *Journal of Speech, Language, and Hearing Research, 43,* 324–339.

Semel, E., Wiig, E. H., & Secord, W. A. (1995). *Clinical Evaluation of Language Fundamentals—3.* San Antonio, TX: Psychological Corporation.

Shapley, K., & Bush, M. (1999). Developing a valid and reliable portfolio assessment in the primary grades: Building on practical experience. *Applied Measurement in Education, 12*(2), 11–32.

Shonkoff, J. P., & Phillips, D. A. (2000). *From neurons to neighborhoods: The science of early child development.* Washington, DC: National Academy Press.

Shulman, B. B., Katz, K. B., & Sherman, T. (1995). Language and assessment: Current issues and anticipated trends. *Diagnostique, 20*(1–4), 53–69.

Silliman, E. R., Bahr, R. H., Turner, C. R., & Wilkinson, L. C. (in press). Language variation and struggling readers. In K. G. Butler & E. R. Silliman (Eds.), *Speaking, reading, and writing in children with language learning disabilities: New paradigms for research and practice.* Mahwah, NJ: Lawrence Erlbaum.

Silliman, E. R., Ford, C. S., Beasman, J., & Evans, D. (1999). An inclusion model for children with language learning disabilities: Building classroom partnerships. *Topics in Language Disorders, 19*(3), 1–18.

Silliman, E. R., Jimerson, T. L., & Wilkinson, L. C. (2000). A dynamic systems approach to writing assessment in students with language learning problems. *Topics in Language Disorders 20*(4), 45–64.

Silliman, E. R., & Wilkinson, L. C. (1991). *Communicating for learning: Classroom observation and collaboration.* Gaithersburg, MD: Aspen.

Singer, B. D., & Bashir, A. S. (1999). What are executive functions and self-regulation and what do they have to do with language-learning disorders? *Language, Speech, and Hearing Services in Schools, 30,* 265–273.

Snell, F., & Brown, M. (2000). *Instruction of students with severe disabilities.* Englewood Cliffs, NJ: Prentice-Hall.

Snow, C. E., Burns, M. S., & Griffin, P. (1998). *Preventing reading difficulties in young children.* Washington, DC: National Academy Press.

Stanovich, K. E. (1999). The sociopsychometrics of learning disabilities. *Journal of Learning Disabilities, 32,* 350–361.

Stanovich, K. E. (2000). *Progress in understanding reading: Scientific foundations and new frontiers.* New York: Guilford.

Strong, C. J. (1998). *The Strong Narrative Assessment Procedure (SNAP).* Eau Claire, WI: Thinking Publications.

Swank, L. K., & Catts, H. W. (1994). Phonological awareness and written word decoding. *Language, Speech, & Hearing Services in Schools, 25,* 9–14.

Tallal, P., Miller, S. L., Jenkins, W. M., & Merzenich, M. M. (1997). The role of temporal processing in developmental language-based learning disorders: Research and clinical implications. In B. Blachman (Ed.), *Foundations of reading acquisition and dyslexia: Implications for early intervention* (pp. 49–66). Mahwah, NJ: Lawrence Erlbaum.

Tager-Flusberg, H. (2001). Putting words together: Morphology and syntax in the preschool years. In J. Berko Gleason (Ed.), *The development of language* (5th ed.). Boston: Allyn & Bacon.

Taylor, R. L. (2000). *Assessment of exceptional students: Educational and psychological procedures* (5th ed.). Boston: Allyn & Bacon.

Templeton, S., & Morris, D. (2000). Spelling. In M. L. Kamil, P. B. Mosenthal, P. D. Pearson, & R. Barr (Eds.), *Handbook of reading research* (Vol. III) (pp. 525–543). Mahwah, NJ: Lawrence Erlbaum.

Thurlow, M. L., House A. L., Scott, D. L., & Ysseldyke, J. E. (2000). Students with disabilities in large-scale assessments: State participation and accommodation polices. *Journal of Special Education, 34,* 154–163.

Tomblin, J. B. (1989). Familial concentration of developmental language impairment. *Journal of Speech and Hearing Disorders, 54,* 287–295.

Tomblin, J. B., & Zhang, X. (1999). Language patterns and etiology in children with specific language impairment. In H. Tager-Flusberg (Ed.), *Neurodevelopmental disorders* (pp. 361–382). Cambridge, MA: MIT Press.

Torgesen, J. K., Alexander, A. W., Wagner, R. K., Rashotte, C. A., Voeller, K. K. S., & Conway, T. (2001). Intensive remedial instruction for children with severe reading disabilities: Immediate and long-term outcomes from two instructional approaches. *Journal of Learning Disabilities, 34,* 33–58, 78.

Torgesen, J. K., & Wagner, R. K. (1998). Alternative diagnostic approaches for specific developmental reading disabilities. *Learning Disabilities Research & Practice, 13,* 220–232.

Treiman, R. (1993). *Beginning to spell.* New York: Oxford University Press.

Treiman, R., & Bourassa, D. C. (2000). The development of spelling skill. *Topics in Language Disorders, 20*(3), 1–18.

Tunmer, W. E., & Chapman, J. W. (1998). Language prediction skill, phonological recoding ability, and beginning reading. In C. Hulme & R. M. Joshi (Eds.), *Reading and spelling: Development and disorders* (pp. 33–67). Mahwah, NJ: Lawrence Erlbaum.

Tyner, K. (1998). *Literacy in a digital world: Teaching and learning in the age of information.* Mahwah, NJ: Lawrence Erlbaum.

Villa, R., & Thousand, J. (1995). *Creating an inclusive school.* Alexandria, VA: Association for Supervision and Curriculum Development.

Wagner, R. K., Torgesen, J. K., & Rashotte, C. A. (1999). *Comprehensive Test of Phonological Processing.* Austin, TX: Pro-Ed.

Wallach, G. P. & Butler, K. G. (1994). Creating communication, literacy, and academic success. In G. P. Wallach & K. G. Butler (Eds.), *Language learning disabilities in school-age children and adolescents: Some principles and applications* (pp. 2–26). Boston: Allyn & Bacon.

Washington, J. A., & Craig, H. K. (2001). Language variation and literacy acquisition in African American students. In J. L. Harris, A. G. Kamhi, & K. E. Pollock (Eds.), *Literacy in African American communities* (pp. 147–168). Mahwah, NJ: Lawrence Erlbaum.

Westby, C. (in press). Beyond decoding: Critical and dynamic literacy for students with dyslexia, LLD, or ADHD. In K. G. Butler & E. R. Silliman (Eds.), *Speaking, reading, and writing in children with language learning disabilities: New paradigms for research and practice.* Mahwah, NJ: Lawrence Erlbaum.

Westby, C. E., & Clauser, P. S. (1999). The right stuff for writing: Assessing and facilitating written language. In H. W. Catts & A. G. Kamhi (Eds.), *Language and reading disabilities* (pp. 259–324). Boston: Allyn & Bacon.

Westling, D. L., & Fox, L. (2000). *Teaching students with severe disabilities* (2d ed.). Upper Saddle River, NJ: Merrill.

Whitmire, K. (2000a). Action: School services. *Language, Speech, and Hearing Services in Schools, 31,* 194–199.

Whitmire, K. (2000b). Cognitive referencing and discrepancy formulae: Comments from ASHA resources. *Newsletter of the Special Interest Division 1, Language Learning and Education, American Speech-Language-Hearing Association, 7*(1), 13–16.

Windsor, J. (1994). Children's comprehension and production of derivational suffixes. *Journal of Speech and Hearing Research, 37,* 408–417.

Windsor, J., Scott, C. M., & Street, C. K. (2000). Verb and noun morphology in the spoken and written language of children with language learning disabilities. *Journal of Speech, Language, and Hearing Research, 43,* 1322–1336.

Witt, J., Elliott, S., Daly, E., Gresham, F., & Kramer, J. (1998). *Assessment of at-risk and special needs children.* Boston: McGraw-Hill.

CHAPTER 6

Planning Language Intervention for Young Children

Amy L. Weiss
University of Iowa

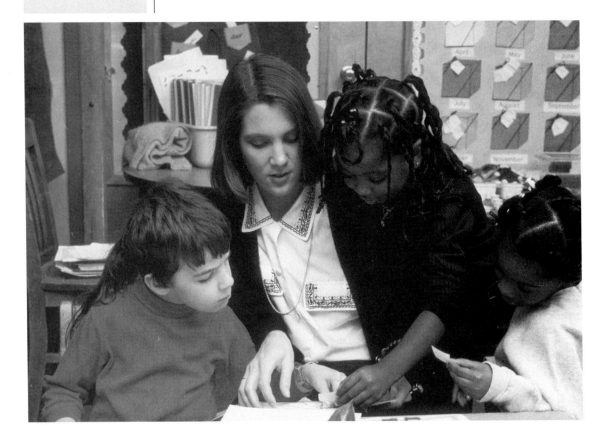

When you finish this chapter you should be able to

- Discuss how SLPs develop language intervention programs for young, preschool age children
- Understand the changes in federal legislation that have mandated provision of services for young children with disabilities and how they have affected the role and responsibilities of SLPs in designing treatment programs for children of preschool age
- Select goal attack strategies and appropriate goals for intervention programs with preschool age children
- Identify a series of intervention techniques that can be used to teach new language forms and functions to young, preschool age children
- Facilitate generalization of language goals from therapeutic contexts to non-treatment settings
- Explain how recent research findings from investigations of treatment efficacy with preschool age children have changed recommendations for best practices in treatment with this population

In this chapter, readers will be challenged to think about language intervention planning and implementation with young children as dynamic processes that are driven by a young client's changing abilities and needs, the clinical skills and experience of speech-language pathologists (hereafter designated as SLPs), and those of additional support personnel, as well as the less easily measured environmental factors that impinge on language development and use, such as caregiver input and the child's opportunities for social interaction with peers. In addition, the alternatives for intervention context will be explored, including suggestions for choosing among those alternatives. A case will also be made for the importance of thorough generalization planning when we first design our treatment protocols; the reader will be introduced to several methods useful for increasing the likelihood that generalization and maintenance of competencies will occur as a result of the language intervention provided. It will also be made obvious to the reader that the general principles of working with young children who have language disorders are really the same general principles used with any population with a communication disorder.

WHAT IS LANGUAGE INTERVENTION?

The Demographics of Early Language Disorder

According to research findings compiled by the American Speech-Language-Hearing Association (2000b), hereafter referred to as ASHA, language disorders are found in approximately 8 to 12 percent of the preschool population. Estimates of the occurrence of specific language impairment (SLI), where other developmental systems (e.g., cognitive, socioemotional, and physical) appear to be intact and functioning within normal limits, average around 7.4 percent of the kindergarten-age population (Tomblin, Records, Buckwalter, Zhang, Smith, & O'Brien, 1997). These percentages are related to the approximately 571,000 students in the age range of 3 to 5 years who were diagnosed with disabilities and who received special education services for the 1997–1998 school year (Office of Special Education Programs, 1999) under the auspices of the Preschool Grants Program that represents Part B of the Individuals with Disabilities Act (IDEA). Additional studies that have examined the development of speech and language in late talkers have reported that a significant proportion of these children, identified prior to their second birthdays and delayed in both expressive and receptive language, remained delayed in language development when 3 years of age (Thal, 1999), and thus carried with them a higher risk for a later diagnosis of a learning disability (Stothard, Snowling, Bishop, Chipchase, & Kaplan, 1998). This latter finding is particularly important because it supports the need for aggressive and comprehensive programs for early identification and intervention of communication problems.

In addition to facing the challenges posed by the numbers of service recipients as intimated above, SLPs have been made increasingly aware over the last couple of decades of the changing makeup of the national caseload in terms of cultural diversity (Cole, 1989; Battle, 1998). More than 10 years ago, Cole (1989) noted that SLPs need to be aware of the multicultural issues that face the profession, among them: (1) there are now more individuals representing minorities on caseloads; (2) more minority children are born at risk for communication disorders; (3) the non-European American presents with different etiologies and prevalences for disorders; (4) there is less normative data available for nonmajority populations; (5) there are different perspectives on the concepts of health and disorder to be addressed in different cultures; (6) there is greater opportunity for conflicts in the intervention context based on cultural differences; (7) there are differences in service delivery preference from the mainstream; and (8) there is a greater incidence of linguistic differences within nonmajority populations. One contribution to why these facts have remained challenges is the stability in the demographics of the ASHA membership. As the 1999 ASHA membership and affiliation counts showed, only 7.6 percent of ASHA members described themselves as belonging to a racial or ethnic minority group. This number remains low when compared with the proportion of racial and ethnic minorities in the United States (17.7 percent), and it represents no appreciable change in the racial or ethnic makeup of the ASHA membership over the past several years (Janota, 1999). Besides identifying themselves as members of the majority culture, the vast majority of ASHA members are also monolingual (Screen & Anderson, 1994), which adds to the difficulty of providing appropriate services to all children with language disorders (ASHA, 1985). As will be discussed later in this chapter, the issue of cultural differences is a critical one in the development of appropriate intervention programming for young children, as it is for all of SLP clients.

The difficulty of providing appropriate service delivery to children who are culturally and linguistically different is national in scope (Goldstein, 2000). Roseberry-McKibben & Eicholtz (1994) reported findings from their national survey investigating how children who were diagnosed as limited English proficient (LEP) were serviced in the schools. They found that although treatment focusing on language was what was most often provided by the more than 1,100 SLPs who replied to the survey, more than 90 percent of them did not speak the language (most often Spanish) spoken by their clients well enough to provide treatment themselves in that language. In addition, the authors noted that more than three-quarters of their respondents indicated that they had not completed any course work designed to prepare them for working with children who were LEP. Clearly, our profession needs to continue to emphasize ways of infusing multicultural information into the curricula of our graduate programs and providing adequate continuing education opportunities so that practitioners can better meet the needs of their diverse clientele.

Why Early Language Intervention Is Needed

Several investigators have studied young children with language disorders over time and determined that disorders of language first identified in childhood often continue to be a part of the social and communicative life of the individual and are not easily outgrown (Aram, Ekelman, & Nation, 1984; Hall & Tomblin, 1978; Stothard et al., 1998; Records, Tomblin, & Freese, 1992). So language disorders in children not only exist, they have the potential to be a problem of long standing for the children themselves, their families, school personnel, SLPs charged with the responsibility of teaching them, and perhaps society as a whole.

Moreover, because the needs for competent language use are pervasive in our daily lives, if a person's language abilities are just functional, that person will likely lead a life that is compromised in some respect. Consider the role played by language in establishing and maintaining relationships between friends, colleagues, and loved ones, or in functioning as a productive member of a society through one's career, civic, and social activities. It is because language is such an integral part of our lives that the development of techniques to augment the language learning abilities of young children who exhibit language disorders is a very important charge to SLPs, caregivers, and others who work with this population.

Ramey and Ramey (1998, pp. 115–117) delineated six principles—mostly intuitive—for enhancing success that emerged from their review of the research literature describing the effectiveness of early intervention provided for children identified as at risk for developmental disorders. SLPs should take note of these principles as good rationales for early initiation of their own work with families who have children with developmental language disorders. These investigators were struck by the converging data that clearly suggested the following:

1. A "principle of developmental timing" suggests that the earlier an intervention is begun and the longer it continues, the more benefit it will have versus intervention programs that are begun later and are of shorter duration.
2. A "principle of program intensity" suggests that programs that are designed to be more intensive in nature, in terms of the amount of contact between the interventionist(s) as well as the degree to which the family participates in the designated program, will be more successful.
3. A "principle of direct versus intermediary provision of learning experiences" suggests that programs that focus directly on delivery of services to children rather than on training parents, or other caregivers to provide the treatment, are more successful.

4. A "principle of program breadth and flexibility" suggests that comprehensive programs that address the needs of the child and family in multiple ways are more likely to yield positive results than a program that takes a more limited perspective of intervention services.
5. A "principle of individual differences in program benefits" suggests that not all children will benefit equally from the services provided and that one strong predictor of which children will benefit more from an intervention is probably the child's status at the beginning of treatment.
6. A "principle of ecological domain and environmental maintenance of development" suggests that unless there is an environmental support system in place to help maintain the skills learned by the child through the intervention program, it is unlikely that the gains made by the child will be maintained over time.

Taken together, these principles provide SLPs with a great deal of direction in terms of their recommendations for programming when young children with diagnosed language disorders or those at risk for developing language disorders are being considered.

A Definition of Language Intervention and Interventionists

According to the 1999 Omnibus Survey conducted by the ASHA (Janota, 1999), the majority of this sample's SLPs who worked in either schools or nonresidential health care settings regularly served children diagnosed with language disorders. Taking the diagnoses of autism/PDD, ADHD, learning disabilities, and "Other" (including in that category children meeting the definition of SLI) into account and considering SLPs in hospitals and residential health care facilities together with those employed in schools and nonresidential health care facilities, 70 percent of their caseloads is made up of children with language disorders. In the school employment setting alone, this average was as high as 95 percent. Thus, SLPs are frequently working with clients with the diagnosis of childhood language disorders.

There have been at least three recent changes in how we perceive our roles and enact them with the population of young children with language disorders. With the advent of collaborative models, the responsibility for language facilitation is often shared with classroom teachers. (See Chapter 3 for more information on this topic.)

In a second and related change, transdisciplinary teaming models are becoming more frequently instituted than the more traditional multidisciplinary and interdisciplinary team approaches, where multiple professionals are involved in the planning and provision of young children's treatment programs. The concept of "role release," indigenous to the transdisciplinary teaming model, allows team members to transcend the typical boundaries of their disciplinary training, where necessary, to provide clients with comprehensive service delivery. For example, SLPs working to facilitate accurate articulatory productions in a child with cerebral palsy may work to reduce the child's hypertonicity before beginning speech activities, a goal usually reserved for the physical therapist. In both situations the roles and responsibilities of SLPs have shifted to meet the demands posed by changes in service delivery models.

The third major change to the role that SLPs play in their treatment of language disorders in young children is in the renewed efforts—mandated by the Individuals with Disabilities Education Act (hereafter IDEA)—to provide family-focused intervention, where the functioning of the child's family unit is viewed as being inextricably tied to the child's treatment and the appropriate context for intervention (Pletcher, 1995). The family systems approach acknowledges that the family's strengths and needs must be accounted for and addressed by the intervention program. Federal law requires that families be included in the planning of the intervention program of their young children, assisting professionals in choosing among possible treatment plans and helping to prioritize goals in treatment, after their involvement in the assessment procedures that yielded the data for intervention planning. (See Chapter 3 for a more comprehensive accounting of how federal legislation has affected service delivery options for the preschool population.)

For the purposes of this chapter, language intervention is defined as the careful planning, manipulation, and implementation of instructional contexts designed to facilitate language learning. Depending on the needs and abilities of the client and his or her family, programs of language intervention will differ in terms of *who* is involved in the intervention, *where* the intervention takes place, *what* the specific goals of the treatment are, and the *degree of structure* imposed on the client within the instructional context.

It is important for student SLPs to recognize that the goal of language intervention, or any type of intervention, is to make itself and the job of the clinician obsolete. That is, the objective of any language intervention program is to eliminate its rationale for existence by demonstrating that the client is ready for dismissal. This can be done in at least two ways. One is to help the client become his or her own clinician through the development of accurate self-monitoring skills. The client must therefore learn strategies to facilitate new learning for examples not specifically taught in a therapeutic setting. That would be a demonstration of generalization. Once the client has demonstrated correct discrimination between acceptable and unacceptable language productions (or effective and ineffective communication), one of the essential competencies necessary for achieving generalization to these new, untrained contexts has been acquired. Once self-monitoring is established, the client can extend learning without the clinician's input.

Another perspective on "planned obsolescence" involves demonstrating that the client has the language competencies typically observed in normally developing individuals similar to the client in age, education, and culture. Here, techniques for future learning do not appear to be as important as being able to show that the client is presently a successful communicator in all settings in which language is used. For some of our clients, particularly those considered to be culturally or linguistically different, this may involve the use of code-switching or changing from one language or dialect system to another as called for by changing communication contexts.

Appropriate dismissal criteria are those that indicate that treatment services can be removed without an appreciable loss of the gains made by the client through therapy and that additional intervention services are not likely to be needed in the future (Fey, 1988; Olswang & Bain, 1985). So, although it is very important to demonstrate generalization, the child's ability to maintain the gains made in treatment over time once treatment is withdrawn is equally critical. Dismissal from treatment is never an irrevocable decision (Fey, 1988), however. Should a client demonstrate an inability to maintain the new competencies learned in treatment following dismissal, reinstatement into treatment is a possible avenue. The 1997 revision of the Individuals with Disabilities Education Act (hereafter IDEA) defined dismissal criteria from speech and language intervention when one or more of the following conditions are met (ASHA, 2000a):

- The child's parents request that the child no longer receive services.
- All objectives set for the child have been met and no further errors require intervention.
- Measurable benefits from treatment can no longer be documented although attempts have been made to modify strategies used.
- The child's educational performance is no longer affected by his or her language disorder.
- Lack of motivation on the part of the child to participate in treatment.
- The presence of circumstances that may be transient or permanent in nature that prevent the child from benefiting from treatment.
- Special education or other related services are no longer necessary for this child to receive educational services in the mainstream.

This chapter serves as an introduction to some of what we *do* know about language intervention with young children and the thinking that takes place when many SLPs formulate plans for a young child with a language disorder.

THE ROLE OF SPEECH-LANGUAGE CLINICIANS IN EARLY LANGUAGE INTERVENTION

The Efficacy of Early Language Intervention

As already noted (Ramey & Ramey, 1998), it is generally agreed that where identification of communication and language disorders is concerned, earlier is better, whether the etiology of the problem is genetic or due to environmental agents (Warren & Kaiser, 1988). Bricker (1986) noted that it is generally accepted that what the child learns early on is needed to support the more sophisticated learning that will follow, and that early intervention allows the opportunity for SLPs as well as other professionals to set up "proper support systems for families and children to inhibit the development of secondary or associated disabilities" (p. 30). Because speech-language disorders have been shown to have both a pervasive and cumulative effect on children's growth and development, waiting to begin intervention may mean that the problem will be significantly greater by the time a program is instituted. Although sometimes unavoidable—either because of lack of availability of services or the need to convince families that language intervention is the best approach—most children stand to lose valuable time in the language-learning process when lengthy delays occur.

Support for the efficacy of early intervention also comes from research studies demonstrating that development during the prelinguistic period is crucial to the acquisition of linguistic competence (Leonard, 1991). In addition, advanced research technologies have allowed investigators to determine that infants know much more about the world around them by the end of the first year of life than had been previously suspected (Rovee-Collier, Lipsitt, & Hayne, 1998). Thus, delays in beginning intervention have the potential effect of putting young children with language disorders even farther behind their normally developing peers than had been previously thought.

There has also been continued interest in the topic of the "late talker" (Kelly, 1998), the child who is delayed in the development of vocabulary and word combinations, sometimes identified as early as 18 months of age but more often identified at about age two (Rescorla, 1989). Although many children identified as "late talkers" go on to catch up with their peers by age three or four, there is still a substantial proportion of children thus identified who continue to demonstrate delays in language development. According to Leonard (1998), most studies point to proportions ranging from 25 to 50 percent of these children. When we look carefully at the studies completed, there are clearly some factors that tend to place the child labeled as a "late talker" at higher risk for ongoing problems, with one of the most common being demonstrated delays in development of *both* receptive and expressive language skills (Olswang, Rodriguez, & Timler, 1998). Leonard (1998) cautioned that it may not yet be possible to make a highly reliable prognosis of which late talkers will go on to demonstrate language disorders throughout their childhoods before the child reaches the age of three, given all of the variability inherent in early language learning. However, he maintained that this cautionary note should not be interpreted as suggesting that intervention for these at-risk children before age three is inappropriate. On the contrary, he suggested, that given the potential for some of these children to fall increasingly behind their peers, early intervention is warranted.

Some language intervention programs for this young population are centered around teaching parents how to interact communicatively with their at-risk or disordered infants and toddlers so that they can capitalize on what the infants are capable of doing (Klein & Briggs, 1987; MacDonald & Carroll, 1992a; Sparks, 1989). Although SLPs must carefully evaluate the infant or toddler in order to carry out this type of program, the focus of direct training will often be primarily on the parents, who will be trained to become the primary therapeutic agents in classroom programs for preschool-age children designed to teach families how best to work with their children to carry over classroom learning into the home environment.

A Continuum of Language Difficulties

Another reason for the burgeoning interest in early language intervention probably came from the recognition that individuals identified in the preschool years as having language disorders are often the same students diagnosed as language learning disabled later on in their academic careers (Aram et al., 1984; King, Jones, & Lasky, 1982). The problem may persist despite the fact that language intervention is provided to many of these children. Findings from follow-up studies of young children who were identified as speech-language disordered consistently demonstrated that the majority of these children were still showing signs of language disorders or additional problems with learning many years after their initial diagnoses. As noted by Maxwell and Wallach (1984), "one myth, that the majority of children 'outgrow' their early language disabilities, is dispelled by this research" (p. 20). Studies of young children identified as language delayed (Rescorla & Schwartz, 1990; Scarborough & Dobrich, 1990) have indicated that catching up to their peers may take longer than once expected.

If language learning difficulties are resistant to change in the long term, how are the lives of our clients affected? Records et al. (1992) studied the quality of life experienced by young adults with life-long language learning disorders. Interestingly, these investigators found that when they were asked about their perceptions of their own life quality, including issues of personal happiness, satisfaction with their lives, and perceived status with regard to education, their occupations, and their families, the subjects' responses were not significantly different from those of a matched control group of young adults with no history of language learning disorders. However, when these two groups of subjects were compared objectively according to income levels and educational achievement, they were clearly different, with the language-disordered group having achieved to a significantly lesser degree. The authors noted that this result led them to conclude that "language impairment seems to be associated with the objective aspects of life, but not with the subjective aspects" (p. 49).

One of the reasons for the long-term effects of language learning difficulties undoubtedly is related to the connection between a child's oral language competencies and acquisition of literacy skills. The connections between the two systems are complicated and are not the same all the way through the developmental process (Wallach & Butler, 1994), so at times spoken language exerts an influence on literacy learning and at other points in the process the development of literacy competencies influences production of spoken text. An example of this is a situation in which a young child, having become familiarized with literate storytelling style through book reading at school, begins to generalize it to accounts of school activities when she is at home. Even when assembling language intervention programs for young children, which are usually focused on expressive oral language production, we should probably keep in mind that we should be purposefully setting the stage for literacy learning at the same time (Catts & Kamhi, 1998).

Snyder (1980) put some of the blame for the long-standing nature of language disorders on the type of intervention services provided. She suggested that the language intervention provided to school-age children diagnosed as language disordered had little effect on making the children sufficiently "mobilized for reading" (p. 40). Specifically, she noted that the ability to make syntactic predictions and inferences were two skills necessary for reading success and that these were not usually addressed in language intervention programs for young children. The author acknowledged that some of the more specific competencies needed to learn reading and writing have been neglected by SLPs who work with preschoolers. More recently, Fey, Catts, and Larrivee (1995) discussed the academic and social demands placed on children in school and suggested ways to prepare preschool-aged children with language impairments for meeting those demands.

Determining the "Wheres" and "Hows" of Language Intervention

As already noted, attitudes and "fashion" with regard to what SLPs call themselves and the clinical services they perform have changed over time (Miller, 1989). Similarly, the settings where speech-language clinicians most commonly perform language intervention have changed. In fact, the changes in typical settings for clinical service have been dramatic over the past several years, in large part due to the substantive changes mandated through federal legislation. This should not be surprising, given that the changes are in keeping with a more general shift in the perception of the role of SLPs as well as increases in the demand for their services. Table 6.1 presents the benefits and drawbacks inherent in three different language intervention settings: (1) the pull-out model, (2) the classroom model, and (3) the collaborative-consultation model. Professionals in the field of speech-language pathology have attempted to address weaknesses in each of the models by developing new models or revising present models, as shown in Figure 6.1.

The Pull-Out Model

Traditionally, SLPs engaged in the "pull-out" model of service delivery for children attending school programs. With classroom programs for preschoolers with disabilities becoming more commonplace, it is likely that this approach has also been used with very young children. In the pull-out model, students are removed from their

TABLE 6.1   **Benefits and Drawbacks of Service Delivery Models**

Model	Benefits	Drawbacks
Pull-out	Child less distracted by classroom activities Child given opportunities to learn/practice in a less threatening, less competitive atmosphere	Setting for language learning is decontextualized May be stigmatizing to child to be withdrawn from class Child misses important class time
Classroom	Clinician experiences child's language difficulties as they happen "Where the action is"	May be distracting to other students or the teacher May be stigmatizing to the child to be observed receiving special assistance
Consultation (general)	Intervention strategies taught to the teacher by the clinician Teacher is primary intervention agent	Teacher may perceive clinician as language expert to deliver intervention services Teacher may perceive self as too busy
Collaborative consultation	Teacher and clinician share mutual respect and mutual responsibility for the child's program	[same as above]

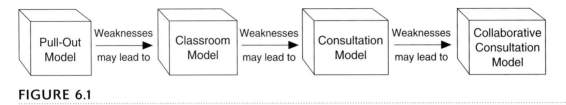

FIGURE 6.1

Relationships among Models of Language Intervention Service Delivery

classrooms to work with SLPs either individually or in groups, usually consisting of other children who exhibit similar problems. Pull-out therapy has typically been performed in small rooms or areas away from the child's classmates and can be used for either individual or group therapy sessions. The rationale for this model probably stemmed from the belief that separating the child(ren) from the rest of the class would provide a quiet location where the specific goals of therapy could be addressed. Not only should there be less opportunity for the child to become distracted, but the therapy provided would not disrupt the classroom program of classmates who do not have language disorders.

One potential "down" side to this approach is that it singles out a child for having a problem and possibly stigmatizes the child as being different from the classmates who stay behind (Brush, 1987). Furthermore, the child is removed from the very setting in which he or she is likely to use the language features being taught. Through the pull-out model, language is often taught without context or at least taught in a rather contrived, unrealistic context. One very important way to ensure generalization—context validity—is eliminated. It should also be noted that for the child receiving therapy in a community clinic or private practice, language intervention can also resemble the decontextualized setting of the pull-out model. Unless steps are taken by SLPs to help the young child recognize that the clinical setting and other frequently experienced settings (e.g., home, school) have some communicative similarities, there is no reason to expect the child to apply the structures and strategies learned in therapy outside of the clinic.

The move away from the pull-out model has been accelerated by legislation mandating that children with disabilities receive appropriate services in the least restrictive environment possible. Specifically, federal law mandates that early intervention services be provided as often as possible in the same natural environments where children without disabilities can be found. Sequestering a child from his or her classmates for language intervention may represent a too restrictive environment, justified only if it is shown to be essential for the success of an individual child's treatment.

Intervention in the Classroom

An appreciation for the social foundations of language development and the need for context support in language learning has led to attempts to remedy the problems posed by the pull-out model. One solution has been to provide speech-language intervention in the classroom itself. Whether a preschool, a kindergarten, or a grade-school classroom, it is the classroom context where language problems, if they exist, are likely to manifest themselves, because it is here that the educational as well as social demands involving language are placed on the child. The classroom is also likely to offer more natural opportunities for conversational exchanges between teachers and students, and between students and their peers. SLPs who provide treatment in the classroom will have a better chance to observe problem situations as they unfold for the child and to provide "on-line" assistance or suggestions for remedying communication breakdowns.

One of the difficulties with a classroom-based approach is that the classroom routine could be affected by the presence of another adult who may be working at cross-purposes with the classroom teacher. That is, the classroom teacher presents information for all of the children, whereas SLPs usually present information that is relevant for just one or maybe a few students. The SLPs' interactions with the child may draw attention to themselves and away from the classroom teacher when attention paid to the classroom teacher would be beneficial for completing class projects. Further, the child with a language disorder is still the recipient of extra assistance in the classroom, and the child or the child's classmates may see this difference in a negative light (Jenkins & Heinen, 1989). So, although working in the classroom eliminates some of the problems presented by the pull-out approach, it may create others for the clients being served.

Collaborative Consultation

A third option is the collaborative consultation model for service delivery (Frasinelli, Superior, & Meyers, 1983). Actually, when we use the term *consultation,* we are referring to a family of possible models for interaction between the SLP and school personnel (Marvin, 1987). By serving as consultants to classrooms, SLPs can eliminate some of the drawbacks to the pull-out and in-class models. In addition, both professionals end up learning more about the other's area of expertise; the classroom teacher should end up learning more about how communication can be facilitated, and the SLPs should learn more about the classroom curriculum and its demands (Prelock, Miller, & Reed, 1995). (See Chapter 3 for a more detailed accounting of the collaborative consultation model of service delivery.)

There is probably an endless variety of ways in which the collaborative consultation model can be implemented. Prelock et al. (1995) described a Language in the Classroom (LIC) program involving collaborative partnerships between speech-language clinicians and classroom teachers. In this particular program, collaborative efforts include assessment, "goal setting, planning, and implementation of intervention for students with communication disorders as well as for those students who are at risk for language and learning problems" (p. 286). In another approach to service delivery, Farber, Denenberg, Klyman, and Lachman (1992) described what they call the Language Resource Room Level of Service, incorporating aspects of "the classroom, a team teaching model, itinerant support, and consultative services" (p. 293). Farber et al. (1992) suggested that with SLPs potentially assuming roles of co-teacher, consultant, or direct service provider depending on programming needs, a greater number of treatment options was possible (p. 293).

No discussion of provision of speech and language services in the classroom would be complete without an acknowledgment of the "bigger picture" of the regular education initiative (REI), more commonly referred to as *inclusion* or *full inclusion* (Wolery & Wilbers, 1994). Following federal legislation mandating the provision of appropriate education to all children in the "least restrictive environment" (P.L. 94-142, 1975; P.L. 99-457, 1986; P.L. 101-576, 1990; and P.L. 105-17, 1997), many state departments of education and individual school districts have interpreted these laws in ways that more or less conform to the notion of the REI, whereby special education and regular education are melded into one (Stainback & Stainback, 1990).

By definition, supporters of full inclusion believe that the "least restrictive environment" is a mainstreamed classroom for all children, regardless of level of ability. That is, as promoters of the full-inclusion standpoint, Stainback, Stainback, and Forest (1989) view the concept of "inclusion" as the logical outcome of the practice of providing children with the least restrictive educational environment; there should be no differentiated, segregated, special education classrooms. However, these authors believe that inclusion is more than just mainstreaming. They note that "an inclusive school is a place where everyone belongs, is accepted, supports, and is supported by his or her peers and other members of the school community in the course of having his or her educational needs met" (p. 3). Within an inclusive classroom model, "the focus is on how to operate supportive classrooms and schools that include and meet the needs of everyone" (p. 4). A more comprehensive discussion of the scope of inclusion theory and practice is provided in Chapter 3.

SLPS' RESPONSIBILITIES FOR LANGUAGE INTERVENTION

A Systems Approach to Evaluating Treatment Outcome

If you take a comprehensive point of view, the responsibility for language facilitation and remediation falls to some extent on everyone who has contact with the child diagnosed with a language disorder. This section presents a synopsis of what parents, classroom teachers, and SLPs are most typically expected to bring to the language intervention table. Obviously, SLPs are trained to provide intervention services. Therefore, it is important for them to have a strong background in language development as well as in the latest procedures for the assessment of young language-disordered individuals (Weiss, Tomblin, & Robin, 1999). An appreciation for the fact that language development represents only one aspect of the growing child's development is also important, as is an understanding of normal cognitive, social-emotional, and physical development patterns. An understanding of learning theory is also essential, along with more specific knowledge of language treatment programs, techniques, and their rationales. Because the study of treatment efficacy is a burgeoning area of research, SLPs should be prepared to continuously update their internalized databases with regard to which strategies for language facilitation have been shown to be both effective and efficient for which types of clients.

Success in the area of language intervention takes more than a wealth of background knowledge, however. There is a clinical art that tempers clinical science. Goldberg (1993) suggests that lists of desirable clinical characteristics typically describe an individual who is "a non-defensive, confident, and accepting individual" (p. 40).

In addition, because the demographics of our nation are changing in substantive ways, along with these changes have gone changes to the distribution of our clients in terms of their cultural backgrounds. Recognizing this pattern, Hanson (1998) suggested that "an appreciation and respect for cultural variations, as well as group and individual differences, is crucial for the interventionist" (p. 5). Lynch (1998) added that interventionists working with families from cultures other than their own will enhance their communicative effectiveness if they focus on the other culture as a potential learning experience and remain open to the different perspectives that will be shared by virtue of working together to develop a workable treatment program.

Along with having basic knowledge about language development and disorders, SLPs should know how to use that information to decide which young children are developing language normally and which ones are not. Once the decision has been made that a problem exists, it must be decided whether language intervention is warranted. Olswang and Bain (1991) described three methods: profiling, the static determination of what a client knows at a particular point in time; dynamic assessment, an analysis of the extent to which a client can benefit from cues and support in the environment; and monitoring (or tracking), a systematic evaluation of progress over time that allows for a prediction of future development, which can be incorporated into the decision-making process to facilitate appropriate recommendations for treatment (p. 255). According to the authors, the two critical determiners for treatment readiness are the exhibition of a significant difference between competencies of different language components, or between linguistic and cognitive competencies; and evidence that the client is ready to make changes in language performance. Specifically, profiling and dynamic assessment are most useful in providing clues as to when to begin intervention, and tracking or monitoring can be used retrospectively to evaluate whether the decision to intervene had been a good one. See also Bain and Olswang (1995); Long and Olswang, (1996); and Olswang and Bain (1996) for additional uses of a dynamic assessment approach to determine when young children are ready to tackle specific expressive language objectives.

If the SLP believes that intervention is warranted, then decisions must be made about a specific plan of action. Many variables must be considered to develop a plan of action for a child. Of course, how communicative the child is, how much language the child already has, and how much of it is typically used will need to be considered. The clinician must also consider how the child best learns, as well as the degree to which the parents and others who have significant contact with the child and the treatment program can be called on to carry over what is learned in treatment into the home environment. A listing of additional questions that should yield useful information for decision-making purposes is presented in Table 6.2.

Clinical Judgment

Information derived from answers to the questions listed in Table 6.2 alone will not be sufficient to develop an appropriate intervention program. Skilled SLPs recognize that good decision making and intervention planning result from a blend of objective information and good clinical "feel" for the therapeutic situation. There is an art to clinical practice that is difficult to specify but that is most likely a product of clinical

TABLE 6.2	Selected Information Needed to Develop a Language Intervention Plan

1. Is the child cooperative and able to comply with structured tasks?
2. Is the child willing to separate from the parent or caregiver to work with the clinician?
3. Are pictures meaningful to the child, or should three-dimensional objects be used?
4. Does the child exhibit both receptive and expressive language disorders?
5. Do any members of the child's immediate family also have a language disorder?
6. Have the parents expressed interest in participating in their child's language intervention program?
   (a) If so, how much time could they reasonably devote to specific activities?
   (b) If so, how knowledgeable are the parents regarding language development milestones?
   (c) If so, is their typical interaction style with their child directive? egalitarian?
7. Does the child show any awareness of the language disorder?
8. Has the child been reported to become frustrated in his/her attempts to communicate?
9. Will intervention activities hold the child's attention for 5 minutes? 10 minutes? 15 minutes?
10. Is the child involved in a classroom program?
   (a) If so, what is the focus of the classroom (e.g., academic, preacademic, daycare)?
   (b) If so, does the child's language disorder compromise the child's interactions with classmates?
   (c) If so, does the child appear to enjoy the classroom experience?
   (d) If so, are there other children in the child's class with language difficulties? other developmental problems?
   (e) If so, has the child's teacher(s) expressed concern about the child's language abilities? willingness to participate in language intervention?

experience melded with the facts of clinical science (Records & Weiss, 1990). Given this subjective portion of clinical judgment, clinicians must guard against falling victim to unsubstantiated biases as they make decisions. Although we are making gains in efficacy research, there is still too little known pointing conclusively to which intervention programs are best suited to which children. Thus, there is a danger in assuming that one intervention plan that appears to have worked well with one child will necessarily work well with all children.

One way to help overcome a tendency toward bias in selecting intervention approaches is to focus on our rationales for choosing certain clinical methods and to maintain a healthy skepticism until supporting data become available (Newhoff, 1995). Continuing to collect objective data to substantiate client progress or lack of progress helps prevent clinicians from becoming too complacent with one or another therapeutic technique. For example, the school-based SLPs in the state of Iowa, in conjunction with the National Outcomes Measurement System (NOMS) sponsored by the ASHA, has worked diligently to develop better criteria for caseload selection as well as dismissal from therapy, the selection of particular service delivery systems for different children, and curriculum evaluation. It is these objective data collected by clinicians across Iowa that are needed nationwide and will eventually assist SLPs in their clinical decision making regarding what works for clients exhibiting different patterns of communication needs.

Flow Charts and Decision Trees Facilitate Decision Making

Some clinicians use flow charts or decision trees with an "if X . . . then Y" perspective to assist in the decision-making process. Several years ago, Yoder and Kent (1988) edited a collection of these decision-making tools that covered a vast range of clinical case types (e.g., child language disorders, adult neurogenic disorders), and situations (e.g., dismissal from treatment, eligibility for treatment). Many SLPs find these particularly helpful to "view" the thinking process that expert clinicians go through as they work through a case step by step. This approach tends to reduce the cognitive load on the individual clinician and allows him or her to benefit indirectly from the experience of SLPs and other professionals who have established themselves as experts in a particular clinical area. For example, in a flow chart designed for SLPs who are planning an intervention program for a child with difficulties in language learning in the absence of detectable problems with the child's hearing, motor, cognitive, or social-emotional development, we would probably want to view a decision-making tree designed by Ellis Weismer (1988), as well as decision-making information suggested by Paul (1995) and Nelson (1998).

What steps would be critical in thinking through a clinical case in terms of planning for intervention? SLPs must take into consideration all of the intake information gleaned from the case history collected from the primary caregiver(s), additional test data collected from other professionals such as audiologists, psychologists, and developmental specialists, and include results from a "comprehensive communication profile" (Ellis Weismer, 1988, p. 42) to determine what language and/or communicative demands are placed on the child in his or her activities of daily living and the degree to which the child is capable of meeting those demands. This profile is likely to yield a relative priority for each language need in terms of the functional communicative weighting it carries. In addition, as part of our input information, we want to include the family in helping us to prioritize concerns about their child's communication performance. They can provide essential information regarding the context-based nature of the communication problem. Is the deficit in communication skills also observed in the home environment?

Note that having the child's hearing assessed is a crucial prerequisite to language testing whenever a language disorder is suspected in a young child. Remember that having psychological testing also serves to determine whether the child can be considered "specifically language impaired." This diagnosis is important because it will likely lead to different intervention planning and at least to different information being transmitted to the family with regard to prognosis and need for additional support services.

The information provided by the intake information will allow SLPs to make the most appropriate choices concerning selection of a test battery that will determine whether a language disorder is present. SLPs should consider the presence of both standardized and nonstandardized test formats, with some observation of the child in as naturalistic a setting as possible included so that a more complete picture of the child's communicative competencies can be formulated.

Following analysis of the results from the test instruments chosen for administration by the SLP, a determination is made, whether by comparison with normative data or in reference to age-appropriate demands on the child's language, about whether the child is capable of meeting expectations for performance. If not, and it is believed that the results of the testing are a fair representation of the child's abilities, the diagnosis of a language disorder is made. It will be important at this time to determine whether this is a problem that is present in both comprehension and production of language—or in one or the other. This information will have a bearing on prognosis as well as on treatment selection.

Following goal selection and the selection of a goal attack strategy, it is critical to gather new information or use what is already known about how the child responds to support in a teaching environment to make changes in behavior. This can be viewed as diagnostic therapy or the dynamic assessment that must precede our first "best guesses" about what will work best in treatment. Included in this step of the flow chart is the determination of ways we can help the child adequately make use of language input provided during intervention. For example, if the child is demonstrating a language problem and has been unable to learn the rule structures of language, then maybe the language input presented has not been sufficiently structured for that purpose. Specific suggestions can be provided about how linguistic input might be altered to achieve greater success. Any alterations of the input signal (e.g., timing, slowed rate of presentation) or the use of emphasis on important language forms or structures and other prosodic cues (Bedore & Leonard, 1995) could make the difference between the child's understanding or misunderstanding of language both in and out of intervention.

It is also important for the clinician to determine the best setting for intervention. Certainly the settings selected will differ according to each child's special circumstances as well as the availability of intervention services. SLPs may be fortunate enough to have many alternatives to choose from or may be relegated to only one option. Obviously, the caregivers are a critical element in the final selection of a placement for the child; it is a good idea for SLPs to remember that working toward consensus with the child's caregivers is an important part of the role of a clinician in a family-centered service delivery model.

Once the initial methods for language input and the intervention context have been determined, the clinician must then choose the specific training technique to be used, and Ellis Weismer (1988) cautioned that clinicians must select the technique carefully, depending on the area of language targeted for intervention. Decisions concerning use of reinforcers, how feedback will be provided, and how generalization and maintenance will be promoted also should be considered at this early point in planning. And remember that although these are not arbitrary decisions, they represent a best guess on the part of the SLPs from his or her observation of this specific client, the SLP's own past clinical experiences, and input from the caregivers, and they may change in time as new data are collected.

The SLP's role as a decision maker does not end with the actual implementation of the intervention program. To determine whether the early decisions made have been appropriate, it is critical for SLPs to systematically collect data that support or refute the contention that progress has been made. If the data show that progress has been made, the intervention program has likely been effective and should be continued. If no measurable progress has been demonstrated, then the clinician will need to return to the beginning steps of the program where goals are selected and procedures developed to troubleshoot the program for errors. Sometimes major changes in the program need to be made, and at other times relatively minor changes need to be made in order to get the client's learning trajectory back on track. Fey (1988) discusses a decision-making tree devoted specifically to dismissal decisions. He systematically addresses the troubleshooting of an intervention program complete with carefully delineated criteria for dismissal where no decision to dismiss is ever irrevocable.

OTHERS WHO SHARE IN THE PROVISION OF LANGUAGE INTERVENTION

It has already been mentioned that to some extent, anyone in contact with a child in need of language intervention can share in the responsibility for intervention. Most individuals who come in contact with the child provide incidental language modeling (input) or opportunities for interaction where language can be used and learned. Because all interactions can potentially provide positive language learning experiences, one of the challenges to beginning student clinicians is to start viewing every interaction with a client in terms of its particular language facilitation possibilities. Given the pervasiveness of language learning contexts, children's parents, other caregivers, classroom teachers, siblings, and peers can and should share in the intervention process to a greater or lesser extent depending on the specifics of the client's needs, abilities, and circumstances. One role that SLPs can play is in teaching these potential language partners how best to serve this function.

There are two aspects of the intervention process with which these "others" are most closely associated. The first is in promoting generalization, either stimulus or response generalization to untrained contexts (Hughes, 1985). The second is in the facilitation of language learning itself, where these more knowledgeable language users consider what the child already knows in creating low-risk language learning experiences (van Kleeck & Richardson, 1988). This is sometimes called **scaffolding** (Bruner, 1985) and is closely related to the concept of **dynamic assessment**, already referred to as a technique to determine readiness for intervention (Olswang & Bain, 1991).

The Role of Parents: Decision Making and Service Delivery

As first mandated by the Education of the Handicapped Amendments of 1986 (Public Law 99-457), parents are viewed as integral members of the team for both the planning and executing of an Individualized Family Service Plan (IFSP), to be drawn up with substantive assistance from professionals representing various disciplines. The implication of this legislation was that parents are deemed highly responsible parties in intervention planning, although of the team's members, they probably do not possess the most information about enhancing the efficacy of language intervention. The need to bring parents into the circle of service providers in a manner that builds mutual respect and consensus for the duration of service delivery has led to a substantial literature on the best ways to accomplish this (Crais, 1991; Pletcher, 1995). Crais (1991) noted that the involvement of parents in service delivery has shifted, which is apparent in the changing terminology used, where terms referring to the family-focused or family-centered nature of treatment are commonplace. She further suggested that all of these approaches share a set of common underlying assumptions, among them "that families are equal partners in assessment and intervention, that families will be encouraged and allowed to choose their own level of involvement in decision making and implementation of both assessment and intervention practices, and that supporting the family in the ways they consider useful is a primary goal of intervention services" (Crais, 1991, p. 2).

SLPs should note that the notion of incorporating parents into the decision-making process, while implemented as a means to empower family members and acknowledge their important role in service delivery, operates as a culturally sensitive phenomenon. That is, when a practitioner from the majority culture is working with families from some nonmajority cultures (e.g., Asian, Hispanic), he or she may be viewed as the expert to whom the child has been brought for the express purpose of deciding on a course of action. If the parents are then asked to take part in the decision-making process by giving and setting priorities, this may signal that the so-called experts are less than competent and the professionals' credibility is diminished. In a general sense, when the speech-language clinician is a member of a different culture from that of the family, it is important to be cognizant of potential misunderstandings brought on by differences in belief systems surrounding health care, child-care routines, wellness management, and so on. Hanson (1998) refers to these misunderstandings as potentials for "cultural clashes" (pp. 4–5).

Lynch (1998) noted that cultures differ in terms of their preferred mode of information transfer, with some cultures exhibiting a preference for explicit transfer through oral language and others preferring to transmit information implicitly by means of the contextual cues inherent in a situation, the relationship that holds between the participants, and nonlinguistic cues (p. 42). This difference in style translates into two culture types, according to the author. There is a "high-context" culture that is observed to be more formal than the "low-context" culture type, which is more informal and which demonstrated a tendency toward more egalitarian interaction (Lynch, 1998). The assumption by SLPs that a family adheres to a particular style of child rearing, for example, but that actually does not match the family's set of beliefs and practices, may result in unintended communications of insensitivity, which are likely to impede the working relationships of the participants. Therefore, it is worthwhile for SLPs to attempt to determine, as early in their interactions as possible, the level of context-based communication that will be comfortable for the family in question. In her paper describing the assumptions made by mainstream SLPs about how families work that make themselves apparent in the suggestions we provide parents for their role in the intervention process, van Kleeck (1994) warns us to remember that there is much cross-cultural variation in terms of the quality and quantity of family routines, or viewpoints regarding who is an appropriate conversation partner for a young child, to give two examples. For SLPs who are likely to recommend that the family spend fifteen minutes each night during their dinner time having the child talk about his day may meet with resistance not because the family is disinterested in helping, but because the assumption of a routine dinner time and discourse focusing on the child are both foreign concepts.

The amount of time that parents spend with their children will vary from family to family, but it is very likely that they spend more time with the child than do SLPs. That means that in addition to their legal role as decision makers for their child, they also are likely to have a great deal of influence over their child's language intervention by virtue of the importance of language input and their frequent presence as language interactants. SLPs should find some way to use the parents' proximity and interest in helping their child who has a language disorder. The parental role in intervention will also vary from parent to parent depending on the parent's facility, willingness or availability to learn intervention techniques, reporting skills for monitoring the child's language use at home, and ability to follow through at home with the therapeutic contingencies used in the clinic. Techniques for making the home environment more like the intervention setting and the intervention setting more like home have been suggested by Hughes (1985) and others to promote generalization outside the treatment setting. Parents are the perfect consultants for putting these suggestions into practice.

It is also important for speech-language clinicians to remember that, as important as the development of speech-language competence is, it may be considered a lower priority than some of the other concerns parents may have. In families where having sufficient food and shelter are daily worries, or catastrophic health issues are present, following through on a language intervention program may take a back seat. Just as it is important not to set children up to fail by instituting impossible goals, it is also important when incorporating parents into an intervention plan not to ask them to do more than can be reasonably expected. Asking a parent to spend a half-hour per night engaged in a specific language task is often too much to ask. Most parents want to be as helpful as possible, but for many such a request would seriously compromise other familial duties, and noncompliance may result.

One approach that might solve this problem is to work with parents on ways to facilitate their child's participation in naturally occurring language "happenings," perhaps during quiet times when the child and parent are the only participants, or when several family members can participate in some group activity. Promoting conversations at mealtimes—when the family does have routine mealtimes—is one suggestion that parents frequently say works well. Here the family members can all serve to reinforce the child's attempts to communicate. Better still, the parents do not have to be put in a position of doling out performance-based rewards or punishments.

Several investigators have studied the effects of having parents serve as conveyers of treatment programs. In one study, Fey, Cleave, Long, and Hughes (1993) compared two techniques for facilitating grammatical productions in children with language impairments, one of which utilized the child's parents for service delivery.

The authors noted that although both the parent-administered technique and a more traditional clinician-administered technique appeared to yield positive results, it was the clinician-administered approach that provided more consistently positive treatment effects. This led the authors to caution their readers that parent-administered programs may require clinicians to monitor change more closely over time and to institute changes to the program if the child's progress falls below what is expected. This conclusion by Fey and colleagues (1993) may provide support for the notion that although parents are generally highly useful resources for implementing some language programs, they do not take the place of trained SLPs. In a similar vein, results reported by Girolametto, Tannock, and Siegel (1993) revealed that parents' subjective judgments of the posttherapeutic improvements of their children bore little relationship to the objective data chronicling pre- to posttherapy changes in the same children's performances. This again suggests that parents are very interested in their children's successes but are unlikely, because of the bias in wanting to see progress as well as their lack of specialized training in speech-language pathology, to take the place of the SLP's eyes, ears, and expertise. When Cleave and Fey (1997) compared the progress made by children who had received clinician-directed treatment versus intervention administered by their parents, they concluded that probably the best treatment would have been a combination of the two, in which the parent program was administered at the same time as the clinic-based treatment was provided.

Other investigators have suggested that parents can be given rather specific goals in terms of providing their children with language learning experiences. Pierce and McWilliams (1993) noted that the parents of children with severe speech and physical impairments who indicated willingness to participate can be given specific suggestions for increasing the literacy and preliteracy experiences of their young children. In a recent study by van Kleeck, Gillam, Hamilton, and McGrath (1997), a direct link was noted between middle-class parents' different methods of reading and discussing books with their preschoolers and the children's later demonstration of more or less abstract language formulation.

The Role of Classroom Teachers in Facilitating Language Learning

Classroom teachers can play an important role in a young child's language intervention program. By understanding their young student's language deficiencies, and usually with some assistance from the speech-language clinician, the teacher can provide frequent language learning experiences in the classroom and make these experiences more relevant to the child's ongoing classroom curriculum (Fujiki & Brinton, 1984).

As the expert on the classroom curriculum, the classroom teacher is a valuable resource for the clinician who is working in the classroom itself or serving as a classroom consultant. Classroom teachers can help to pinpoint the situational demands on language that occur during the classroom routine, and they are in a good position to monitor the child's successes and failures in generalizing the language features targeted in intervention. Teachers also have the knowledge and expertise to facilitate success in the classroom. For example, by periodically changing the child's seating arrangement to promote interactions with a variety of classmates (some of whom may be more willing to interact with a child who has a language disorder than others), the child may have more opportunities to practice and perfect new communication skills. The classroom teacher should have expert understanding of the classmates' social dynamics, and this information can be used to advantage by those planning language intervention.

The Role of Classmates in Facilitating Language Learning

Young, normally developing children seem to learn quickly which of their classmates have difficulties with communicating. This has been demonstrated by their ability and willingness to accommodate their own language to the less sophisticated abilities of their classmates (Guralnick & Paul-Brown, 1977). It is also clear that normally developing children are preferred when a peer wants to initiate contact or when children in a classroom are asked to indicate with whom in the classroom they would prefer to play (Craig & Washington, 1993; Rice, 1993; Rice, Sell, & Hadley, 1991). Further, when children with language difficulties do communicate, they tend to do so with adults, perhaps because historically they have found more acceptance in such interactions.

Rice, Hadley, and Alexander (1993) suggested that data describing the interactions of preschool-age children with different abilities within classroom settings point to a pattern of social consequence for children with language impairment or limitations in language use. That is, if a child demonstrates limited language abilities, he or she will be less likely to be involved in experiences that will facilitate peer initiation abilities or to practice the language competencies that are needed to develop friendships. Furthermore, when a child discovers that he or she is not a likely candidate for friendships with classmates, there is probably less motivation for the child to work to develop those needed language skills. After a short period of time in classrooms where young children with disabilities are mainstreamed, it is not unusual for the normally developing children to ignore their classmates with language impairments in favor of interacting with their normally developing peers (Snyder, Apolloni, & Cooke, 1977). With very young children, some of this behavior results from immature socialization skills, but with older children it seems that the children are being ignored because of their poor language skills. As Craig (1993) noted with reference to children with specific language impairment, "it appears that the amount of their peer interaction is limited and that, when it does occur, it probably is reduced in quality compared to that of children with normal language development" (p. 214).

Children from nonmajority cultures may present both language and socialization challenges to the speech-language clinician (Damico & Damico, 1993). Given that so much important language learning is closely tied with the development of children's social skills, it is important for SLPs (as well as the classroom teacher) to learn how to assist the culturally different children in their classrooms "in becoming more empowered in their social and educational contexts" (p. 241).

These findings lead us to believe that SLPs and classroom teachers must not assume that beneficial language learning interactions take place between all children in classrooms; instead, they need to figure out ways to facilitate the opportunities for interaction both inside and outside of the classroom. Rice (1993) additionally suggested that teachers and others not only redirect the requests and statements made to adults by children with language difficulties to classmates, but also teach the children specific strategies to do so. This technique makes it less likely that the child with limited language abilities will use the adults in the classroom as the "default" interactant. Schuele, Rice, & Wilcox (1995) described a method of redirection training that they found enabled a higher degree of successful and generalized interactions between normally developing preschoolers and their classmates diagnosed with SLI. Hadley and Schuele (1998) also discussed ways in which SLPs could set treatment objectives to utilize the social structure of the classroom to encourage peer interactions between children of different language abilities.

In another approach to capitalizing on the benefits of peer interaction, Goldstein, English, Shafer, and Kaczmarek (1997) developed what they called a "peer-mediated" treatment program. Here the goal was to focus on increasing the abilities of the normally developing children to determine when their classmates with language impairments were attempting to communicate with them so that they could be more helpful in making those communicative interactions successful ones. As a result of this program, the investigators observed an increase in the amount of social integration between their groups of children who were normally developing and those with disabilities. Furthermore, generalization of these skills across children was observed.

Even in classroom situations where language "models" are employed, it cannot be taken for granted that these children, by virtue of their language normal status and presence in the classroom, are providing adequate language modeling for their classmates with limited language. Weiss and Nakamura (1992) investigated the extent to which normally developing children serving as "model" children in a class of language-disordered children interacted with their classmates. They found that two of the three model children spent minimal time with their peers who had language disorders. Unfortunately, the underlying purpose of this classroom's reverse mainstreaming plan was to promote interactions between the models and their classmates so that those with language disorders would benefit from competent language input provided by the models. The authors recommended that teachers should take the lead in putting groups of child conversants together and give them less opportunity to form their own interactant groups based on language competencies.

Taking this thought one step further, Venn, Wolery, Fleming, DeCesare, Morris, and Cuffs (1993) reported on the use of a mand-model procedure to teach normal classroom peers to interact with their classmates who had language disorders. Not only did the normal classmates easily learn to incorporate the mand-model appropriately, but the children with disabilities with whom they were paired increased both the frequency of their responses to their peers and in the production of their own unprompted requests!

FACILITATING LANGUAGE CHANGE

The Connection of Theories to Treatment

SLPs need methods for critically assessing and choosing among the many approaches to language intervention that are possible. Johnston (1983) proposed that, to develop intervention procedures that work, SLPs must determine their own theory of language development as well as disorders and design treatment approaches, or select from among those already available, that are consistent with those beliefs. The development of intervention strategies for children demonstrating disorders in language have paralleled the changes in the theories proposed to explain child language acquisition. Although changes in therapeutic approaches have lagged somewhat behind major shifts in perspectives on language acquisition theory, a review of the history of language intervention reveals strong connections between the two (McLean, 1983).

For example, SLPs who adhere to a social-interactionist viewpoint typically have placed emphasis on early intervention services by suggesting that children begin to learn important pieces of the language puzzle long before they produce their first words. Sometimes medical or social problems upset the possibility for natural caregiver–child interactions, as may be the case with prolonged hospitalizations following premature birth or other birth complications. SLPs may be asked to analyze infant behaviors and abilities to develop a program demonstrating to family members how to capitalize on their infant's limited capabilities for early communication (Ensher, 1989; Sparks, 1989). Similarly, the importance of early-childhood special programs for children developing more slowly than their peers has received support due to the popularity of the social-interaction approach. The passage of P.L. 99-457, which first mandated services to children ages 3 to 5 who have disabilities, was probably an outcome of the interest in the language learning that goes on during the preschool years and the recognition that the presence of language-based activities in the child's social milieu can provide opportunities for the learning and practice of language in context.

In addition, the transition of service delivery to a collaborative consultation model from the more traditional pull-out model of therapy could also be traced to adherence to the social-interaction approach. The language milieu in the classroom has been shown to be quite different from that in the home environment. To be successful conversationalists in school, children need to learn the rule systems of both, determining where they are similar and where they are different. For example, there are constraints to turn taking in the classroom that may not exist in the child's home speaking environment. Instead of learning discourse conventions of the classroom in a third setting, the therapy room, treatment in the classroom itself provides immediate occasions for using the new structures and strategies targeted in therapy.

Getting Started

The role of SLPs in facilitating language change with young children proceeds from a series of decisions, and these decisions follow a logical, scientific progression not unlike those made by SLPs working with other populations of individuals presenting with communication disorders. The first major decision involves a "best guess" about where to begin in therapy; this will come from the results of both standardized and nonstandardized tests and measures completed during the child's diagnostic evaluation. Added to this will be the observations of parents and other caregivers who will be able to contribute information relevant to how well the child can use the language he or she does have to best advantage, and who will also be able to provide input with regard to the language demands in the child's life. Along with determining whether a problem exists, the clinician should determine the scope of the problem and how the child can best learn language. Often these last two features of the case are not determined until after a period of diagnostic therapy or within the framework of dynamic assessment procedures (Goldberg, 1993; Olswang & Bain, 1991; Weiss et al., 1999).

During diagnostic therapy, a variety of materials can be employed, and different combinations of input stimuli are emphasized while the child's performance is carefully monitored for changes. Questions concerning the breadth of the problem and most useful methods for remediation are important and need to be answered by the clinician because their answers will furnish useful insights for designing treatment plans that have a greater chance of success. Answers to these questions supply the "how" of the therapy plan's implementation. Here are four examples:

1. *What presentation methods facilitate the child's ability to demonstrate new language targets?* That is, should the targets be embedded in a story retelling task, or should sentence contexts be used? If the child is supplied with opportunities to produce targeted structures in natural conversation exchanges, will the child tend to take advantage of these with little prompting?

2. *How much stimulus support does the child need to be successful?* For example, are auditory cues alone sufficient to result in production of the targeted language structures, or are combinations of auditory and visual cues necessary? Does the child benefit from orthographic cues (letter symbols), or are these confusing? For some young children, orthographic cues may not be meaningful and may present more of a hindrance than a help.

3. *Is the child willing to risk being wrong?* Does the child refuse to incorporate newly targeted structures and forms unless provided with imitative prompts so that he is left with little guesswork when formulating language? Or is this young child willing to try to incorporate new language targets into his own spontaneous language? If the latter is true, under what circumstances is spontaneous usage more likely to occur?

4. *What motivates the child to improve language performance?* Does the child demonstrate any awareness of her own difficulties in being understood or in understanding others? When placed in a situation where a communication breakdown is likely to occur, and then occurs, does the child exhibit any understanding of what happened? What strategies does the child use, if any, to remedy a breakdown in communication?

Obviously, along with the "hows," the "whats" of the therapy plan also need to be determined. Goals that emerged from formal testing and therefore appear to be appropriate should be targeted in baseline testing before their final selection. That is, several trials containing a number of examples of the potential structure or forms to be targeted for therapy should be administered so that the clinician can determine whether test results were artifacts of the testing process, of the test itself, or truly represent the child's specific deficits. Sometimes baseline trials are administered in one session; sometimes they are administered over the course of several days. The point is that a stable baseline of the child's performance should be established so the clinician knows the child's level of competence before therapy begins. Failure to have this information leaves open the possibility that time will be wasted either by targeting "goals" already established and leaving other appropriate goals untargeted, or by incorrectly crediting the child's miraculous progress to the therapy program. See Hegde (1993) for a detailed discussion of the implementation of baseline testing.

Selecting Goal Attack Strategies

If the goals are shown to be appropriate, the SLP's next step is to designate a goal attack strategy (Fey, 1986) that will provide a framework for the intervention program. A **goal attack strategy** is a pattern of goal sequencing and emphasis used in a treatment program when more than one goal will be targeted. Fey (1986) noted that selecting a goal attack strategy is an important decision worthy of careful consideration because different types of clients, different types of goals, and different philosophies fit better into different goal attack strategy types. To make this selection, SLPs need to answer several pertinent questions in light of the goal attack strategies available:

1. What characteristics of the language learner may render one or another of the strategies more or less successful?
2. Will the specific goals selected for the child have a particular impact on attack strategy chosen?
3. What is the theory of the clinician with regard to language learning?

Fey (1986) described three different goal attack strategies: vertical, horizontal, and cyclical. In the **vertical goal attack strategy,** one goal is worked on until a predetermined criterion level of performance is reached. This criterion may have been set by the clinician at 80, 90, or 100 percent correct. Percentage level criteria are arbitrary but typically are set at a level the clinician believes will ensure adequate learning by the child for generalization of that goal, maintenance of that skill without further treatment, or success at the next higher level of difficulty. When the criterion performance level is met, the next goal becomes the focus of treatment. Entire sessions are often devoted to the teaching of one goal, and it is likely that this goal will remain the focus of intervention for a considerable period of time. Because of the intensive nature of the vertical strategy, some children are less likely to become distracted or confused when it does come time to change goals. This approach is believed to be less cognitively demanding and ensures concentrated practice on one goal, which the child learns well before moving on to the next. A potential negative feature of the vertical strategy is that the child may become bored during a session due to its narrow focus. Another is that the child may have more difficulty seeing generalities across different speech-language behaviors. The child may not recognize the shared features of goals 1 and 2 because work on these goals is separated in time. Because generalization may thus be impeded, some clinicians suggest that the vertical approach is the least time efficient of the three for many children in certain clinical situations.

The **horizontal goal attack strategy** prescribes work on more than one goal in the same session. These goals may be closely related to each other (e.g., all conversation act types) or quite dissimilar (e.g., plural morpheme -s, tag questions, and responses to clarification requests). The underlying principle is that this strategy better reflects normal language learning because many different language forms and structures are experienced and learned at the same time. The horizontal strategy may be more time efficient because general insights and skills in language learning gained from working on goal 1, such as learning to monitor self-performance, may benefit progress on goal 3. Children known to be distractible may not be considered good candidates for this strategy, because they might not recognize when a different goal, with different expectations for acceptability, is being targeted. It will also take more time for individual goals to become well learned or to become routine, because less time is devoted to each. For children who have particular problems with language learning, overlearning may be necessary for success, and for them the vertical goal attack strategy may be a wiser selection.

In the **cyclical goal attack strategy,** a number of different goals are worked on with a particular time unit of treatment (e.g., month, semester, or school year), but unlike the horizontal goal attack approach, each goal is presented individually, in its own session. After each of the goals has been worked on sequentially over the time frame of interest, the targets in the cycle are reevaluated and the cycle is revised (goals may be added or subtracted) or repeated if need be. Cyclical approaches suggest that much of the child's learning takes place when the clinician is not present. The child takes what is learned in the therapy setting, considers it, and practices it when outside of therapy. Therefore, intensive ongoing client–clinician contact often duplicates effort or wastes time because its benefits may be easily derived by the child alone, provided that the clinician has successfully taught the necessary tools for learning language. According to proponents of the cyclical goal attack strategy, true changes in language competencies occur only after the child has figured out how to incorporate new language targets into his repertoire over time.

Figure 6.2 lists some of the variables a clinician must consider when selecting a goal attack strategy. Also, see Weiss (2001) for a comparison of how the three goal attack strategies could be used for the targeting of goals typical to the young child with a language impairment.

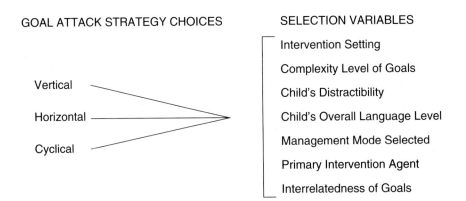

GOAL ATTACK STRATEGY CHOICES

SELECTION VARIABLES

Vertical

Horizontal

Cyclical

Intervention Setting

Complexity Level of Goals

Child's Distractibility

Child's Overall Language Level

Management Mode Selected

Primary Intervention Agent

Interrelatedness of Goals

FIGURE 6.2

Variables Involved in Goal Attack Strategy Selection

Selecting Intervention Settings

Beginning SLPs often fail to recognize that many of the decisions dealing with the disposition of a treatment plan need to be *tentatively* decided at the beginning stages of treatment. That is, the clinician needs to know where the young child with a language disorder uses language and then plan treatment so that the child's new language competencies will be incorporated in an ever-widening set of daily circumstances. In short, the clinician should start therapy having already made some decisions concerning where therapy should take place, with whom, and the amount of structure to be imposed. In addition, there should be some general plan for increasing the "degree of difficulty" for the child as progress is made. One conceptualization for making these sorts of decision was described by Fey (1986) as a "naturalness continuum" (Figure 6.3).

Common sense dictates that for language intervention to be considered successful, the goals targeted for intervention must be apparent in the child's spontaneous language repertoire. So, at some point in the intervention process, SLPs will need to be sure that the therapeutic environment closely resembles the child's natural environment, or vice versa (Hughes, 1985). If this is not done, generalization of newly learned language competencies to the child's activities of daily living may not be easy. Some SLPs wait until the closing stages of intervention before introducing activities aimed specifically at promoting generalization. Others develop intervention programs that account for the generalization of language goals from the very start

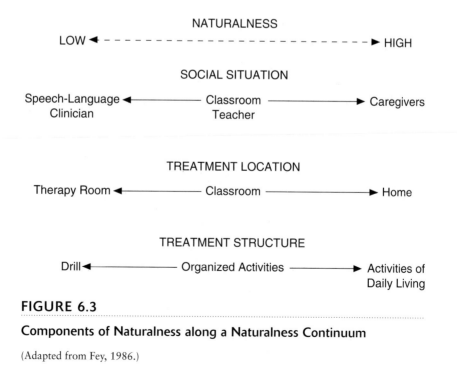

FIGURE 6.3

Components of Naturalness along a Naturalness Continuum

(Adapted from Fey, 1986.)

of treatment. Growing sentiment in the field of speech-language pathology supports the latter approach.

As shown in Figure 6.3, Fey (1986) delineated three features of naturalness on his naturalness continuum: the activity by the clinician, the physical context used for intervention, and the social context in which the intervention transpires. For each of these parameters, he suggested that a continuum exists, ranging from more to less naturalness. Taken together, the relative naturalness of the therapy plan can be estimated. A treatment program that incorporates daily activities in the child's home with parents would be perceived as possessing a very high degree of naturalness. That means that the therapeutic setting closely resembles a *non*therapeutic setting. When the child achieves success in this type of a treatment milieu, the clinician can be more comfortable that the transition to generalization will be accomplished with less directed effort. If the child already views the two settings as similar, he or she should view the opportunities and requirements for language use as similar as well.

Just because a highly natural treatment setting appears to have a major advantage for generalization purposes does not mean that all intervention programs should be designed in the same way. As with selecting the most appropriate goal attack strategy for a particular child, there are client characteristics that may steer the clinician to one or another location along the naturalness continuum at one time in treatment or another. Imposing more structure and very little naturalness in the therapy setting on some children early on may better ensure that they learn new structures. However, generalization will eventually need to be addressed in the therapy program for these children as well. To some degree, an increase in naturalness will have to be incorporated.

Selecting Management Modes: One Example

One way for SLPs to arrive at a general framework for intervention planning is by looking carefully at the essential component parts of therapy and assembling them logically and creatively according to the child's needs and the clinician's own philosophy of management. Most SLPs can tell you that "drill" is more structured than "play," but the specifics of how the two treatment methods differ and in what ways they are similar are less widely understood. By understanding these specifics, we have a better chance of matching a child to an appropriate treatment approach and knowing which components may need to be altered when and if a change in our initial therapy plan becomes necessary.

In their germinal article discussing therapy modes useful in the management of young children with phonological disorders, Shriberg and Kwiatkowski (1982) described four categories of treatment components:

1. *Target responses:* including what the clinician intends the target response to be, and the client's actual response.
2. *Training stimuli:* the stimuli that will be used to elicit responses from clients, that may be presented individually or in sets; and the termination criterion for moving on to high degrees of difficulty in the treatment plan.

3. *Instructional events:* the clinical teaching we do is referred to as an **antecedent instructional event** while the feedback we provide to our clients following their responses is referred to as a **subsequent instructional event.**
4. *Motivational events:* are employed to "accelerate learning by heightening a child's receptivity to all instructional events" (Shriberg & Kwiatkowski, 1982, p. 245) and can be incorporated as antecedent motivational events prior to the client's attempts at a response, or as subsequent motivational events, also referred to as **reinforcement.**

The authors arranged these component parts into four different management modes, called **drill, drill play, structured play,** and **play.** The modes exist along a continuum from "most structured" (drill) to "least structured" (play). It should also be noted that as one moves from the more structured end of the management mode continuum to the less structured end, the treatment focus moves from being clinician centered to being client centered (which in this case is also child centered). That is, on the less structured end of the continuum, the child exerts more influence on the pace and focal point of therapy, whereas on the clinician-centered end of the continuum the SLPs are in control of therapeutic focus and pace.

By incorporating the components described by Shriberg and Kwiatkowski (1982) as the entire set of options for the four modes, we can observe the ways in which the four management modes are related to one another. Figure 6.4 illustrates these differences. Note that structured play and play are quite similar, as are drill play and drill. For example, drill and drill play are identical with one exception. In drill play there is an antecedent motivational event that is missing in drill. That is, something is added to the drill play approach to increase the likelihood that the child will comply with the task. The antecedent motivational event, then, represents a small shift away from the most structured end of the continuum. In both of these modes, drill and drill play, there is a subsequent motivational event (a reinforcer), but this will be presented only in cases where the child's actual response is equivalent to the response definition delineated. Said another way, the child is not being reinforced for willingness to participate; the reinforcer is tied directly to the adequacy of the response.

As the structured nature of the management mode decreases, there is less emphasis on the antecedent instructional event. This means that formalized teaching of the target becomes a less important part of the treatment. For example, in the play management mode, the definition of an acceptable response and the criterion needed for terminating therapy are not even brought to the child's attention in therapy. This is quite a contrast to the way proponents of drill view therapy, but this management mode is considered equally viable and is more appropriate than drill for certain children in certain therapeutic situations. In structured play, which is closer to the clinician-centered end of the continuum than play, the child is presented with information about response definition if he is interested in that information. What is more important in structured play is that the clinician will spend time emphasizing the enjoyableness of the therapy activity.

In follow-up work with this model, Shriberg and Kwiatkowski (1982) reported the results of studies that incorporated their taxonomy in the treatment of twenty-two children with phonological disorders. Their findings indicated that the drill and

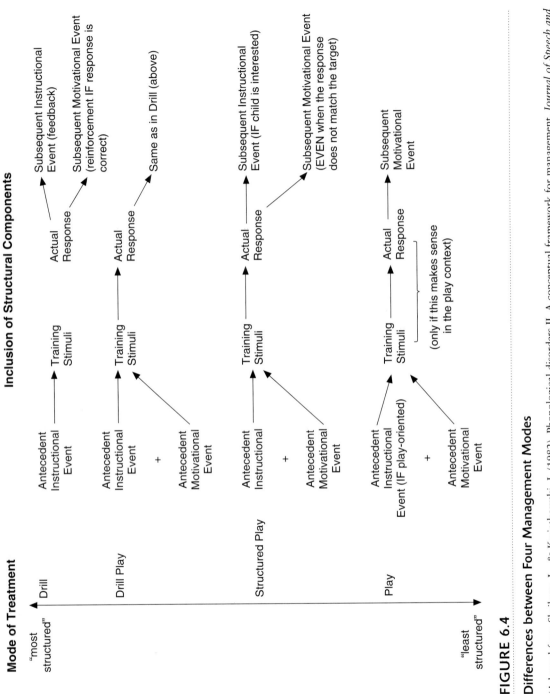

FIGURE 6.4

Differences between Four Management Modes

(Adapted from Shriberg, L., & Kwiatkowski, J. (1982). Phonological disorders II. A conceptual framework for management. *Journal of Speech and Hearing Disorders, 47,* 242–256.)

drill play modes were more effective and efficient than were the structured play and play modes. SLPs who had participated in the studies reported that they believed drill play was the most effective and efficient mode, and not surprisingly they preferred to use the drill play approach, although they believed that their clients preferred drill play, structured play, or play over drill. One small study focused on determining the specific client characteristics that would better match with one or another management mode, but unfortunately this investigation yielded inconclusive results.

Using Information about Caregiver–Child Interactions in Therapy

Once the goals for therapy have been selected and arranged according to the chosen goal attack strategy, and the management mode has been developed, the clinician must decide how interactions with the child will teach or facilitate the learning of these goals. Research based on how caregivers and young children interact serves as a basis for some language therapy techniques; these techniques are sometimes called **experiential language intervention techniques.** Researchers have noted recurring patterns of language use, usually from research with *mother*–child dyads, and have hypothesized that these play an important role in facilitating infants' developing linguistic competence. It has been suggested that these patterns should have a similar effect on the child who is not learning language normally. Therefore, patterns such as expansion, expatiation, modeling, and scaffolding have been discussed in the literature of language development as well as that of language intervention (Connell, 1982; Leonard, 1981; Ratner & Bruner, 1978; Snow, 1986; Weiss, 1981). In terms of management mode, most of the natural caregiver–child techniques fit better with the less structured modes—structured play and play—because they are usually embedded within conversation contexts.

This is probably an appropriate point to insert a cautionary note having to do with the cultural biases inherent in the caregiver–child research used as a basis for much of this branch of language intervention. The vast majority of research done on caregiver–child interventions has been done with families from the mainstream culture. As a result, it is very likely (and in fact we know this to be true) that there are significant enough cultural differences from one culture to another in terms of child-rearing practices, view of children's talking with adults, and so on, that the techniques to be described may not be typical for many of the clients we see professionally.

van Kleeck (1994) reported on a number of the cultural differences that could lead to misunderstandings when we as SLPs attempt to teach caregivers how to interact "appropriately" with their children for therapeutic purposes. For example, in some cultures, in which young children are not encouraged to initiate conversations with their elders, teaching parents strategies for responding to their child's initiations probably would not be a particularly fruitful approach. Even the assumption that the mother—or father—is the child's primary caregiver and thus primary language partner may be erroneous. In cultures where large, extended families tend to be the rule rather than the nuclear family, it may be a grandmother, aunt, or older sibling who has the role of primary caregiver.

Adopting caregiver–child interaction techniques in therapy has also been challenged by some SLPs. Their view is that because most caregivers engage their young children in similar types of language interaction, the language-disordered child has probably already been exposed to these techniques. If the usual type of caregiver–child interaction patterns had been sufficient to effect language development for the child, they would have done so. Opponents to using natural caregiver–child interaction techniques suggest instead that more directive bombardment with examples of acceptable structures in natural conversation contexts is needed. They believe that, by definition, the child diagnosed as having a language disorder probably possesses some sort of deficit that makes it more difficult to benefit from natural interaction patterns. Thus, reliance on these natural intervention techniques alone has no reasonable chance for success. Despite this controversy, experiential language intervention techniques have been widely used and deserve consideration.

Remember that experiential language intervention techniques have their roots in natural caregiver–child interactions for mainstream populations and that their use in therapy should not seriously compromise the naturalness of the treatment. Although the manner in which they are presented by the clinician is prescribed, in practice they are supposed to sound less like a contrived script and more like the normal course of conversational events. The following techniques are commonly used in programs that emphasize conversation development in children who are severely limited in their ability to express themselves (MacDonald & Gillette, 1984; Weiss, 1981).

Imitation

The clinician's use of imitation appears to accomplish several things. First, it has been hypothesized that it validates the acceptability of the child's own production. It also gives the child an opportunity to imitate for emphasis by copying what the clinician said. That is, the child may believe that if the clinician repeated what he said first, it must be acceptable. When the child is expected to imitate the clinician, it represents a less risky attempt at contributing to a conversation. Remember that children with language impairments often know that language is not their strong suit and so being a risk taker in terms of language use is not a typical pattern. Although imitation has been used widely in operant programs as the main means for eliciting decontextualized responses from clients, the discussion here refers to a less structured use. Imitation occurs frequently in language samples collected from normally developing children and their caregivers (Cross, 1978).

Definitions of what constitutes an imitation differ. Imitations may refer to a verbatim reiteration of what was said or only part of it (a partial imitation). An imitation called for by the clinician may require an immediate imitation or a delayed imitation, where either a pause or some intervening dialogue is imposed. Imitation by the clinician also serves as a topic maintainer, letting the child know that the clinician acknowledges the topic established by the child.

Expansion

Expansion refers to the clinician's embellishment of a young child's immature production so that it reflects the adult version of what the child was attempting to produce. Sometimes this is tricky because it is not always clear what the child's intention was. The clinician is not supposed to extend the boundaries of the child's original production, so if the child produced "kitty go," for example, an appropriate expansion would be "The kitty goes." To extend beyond the verb (e.g., "The kitty goes in the car") would constitute the use of expatiation, a slightly different experiential language intervention technique.

The clinical assumption is that expansion, like imitation, provides some useful feedback to the child. Here the message is not necessarily that the child's contribution was acceptable, but that its value as a contribution to the conversation structure has been acknowledged. That is, the clinician has accepted the child's contribution as a turn that served to initiate, maintain, or bring to a close an already established topic. Furthermore, the clinician has modeled a more acceptable version of the child's production, possessing the same communicative intention but with a different surface structure.

Back to the "tricky part" of expansion use: unless the clinician carefully uses the linguistic and nonlinguistic information available from the context of the ongoing conversation—for example, what was happening at the time of the child's utterance, what constituted the clinician's linguistic turn just before the child spoke—the clinician may misinterpret what the child was attempting to convey and the child may not have the ability or willingness to correct the adult.

Expatiation

Expatiation is closely related to expansion in that the clinician produces an adult-appropriate version of what the child was attempting to produce. However, in expatiation, the clinician's version of the child's utterance extends beyond the apparent limits of the child's original utterance. Again, the clinician must carefully consider the context of the child's utterance to produce something that reflects the child's intent. If the main goal of expressive language development is to enable the child to encode the relationships among the people, places, things, and events in the world, then what is said must match closely the child's own perceptions. This is not always easy to do, especially when SLPs operate in situations where contextual information can be compromised, as in a therapy room.

Recasting

Recasting is a technique for providing new linguistic information to a child by producing a "new linguistic structure embedded within a partial repetition of the child's own prior utterance" (Camarata, 1995, p. 72). Similar to the description of expansions and expatiations provided above, recasts are required to be produced immediately after production of an incorrect (or incomplete) child utterance and they must provide the child with added linguistic information relative to how the child can more accurately use the language structure he or she attempted. So, for example, if the child said, "More cookie," the adult might recast that utterance by saying, "You want more cookies." According to Nelson and his colleagues (Nelson, Camarata, Welsh, Butkowski, & Camarata, 1996), recasts represent "rare events" in child–caregiver conversations, but when they do occur with sufficient frequency, they can facilitate the development of new language structures in a child's repertoire.

Modeling

Definitions of the modeling technique abound. For our purposes, a very broad definition has been adopted. Modeling can be thought of as an utterance that attempts to demonstrate one viable linguistic option that could be used in that situation. Unlike imitation, expansion, and expatiation, the basis for the modeled utterance does not have to be something said by the child.

Sometimes the clinical expectation in modeling is that the child will imitate the clinician's production. In other clinical applications, modeling provides the child with examples of the acceptable target structure, either in a structured setting or within quasi-natural conversation, and no response from the child is expected. What is expected is that the child will listen carefully and observe how the clinician's utterances "work" in the situation. In still others, reinforcers are given to the speaker-model for acceptably modeled utterances. Sometimes the speaker is a third participant (Leonard, 1975), and the client is asked to consider all of the examples provided and then determine what made some of the modeled utterances acceptable and others unacceptable. In this way, the child is led along a path of rule induction.

In some language intervention programs, self-talk and parallel talk are described as separate techniques, but under the broad definition used here, they are both more specific types of modeling. **Self-talk** refers to the clinician's monologue about what she is doing. **Parallel talk** refers to the clinician's running commentary describing what the child is doing. Neither situation necessitates that the child says anything in response. Instead, it is hypothesized that the client is being provided with opportunities to match ongoing activity with appropriate linguistic encoding in a nonthreatening manner.

Scaffolding

Bruner (1985) and others have used the term *scaffolding* to describe a pattern of interaction noted in mother–child dyads. It is a description of what Vygotsky may have been referring to when he suggested that children learn through the assistance of competent confederates (Bruner, 1985). Caregivers become well versed in their children's abilities, whether language or motor skills, so that when they request action or information from their children they can predict whether their child will be able to comply successfully. It has been generally observed that most parents want to see their children succeed. Knowing their child's capabilities is useful not only because caregivers like to have their children "show off," but also because they want to be able to *reasonably* increase the degree of difficulty in the tasks they request of their children. In this way, they can maintain the challenge of the interaction (and thus their child's attention) and promote success at the same time. These two characteristics of a language task will help to ensure their child's continued participation and learning (Kirchner, 1991).

This sort of scaffolding interaction has been demonstrated in repetitions of storybook readings observed between young children and their caregivers. Often children request readings of the same book night after night. When examples of these separate readings were analyzed in a controlled study, Snow and Goldfield (1983) found that the dialogue between caregiver and child changed as the child became more familiar with the book. Specifically, the mother in the study was asking new and more challenging questions of her child when she was reasonably sure the child would be able to answer correctly.

Scaffolding also serves as a useful metaphor for speech-language intervention. That is, treatment goals should always represent achievements still beyond the child's easy grasp. If they are too easily achieved or cannot be achieved, the goals are inappropriate. Reaching an easily achieved goal does not represent true growth, and improbably difficult goals only frustrate the child. Prerequisite skills for achieving selected goals should be in place, making the eventual reaching of the goal reasonable with sufficient teaching and practice. Competent SLPs constantly monitor their clients' performances for evidence that tasks and goals have been chosen appropriately.

S.O.U.L.

S.O.U.L (Silence, Observation, Understanding, and Listening) is a technique developed in conjunction with the INREAL (Inclass Reactive Language Therapy) program (Weiss, 1981) to establish an empathetic relationship with the child. The four portions of S.O.U.L. are part of the general reactive approach espoused by INREAL proponents, who are taught to "follow the child's lead" rather than impose structure on the client. Remaining silent at least initially in your dealings with a young child, observing what the child is able to do and is interested in, attempting to make sense of the observations you have made, and listening to what the child says whether or not you are involved in the conversation should permit you and the young child to get to know each other. According to the INREAL approach, that is the way an adult earns the right to enter into a therapeutic relationship with a child (Weiss, 1981). See Table 6.3 for examples of these six techniques carried out in context.

TABLE 6.3	Dialogue Excerpts Illustrating Language Intervention Techniques

Setting: A preschool classroom at snacktime. A speech-language clinician and a child with a language disorder are seated next to each other. They talk while consuming grape juice and celery sticks spread with peanut butter.

S.O.U.L.: Before joining the child at the snack table and engaging the child in conversation, the clinician spent several minutes silently observing the child. Listening carefully, the clinician realized that the child had some concerns about the snack. He had never eaten celery before and was told by his teacher that he had to at least try some. The child appeared to be quite apprehensive as the clinician approached.

Imitation
CHILD: Don't want more juice.
CLINICIAN: Don't want more juice?

Expansion
CHILD: That crunchy one. (*referring to celery*)
CLINICIAN: You're right. That's a crunchy one.

Expatiation
CHILD: Gimme more uh that.
CLINICIAN: Give me some more of that celery because it's *good*.

Modeling (parallel talk)
CLINICIAN: You've licked all the peanut butter out of that celery stalk. Now you're chewing that celery very carefully. Oh, you're done with it.

Scaffolding
CLINICIAN: That peanut butter is crunchy. That celery is crunchy. That snack is crunchy. That peanut butter is _____ .
CHILD: Crunchy.
CLINICIAN: Yeah. It sure is. Tell me about that celery.
CHILD: Celery is crunchy.

CURRENT INTERVENTION APPROACHES

This section is divided into four parts, each of which reflects an aspect of the current intervention literature. In one, Fey's (1986) assertiveness-responsiveness scheme will be explained in some detail because it presents an underlying focus on intervention that is functionalist; in other words, it is pragmatic in its orientation and thus very current in its approach. Second, approaches useful in treatment focusing on caregiver–child interactions will be discussed (MacDonald & Carroll, 1992a, 1992b). The third portion of this section is the topic of treatment efficacy research where treatment approaches have been compared. This has continued to represent a burgeoning part of the work done in the area of language intervention for young children, and we will deal with some of the most recent findings in this very necessary area of research endeavor. In the final portion, several approaches—one new and two that have been discussed for a number of years—will be presented.

Fey's Assertiveness-Responsiveness Scheme

In his text, *Language Intervention with Young Children,* Fey (1986) described four different types of language-impaired children, a method used to delineate these types, and a suggested prescription for planning appropriate intervention based on the characteristics of each. A traditional approach would have been to take the child's production of language form as the basis of the classification system by prioritizing analysis of syntax and morphological performance. Instead, Fey suggested that the child's ability to *use* the language he has in his productive repertoire is the key for delineating impairment type. This is clearly a functional approach to clinical intervention, as evidenced by the fact that the author strongly encourages that data used for diagnostic decision making be collected in a number of natural speaking situations where the child interacts with different co-conversationalists. The child's home and classroom environments should both be carefully scrutinized so that conversational competencies exhibited by the language-impaired child in the clinic do not bias the diagnosis of impairment type.

Fey (1986) used two distinctive features of conversational participation as his primary diagnostic variables: conversational assertiveness, a reference to the child's propensity or ability to take a turn in a conversation even when one has not been specifically solicited by the child's co-conversationalist; and conversational responsiveness, the child's propensity or ability to provide appropriate responses to the requests made by the child's conversation partner. If the child exhibits the feature, it is assigned a positive value; if the child does not exhibit the feature, it is assigned a negative value. Four combinations of the two features and their respective values are possible, each describing a different type of language impairment:

Conversational Characteristics	*Description of Child*
+ Assertiveness, + Responsiveness	"Active conversationalist"
– Assertiveness, + Responsiveness	"Passive conversationalist"
+ Assertiveness, – Responsiveness	"Verbal noncommunicator"
– Assertiveness, – Responsiveness	"Inactive communicator"

Methods for analyzing assertiveness and responsiveness with a child's language sample using a coding system designed to analyze both utterance-level contributions and topic management as well as cautions for making diagnoses of each of these four language impairment types are carefully delineated by the author. Note that each of the four "types" really describes a prototype, so that some children may not neatly fit into one or another of these groups but fall somewhere between.

Once the child has been described as generally exhibiting one or another of these impairment/language use types, intervention programming goals based on the child's conversational characteristics can be implemented (Fey, 1986, p. 99). The basic premise for devising intervention plans for each of these four separate groups is that the general goals for each impairment type are closely related to how the child does and does not use language in conversations. For example, consider a child who has been diagnosed as an active conversationalist by demonstrating that he is assertive and responsive in conversations. This means that the child places himself in situations where conversations are occurring and participates in them even though the language form or content used may not be as sophisticated as would be expected, given the child's age. Nevertheless, this child has demonstrated an appreciation for the assertiveness and responsiveness expected of a conversational partner. It is also likely that the child will recognize the conversational utility of learning new forms. In fact, this is a child for whom spontaneous generalization to using newly trained forms in conversation may occur because the underlying knowledge of conversational speech acts is present and put into practice.

Table 6.4 contains a delineation of basic intervention goals for the four classifications of language-impaired children described by Fey (1986). As shown in the table, active conversationalists have demonstrated use of a number of different conversation acts (requests for information, comments, response for clarification, etc.) but need new structures to fulfill them in conversation. According to Fey (p. 99), these children will also need opportunities to recognize that forms already in their repertoire may satisfy a number of different conversational acts (goal 2). In contrast to active conversationalists, inactive communicators demonstrate a lack of both assertiveness and responsiveness in conversation. These children need to learn their roles in conversation first, before specific forms are targeted. Unlike with active conversationalists, it cannot be assumed that these children have an underlying appreciation for conversational act usage.

It is helpful to view the basic goals outlined by Fey as a general umbrella under which more client-specific goals can be listed. Once the classification of the child has been established, treatment may begin because the clinician then has a better understanding of the conversational role(s) typically played by the child and what the child's conversational needs are. Note that conversational competence is the goal for all clients served by this approach.

Use of a Conversational Framework for Treatment

As noted earlier in this chapter, the incorporation of parents into treatment programs is not necessarily a new focus for language interventionists working with young children. Caregivers presumably spend a significant amount of time with their children,

TABLE 6.4	Goals Suggested for Children Exhibiting Fey's Patterns of Language Use

Impairment Type	Goals
Active conversationalist (+ assertive, + responsive)	1. New content-form interactions are trained for use with conversation acts already acquired. 2. Child will use old forms to express different conversation acts.
Passive conversationalist (– assertive, + responsive)	1. Child will make more frequent use of acquired assertive conversation acts in social contexts. 2. Child will increase the variety of requestive conversation acts used. 3. New linguistic forms will be learned to express assertive conversation acts.
Verbal noncommunicators (+ assertive, – responsive)	1. The child's responses will demonstrate more relatedness to assertives produced by the co-conversationalist. 2. Topically related utterances will be produced more often. 3. Referents will be indicated more clearly.
Inactive communicators (– assertive, – responsive)	1. Both verbal and nonverbal social bids will occur more frequently in many different social contexts. 2. Add goals for the passive conversationalist.

Source: Adapted from Fey (1986).

involved in daily routine activities that can be used as background for a foreground of language-learning opportunities. MacDonald and Carroll (1992a, 1992b) have delineated a systematic approach for teaching parents, as well as whoever else typically interacts with children, how to facilitate conversational exchanges with young partners who are very limited in how they can make conversational contributions. Their overriding rationale for this program is that when a child with a language disorder can communicate successfully with adults, all developmental areas will benefit, not just the development of the child's communication skills (p. 47).

MacDonald and Carroll (1992a) refer to their approach as the ECO model, signifying that when involving young children with language deficits in conversations it is important also to involve "their social ecology, including the relationships and play contexts" and to remember the framework supplied by the scaffolding technique, discussed above, where a more knowledgeable interactant provides assistance to the degree needed to ensure the less competent participant's success. In this case, all potential language-competent conversation partners can serve as the supportive, enabling participants for the child with language disorders. Notice how the heart of the intervention is in the most social of venues: conversation.

The authors suggest that it is important to teach children to be initiators in their conversational interactions as well as to be adequate responders. Remember from the discussion of work reported by Rice and colleagues (1993) that children with language deficits rarely initiate and only infrequently are they selected to receive the social/conversational bids of their peers. It was this finding that led Rice and her colleagues to suggest that classroom teachers intervene directly to redirect the children's adult-directed conversation turns to their classmates. MacDonald and Carroll's (1992a, 1992b) program may represent a prerequisite step in this process inasmuch as it focuses more directly on adult–child communications. It provides guidance for adults who want to figure out how to increase the likelihood that children with limited language will be successful communicators in these interactions. Part of the battle may first involve increasing the likelihood that the child will be willing to communicate with the adult.

The following five interactive styles of communication are suggested by Mac-Donald and Carroll (1992a) as successful for facilitating communication with young children. Adults are told that *balance,* as it relates to the egalitarian nature of sharing the responsibility for conversation, should be a goal. That is, neither partner should be expected to carry the burden of the conversation; similarly, no one participant should dominate the conversation. Adults are also told to promote *responsiveness,* meaning that as rudimentary as a child's early attempts at conversation turn taking are, efforts should be made by the adult to fit these turns within a meaningful conversation framework. It is also important for the adults to *match* the child's current linguistic repertoire with the expectations for conversation participation. This should ensure a maximum of participation on the part of the child because he or she will be less likely to feel overwhelmed with the conversation task and more likely to risk participation. Another interactive style is that of *nondirectiveness,* meaning that the child's lead is followed by the adult where the former clearly has a topic or focus. In addition, nondirectiveness has to do with the adult's demonstrated willingness to allow the child to direct the interaction (i.e., changing or shading topics). Finally, *emotional* attachment refers to the stage of participation in the dyad when the adult begins to converse with the child because the activity is rewarding in and of itself, rather than because the particular conversation serves as a means to an end.

Note that the Hanen program, developed by Manolson and colleagues in Toronto, as well as the INREAL program developed by Weiss and her colleagues in Colorado, take much the same tack. That is, the child with a language disorder is viewed as part of a communication dyad, most often with a primary caregiver, that needs repair to function optimally. With conversation as its basis, participants—both child and adult—are taught how to communicate more successfully within the limitations imposed by the child's deficient language repertoire. In all cases, caregivers are trained to become more reactive to their children's language attempts.

Recent Findings in Intervention Research

There appear to be at least two main focuses for research involving language intervention with young children. In one branch of the research literature, investigators are attempting to determine whether one service delivery mode is more efficacious than another (Wilcox, Kouri, & Caswell, 1991). In the other branch of intervention research, investigators are comparing two or more treatment methods to determine which work, which may work better, and if there is a differential effect of the treatments, which children seem to benefit more from which treatment (Ellis Weismer,

Murray-Branch, & Miller, 1994). Related to this second focus are studies that have attempted to study the relationships that may exist between treatments provided for phonological or grammatical deficits (Tyler & Sandoval, 1994).

A Comparison of Classroom versus Individual Intervention

Wilcox et al. (1991) reported the results from a study of 20 children roughly between a year and a half and four years of age who were learning their first vocabularies. All of the children had been diagnosed with language delays; half received treatment within a classroom setting and half received individual treatment. Treatment measures of vocabulary growth indicated that neither service delivery situation had yielded superior results until the investigators looked at the children's abilities as measured by generalization to their home environments. Specifically, the children taught the new targeted vocabulary items in the classroom were significantly more likely to generalize these vocabulary words to the home environment than were the children who had received individual (pull-out) instruction. Therefore, the researchers concluded that for the purpose of early vocabulary training, the classroom environment is not only a viable location for service delivery but it is also a superior one.

In another, more recent study that looked at differences between service delivered within the classroom and outside of the classroom setting, Roberts, Prizant, and McWilliam (1995) focused on the communication dynamics of the clinician–client dyads in both venues. Although they looked carefully at a number of potential differences in conversation behaviors, only two reached significance. Their findings revealed that during the within-class interactions, children were less responsive to the clinicians, showing a significantly greater degree of compliance during the out-of-class sessions. On the other hand, their SLPs tended to contribute more turns to conversations conducted during out-of-class sessions than those held within the classroom. Given that only these two differences were discovered, the authors suggested that decisions concerning selection of in-class versus out-of-class service delivery should be made on the basis of more than just these differences in communication dynamics. They argued that their findings did not allow them to conclude that a higher degree of treatment efficacy could necessarily be related to a particular service delivery model.

Treatment Efficacy: Selecting among Treatment Options

Ellis Weismer and colleagues (1994) attempted to determine the effects of two procedures—modeling only, and modeling with an evoked production—on teaching new vocabulary items to three young children identified as late talkers. Two of the three subjects demonstrated learning that could be attributed to the treatment procedures, but interestingly, one of the two children appeared to benefit from one of the techniques and the other benefited from the other technique. Unfortunately, attempts to utilize dynamic assessment methods to determine if it might have been possible to predict ahead of time which subject would do better with which treatment technique failed to yield helpful results. The third subject did not appear to make gains from implementation of either treatment method.

In a study by Camarata, Nelson, and Camarata (1994), two methods, one employing imitation and one employing conversational recasting, were employed to teach a number of different grammatical structures to young children diagnosed with specific language impairment. Although both of the techniques appeared to be effective in facilitating the subjects' productions of the majority of the targeted structures, the conversational recasting procedure was more facilitative when both spontaneous productions of the trained targets and generalized, spontaneous productions of untrained structures were considered. These findings suggest that a method that is less structured and more naturalistic may be better able to foster generalization, specifically to conversational settings.

In a study utilizing the techniques of verbal routines and expansions, Yoder, Spruytenburg, Edwards, and Davies (1995) found that their four subjects, who ranged in age from two years to four and a half years, made gains as measured by mean length of utterance (MLU) over the duration of the treatment. However, looking retrospectively at the results, which included assessing generalization across trainers, interaction styles, and modalities, the authors noted that the children in the earlier stages of language development appeared to make greater gains than those subjects who were in the later stages, which may have had to do with the measure of progress chosen (MLU), which is less sensitive to gains in language development after the MLU reaches 3.0.

Remember that we already discussed Fey and his colleagues' work comparing the performance of parents and clinicians in providing treatment (Cleave & Fey, 1997) and the differences in recasting production by parents of children with language impairments versus the recasting production of parents with normally developing children (Fey, Krulik, Loeb, & Proctor-Williams, 1999). Both studies yielded useful clinical implications. In the first study, both parents and clinicians were trained to provide treatment using focused stimulation and cyclical goal attack strategies. Although both groups of children improved, the authors concluded that a combination of clinic-based services and parent programs would have gleaned the most positive results. In the latter study, Fey et al. (1999) observed no appreciable differences between the quality and quantity of recasting provided by the two groups of parents to their differently abled children which led the investigators to conclude that their language-impaired subjects probably needed the benefit not only of more recasting but recasting that was more focused on their language needs.

Differential Effects of Phonological and Language Treatment

Fey, Cleave, Ravida, Long, Dejmal, and Easton (1994) were interested in examining the effects of two grammar-focused treatment programs on the phonological abilities of their group of subjects, all of whom were diagnosed with deficits in both grammatical and phonological development. Given that phonology is a bona-fide component of language, exploring the potential connectedness for treatment purposes between syntax and phonology makes sense but represents an area where there is little information for clinicians. Despite the fact that both treatment procedures were shown to have had a positive effect on facilitation of the subjects' grammar performance, there were no obvious effects on the children's phonological skills. The authors concluded that their results do not support a shared effect between language treatment focused on grammar and phonological gains, and that difficulties with the speech sound system should be addressed directly with preschool-aged children.

In a study similar in focus, Tyler and Sandoval (1994) reported the findings of their treatment study from preschool-aged subjects who were diagnosed with both language and phonological deficits. There were three possible treatment methods received by the subjects, and they yielded significantly different results. Specifically, subjects who were recipients of direct intervention on their phonology targets ended up demonstrating moderate gains for both their phonology and language goals; those who were recipients of language treatment only showed some small language gains but little improvement in their phonology targets. Those subjects who were the recipients of a combined program focusing on both language and phonology demonstrated appreciable positive gains in both areas. The authors suggested that in most cases, if you can only focus on one of the two treatment areas, treating phonology is more likely to provide you with carryover effects to language than the other way around. However, when children are observed to have deficits in both areas, the most efficacious route would probably be to treat both phonology and language at the same time. Tyler and Sandoval (1994) noted that it was their least severely involved subjects who benefited the most from combined speech and language treatments.

A Language Intervention Focusing on Temporal Processing: Fast ForWord

One of the proposed etiologies for the language problems experienced by children with the diagnosis of specific language impairment is the presence of an auditory/perceptual deficit that renders the child at a disadvantage for processing rapidly changing auditory information such as the acoustic parameters that signal sound transitions in speech (Watkins, 1994). The Fast ForWord training program (Scientific Learning Corporation, 1998) as developed by Tallal, Merzenich, and their colleagues, is an attempt by the authors to retrain the child's brain so that the rapid temporal processing necessary for decoding linguistic input can be accomplished in a normal manner. This computer-based program is a series of games that includes acoustically altered stimuli where speech signal duration is lengthened and speech sound transitions are amplified; these alterations of stimuli are gradually diminished as the child demonstrates more success with the more rapidly presented acoustic information.

This training methodology has received a great deal of publicity due to the claims made by the publisher and the authors regarding the overwhelming success experienced by children who have used the program. According to Gillam (1999), however, there are a number of reasons why SLPs should approach a recommendation to adopt this program with caution. He noted that despite their reported successes with children in a couple of smaller studies (with twenty-two and seven children, respectively) and one larger field study (with data collected from 500 children who had received their training from more than fifty different professionals who had been trained in the Fast ForWord procedure), there are many questions about the efficacy of this approach. First and foremost, Gillam questions the basic assumptions of the program, that language impairment is caused by temporal processing deficits and the claim that the Fast ForWord program can actually change brain structure and functioning. Further, although he reports that there are some children who have apparently made significant gains as judged by pre- and posttesting on the instruments selected by the program's authors, he wonders to what extent these children also demonstrate truly different and improved communicative use of language in activities of daily living. Veale (1999) provides readers with her own critical assessment of Fast ForWord, with an emphasis on the subject selection criteria that have been employed and probably should be employed when deciding whether this is an appropriate program to try with a particular client. Both authors are hesitant to endorse this approach in view of the obvious lack of scientific data to support its basic claims.

INTERVENTION WITH CHILDREN FROM MULTICULTURAL POPULATIONS

Providing language intervention services to children from nonmajority populations can represent a challenge to the speech-language clinician, who may not share the same cultural background and/or first language with the client. Wyatt (1997) noted that SLPs should think carefully about the potential points of bias in the construction of intervention programs or selection of appropriate assessment tools to ensure quality service delivery for all of their clients—even those with whom they share cultural background and language.

For example, as Terrell and Hale (1992) noted, cultural differences may be manifested as differences in individual learning styles. It is important for SLPs to determine what that learning style difference is and how it can be best utilized for language learning purposes. Certainly it is true that paying attention to how our clients learn best should always be of paramount concern to speech-language clinicians. One major difference in learning style that SLPs should be aware of is that of low- versus high-context learning styles (Paul, 1995). Children raised in the majority culture tend to adopt a **low-context learning style,** meaning that they rely a great deal on explicit, verbal messages to learn new material, and often the teaching that occurs is decontextualized. On the other hand, the child who adopts a **high-context learning style**—and many of these children are from nonmajority populations—depends more on observation of the teacher and other nonlinguistic information than on the verbal information provided.

When interacting with children from cultures other than one's own, it is critical that the clinician convey both "respect for and appreciation of the child's L1 and culture" (Roseberry-McKibben, 1994, p. 84). Given a family system's approach to treatment management for young children, it is very likely that the parents and/or the child's extended family will be involved with the treatment program. Therefore, it will be necessary to determine the family's attitude toward intervention provided by someone from outside their cultural milieu—because statistically this is likely to be the case, given ASHA's membership demographics—and more generally, how the family approaches the notion of a disorder of communication and treatment for same. Knowing something of the family's cultural beliefs and attitudes about child rearing, family members' roles and responsibilities, illness and disease, will facilitate appropriate communication exchanges between the clinician and the family.

We will assume that the readers of this chapter are well aware of the language difference versus language disorder issue, that we should not be providing speech-language therapy for children demonstrating normal development in their first language although they may not be competent English language speakers (ASHA, 1983). For those readers who may want some good references that specifically address intervention with nonmajority populations, several useful references are provided in the Suggested Readings at the end of this chapter.

For children with bona-fide language disorders in their first language, treatment should be provided in that first language. Unfortunately, most SLPs are not bilingually competent to do so (ASHA, 1985), which means that provision of services may need to rely on the teaming of monolingual SLPs with someone who does possess linguistic competence in the child's first language. This person may already be a member of the child's treatment team (e.g., a resource room specialist), or may be a paraprofessional person hired because of bilingual competence. When the speech-language clinician works "through" another person, the type of working relationship that develops may range from one similar to the collaborative consultation model discussed to one that is very directive, as in the case of the paraprofessional.

FACILITATING GENERALIZATION

Generalization is such an important topic in the consideration of language intervention that it deserves its own section for discussion. Generalization is the hallmark of a successful intervention program and serves as one of the best ways, if not the best way, for SLPs to demonstrate the benefits of the programs they execute. As already mentioned, the seasoned clinician will develop a language intervention program with generalization in mind and not "train and hope" (Hughes, 1985, p. 1) that it will occur. If generalization did not occur, language intervention programs would be interminably long because clinicians would have to teach every possible occurrence of every goal.

Generalization is usually described as the use of trained responses in untrained situations. It is evidence that the child actually learned something in intervention that is transferable beyond the treatment setting, although, as will be discussed, that "something" may not always be what was intended by the clinician! Note the use of the term *response* here. Much of the work done concerning generalization has come out of the learning theory tradition, with its historical roots in behaviorism. Therefore, the child's participation in language exchanges is most often viewed as a response to the stimuli presented by the world at large, whether by the parent, teacher, peer, sibling, or speech-language clinician.

Generalization Types

There are two basic types of generalization: stimulus generalization and response generalization, and the possibilities for both occurring should be considered. **Stimulus generalization** refers to the use of trained responses in: (1) a new setting (e.g., at school when the intervention took place at home, or in the playground at school when intervention occurred in the classroom), (2) with new people (e.g., with the classroom teacher when an SLP provided intervention, with a classmate when the classroom teacher provided intervention, or with a new clinician during the spring semester when the child had been taught the goal by last fall's clinician), and (3) with new materials (e.g., the child responds to the clinician's use of pictures when only object stimuli had previously been used in intervention, or the child who was taught narrative skills in intervention using sequencing cards now displays those skills when shown a videotape). In each case, the child exhibits command over language goals that had been taught in a different situation.

Response generalization refers to learning that has transcended a language complexity level or that has extended to untrained examples at the same level of complexity. For example, if a language goal was targeted at the sentence level and the child demonstrates production (or comprehension) of that goal in text (e.g., a narrative or an expository paragraph), response generalization has been achieved. Similarly, if in spontaneous interactions with the clinician the child uses request forms that were never specifically targeted in therapy, response generalization has occurred, provided that different request types had been targeted in therapy. If the new request forms in this last example were produced in conversation with the child's classroom teacher, both response and stimulus generalization could be said to have occurred. That is, new response types were produced (response generalization), and they were produced with a new person (stimulus generalization). Table 6.5 lists some of the differences between stimulus and response generalization.

Why Attempts to Teach Generalization Fail

When generalization does not occur, there are several probable explanations. The fact that the clinician has an agenda to enhance generalization through teaching does not mean that the agenda has been conveyed to the child. What may seem perfectly well connected, logical, and rule based to a competent adult language user may not be quite as logical when perceived by a young child with a language disorder.

TABLE 6.5	Example Showing Differences between Stimulus and Response Generalization

Scenario: Child, age 5, receives language intervention at school twice weekly in individual sessions. The clinician uses picture cards with action illustrations to prompt child to form past tense of verbs. Child enters the house and announces: "Mom, I walk*ed* home with Joe."

Stimulus generalization	*Response generalization*
Use with:	Use at a different language complexity level
a new person (with mother),	(in a sentence, not a single word)
or	*or*
in a new setting (at home)	Use of an untrained example at the same
or	language complexity level (*walked* was
new materials (spontaneous production)	never targeted)

In the case of response generalization, what we are really hoping to convey to our young clients is that we are teaching them general rules that can be applied in multiple settings. We do this by teaching a subset of examples that are drawn from all possibilities and that we hope are good, representative examples. Sometimes we use only a few examples of the targeted rule; this has been referred to as "training deep" (Elbert & Gierut, 1985). For some children, the commonality that exists among these few examples cannot be understood. So, in some cases where generalization does not occur, training too deeply may be the problem.

At other times we may make use of too many examples, and the rule may be lost on the young child. Using a large number of exemplars has been referred to by Elbert and Gierut (1985) as "training broad." Training broad may be the problem standing in the way of generalizations for some children in some language learning situations. SLPs sometimes must struggle to find that "just right" mixture where we do not burden the child with too many examples or undercut his or her ability to find the general rule by providing too few examples. Sometimes, too, the examples are poor or nonrepresentative, and that may be another reason why generalization fails to occur.

Some empirical data have been reported to assist clinicians in making these kinds of choices. Elbert, Powell, and Swartzlander (1991) noted that the number of exemplars needed for generalization to occur varied significantly among their nineteen phonologically impaired subjects. The majority of these children needed three exemplars (59 percent), but 14 percent required ten exemplars to reach the generalization criterion specified by these investigators. It might stand to reason that the child with a language impairment who has difficulty with the manipulation of language symbols would have more difficulty discerning common patterns in words, phrases, and sentences that would call for them to be treated in common ways without extensive practice with a large number of examples.

Response Sets

Another possibility for explaining generalization failure has to do with not knowing the appropriate response set for the examples taught. A **response set** is the extension of a language rule that can be reasonably expected.

For example, few SLPs would expect that by targeting -*ing*, the present progressive morpheme, one could logically expect the client to then generalize to learning to correctly use nominative and objective case pronouns correctly—for example, *he* versus *him*. Because these two goals seem to be entirely unrelated, generalization between them appears to be unlikely. What about teaching the initial /s/ sound and testing for generalization to the final /s/? That seems to be logical and could be expected, although there are a number of possible mitigating variables. If it turned out that probe testing revealed generalization to final /s/, it could be said that for that child initial /s/ and final /s/ belonged to the same response set. If not, then we could conclude that at least at this point the child does not see the connection or generalizability between the two.

This discussion of response set is important because it is possible to become overzealous in the quest for generalization and to expect generalization where generalization is not likely to occur. SLPs must remember to try to take the child's perspective and to keep the expectation for generalization from exceeding what is reasonable. Children who have language disorders have already experienced too much failure. Often, their failure to generalize can be traced back to the clinician's own faulty planning. More specifically, the child's failure to generalize could be the result of expecting generalization where none should be expected; using exemplars in intervention that are poor representatives of the rule, principle, or construct being taught; using too few or too many examples; or not having spent enough time in intervention to expect generalization learning to have occurred in the first place.

Planning for Generalization

As stated throughout this chapter, SLPs must plan strategies for generalization from the very start of intervention planning. Remember that to some extent concerns about generalization and context-appropriate treatment led to the movement toward classroom-based language intervention. Providing intervention in a context (the classroom) where newly taught gains in language competencies could be utilized frequently should make it more likely that generalization to the classroom will occur *without* the presence of the clinician. Opportunities for using the new language abilities should occur whether the clinician is present or not. SLPs who want to encourage generalization will be wise to spend substantial time pointing out to the child what the identifying characteristics of these opportunities are.

Hughes's (1985) text, *Language Treatment and Generalization*, contains many thoughtful and thought-provoking suggestions for generalization planning. The author presents two sets of these suggestions, one for making therapy more like natural environments (p. 157) and one for making the natural environment more like therapy (p. 158). In each case, the clinician attempts to give the client a broader perspective of where it is appropriate to use his new language skills. For example, Hughes suggests that SLPs should experiment in the therapy setting by transferring from contrived consequences to more natural consequences or prompts that might occur in activities of daily living, as well as suggesting to the child's caregivers that they use the same prompts used in the treatment setting by the clinician when they are at home with the child.

Apropos of this last suggestion, it is not uncommon to hear a young, noncompliant child tell a parent who is trying to do carryover work in the home: "I don't do that with you. I do that with [name of child's speech-language clinician]." In these cases, the child appears to categorize language functioning according to setting. Certain language is used in one setting and not in another. If the child "knows" this, then we may have fostered it, and we will have to spend time presenting counter evidence to *un*teach it.

SLPs should also recognize that some goals will be more easily generalized than others, due to the inherent, functional nature of the goal. These more easily generalized goals should be considered priorities in intervention, because they may assist the young child in understanding the gist of generalization. Consider, for example, the goal of demonstrating consistent production of request forms (e.g., "Can I have that?") versus the goal of spontaneously producing superlative adjective forms (e.g., fluffiest). Being able to produce a variety of request forms (e.g., "What did you say?" "Tell me another story" "Do you know where Mark is?") will permit a child to specifically request the information or action desired. Request forms are produced frequently in conversations and allow speakers to exert some control over an ongoing conversation and the immediate world. On the other hand, having a firm grasp on how to form superlative adjective forms is less functional. Superlative adjective forms are neither as common nor as critical to communication as the request form.

Last, as the child begins to grasp the specified language goal within a task or intervention structure, generalization can be facilitated if the speech-language clinician begins to systematically alter the teaching situation. Hughes (1985) referred to this as "teaching loosely" (p. 160). Within the teaching phase of intervention, the clinician adds some change to the proceedings. Perhaps this will mean that another person, maybe a parent, begins to sit in on the treatment sessions. It could mean that feedback is given on every other attempt at the teaching task made by the child, so that the intervention more closely resembles life outside the therapy room. Outside the therapy room, it is rare indeed to receive a pat on the back for a well-constructed sentence! Regardless of how the clinician attempts to loosen up the intervention process, the result should be the same: intervention that more closely resembles something other than intervention.

A Final Word on Generalization

These basic suggestions for promoting generalization apply whether intervention takes place in or outside a classroom and whether a teacher collaborated with the speech-language clinician or the speech-language clinician provides direct service delivery. The variables involved in enhancing generalization (e.g., settings, providers, targets for generalization) will differ from case to case depending on how the intervention was originally devised. However, no matter what the format of the language intervention, there is no excuse for not promoting generalization from the very first intervention session.

SOME THOUGHT-PROVOKING QUESTIONS FOR THE FUTURE

When we consider language intervention for young children, it seems we continue to leave at least two critical questions unanswered. The first has to do with our ability as professionals to predict language learning outcomes, and the second can be best described as an issue of treatment efficacy. That is, we need to be better able to predict on the basis of their earliest behaviors which children, who present themselves as at risk for language learning problems, will actually experience difficulties and what will be the magnitude of those problems. The logical concomitant question has to do with how we then go about selecting the most efficient and most effective treatment plan for each individual client.

Note that the twin questions of enhancing our powers of predictability and the efficacy of the treatment we provide both carry with them sets of underlying assumptions. The predictability question, for example, presupposes the availability of valid and reliable measures for evaluating a child's early language, social, and motor behaviors and the existence of adequate information concerning how these behaviors relate to normal developmental expectations. Questions of efficacy also have several underlying assumptions. In order to select an efficacious treatment plan, preliminary studies will first have to establish that each option is efficient and effective in its own right. Additional research will then have to determine which intervention plans are best suited to individual children based on carefully constructed profiles of each child's language learning strengths and weaknesses.

Answering questions that will allow us to serve as reliable predictors of future speech and language performance as well as provide the most efficient and effective intervention for our clients represents a challenge to clinicians and researchers alike. In fact, it is likely that it will take many years to be able to approach a comprehensive answer to either one. However, the answers to these questions are not luxuries. Rather, they are necessary if we are to continue to provide our clients with the best possible clinical services.

SUMMARY

This chapter described the speech-language pathologist's role in the development of language intervention programs for young children. It is important to understand the challenging nature of the decisions the clinician must make along the way, the different options available for selection, and the rationales behind those selections. Given the changing demographics of the young clients we serve as speech-language clinicians, it is additionally important that we acknowledge the ways in which cultural differences should affect the treatment choices we make.

Further, an understanding of the different theories of language acquisition allows the speech-language clinician to appreciate the evolution of the speech-language clinician's role in the therapeutic process itself. Specifically, many SLPs have moved from viewing themselves as language "trainers" to language "facilitators." This change can be credited directly to belief in the child as an active participant in the language development process and the view that learning language involves the learning of a generative rule system.

Language intervention may be accomplished in many different settings. SLPs should acknowledge the benefits and drawbacks to each service delivery model in terms of client progress. In addition, the roles of the classroom teacher and the child's parents in the successful completion of the language intervention program should be considered. It is rarely the case that language intervention for a child can afford to be viewed as the responsibility of SLPs alone.

Finally, the concept of generalization is one of the most essential to the development of appropriate language intervention procedures. Because language is generalizable, we are able to assume that a small and carefully chosen subset of all of the possible examples of a goal form or structure will be sufficient to teach a more general rule. For language intervention programs to work, SLPs must pay close attention to how they expect the children to generalize their learning from the first intervention contact. Troubleshooting the expected course of generalization from the very first planning stages will allow SLPs a greater chance for succeeding in increasing the language competence of the young child with a language disorder.

STUDY QUESTIONS

1. How do parents and classroom teachers serve indispensable functions in the success of language intervention programs developed for young children and their families?
2. Assume that SLPs have the luxury of determining which service delivery model will be used in each of the cases on their caseloads. Delineate the pros and cons of choosing a pull-out, classroom-based, or collaborative consultation service delivery model.
3. If generalization is essential to the success of any language intervention program, SLPs should account for it as early as possible in their planning. List five general strategies for enhancing the generalization observed in a young language-disordered child. Indicate the child's age, a particular goal for consideration, and the service delivery model through which the child receives language intervention.
4. You are planning a language intervention program for a young child from a culture other than your own. What information would you want to have before developing a plan that will assist you in designing an appropriate program? What information would you be able to collect during a diagnostic therapy phase that would help you to fine-tune your treatment approach?
5. What is the nature of the information collected during the evaluation/assessment phase of service delivery to a young child with language needs that would help you to develop an appropriate beginning treatment plan for this child?

SUGGESTED READINGS

Fortunately for those of us who practice in the area of speech-language pathology, the literature pertinent to the planning of language intervention with young children is a burgeoning one, with excellent new sources of information available almost continually. What follows is a listing of what I believe to be some of the best sources of information currently available.

Fey, M. (1986). *Language intervention with young children*. Boston: Allyn & Bacon.

Fey, M., Windsor, J., & Warren, S. (Eds.), (1995). *Language intervention: Preschool through the elementary years*. Baltimore: Paul H. Brookes.

Leonard, L. (1998). *Children with specific language impairment*. Cambridge, MA: MIT Press.

Lynch, E., & Hanson, M. (1998). (Eds.), *Developing cross-cultural competence: A guide for working with young children and their families*. Baltimore: Paul H. Brookes.

MacDonald, J., & Carroll, J. (1992). Communicating with young children: An ecological model for clinicians, parents, and collaborative professionals. *American Journal of Speech-Language Pathology, 1*(4), 39–48.

van Kleeck, A. (1994). Potential cultural bias in training parents as conversational partners with their children who have delays in language development. *American Journal of Speech-Language Pathology, 3*, 67–78.

REFERENCES

American Speech and Hearing Association (1983). Social dialects: A position paper. *ASHA, 25*(1), 23–24.

American Speech and Hearing Association (1985). Clinical management of communicatively handicapped minority language populations. *ASHA, 27*, 29–32.

American Speech-Language-Hearing Association (2000a). *IDEA and your caseload: A template for eligibility and dismissal criteria for students ages 3 to 21.* Rockville, MD: ASHA Action Center.

American Speech-Language-Hearing Association (2000b). *Prevalence of communication disorders in the United States.* Rockville, MD: ASHA Science and Research Department.

Aram, D., Ekelman, B., & Nation, J. (1984). Preschoolers with language disorders: 10 years later. *Journal of Speech and Hearing Research, 27*, 232–244.

Bain, B., & Olswang, L. (1995). Examining readiness for learning two-word utterances by children with specific expressive language impairment: Dynamic assessment validation. *American Journal of Speech-Language Pathology, 4*(1), 81–91.

Battle, D. (1998). Communication disorders in a multicultural society. In D. Battle (Ed.), *Communication disorders in multicultural populations* (2d ed.) (pp. 3–29). Boston: Butterworth-Heinemann.

Bedore, L., & Leonard, L. (1995). Prosodic and syntactic bootstrapping and their clinical applications: A tutorial. *American Journal of Speech-Language Pathology, 4*(1), 66–72.

Bricker, D. (1986). An analysis of early intervention programs: Attendant issues and future directions. In R. Morris and B. Blatt (Eds.), *Special education: Research and trends* (pp. 28–65). New York: Pergamon.

Bruner, J. (1985). Vygotsky: A historical and conceptual perspective. In J. Wertsch (Ed.), *Culture, communication, and cognition: Vygotskian perspectives.* Cambridge, UK: Cambridge University Press.

Brush, E. (1987, November). Public school language, speech and hearing services in the 1990's. Paper presented to the annual convention of the American Speech-Language-Hearing Association, New Orleans.

Camarata, S. (1995). A rationale for naturalistic speech intelligibility intervention. In M. Fey, J. Windsor, & S. Warren (Eds.), *Language intervention: Preschool through the elementary years* (pp. 63–84). Baltimore: Paul H. Brookes.

Camarata, S., Nelson, K., & Camarata, M. (1994). Comparison of conversational-recasting and imitative procedures for training grammatical structures in children with specific language impairment. *Journal of Speech and Hearing Research, 37*, 1414–1423.

Catts, H., & Kamhi, A. (Eds.). (1998). *Language and reading disabilities.* Boston: Allyn & Bacon.

Cleave, P., & Fey, M. (1997). Two approaches to the facilitation of grammar in children with language impairments: Rationale and description. *American Journal of Speech-Language Pathology, 6*(1), 22–32.

Cole, L. (1989). E pluribus pluribus: Multicultural imperatives and the 1990s and beyond. *ASHA, 31*, 65–70.

Connell, P. (1982). On training language rules. *Language, Speech and Hearing Services in Schools, 13*, 231–248.

Craig, H. (1993). Clinical forum: Language and social skills in the school-age population, social skills of children with specific language impairment: Peer relationships. *Language, Speech, and Hearing Services in Schools, 24,* 206–215.

Craig, H., & Washington, J. (1993). Access behaviors of children with specific language impairment. *Journal of Speech and Hearing Research, 36,* 311–321.

Crais, E. (1991). *A practical guide to embedding family-centered content into existing speech language pathology course work.* Chapel Hill, NC: Carolina Institute for Research in Infant Personnel Preparation.

Cross, T. (1978). Mothers' speech adjustments: The contribution of selected child listener variables. In C. Snow & C. Ferguson (Eds.), *Talking to children: Language input and acquisition.* Cambridge, UK: Cambridge University Press.

Damico, J., & Damico, S. (1993). Language and social skills from a diversity perspective: Considerations for the speech-language pathologist. *Language, Speech, and Hearing Services in Schools, 24,* 236–243.

Elbert, M., & Gierut, J. (1985). *Handbook of clinical phonology.* San Diego, CA: College-Hill.

Elbert, M., Powell, T., & Swartzlander, P. (1991). Toward a technology of generalization. How many exemplars are sufficient? *Journal of Speech and Hearing Research, 34*(1), 81–87.

Ellis Weismer, S. (1988). Specific language learning problems. In D. Yoder & R. Kent (Eds.), *Decision making in speech-language pathology.* Toronto: B. C. Decker.

Ellis Weismer, S., Murray-Branch, J., & Miller, J. (1994). A prospective longitudinal study of language development in late talkers. *Journal of Speech and Hearing Research, 37,* 852–867.

Ensher, G. (1989). The first three years: Special education perspectives on assessment and intervention. *Topics in Language Disorders, 10*(1), 80–90.

Farber, J., Denenberg, M., Klyman, S., & Lachman, P. (1992). Language resource room level of service: An urban school district approach to integrative treatment. *Language, Speech, & Hearing Services in Schools, 23,* 293–299.

Fey, M. (1986). *Language intervention with young children.* Boston: Allyn & Bacon.

Fey, M. (1988). Dismissal criteria for the language-impaired child. In D. Yoder & R. Kent (Eds.), *Decision making in speech-language pathology.* Toronto: B. C. Decker.

Fey, M., Catts, H., & Larrivee, L. (1995). Preparing preschoolers for the academic and social challenges of school. In M. Fey, J. Windsor, & S. Warren (Eds.), *Language intervention: Preschool through the elementary years* (pp. 3–34). Baltimore: Paul H. Brookes.

Fey, M., Cleave, P., Long, S., & Hughes, D. (1993). Two approaches to the facilitation of grammar in children with language impairment: An experimental evaluation. *Journal of Speech and Hearing Research, 36,* 141–157.

Fey, M., Cleave, P., Ravida, A., Long, S., Dejmal, A., & Easton, D. (1994). Effects of grammar facilitation on the phonological performance of children with speech and language impairments. *Journal of Speech and Hearing Research, 57,* 594–607.

Fey, M. Krulik, T., Loeb, D., & Proctor-Williams, K. (1999). Sentence recast use by parents of children with typical language and children with specific language impairment. *American Journal of Speech-Language Pathology, 8*(3), 273–286.

Frasinelli, L., Superior, K., & Meyers, J. (1983). A consultation model for speech and language intervention. *ASHA, 25*(11), 25–30.

Fujiki, M., & Brinton, B. (1984). Supplementing language therapy: Working with the classroom teacher. *Language, Speech and Hearing Services in Schools, 15*, 98–109.

Gillam, R. (1999). Computer-assisted language intervention using Fast ForWord: Theoretical and empirical considerations for clinical decision making. *Language, Speech, and Hearing Services in Schools, 30*(4), 363–370.

Girolametto, L. Tannock, R., & Siegel, L. (1993). Consumer-merited evaluation of interactive language intervention. *American Journal of Speech-Language Pathology, 2,* 41–51.

Goldberg, S. (1993). *Clinical intervention: A philosophy and methodology for clinical practice.* New York: Macmillan.

Goldstein, B. (2000). *Cultural and linguistic diversity resource guide for speech-language pathologists.* San Diego, CA: Singular/Thomson Learning.

Goldstein, H., English, K., Shafer, K., & Kaczmarek, L. (1997). Interaction among preschoolers without disabilities: Effects of across-the-day peer intervention. *Journal of Speech, Language, and Hearing Research, 40*(1), 33–48.

Guralnick, M. & Paul-Brown, D. (1977). The nature of verbal interactions among handicapped and non-handicapped preschool children. *Child Development, 48,* 254–260.

Hadley, P., & Schuele, M. (1998). Facilitating peer interaction: Socially relevant objectives for preschool language intervention. *American Journal of Speech-Language Pathology, 7*(4), 25–36.

Hall, P., & Tomblin, J. (1978). A follow-up study of children with articulation and language disorders. *Journal of Speech and Hearing Disorders, 43,* 227–241.

Hanson, M. (1998). Ethnic, cultural, and language diversity in intervention settings. In E. Lynch & M. Hanson (Eds.), *Developing cross cultural competence: A guide for working with young children and their families* (2d ed.) (pp. 3–22). Baltimore: Paul H. Brookes.

Hegde, M. (1993). *Treatment procedures in communicative disorders* (2d ed.). San Diego, CA: College-Hill.

Hughes, D. (1985). *Language treatment and generalization: A clinician's handbook.* San Diego, CA: College-Hill.

Janota, J. (1999). *ASHA omnibus survey.* Rockville, MD: American Speech-Language-Hearing Association.

Jenkins, J., & Heinen, A. (1989). Students' preferences for service delivery: Pull-out, in-class, or integrated models. *Exceptional Children, 55*(6), 516–523.

Johnston, J. (1983). What is language intervention? The role of theory. In J. Miller, D. Yoder, & R. Schiefelbusch (Eds.), *Contemporary issues in language intervention* (ASHA Reports No. 12). Rockville, MD: American Speech-Language-Hearing Association.

Kelly, D. (1998). A clinical synthesis of the "late talker" literature: Implications for service delivery. *Language, Speech, and Hearing Services in Schools, 29*(2), 76–84.

King, R., Jones, C., & Lasky, E. (1982). In retrospect: A fifteen-year follow-up report of speech-language disorders in children. *Language, Speech and Hearing Services in Schools, 13,* 24–32.

Kirchner, D. (1991). Using verbal scaffolding to facilitate conversational participation and language acquisition in children with developmental disorders. *Journal of Childhood Communicative Disorders, 14,* 81–98.

Klein, M., & Briggs, M. (1987). Facilitating mother–infant communicative interaction in mothers of high-risk infants. *Journal of Childhood Communicative Disorders, 14,* 81–98.

Leonard, L. (1975). Modeling as a clinical procedure in language training. *Language, Speech, and Hearing Services in Schools, 6,* 72–85.

Leonard, L. (1981). Facilitating linguistic skills in children with specific language impairment: A review. *Applied Psycholinguistics, 2,* 89–118.

Leonard, L. (1983). Discussion: Part II: Defining the boundaries of language disorders in children. In J. Miller, D. Yoder, & R. Schiefelbusch (Eds.), *Contemporary issues in language intervention* (ASHA Reports No. 12). Rockville, MD: American Speech-Language-Hearing Association.

Leonard, L. (1991). New trends in the study of early language acquisition. *American Speech-Language-Hearing Association, 33*(4), 43–44.

Leonard, L. (1998). *Children with specific language impairment.* Cambridge, MA: MIT Press.

Long, S., & Olswang, L. (1996). Readiness and patterns of growth in children with SELI. *American Journal of Speech-Language Pathology, 5*(1), 79–85.

Lowenthal, B. (1987) Public Law 99-457: An ounce of prevention (ERIC Document 293 300).

Lynch, E. (1998). Developing cross-cultural competence. In E. Lynch & M. Hanson (Eds.), *Developing cross-cultural competence* (2d ed.) (pp. 47–89). Baltimore: Paul H. Brookes.

Lyngaas, K., Nyberg, B., Hockenga, R., & Gruenewald, L. (1983). Language intervention in the multiple contexts of the public school setting. In J. Miller, D. Yoder, & R. Schiefelbusch (Eds.), *Contemporary issues in language intervention* (ASHA Reports No. 12). Rockville, MD: American Speech-Language-Hearing Association.

MacDonald, J., & Carroll, J. (1992a).Communicating with young children: An ecological model for clinicians, parents and collaborative professionals. *American Journal of Speech-Language Pathology, 1*(4), 39–48.

MacDonald, J., & Carroll, J. (1992b). A social partnership model for assessing early communication development: An intervention model for preconversational children. *Language, Speech, & Hearing Services in Schools, 23,* 113–124.

MacDonald, J., & Gillette, Y. (1984). Conversation engineering: A pragmatic approach to early social competence. *Seminars in Speech and Language, 5,* 171–183.

Marvin, C. (1987). Consultation services: Changing roles for SLPs. *Journal of Childhood Communication Disorders, 11,* 1–15.

Maxwell, S., & Wallach, G. (1984). The language learning disabilities connection: Symptoms of early language disability change over time. In G. Wallach & K. Butler (Eds.), *Language learning disabilities in school-age children.* Baltimore: Williams & Wilkins.

McLean, J. (1983). Historical perspectives on the content of child language programs. In J. Miller, D. Yoder, & R. Schiefelbusch (Eds.), *Contemporary issues in language intervention* (ASHA Reports No. 12). Rockville, MD: American Speech-Language-Hearing Association.

Miller, L. (1989). Classroom-based language intervention. *Language, Speech and Hearing Services in Schools, 20,* 153–169.

Nelson, C., & Blakeley, R. (1989). Clinicianship: What is it? *Seminars in Speech and Language, 10*(2), 102–112.

Nelson, K., Camarata, S., Welsh, J., Butkovsky, L., & Camarata, M. (1996). Effects of imitative and conversational recasting treatment on the acquisition of grammar in children with specific language impairment and younger language-normal children. *Journal of Speech and Hearing Research, 39*, 850–859.

Nelson, N. (1998). *Childhood language disorders in context: Infancy through adolescence* (2d ed.). Boston: Allyn & Bacon.

Newhoff, M. (1995). So many fads, so little data. *Clinical Connection, 8*(3), 1–5.

Odom, S., & McEvoy, M. (1988). Integration of young children with handicaps and normally developing children. In S. Odom & M. Karnes (Eds.), *Early intervention for infants and children with handicaps*. Baltimore: Paul H. Brookes.

Olswang, L., & Bain, B. (1985). Monitoring phoneme acquisition for making treatment withdrawal decisions. *Applied Psycholinguistics, 6*, 17–37.

Olswang, L., & Bain, B. (1991). Clinical Forum: Treatment efficacy: When to recommend intervention. *Language, Speech, and Hearing Services in Schools, 22*, 255–263.

Olswang, L., & Bain, B. (1996). Assessment information for predicting upcoming changes in language production. *Journal of Speech and Hearing Research, 39*(2), 414–423.

Olswang, L., Rodriguez, B., & Timler, G. (1998). Recommending intervention for toddlers with specific language learning difficulties: We may not have all the answers, but we know a lot. *American Journal of Speech-Language Pathology, 7*(1), 23–32.

Office of Special Education Programs (1999). *21st annual report to Congress on the implementation of the Individuals with Disabilities Education Act*. Washington, DC: U.S. Department of Education.

Paul, R. (1995). *Language disorders from infancy through adolescence: Assessment and intervention*. St. Louis: Mosby-Year Book.

Pierce, R., & McWilliams, P. (1993). Emerging literacy and children with severe speech and physical impairments (SSPI): Issues and possible intervention strategies. *Topics in Language Disorders, 1*(2), 47–57.

Pletcher, L. (1995). *Family-centered practices: A training guide*. Raleigh, NC: ARCH National Resource Center.

Prelock, P., Miller, B., & Reed, N. (1995). Collaborative partnerships in a language in the classroom program. *Language, Speech, and Hearing Services in Schools, 26*, 286–292.

Ramey, C., & Ramey, S. (1998). Early intervention and early experience. *American Psychologist, 53*, 109–120.

Ratner, N., & Bruner, J. (1978). Games, social exchange and the acquisition of language. *Journal of Child Language, 5*, 392–401.

Records, N., Tomblin, J., & Freese, P. (1992). The quality of life among young adults with histories of Specific Language Impairment. *American Journal of Speech-Language Pathology, 1*(2), 44–53.

Records, N., & Weiss, A. (1990). Clinical judgment: An overview. *Journal of Childhood Communication Disorders, 13*(2), 153–165.

Rescorla, L., & Schwartz, E. (1990). Outcome of toddlers with specific expressive language delay. *Applied Psycholinguistics, 11*, 393–407.

Rice, M. (1993). Social consequences of specific language impairment. In H. Grimm & H. Skowranek (Eds.), *Language acquisition problems and reading disorders: Aspects of diagnosis and intervention* (pp. 111–128). New York: de Gruyter.

Rice, M., Hadley, P., & Alexander, A. (1993). Social biases toward children with speech and language impairments: A correlative causal model of language limitation. *Applied Psycholinguistics, 14,* 445–471.

Rice, M., Sell, M., & Hadley, P. (1991). Social interactions of speech and language impaired children. *Journal of Speech and Hearing Research, 34,* 1299–1307.

Roberts, J., Prizant, B., & McWilliam, R. (1995). Out-of-class versus in-class service delivery in language intervention: Effects on communication interaction with young children. *American Journal of Speech-Language Pathology, 4*(2), 87–94.

Roseberry-McKibben, C. (1994). Assessment and intervention for children with limited English proficiency and language disorders. *American Journal of Speech-Language Pathology, 3*(3), 77–88.

Roseberry-McKibben, C., & Eicholtz, G. (1994). Serving children with limited English proficiency in the schools: A national survey. *Language, Speech, & Hearing Services in Schools, 25,* 156–164.

Rovee-Collier, C., Lipsitt, L., & Hayne, H. (Eds.). (1998). *Advances in infancy research 12.* Stamford, CT: Ablex.

Scarborough, H., & Dorbrich, W. (1990). Development of children with early language delay. *Journal of Speech and Hearing Research, 33,* 70–83.

Schuele, M., Rice, M., & Wilcox, K. (1995). Redirects: A strategy to increase peer initiations. *Journal of Speech and Hearing Research, 38*(6), 1319–1333.

Screen, R., & Anderson, N. (1994). *Multicultural perspectives in communication disorders.* San Diego, CA: Singular.

Shriberg, L., & Kwiatkowski, J. (1982). Phonological disorders II: A conceptual framework for management. *Journal of Speech and Hearing Disorders, 47,* 242–256.

Snow, C. (1986). Conversations with children. In P. Fletcher & M. Garman (Eds.), *Language acquisition* (2d ed.). New York: Cambridge University Press.

Snow, C., & Goldfield, B. (1983). Turn the page please: Situation-specific language acquisition. *Journal of Child Language, 10,* 551–569.

Snyder, L. (1980). Have we prepared the language disordered child for school? *Topics in Language Disorders, 1*(1), 29–45.

Snyder, L., Apolloni, T., & Cooke, T. (1977). Integrated settings at the early childhood level: The role of non-retarded peers. *Exceptional Children, 43,* 262–266.

Sparks, S. (1989). Assessment and intervention with at risk infants and toddlers: Guidelines for the speech-language pathologist. *Topics in Language Disorders, 10*(1), 43–56.

Stainback, S., Stainback, W., & Forest, M. (Eds.). (1989). *Educating all students in the mainstream of regular education.* Baltimore: Paul H. Brookes.

Stainback, W., & Stainback, S. (1990). *Support networks for inclusive schooling: Independent integrated education.* Baltimore: Paul H. Brookes.

Stothard, S., Snowling, M., Bishop, D., Chipchase, B., & Kaplan, C. (1998). Language impaired preschoolers: A follow-up into adolescence. *Journal of Speech, Language, and Hearing Research, 41*(2), 407–418.

Terrell, B., & Hale, J. (1992). Serving a multicultural population: Different learning styles. *American Journal of Speech-Language Pathology, 1*(2), 5–8.

Thal, D. (November, 1999). Early identification of risk for language impairment: Challenges for the profession. A seminar presented at the annual convention of the American Speech-Language-Hearing Association, San Francisco.

Tomblin, J. B., Records, N., Buckwalter, P., Zhang, X., Smith, E., & O'Brien, M. (1997). Prevalence of specific language impairment in kindergarten children. *Journal of Speech, Language, and Hearing Research, 40,* 1245–1260.

Tyler, A., & Sandoval, K. (1994). Preschoolers with phonological and language disorders: Treating different linguistic domains. *Language, Speech, and Hearing Services in Schools, 25,* 215–234.

van Kleeck, A. (1994). Potential cultural bias in training parents as conversational partners with their children who have delays in language development. *American Journal of Speech-Language Pathology, 3,* 67–78.

van Kleeck, A., Gillam, R., Hamilton, L., & McGrath, C. (1997). The relationship between middle class parents' book-sharing discussion and their preschoolers' abstract language development. *Journal of Speech, Language, and Hearing Research, 40*(6), 1261–1271.

van Kleeck, A., & Richardson, A. (1988). Language delay in the child. In N. Lass, L. McReynolds, J. Northern, & D. Yoder (Eds.), *Handbook of speech-language pathology and audiology.* Toronto: B. C. Decker.

Veale, T. (1999). Targeting temporal processing deficits through Fast ForWord©: Language therapy with a new twist. *Language, Speech, and Hearing Services in Schools, 30*(4), 353–362.

Venn, M., Wolery, M., Fleming, L., DeCesare, L., Morris, A., & Cuffs, M. (1993). Effects of teaching preschool peers to use the mand-model procedure during snack activities. *American Journal of Speech-Language Pathology, 2*(1), 38–46.

Wallach, G., & Butler, K. (1994). Creating communication, literacy, and academic success. In G. Wallach and K. Butler (Eds.), *Language learning disabilities in school age children and adolescents: Some principles and application* (pp. 2–26). New York: Macmillan.

Warren, S., & Kaiser, A. (1988). Research in early language intervention. In S. Odom & M. Karnes (Eds.), *Early intervention for infants and children with handicaps.* Baltimore: Paul H. Brookes.

Watkins, R. (1994). Specific language impairments in children: An introduction. In R. Watkins & M. Rice (Eds.), *Specific language impairments in children* (pp. 1–15). Baltimore: Paul H. Brookes.

Weiss, A. (2001). *Preschool language disorders resource guide: Specific language impairment.* San Diego, CA: Singular/Thomson Learning.

Weiss, A., & Nakamura, M. (1992). Language-normal children in preschool classrooms for children with language impairments. *Language, Speech and Hearing Services in Schools, 23,* 64–70.

Weiss, A., Tomblin, J., & Robin, D. (1999). Language disorders. In J. Tomblin, H. Morris, & D. Spriesterbach (Eds.), *Diagnosis in speech-language pathology* (2d ed.) (pp. 129–173). San Diego, CA: Singular.

Weiss, R. (1981). INREAL intervention for language handicapped and bilingual children. *Journal of the Division of Early Childhood, 4,* 40–51.

Wilcox, M., Kouri, T., & Caswell, S. (1991). Early language intervention: A comparison of classroom and individual treatment. *American Journal of Speech-Language Pathology, 1*(1), 49–62.

Wolery, M., & Wilbers, J. (Eds.). (1994). Including children with special needs in early childhood programs. *Research Monograph of the National Association for the Education of Young Children, 6,* Washington, DC: NAEYC.

Wyatt, T. (1997). Assessment issues with multicultural populations. In D. Battle (Ed.), *Communication disorders in multicultural populations* (2d ed.) (pp. 379–425). Boston: Butterworth-Heinemann.

Yoder, D., & Kent, R. (1988). *Decision making in speech-language pathology.* Philadelphia: B. C. Decker.

Yoder, P., Spruytenburg, H., Edwards, A., & Davies, B. (1995). Effect of verbal routine contexts and expansions on gains in the mean length of utterance in children with developmental delays. *Language, Speech, and Hearing Services in Schools, 26,* 21–32.

Zigler, E., & Hall, N. (1995). Mainstreaming and the philosophy of normalization. In J. Kauffman and D. Hallahan (Eds.), *The illusion of full inclusion.* Austin, TX: Pro-Ed.

CHAPTER 7

Language Intervention in School Settings

Nickola Wolf Nelson
Western Michigan University

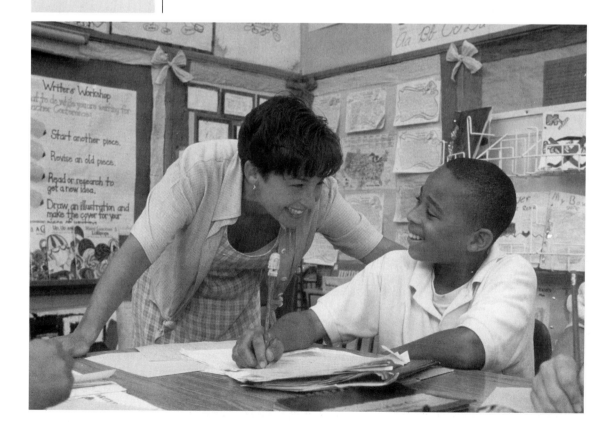

- List and describe a variety of roles and service delivery models for school practitioners and their benefits
- List and describe key features of major legislation (IDEA and Section 504) that influence school service delivery
- Compare and contrast IEPs and IFSPs
- Understand the importance of contributing to the development of guidelines and strategies for implementing policy
- Describe three models of team process set in the broader context of strategies and benefits of collaborative practices
- Use four steps to conduct curriculum-based language assessments and to set curriculum-relevant goals for intervention in collaboration with students, parents, and teachers
- Describe the importance of communication skills to participation and the importance of participation to the development of communication skills for all children

OBJECTIVES

ROLES AND BENEFITS OF WORKING IN SCHOOL SETTINGS

Although school settings are not the only settings for working with children with language and communication disorders, they are particularly important ones. This is because of their many advantages for helping children with special needs develop the language, learning, and communication skills necessary to become full participants in society.

School settings present special opportunities because of the proximity to teachers and the curriculum of general education. Working in the same agencies, speech-language pathologists (SLPs) have rich opportunities to collaborate with teachers to work toward mutual goals for students with disabilities. Together, they can target students' higher-order language skills for understanding the language of the curriculum and expressing themselves within it. SLPs working in school settings also have rich opportunities to scaffold social-interaction discourse as students interact with peers in real academic and social contexts, rather than having to simulate such interactions in isolated clinic rooms. This enhances opportunities to make significant life-altering changes for children with language and communication needs.

This chapter addresses these opportunities and reviews the procedures, including those guided by federal legislation, that school-based communication specialists use when working with children across the age span from infancy through adolescence. Case examples are woven throughout to illustrate the practices discussed.

The chapter begins with an overview of the varied roles that speech-language pathologists play in school settings, as shown in Table 7.1. The table uses the categorization scheme of the American Speech-Language-Hearing Association (1999a), with the addition of a role for advocacy and leadership. Aspects of these roles are explained in further detail throughout the chapter.

TABLE 7.1	**Roles and Responsibilities of School-Based Speech-Language Pathologists**

Intervention Assistance Team/Child Study Team Member

Prevention: Providing inservice training, disseminating information, consulting with parents and teachers about best practices for fostering normal development and preventing disorders

Identification: Soliciting appropriate referrals, screening, providing prereferral interventions, following up on referrals and obtaining consent for evaluation

Interdisciplinary Assessment/Evaluation Team Member

Assessment: Forming an assessment plan, collecting data using interview and observation strategies to understand the problem from the perspectives of participants, and using valid standardized and nonstandardized assessment procedures to gain insights about the dimensions of the problem

Evaluation: Interpreting assessment data regarding the child's strengths, needs, and emerging abilities; using the data to make diagnostic decisions about whether the child has a disorder and whether it affects educational performance; forming preliminary recommendations about how to respond to the areas of concern

IEP Team Member

Eligibility determination: Meeting with the team to decide whether the child has a disorder that affects educational performance and makes the child eligible for special education and/or related services under local, state, and federal policy; considering multiple factors related to the child's need for services (ASHA, 1989b)

IEP/IFSP development: Collaborating with the team to design an Individualized Education Program (IEP) or, in the case of an infant, toddler, and in some states, preschooler, Individualized Family Service Plan (IFSP) that meets local, state, and federal requirements (Polmanteer & Turbiville, 2000)

Caseload management: Coordinating the IEP/IFSPs for all children on the caseload; scheduling services in a manner that meets the requirements of the IEP/IFSPs and leaves time for assessment, evaluation, and other responsibilities; advocating to superiors when the caseload size grows too large to meet those needs; keeping track of needs for reevaluation, transition, dismissal (ASHA, 1993)

Educational Team Member

Intervention for communication disorders: Providing intervention services in the IEP/IFSP designed to reduce the child's impairment, functional limitation, or disability within any of the areas in the SLP's scope of practice—communication, language (spoken or written), speech (articulation/phonology, fluency, voice/resonance), or swallowing (and feeding); consulting and collaborating with others to provide educationally relevant services; planning, managing, delivering, and evaluating intervention (ASHA, 1990, 1996, in press)

Intervention for communication variations: Consulting and collaborating with preschool and elementary school teachers and other school personnel to develop a school environment in which cultural and linguistic diversity are respected and addressed within the curriculum, and in which instructional approaches, materials, and activities are appropriate for the child's cultural and linguistic differences; recommending classroom and curriculum modifications for students with limited English proficiency and helping students who are eligible for services develop a command of the structure, meaning, and use of English (ASHA, 1985, 1990, 1993, 1998a)

(continued)

TABLE 7.1	*(continued)*

Intervention for students requiring technological supports: Recommending augmentative and alternative communication and other assistive technology, computer supports, and classroom adaptations that will improve communication and participation opportunities for students with communication, speech, or language impairments; assisting with obtaining systems, instructing others regarding programming, and updating systems as needed (ASHA, 1998b; Crandell & Smaldino, 2000; Nelson & Soli, 2000)

Counseling/consulting for students not eligible for direct services: Counseling students and families regarding how to address communication needs and increase participation; providing information, seeking information from others, supporting families and students in efforts to achieve their goals, making referrals to others when appropriate

IEP Team

Reevaluation: Determining whether there is a need to reevaluate children on the caseload at least once every three years; obtaining informed parental consent to do so; and performing the reevaluation

Transition: Preparing for and assisting children to make successful transitions at multiple points—from special education to general education; between early intervention, preschool, elementary, and secondary programs; or from high school to postsecondary activities, including employment, vocational training, military, community college, or four-year college

Dismissal: Beginning to discuss dismissal criteria during eligibility team meetings; explaining that students may be dismissed at certain points in their educational sequences, but readmitted later if necessary; determining when the student no longer needs special education or related services using local, state, and federal policies

Other SLP Roles

Supervision: Supervising colleagues completing their clinical fellowship years, speech-language pathology assistants (ASHA, 1996), university practicum students, and school-approved community volunteers

Documentation and accountability: Providing required and appropriate documentation at all levels of the clinical cycle for students and families, federal, state, and local agencies, and third-party insurance payers, such as Medicaid

Advocacy and leadership: Working with colleagues in the discipline at the local, state, and federal level to design and modify policies that influence the provision of services to children with communicative, speech, and language disabilities in school settings; collaborating with colleagues across disciplines to lead and implement school reform efforts to expand and maximize the education and communication participation opportunities for all students

Source: Based on ASHA, 1999a, with revisions and additions.

LEGISLATIVE INFLUENCES ON SCHOOL SERVICE DELIVERY

Public policies generated at local, state, and federal levels influence how service is provided in any setting, including schools. In the United States, the primary legislation that governs school services is the Individuals with Disabilities Education Act (IDEA97; Public Law 105-17, 1997). This legislation, which was passed first by the 94th Congress in 1975 as the Education for All Handicapped Children Act (Public Law 94-142), was not the original legislation with major implications for serving children with special needs in public schools. Public Law 94-142 as it was known for many years, followed a piece of civil rights legislation passed by the 93rd Congress: Section 504 of the Rehabilitation Act. Table 7.2 shows the legislative history of these and related pieces of federal policy.

TABLE 7.2	Recent Federal Legislation Related to School-Based Practices

Congress	Years	Law	Brief Description
93rd	1973–1974	Sec. 504	The Rehabilitation Act of 1973 established a requirement for nondiscrimination on the basis of disability among agencies that accept federal funds.
94th	1975–1977	P.L. 94-142	The Education for All Handicapped Children Act first established the right to Free Appropriate Public Education with IEPs.
99th	1985–1986	P.L. 99-457	The Education of the Handicapped Act Amendments of 1986 added options for serving infants and toddlers.
100th	1987–1988	P.L. 100-407	The Technology-Related Assistance for Individuals with Disabilities Act defined assistive technology to include both services and devices.
101st	1989–1990	P.L. 101-336	The Americans with Disabilities Act (ADA) extended the provisions of Section 504 of the Rehabilitation Act by requiring agencies to make reasonable accommodations to enable otherwise qualified people to be hired or to keep their positions when they have disabilities and to ensure that new or renovated structures (including schools) meet specific accessibility guidelines for people with disabilities.
		P.L. 101-476	Changed the name of the EHA to the Individuals with Disabilities Education Act (IDEA); added autism and TBI categories and transition services.
102nd	1991–1992	P.L. 102-119	Added assistive devices to IDEA and indicated that 3- to 5-year-olds could have either an IFSP or an IEP.
105th	1996–1997	P.L. 105-17	Made major revisions to IDEA and generated new regulations; infant and toddler services (formerly Part H) became Part C.

A third piece of legislation, which also affects service delivery in school settings, although less than the other two, is the Technology-Related Assistance for Individuals with Disabilities Act of 1988 (P.L. 100-407, amended in 1994). The "Tech Act," as it is generally known, established a definition of assistive technology as "any item, piece of equipment or product system, whether acquired commercially off the shelf, modified or customized, that is used to increase, maintain, or improve functional capabilities of individuals with disabilities" [Chapter 33, Sec. 1401(25)]. This act and its amendments established incentives for states to develop consumer-responsive comprehensive statewide programs of technology-related assistance for individuals of all ages with disabilities. Its regulations provide rules for applying for and spending federal funds under this program, with a special emphasis on programs serving children and youth.

Although it is usually thought of as legislation affecting adults, the Americans with Disabilities Act (ADA; P.L. 101-336), passed in 1990, also affects school service delivery. The ADA extended the provisions of Section 504 by requiring agencies to make reasonable accommodations to ensure accessibility, and particularly, that new or renovated structures (including schools) should meet specific accessibility guidelines for people with disabilities. This includes not only responsibility to ensure physical access for individuals who use wheelchairs, but also responsibility to ensure adequate acoustic qualities of classrooms so that children with hearing impairments and language and learning disabilities can have access to the language of instruction (Sieben, Gold, Sieben, & Ermann, 2000; Sorkin, 2000; Smaldino & Crandell, 2000).

Section 504 of the Rehabilitation Act of 1973

The first in this series of important legislation, Section 504, made it illegal for agencies receiving financial assistance from the federal government—including public elementary, secondary, and postsecondary schools—to discriminate or deny benefits on the basis of disability. Public schools could no longer tell parents that their children were too handicapped to attend public schools. Subsequent passage of P.L. 94-142 in 1975 established regulations and expectations to guide service delivery, which became mandatory across the United States in 1979. The law and regulations have been updated periodically since, most recently as IDEA97. Section 504 continues to influence school service delivery as well. Section 504, however, carries no funds to pay for its provision, whereas IDEA does.

Children who do not qualify for special education services under IDEA, but who have other physical or mental impairments that substantially limit one or more of their major life activities, such as attention deficit hyperactivity disorder, can have a Section 504 Plan. These plans are designed to meet individualized needs by providing "reasonable accommodations" in the way instruction is delivered. Evaluations under Section 504 must be conducted with procedures that are: (1) validated for the specific purpose for which they are used, (2) administered by trained personnel, (3) tailored to assess specific areas of educational need, and (4) selected to ensure that, when a test is administered to a student with impaired sensory, manual, or speaking skills, the test results accurately reflect the student's aptitude or achievement rather than reflecting the student's impairment. These are similar to requirements for individualized assessment under the IDEA.

Individuals with Disabilities Education Act

Similar due process rights are guaranteed under the IDEA. The primary purpose of IDEA since its original passage as P.L. 94-142, however, has been to ensure that all children with disabilities have access to a *free appropriate public education* (FAPE) in the *least restrictive environment* (LRE).

The IDEA has four major parts. **Part A** includes definitions and general provisions; **Part B** specifies how services are to be provided to preschool and school-age students; **Part C** specifies requirements for service provision to infants and toddlers and their families; **Part D** includes provisions for supporting research, personnel preparation, technical assistance, support, and dissemination of information for improving the education of children with disabilities. This section of the chapter places the roles and responsibilities for school service delivery, which are summarized in Table 7.1, into the context of the rules and regulations of the IDEA, mostly from Parts B and C.

Definitions

In Part A [Sec. 602(8)], the IDEA defines "free appropriate public education" as meaning "special education and related services" that:

(A) have been provided at public expense, under public supervisions, and without charge;
(B) meet the standards of the State educational agency;
(C) include an appropriate preschool, elementary, or secondary education in the State involved; and
(D) are provided in conformity with the individualized education program.

SLP services may be considered either special education or related services, depending on the state and situation, whereas most other services are either one or the other. Audiological services, for example, are always considered a "related service." **Special education** is defined as "specially designed instruction, at no cost to the parents, to meet the unique needs of a child with a disability, including instruction conducted in the classroom, in the home, in hospitals and institutions, and in other settings" [Sec. 602(26)]. **Related services** "means transportation, and such developmental, corrective, and other supportive services (including speech-language pathology and audiology services, psychological services, physical and occupational therapy)" [Sec. 602(22)]. In some cases, the distinction as to whether SLP services are considered instruction or related services is made on the basis of whether the child has another diagnosis in addition to speech-language impairment. In these cases, SLP services often are considered "related services," although the rules vary from state to state.

Serving Infants and Toddlers Under IDEA

Part C describes provisions for services to meet the needs of **infants and toddlers with disabilities**. Governors of many states have appointed education agencies (otherwise, health agencies) to lead the implementation of Part C of the IDEA with infants, toddlers, and their families. SLPs employed by schools, therefore, are often responsible for helping families whose infants and toddlers have developmental needs, because those needs almost always include communication (Polmanteer & Turbiville, 2000). Lead agencies also have the responsibility to actively seek and find infants and toddlers whose families need assistance. Any parents who are concerned about their children's development may consult their local school system. School-based SLPs also work with hospital-based SLPs and audiologists who provide neonatal hearing screening programs. Such teams help families obtain appropriate amplification for their young children if needed and assist parents to maximize early communication opportunities.

Identification, Assessment, and Evaluation under Part C. Part C of IDEA97 requires states to provide services to any child under 3 years of age who "needs early intervention services" because the child:

  (i) is experiencing developmental delays, as measured by appropriate diagnostic instruments and procedures in one or more of the areas of cognitive development, physical development, communication development, social or emotional development, and adaptive development; or

  (ii) has a diagnosed physical or mental condition which has a high probability of resulting in developmental delay. [Sec. 632(5)(A)]

It is up to the states to design procedures and quantitative criteria for determining which children actually have a "developmental delay" or "established risk." In addition to providing these required services, states have the *option* to provide services to "at-risk" infants and toddlers, who are defined under Part C as "an individual under 3 years of age who would be at risk of experiencing a substantial developmental delay if early intervention services were not provided to the individual" [Sec. 632(1)].

The National Early Childhood Technical Assistance System (NECTAS) surveyed the fifty states and other U.S. jurisdictions with responsibility for implementing Part C of the IDEA. Shackelford (2000) reported that:

The task of defining the eligible population has been a challenge for states. Eligibility criteria influence the numbers and types of children needing or receiving services, the types of services provided, and ultimately the cost of the early intervention system. Over the years, several states have revised their definitions: some have narrowed their eligibility criteria and others have expanded them. Soon after the creation of the Early Intervention Program under IDEA, many states were interested in serving children at risk, but fears of highly increased numbers of eligible children and, therefore, highly increased costs, reduced the number of states that included children at risk in their eligibility definition. Several states that are not serving children at risk under their definition indicate that they will monitor the development of these children and refer them for early intervention services as delays are manifested. (p. 1)

The role of the SLP is to diagnose the level of communication development, which is one of the five areas to be considered—the others being cognitive development, physical development, social or emotional development, and adaptive development. At this age, developmental delays are considered significant if they can be documented "in one or more of the areas." The areas are not generally referenced against cognitive development, as often occurs for older children, but against chronological age. Several states specify quantitative criteria, such as 30 percent below age norms or six months' delay. Others are based in standard deviations (SD) below the mean, such as 1.5 (or 2) S.D. in one area, or 1.0 (or 1.5) S.D. if two or more areas are involved.

As noted in Chapter 4, the assessment and evaluation roles with infants and toddlers require working as members of teams, which include parents, to select appropriate tools and to administer standardized and nonstandardized instruments across developmental areas. The requirement is for a "multidisciplinary assessment of the unique strengths and needs of the infant or toddler and the identification of services appropriate to meet such needs" [Sec. 636(a)(1)]. In addition, the team must conduct "a family-directed assessment of the resources, priorities, and concerns of the family and the identification of the supports and services necessary to enhance the family's capacity to meet the developmental needs of the infant or toddler" [Sec. 636(a)(2)]. The team then evaluates the results and makes decisions about eligibility, or, if not, consults with parents about how to address their immediate concerns and to monitor the child's development over the coming months and years.

It is most effective if this process includes a family visit, in which the child is observed in his or her home environment (Prelock, Beatson, Contompasis, & Bishop, 1999), and providers can get to know families as "families" before they know them as "clients." They can use such broad questions as, "Why did you take _____ to Child Find?" to understand the family's general concerns. Providers also should be prepared to listen to more specific concerns of the family, such as being unable to eat at a fast-food restaurant because of the child's disruptive vocalizations and other behaviors, or needing a new babysitter so the child will have children her own age to play with (Polmanteer & Turbiville, 2000). These concerns should be written in the words of the family and not the jargon of the providers.

Using Individualized Family Service Plans (IFSPs) to Guide Intervention.   For infants or toddlers who are found eligible under a state's criteria, Part C specifies the development of Individualized Family Service Plans (IFSPs). IFSPs define the service unit as the family rather than the child. Development of IFSPs requires decisions to be made about a family's service needs and mandates family representation in the decision making process. The content of IFSPs includes statements of: (1) the infant's or toddler's present levels of development; (2) the family's resources, priorities, and concerns; (3) major outcomes expected, with "criteria, procedures, and timelines used to determine the degree to which progress toward achieving outcomes is made and whether modification or revisions of the outcomes or services are necessary"; (4) "early intervention services necessary to meet the unique needs of the infant or toddler and the family, including the frequency, intensity, and method of delivering services"; (5) the "natural environments in which services shall appropriately be provided, including a justification of the extent, if any, to which the services will not be provided in a natural environment"; (6) projected dates of initiation of services and anticipated duration; (7) identification of the family service coordinator, and (8) steps to be taken to support the transition to preschool or other educational levels. IFSPs must be revised at least every six months (compared with twelve months for IEPs). An example IFSP appears in Figure 7.1.

INDIVIDUALIZED FAMILY SERVICE PLAN (IFSP)

Referral Date 2-11-01

Today's Date 2-12-01

Person Referring D. Smith

Agency Initiating IFSP Public School

Child Information			Social Security # 111-11-1111	
Child's Legal Name Janna Johnson		Nickname Janna	Date of Birth 11-1-99	Sex M/Ⓕ
Address 123 Main Street, Any town, USA		Phone (home) 555-5555		Phone (daycare) 555-5554
Address		Medical Insurance # 123456789		
School District of Residence Any town Schools	County Any town		Ethnic Heritage African Am.	Native Language English

Name	Relationship to Child	Birth date (Optional)	Address	Phone (home)	Phone (work)
Mike Johnson	Father	3-15-71	Same as above	Same	555-1212
Sharika Johnson	Mother	8-29-71	Same as above	Same	555-1234
Issac Johnson	Brother	7-13-97	Same	Same	-----

If parent/guardian needs an interpreter, give language:

Agencies and Persons Working with the Family (Fill in anytime)

Start Date	Agency	Contact Person(s)	Phone	Type of Service or Title	End Date	Send Copy of IFSP?
11-5-99	Health Services Hosp.	Isabel Jones	222-2222	Audiologist		X
1-5-00	Any town Public School	Diane Smith	333-3333	Speech Language Pathologist		

Child's Strengths and Needs

Child's Name Janna Johnson	Birth Weight 7.2	Birth date 11-1-99	Number of Wks premature NA

Area	Present level of Development		Date	Name/Type of Evaluation	Person Doing Evaluation	Agency
	Parent Input	Professional Input				
General	Very expressive, and "laid back." A good baby	Speech therapy, Continued hearing impaired services after a cochlear implant	1-15-01	Cognitive screening	Developmental Psychologist	Any town Schools
Hearing	Doesn't respond to sound but does to gestures	Profound bilateral hearing imp.	11-5-99 12-15-99	Neonatal screening ABR	Audiologist	Health Services Hospital
Communication	Follows eyes, coos and makes sounds	Age appropriate so far		Rossetti Infant-Toddler Scale	SLP	Any town Schools

Child Eligibility

Part C of IDEA	☒ Yes	☐ No	☐ Unknown	(Based on: Established Condition **deafness**	Developmental Delay _____

FIGURE 7.1

Example of an Individualized Family Service Plan

Service Plan

Service Coordinator D. Smith				Services Coordinator Phone # 333-0300			

| ☐ Interim | ☒ Initial | ☐ Review | ☐ Annual | ☐ Transition (90 days before entry into new program or third birthday—whichever comes first.) |

OUTCOMES	WHO & WHAT	WHERE, WHEN & HOW	DATE SERVICE		PAYOR	REVIEW
What would we like to have happen, by when, and how will we know when it happens.	What service or activity is needed and Who will do it.	When will the services occur, How often, How long each time, Individual or Group.	Begins	Ends	Who will pay for it	Date/ Rating/ Comments
1) Cochlear implant (3-5-01)	1) Univ. Hospital	1) Implant programming	3-15-01 2-17-01	When complete	Private insurance + Medicaid	
2) Understand and say words by age 2 (at least 50)	2) Speech/Lang Pathologist, Speech language therapy	2) Parent-toddler group 60 min. 2x/week; 20-30 min. Individual Tx with family	1-18-00 11-1-99		Public School	
3) Take part in family discussions by age 3 (make comments and ask Qs)	3) Hearing Impaired Teacher Consultant	3) Home Visit 1x/month: 45 min Individual Tx		Ongoing	Public School	
4) Play normally with other children by age 4	4) Early Intervention Coordinator	4) Weekly home or clinic consultation by HI Consultant.			Public School	

Providing family-centered service in "natural environments" involves working with whole families using culturally sensitive practices to foster the communicative development of infants, children, or adolescents. Family-centered practices begin by discovering and addressing the general concerns and communicative needs identified by the family. This is crucial for setting appropriate and meaningful goals, using everyone involved with the child to maximize progress toward those goals and to realize changes in communicative functioning across contexts.

When working with infants and toddlers, this service should be provided in "natural environments," which might include homes, day-care centers, or other places where children of this age would be found naturally. SLPs consult with families and other early intervention team members to maximize communicative development for eligible children. For example, they may work with families to alleviate feeding concerns and to help families become attuned to their infant's early communicative signals, thus setting up healthy reciprocal communicative interactions in the critical early months of life. They may assist families with toddlers to develop child-centered and play-based communication facilitation strategies. In the IFSP in Figure 7.1, the focus is on helping the child with a profound hearing loss make use of a cochlear implant and communicative interactions to maximize language learning experiences.

The IFSP team members should be chosen to maximize the comfort level and participation of the family. If the team includes only the mother of the child, the family service coordinator, and one or more representatives of agencies providing services to the family, the mother is likely to have the intimidating sensation of being alone in a group of experts. By contrast, if others who share the family's culture and concerns join in the discussions, such as other members of the family (fathers, siblings, grandparents), friends, or other parents of children with disabilities, the plan may be more comprehensive and truly attuned to the family's concerns and priorities (Polmanteer & Turbiville, 2000).

Several features differentiate service delivery under IFSPs and IEPs. The IFSP is more flexible in that it is a service delivery plan rather than a treatment plan and can address issues beyond those related to a child's educational needs. It specifies the services to be provided, with multiple agencies potentially involved and responsible, and at least one "outcome" for the child. Family outcomes also may be specified, if desired by the family. Contrasting with IEPs, treatment goals and objectives are not part of the IFSP per se, but are developed by the various service providers named in it, with the aim toward achieving the targeted outcomes on the IFSP.

Child-centered outcomes are generally easier for teams to write than family-centered ones, especially if the family has been only a marginal part of the assessment process. When family-centered outcomes are included, they should *not* be written as tasks for the family to complete, such as "Mrs. Jones will have Jessica dressed and ready for the school bus every day," but should address family concerns in family members' own words. Family outcomes can address broad concerns that do not have to have immediate relevance to the specific disability, but they should include "so that" statements to convey their general relevance—for example, "We want to find another place to live so that we won't have to worry about the roof leaking," or "We want to know about any groups for brothers and sisters in our town so that Jeremy's sisters will know about his disability" (Polmanteer & Turbiville, 2000, p. 6).

Serving Preschool-Age Children

Children between 3 and 5 years of age may have either IFSPs under Part C or IEPs under **Section 619** of Part B, depending on a state's organizational system. Service delivery to children between 3 and 5 years of age used to be optional, but it is now required for children with established risks or developmental delays, as it is for infants and toddlers. The identification, assessment, evaluation, and intervention procedures for serving preschool-age children are similar to those for infants and toddlers. Under Part C, children from birth through age 8 may be identified as having "developmental delay" (rather than a specific disability). In most states, starting at age 5 years, or at least by age 8, students must meet a set of criteria as having a speech-language disability to be eligible for speech-language intervention services. Assessment practices should be comprehensive and provide answers to the question, "What to do next?" (Warner & Nelson, 2000).

"Natural environments" for preschool-age children served under IFSPs include homes, child-care settings, and special education and/or general education preschools, including Head Start classrooms. The equivalent of natural settings for children served under IEPs is what the IEP team determines to be the least restrictive environment for the child. For 3 to 5 year olds, preschool classrooms offer particularly rich environments for working on combined communication, language, play, and social-interaction skills. SLPs can use any of the service delivery options described in Table 7.3 to work with preschool-age children.

Family-centered practices are important for preschool-age and kindergarten-age children, whether they are served with IFSPs or IEPs. Prelock and her associates (1999) described an interdisciplinary team model for serving rural families in which they saw Alicia, a child whose teachers reported limited verbal communication, restricted play schemes, and inability to interact socially with peers. Alicia's parents were confused by this description because it did not fit the child they saw at home. When members of the team listened to the parents and observed Alicia at home, they saw a different child too—one who used complete sentences to request information and make comments, who used language to initiate interactions with her sister, and who engaged in imaginative play with her favorite toys in her bedroom. If the team had not listened to Alicia's parents and made this visit, their views of Alicia's strengths and needs would have been inaccurate. Having more information made it possible to design an appropriate intervention plan.

Serving School-Age Children and Adolescents

Part B of IDEA regulates the provision of services for children with disabilities from ages 6 through 21 years. The law and its regulations guide all of the activities from identification through dismissal or transition and follow-up monitoring when appropriate. Students with any of the disabilities listed in the IDEA97 definition may need speech-language assessment and intervention services.

Identification, Assessment, and Evaluation under Part B.

Before a child can receive services under Part B of IDEA, a "full and individual initial evaluation" must be conducted. Prior to evaluation, the agency proposing to conduct it must obtain informed consent from the child's parent. This means conveying rights and due processes guaranteed by IDEA to parents in a manner and language that parents can understand.

In conducting an initial evaluation to determine eligibility, the multidisciplinary team must:

(A) use a variety of assessment tools and strategies to gather relevant functional and developmental information, including information provided by the

TABLE 7.3   Service Delivery Options (From Least to Most Restrictive)

Consultation Service

For children

- Whose needs can be met through collaborative consultation with parents, teachers, and others, and
- Who do not need weekly scheduled, direct contact with the SLP, or
- Who are receiving direct services but need consultation services as well

They may be children

- Who are infants/toddlers at risk and whose families need consultation about early development and how to foster it, or
- Who need prereferral teacher assistance to determine whether the student's needs can be met with modifications in usual procedures, or whether a formal evaluation is needed, or
- Who need instructional consultation so that their preschool or school-age teachers will understand their special needs and make accommodations or instructional modifications to meet those needs, or
- Who need monitoring in natural contexts before or after direct treatment to observe whether they are demonstrating previously established speech, language, and communication skills

Home- or Community-Based Service

For children

- Who are infants/toddlers and who need direct services and consultation within the family unit, or
- Who are children and adolescents with communication goals that are best met in home and community

They may be children or adolescents

- Whose pragmatic communication needs are most likely to be met and generalized when targeted in home and community settings
- Whose special education curriculum focuses on functional community-centered interactions
- Whose community-based goals are set in work-study or vocational contexts

Classroom-Based Service

For children

- Whose speech, language, and communication development needs can be met best by working with them in their general education classrooms, or
- In their special education classrooms, or
- Through a combination of service delivery models, including classroom-based service and pull-out service aimed at meeting general curricular goals

They may be children

- Who can almost but not quite meet the language and communication demands of their classrooms, or
- Who have severe disabilities, but are included full time in general education classrooms, and who need direct scaffolding to support their communication in the classroom academic and social interactions

Within the classroom-based model, the service may be delivered through

- Whole class, small group, or individual instruction, and
- Team teaching (co-teaching), in which SLP and teacher share responsibility for planning and delivering instruction
- Complementary instruction, in which the SLP designs a lesson within a lesson (e.g., note taking) to complement the classroom teacher's content instruction
- Supportive instruction, in which the SLP develops specialized instruction, grouping, or strategy instruction in support of class lessons and delivers them in the classroom
- Pull-in instruction, in which the SLP works with children with multiple or severe disabilities who are "pulled in" from special education placements for selected general education activities

Pull-Out Service

For children and adolescents

- Who need specialized speech-language instruction that cannot be delivered readily in the classroom to learn such specific skills as how to articulate a phoneme, speak fluently, or use a healthy voice, or to learn basic language skills that cannot be efficiently or effectively addressed in the general education classroom

- Who prefer to receive intervention in settings apart from their general education peers, because such services would be conspicuous and embarrassing to the student or distracting to others

Within the pull-out model, service may be delivered
- Through small group, or individual instruction, and
- On varying schedules (one, two, three, or more times per week) designed to optimize new skill learning (e.g., by maximizing talking time) while avoiding pulling them from important general curricular or extracurricular experiences
- Using curriculum materials drawn from the general education classroom for the content and context for intervention activities
- In combination with any of the other models
- With the goal to return to classroom-based services, followed by follow-up monitoring, as soon as possible

Self-Contained Classrooms

For children
- Who are in their school-age years and who, because of severe primary speech-language impairments, need a language-learning classroom for one or more years with specially designed instruction all day long from an SLP serving as classroom teacher (depending on state certification policies) to learn basic oral and written language skills and how to use language to learn while preparing for transition to a general education classroom and instruction
- Who have other primary disabilities and need a special education classroom with specially designed instruction from a special education teacher all day long for one or more years to prepare them for participating in general education classrooms and instruction, in which case SLPs may provide classroom-based services in collaboration with the special education teacher using any of the models described previously
- Who have severe speech-language impairments and/or other disabilities and who need part-day resource room placements, but who need to be included in a general education classroom during the rest of the day, perhaps receiving classroom-based SLP services in both placements, or who may receive pull-in services in the general education classroom during selected activities
- Who need a daily alternative language arts class in elementary, middle, or secondary school, in which an SLP provides intensive direct instruction to help them learn the oral and written language, critical thinking, executive functioning, pragmatics, and study skills to function successfully in other classrooms and for transition to general education language arts instruction (Anderson & Nelson, 1988)

Separate School or Facility

For children
- Who need intensive specially designed instruction in a center-based program separate from the school they would be attending if they had no disability
- Whose parents wish them to be educated in a residential school with children with similar characteristics, such as deafness, so that they can participate in a community of learners who communicate with American Sign Language, or to meet some other unique need
- Whose behavioral or emotional needs are severe and who require specially trained staff who can assure their safety and those of classmates (e.g., residential programs for children or adolescents with mental health needs or juvenile treatment centers for adjudicated youth)

Within center-based or residential programs
- SLP services may be delivered using any of the models described above
- Activities should focus on pragmatic communication skills as well as other speech-language needs and should be designed to prepare students for transition to situations in which they will participate with individuals without disabilities

Sources: Based on Anderson & Nelson, 1988; ASHA, 1989a, 1990, 1996, 1998b, 1999a, 1999b; Beck & Dennis, 1997; Buttrill, Niizawa, Biemer, Takahashi, & Hearn, 1989; Ehren, 2000; Elksnin & Capilouto, 1994; Ferguson, 1991; Merritt & Culatta, 1998; Prelock, Beatson, Contompasis, & Bishop, 1999; Prelock, Miller, & Reed, 1995.

parent that may assist in determining whether the child is a child with a disability, and the content of the child's individualized education program, including information related to enabling the child to be involved in and progress in the general curriculum or, for preschool children, to participate in appropriate activities;

(B) not use any single procedure as the sole criterion for determining whether a child is a child with a disability or determining an appropriate educational program for the child; [Sec. 614(b)(1)]

The agency also must ensure that "(A) tests and other evaluation materials used to assess a child under this section—(i) are selected and administered so as not to be discriminatory on a racial or cultural basis; and (ii) are provided and administered in the child's native language or other mode of communication, unless it is clearly not feasible to do so" [Sec. 614(b)(3)]. This means when making the determination of eligibility, it is also important that the child be "assessed in all areas of suspected eligibility." This means that the SLP should be involved in the assessment process if there is a possibility that speech-language services might be needed.

To be eligible for services under Part B of IDEA, evidence must be gathered to document that students need special services in order to benefit from their educational experiences. According to IDEA (Part A), "In general, the term 'child with a disability' means a child—

(i)   with mental retardation, hearing impairments (including deafness), speech or language impairments, visual impairments (including blindness), serious emotional disturbance (hereinafter referred to as "emotional disturbance"), orthopedic impairments, autism, traumatic brain injury, other health impairments, or specific learning disabilities; and

(ii) who, by reason thereof, needs special education and related services. [Sec. 602(3)(A)]

The primary identification challenge facing school SLPs is to find and work with students who need special assistance to acquire communication skills at levels commensurate with their peers. At times, questions are raised about whether children with speech impairments involving voice, stuttering, or articulation should qualify for school services. According to this federal definition, they do if they need special education and related services to benefit from their education. Oral communication (along with written communication) is a basic skill. Furthermore, education takes place through the process of communication. If students have difficulty using oral communication in educational contexts, or have difficulty in any way accessing their education through communication, the case generally can be made that they need special services to improve that communication. Thus, they should qualify for services as speech-language impaired. Federal interpretation of the rules has clarified that it is not necessary for students to have academic difficulties or low grades to qualify for services (ASHA, 1999b).

The assessment process for students with suspected multiple disabilities should yield information about all areas of concern. This may require input from specialists in several disciplines. In addition to parents and at least one general education teacher, evaluation and IEP teams for these students might include special education teachers, occupational therapists, physical therapists, social workers, psychologists, and school counselors, each of whom may administer formal tests. The evaluation report should represent the collective results of the professional team, as well as input of parents and general educators. At a collaborative meeting, this interdisciplinary group determines the student's category of eligibility.

Students with multiple difficulties each have a primary eligibility, such as specific learning disability, cognitive disability, autistic spectrum disability, hearing impairment or deafness, or emotional/behavioral disability. Speech-language disability often becomes a secondary category of eligibility for such students, so that speech-language intervention is described as a "related service" rather than as an instructional program, as discussed previously.

As they do for infants and toddlers, states and local educational agencies further define the criteria for determining who has a disability under Part B of IDEA. It is the IEP team that makes this determination. Threshold criteria for formal assessment results generally specify how far scores must be from the range of "normal" for a particular referent group. For articulation, most states specify the child's age and number of affected phonemes and contexts to justify eligibility. When valid standard test scores are available, threshold requirements usually specify that scores should be more than one (often 1.3 to 1.5, or sometimes 2) standard deviations below the mean. It is not just the score itself, but the range indicated by the test's *standard error of measurement* (SEM) that is used to differentiate such discrepancies. Not all test manuals report SEM, but when available, the high end of the range within which a particular score is predicted to fall (rather than the actual score) must be below the threshold.

In some cases, discrepancy criteria are relative to children of the same *chronological age* (CA); in others, the referent group is children of the same cognitive or *mental age* (MA). Mental age referencing, also called "cognitive referencing," is required for diagnosis of learning disability or specific language impairment. "Cognitive discrepancy" criteria for identifying language impairment in general also appear, however, in many state policies (31 of 50 states, according to Casby [1992]). The problem with such practices is that they have no research-based validity, they violate the spirit of IDEA to identify all children who need special services to benefit from general education, and they seem primarily to serve a gatekeeping function to keep too many children with mental retardation or low-normal cognitive skills from qualifying for language intervention services. The research evidence that calls the validity of cognitive referencing practices into question includes findings that:

- Language tests and cognitive tests measure many of the same abilities (Cole, Dale, & Mills, 1990; Francis, Fletcher, Shaywitz, Shaywitz, & Rourke, 1996).
- Different combinations of tests yield different results (Cole, Dale, & Mills, 1990; Cole, Mills, & Kelley, 1994).
- Test relationships vary across developmental periods so that the same child may qualify at one point but not another (Cole, Dale, & Mills, 1992).
- Both language and cognitive tests are biased for a student whose cultural and linguistic background differs from that of the test's normative population (Battle, 1993; Taylor & Payne, 1983).
- Contrary to the assumption that a student cannot benefit from intervention if there is no cognitive discrepancy, research evidence has shown that preschool

children with and without cognitive deficits can benefit equally from language intervention (Cole & Harris, 1992; Fey, Long, & Cleave, 1994).

One of the roles for school-based SLPs described in Table 7.1 involves advocacy and leadership. As states revise their eligibility criteria, the gatekeeping function of cognitive criteria hopefully will be abandoned. Research evidence also suggests that current identification practices are more likely to identify speech and expressive language problems than receptive language problems and more likely to identify boys as having special needs than girls (Zhang & Tomblin, 2000). Professionals are working to find more valid methods for identifying children who need language intervention services so that they can develop and benefit from their educational experiences. School-based SLPs have a responsibility to contribute to this process so that all children who need and can benefit from services will be served.

Using Individualized Education Programs (IEPs) to Guide Intervention.   After a student's eligibility is established, the student's Individualized Education Planning (IEP) team plans an intervention program. The members of the IEP team are:

(i)   the parents of a child with a disability;

(ii)   at least one regular education teacher of such a child (if the child is, or may be, participating in the regular education environment);

(iii)   at least one special education teacher, or where appropriate, at least one special education provider;

(iv)   a representative of the local education agency who—

    (I)   is qualified to provide, or supervise the provision of specially designed instruction to meet the unique needs of children with disabilities;

    (II)   is knowledgeable about the general curriculum; and

    (III)   is knowledgeable about the availability of resources of the local educational agency;

(v)   an individual who can interpret the instructional implication of evaluation results, who may be a member of the team described in clauses (ii) through (vi);

(vi)   at the discretion of the parent or the agency, other individuals who have knowledge or special expertise regarding the child, including related services personnel as appropriate; and

(viii)   whenever appropriate, the child with a disability. [Sec. 614(d)(B)]

For students with speech-language impairments, the SLP may serve multiple roles—as the representative of the local education agency who is knowledgeable about the system, the special service provider, *and* the individual who can interpret the instructional implications of evaluation results. In such cases, the general education teacher and parent are still required members of the team. Other teams are larger, but professionals should take care not to overwhelm parents and students. IEP meetings may not be the best place for students to participate in the planning process, depending on the number of people involved, but they should be actively involved as soon as possible. That is, at some point IEP goals should be negotiated with students and written in student-friendly language to build a sense of ownership for them and to enhance the intervention process.

During the IEP meeting, when official intervention goals are outlined, the type and frequency of services to address the goals also are specified. The intended outcome of intervention is successful participation in the general education curriculum. Modifications and accommodations to that curriculum also are outlined, with care so as not to oversimplify expectations at the sacrifice of students' opportunities to progress in the general curriculum and participate with peers. Again, it is important for families and teachers to join in the planning process. IEPs must include:

> (i)　a statement of measurable annual goals, including benchmarks or short-term objectives, related to—
> > (I)　meeting the child's needs that result from the child's disability to enable the child to be involved in and progress in the general curriculum; and
> > (II)　meeting each of the child's other educational needs that result from the child's disability. [Sec.614(1)(1)(A)]

For many students with communication difficulties, this means that IEPs will include goals and objectives aimed at connecting oral and written language abilities with the increasingly complex communication demands of the general curriculum. For students with severe disabilities, this may involve efforts to keep them included or active in general curricular activities, but with modified expectations.

Service delivery requirements for IEPs must include:

> (iii)　a statement of the special education and related services and supplementary aids and services to be provided the child, or on behalf of the child, and a statement of the program modifications or supports for school personnel that will be provided for the child—
> > (I)　to advance appropriately toward attaining annual goals;
> > (II)　to be involved and progress in the general curriculum in accordance with clause (i) and to participate in extracurricular and other nonacademic activities; and
> > (III)　to be educated and participate with other children with disabilities and nondisabled children in the activities described in this paragraph. [Sec.614(1)(1)(A)]

The essence of a school-based program of service delivery is the provision of services to help students acquire the communicative skills for participating in important life contexts. Describing "supplementary aids and services" requires the team to consider the need for assistive technology and other supports. Such decisions may address a variety of needs, one of which is the need for augmentative and alternative communication technology and services.

Occupational and physical therapists have important roles for students with assistive technology needs, positioning the student and exploring means of accessing switches or scanning devices. SLPs work with families and teachers to determine such things as the level of symbolic communication and students' communication needs for participating in the general curriculum. This collective information is used to make decisions regarding use of objects, pictures, or symbols to support students' social communicative and learning needs.

In addition, the IEP team must consider the LRE requirements, which specify that, whenever appropriate, children with disabilities must be educated with children who have no disabilities. It is the IEP team's responsibility to consider how to keep the student in the least restrictive environment (LRE) while meeting the student's individualized needs. IDEA specifies that each public agency shall ensure:

(1) That to the maximum extent appropriate, children with disabilities, including children in public or private institutions or other care facilities, are
educated with children who are nondisabled; and

(2) That special classes, separate schooling, or other removal of children with
disabilities from the regular educational environment occurs only when the
nature or severity of the disability is such that education in regular classes
with the use of supplementary aids and services cannot be achieved satisfactorily. [Sec.(a)(1)(C)(iv)]

The group process in considering LRE for a particular student might start with
a discussion of supports that would be necessary to keep the student in a full-time
placement with normal-learning peers. If all of the student's needs could not be met
in such a placement, alternatives along a continuum of more restrictive services might
be selected as more appropriate to maximize success. Such a program is operationally
defined as least restrictive for that student.

The continuum of placements described in Table 7.3 applies here. Although
pull-out therapy for a specified number of sessions per week (often twenty to thirty
minutes in length) is the most frequently used service delivery model in school
programming, it should not be selected automatically (ASHA, 1999a, 1999b).
On the continuum described in Table 7.3, the least restrictive program (on the surface) would involve consultation services but with no separation from family, peers,
or the general curriculum. Next on the LRE continuum would be classroom-based
services or services in other natural environments where the child would be found if
no disabilities existed. Pull-out services would be further on the continuum. Self-
contained classrooms in the student's home school would be more restrictive yet, and
self-contained classrooms in a separate school or "center program" would be considered the most restrictive (Nelson & Staskowski, 2000). Any of these service delivery
options, however, could be found by an IEP team to be least restrictive for a particular child.

Determining the most appropriate goals for a student with multiple disabilities
requires collaboration as well, with all members of a team working together, each
adding input from diverse areas of expertise and listening to the observations of
others. When goals are written collectively, opportunity exists for all specialists to facilitate the student's growth. For example, the teacher can emphasize communication
during classroom interactions using strategies the SLP models. The teacher then can
help the SLP know which strategies were more or less successful, so that adjustments
can be made in other aspects of intervention. The social worker can emphasize the
communicative goals during her session on social skills, and the physical or occupational therapist can facilitate communication during therapy. At the same time, the
SLP is aware of other goals the student is working toward and can facilitate their development as well.

When children have severe developmental disabilities, SLPs serve on teams that
are established early in the student's school career or even in infancy. Special education programs often have SLPs and physical and occupational therapists who work
together to coordinate services. When augmentative and alternative communication
systems are needed, SLPs may lead teams to select technology supports and instructional strategies (ASHA, 1991, 1998b).

In the role of providing documentation and accountability, the school-based SLP is required by the IDEA to provide parents with reports on their children's progress on IEP goals. These reports must be sent home at least as frequently as report cards are sent for all students. The information should be in language that will be understandable to parents. Qualitative descriptions of a student's demonstration of language skills within the general education curriculum are particularly appropriate. It also may be possible to describe advancing skills in quantitative terms, such as the number of comments a student makes in a group discussion, or numbers of different words or complex sentences in written language probes. Broader outcomes, such as fewer requests for repetition of directions in the classroom, or evidence of increasing self-confidence by approaching groups of children on the playground, for example, are also important to document. IEPs must be revised at least once per year.

OPPORTUNITIES ENHANCED BY WORKING IN SCHOOL SETTINGS

Collaboration, curriculum-based relevance, and participation are three characteristics that hallmark successful service delivery for infants, toddlers, children, and adolescents with language and communication disorders. To some extent they are encoded in policy, in that each is required under the rules and regulations of the Individuals with Disabilities Education Act, but even more, they are dictated by best practice. Speech-language pathologists (SLPs) and special educators who maximize these characteristics in practice have powerful possibilities to influence the development of children's lives in positive directions. Working in school settings enhances their opportunities to do so.

Collaborative Partnerships and Team Models

Collaboration is a key to successful service delivery in any setting (see Chapter 3), but particularly in schools (Coufal, 1993; Ferguson, 1991; Secord & Wiig, 1990; Simon & Myrold-Gunyuz, 1990). When individuals collaborate, they work together to achieve a common goal. Collaborative partnerships do not form automatically, however. They require nurturing. Collaborative relationships may exist among individuals, as they do in parent–professional or co-professional relationships, or they may exist among relatively more structured teams of professionals working together to solve a common problem (McCormick, 1990).

Key characteristics of good collaborative relationships are mutual goal setting and openness to consultation across professional boundaries. Collaborative consultation is defined as

> an interactive process that enables teams of people with diverse expertise to generate creative solutions to mutually defined problems. The outcome is enhanced, altered, and produces solutions that are different from those that the individual team members would produce independently. (Idol, Paolucci-Whitcomb, & Nevin, 1986, p. 1)

Collaboration works best when teams of parents, professionals, and students start with mutual identification of problems they will address as a team. When SLPs, family members, teachers, and other professionals collaborate, they draw on their diverse expertise about the child to build a comprehensive picture of the family's culture, values, and hopes; aspects of the curriculum or early development that are particularly challenging for the child; and the child's communicative needs and strengths.

Collaborative Goal Setting Models

Goal setting models might be characterized as **competitive, individualistic, or cooperative** (Johnson & Johnson, 1975). At times, groups of parents and professionals who are supposed to be working as teams find themselves working at cross-purposes instead. When this occurs, it helps to acknowledge that a competitive model of goal setting is at work (Nelson, 1998).

A model based on **competitive goal setting** is one in which some team members perceive that they will achieve their goal only if others fail to achieve theirs. This contrasts with the model of **individualistic goal setting**, in which team members set goals in relative isolation of one another. Both contrast with the more desirable model of collaborative or **cooperative goal setting**, in which mutual goals are established and each member perceives that his or her goals can be met only if the other members of the team also achieve theirs. Once a team having difficulty has acknowledged that the members cannot agree on goals at one level—for example, whether to retain the child or promote her to the next level—they can agree to disagree on that goal for the moment. They can then focus instead on areas where they *can* agree, such as how to help the child gain more success and independence within the general education curriculum at her current grade level.

Team Models

Teams also may work in one of several structural models—**multidisciplinary, interdisciplinary**, and **transdisciplinary** (represented graphically in Figure 7.2). Many factors influence which model is used for a particular student. One model is not necessarily better than the others. Although higher degrees of communicative interaction and collaboration are generally desirable, each model has advantages and drawbacks within certain situations.

Multidisciplinary teams comprise individuals working together from their own professional identities, each completing a separate assessment and treatment plan, and communicating with other team members on an intermittent basis. Some multidisciplinary teams use the individualistic model of goal setting out of necessity, due to high caseloads and separate agencies of employment. In other cases, professionals fail to take full advantage of interdisciplinary communication opportunities that do exist. For example, school-based team members may communicate with each other only fleetingly, then use that "tool" of multidisciplinary collaboration, the stapler, to compile their separate reports into a "multidisciplinary evaluation team report." In such cases, when the team meets with parents for the first time, each sharing separate results and recommendations, many parents feel disenfranchised and overwhelmed by the process. When one parent shared her frustration about not being a member of the team by saying, "You listen to me politely, but you never write it

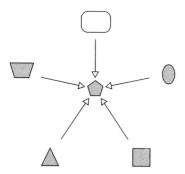

Multidisciplinary Team Model

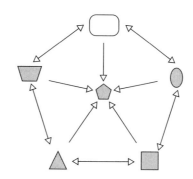

Interdisciplinary Team Model

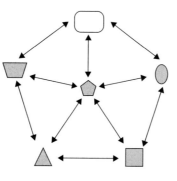

Transdisciplinary Team Model

FIGURE 7.2

Three Models of Team Interaction

Each model has the child and family at the center and professionals from multiple disciplines represented by varied shapes and shading.

down," her child's Individualized Education Planning team did pay attention. They began to treat her as a true collaborative partner, soliciting her written comments as well as her oral input at meetings and using that input in establishing goals for her child (Nelson, 1998).

Interdisciplinary teams use established channels to facilitate communication in multiple directions, sometimes guided by a case manager who coordinates services. The family service coordinator for an Individualized Family Service Plan (under Part C of the IDEA), for example, might arrange for the school-based SLP to visit the home of a toddler with severe developmental delays and then leave a voice-mail message about preliminary findings for other team members. This would allow the occupational therapist and developmental psychologist to fine-tune their own assessment activities on subsequent home visits. Then the team might confer about results and implications that cross their professional domains and establish goals mutually with parents. Teams that use an interdisciplinary structure are in position to produce a truly integrated assessment report incorporating their various findings.

Transdisciplinary teams involve active sharing of information and skills across disciplines in multiple directions. Transdisciplinary teams have three unique features: (1) **joint functioning,** which involves the performance of assessment and intervention functions together as much as possible; (2) **continuous staff development,** in which members train and receive training from each other in reciprocal interactions; and

(3) **role release,** in which team members not only share information with each other, but assist each other to perform functions usually reserved to their own disciplines (Lyon & Lyon, 1980). Members of transdisciplinary teams might work together to design assessment activities for a toddler or preschooler, teaching each other aspects of their various professional roles as they work. In performing "arena assessments," one transdisciplinary team member acts as primary interactant with the child while other team members watch and suggest new questions or modifications in the activities, as needed. After the assessment activities, team members confer to evaluate the results and develop a unified plan. Linder's (1993) Transdisciplinary Play Based Assessment is designed using this model.

Transdisciplinary teams work best when the same group of professionals works together over an extended period of time. Such teams can develop specialized knowledge for working with children of a particular age group (e.g., infants and toddlers) or disability type (e.g., autism spectrum). The arena assessment model also has limitations, however, in that it takes skill not to overwhelm children when surrounded by multiple professionals looking on, even at a distance. It is also difficult for professionals to gain intimate knowledge of a child's strengths and needs in some areas without direct contact with the child.

Collaborative Roles across the Age-Span

School-based SLPs, like all SLPs, serve many roles in meeting their professional responsibilities—from prevention and prereferral through identification, assessment, intervention, and reevaluation, to supervising, documenting, and advocating. Any of these roles may be fulfilled in collaboration with others. Collaborative relationships vary not only with professional roles, but also with the age levels of children served.

Roles for Working with Infants/Toddlers and Families.   Collaboration with parents and health-care providers is particularly essential for providing family-centered services for infants and toddlers (Polmanteer & Turbiville, 2000; Prelock et al., 1999; see also Chapter 4). For example, the birth of a baby with a cleft lip and palate might trigger a referral phone call (with the parents' permission) from the neonatal specialist or hospital-based SLP to a school-district's infant assessment team. The SLP will then collaborate with hospital personnel and the infant's parents as they address concerns about feeding (Arvedson, 2000) and help the family consider and understand the implications and possibilities of surgical interventions in their future. Once the parents' earliest fears and concerns are addressed, the SLP can collaborate with them regarding early communication issues (Nelson, 1998). For example, after collaborating with the mother to adjust feeding equipment, positioning, and strategies, and working together to find the infant's most alert and contented times, the mother and SLP can look for opportunities to maximize the pleasurable eye contact and prelinguistic turn taking of early communicative interactions.

Roles for Working with Preschoolers, Families, and Teachers.   At the preschool level, parents remain the most important collaborative partners in identifying and evaluating children with special needs (see Chapter 3), but collaboration with preschool teachers is also critical to helping children meet developmental expectations and prepare for school. SLPs working collaboratively with preschool teachers and other professionals and paraprofessionals can maximize the opportunities for children to acquire language concepts and forms and to use them pragmatically to perform varied communicative functions. For example, teachers and SLPs might collaborate to schedule "concepts of the week" to be emphasized in circle time and in home programs. They also might collaborate to select key words and phrases that include each child's phonological targets. SLPs can then model ways to cue children to produce their target phonemes, and teachers can emphasize opportunities to use key words and phrases in functional contexts.

Roles for Working with School-Age Students, Families, and Teachers.   During the school-age years, teachers—both special and general education—remain critical collaborative partners for meeting students' needs. Teachers are particularly important partners for identifying language-related problems within the general education curriculum and designing interventions to address them (Bashir, Conte, & Heerde, 1998; DiMeo, Merritt, & Culatta, 1998; Prelock, 2000).

Prelock, Miller, and Reed (1995) described collaborative partnerships for working on language in the classroom. They noted that a typical collaborative team met once every two or three weeks and planned for a two- to three-week unit in thirty to forty minutes. "Initially, most teams met weekly for 30 minutes to plan single lessons. As teams became more time efficient and comfortable in their collaborative interactions, the need for weekly planning meetings decreased" (pp. 288–289). Ebert and Prelock (1994) found that teachers in nonparticipating classrooms tended to underestimate the communicative and cognitive abilities of children with language disorders; whereas teachers who were trained to collaborate "appeared to be more aware of the interference of communication problems on learning and made appropriate adaptations" (p. 213).

Such collaborative relationships are essential to ensuring curriculum-based relevance as well. For example, in the writing lab approach (Nelson, Van Meter, Chamberlain, & Bahr, in press), SLPs, general education teachers, and special education teachers work together in the classroom to help all students develop oral and written language skills in the context of a computer-supported writing process approach. They establish mutual goals, teach each other aspects of their roles, and get to know all of the students' special needs. This model can maximize the opportunities for teachers to scaffold students with disabilities to use emerging communication skills even when the SLP is not in the classroom (DiMeo, Merritt, & Culatta, 1998).

As students transition from high school to higher education or work, their future success will depend on their ability to assume ownership for acquiring new skills; for judging when, how, and to whom to explain their disabilities; and for advocating for accommodations that will allow them to perform competitively with their peers. SLPs can play important collaborative roles in working with them, their high school and employment counselors, and their parents to design transition plans.

Making Collaboration Work

Increasing the levels of collaboration and communication across disciplines requires a number of factors. If members do not value the perspectives of others, teams are unlikely to work collaboratively no matter what their structure or resources. Some practical factors also limit the opportunities for collaboration. Chief among them is the big "T" factor—time.

Particularly in the early stages of development, teams require time to build their relationships and routines. Supportive administrators, such as special education directors and building principals, can set the tone and help teams find time to meet. Teachers are also more likely to find the time to meet when they see SLPs as helping them meet their goals. Conversations about shared students are a good place to start. Collaborative relationships with parents begin when SLPs invite them to share their concerns during initial contacts. At any point, the secret of successful collaborative consultation is this—working with others to establish *mutual goals* based primarily in their needs (not the SLP's), and then working together to achieve them.

Curriculum-Based Relevance

Underlying each of the disability-related goals of prevention, identification, assessment and evaluation, intervention, and monitoring are the general-curricular goals of schooling in general. Society's goal is to educate children to be productive, socially responsible citizens who can read and write, work with mathematical concepts, use scientific and social systems knowledge to solve problems, and ultimately, be productively employed.

In spite of the importance and pervasiveness of these goals for most children, they are often forgotten for children with special education needs. In part, this has resulted from widespread use of a medical model, in which SLPs and other special educators diagnose language and communication disorders and treat them in isolation. Such an approach does not include a comprehensive picture of what the child needs to participate in the general education experience. When intervention objectives are derived exclusively from the results of standardized tests used to determine eligibility, they may bear limited relevance to the child's need to learn within the general education curriculum.

When one considers that communication is essential for gaining access to the general education curriculum and participating as a full member of the classroom, it is hard to imagine that a child's needs could be met without addressing such goals. In many cases, education is delivered entirely through language—both spoken and written. Communication skills are always involved. Students who lack the basic language skills to learn through the language of their teachers or textbooks have significant functional limitations that should be a primary focus of treatment.

Curriculum-based language assessment (CBLA) (Nelson, 1989; Prelock, 1997) is best suited to the purpose of assessing the needs of children with language problems to be involved and progress in the general curriculum. It differs from other forms of curriculum-based measurement (CBM) in purpose and strategy.

CBM can include "*any* procedure that directly assesses student performance within the course content for the purpose of determining that student's instructional needs" (Tucker, 1985, p. 200). It is designed to answer the question of whether a child has learned the curriculum. For example:

- The number of words read aloud in one minute can serve as a valid and reliable index of the child's growing skill in reading ability (Deno, Mirkin, & Chiang, 1982; Fuchs, Fuchs, & Maxwell, 1988; Jenkins & Jewell, 1993).

- The number of words produced and spelled correctly within short writing samples can serve as indicators of growth in written language at the elementary level (Deno, Marston, & Mirkin, 1982).
- The number of correct word sequences minus incorrect ones can serve a similar purpose for middle and secondary school students (Espin, Shin, Deno, Skare, Robinson, & Benner, 2000).

The strength of such measures is that they are quick and can be repeated frequently. The limitation is that they do not provide much information about what to do if a student is not making progress.

That is where the advantages and differences of CBLA becomes apparent. CBLA is defined as the "use of curriculum contexts and content for measuring a student's language intervention needs and progress" (Nelson, 1989, p. 171). It is designed to answer the question of whether a child has the *language skills* to learn the general education curriculum. This is accomplished by first selecting which curriculum contexts and content to use in the assessment.

When thinking about the demands of the general education curriculum, it is helpful to think of that curriculum as having more than one aspect. Nelson (1998) described six kinds of general education curriculum that might be considered when performing curriculum-based language assessment and intervention (see Table 7.4). Areas of greatest significance within one or more of these curricula are selected in collaboration with teachers, parents, and the student him- or herself. It is not necessary to assess language across the entire curriculum, just to identify areas of greatest concern as the best place to start, and it is the key participants who are in the best position to identify them. Interviews can be used for this purpose, or the group can sit down together to discuss those areas collaboratively. When common areas emerge, further probing is used to pull out specific curricular materials and tasks with which the student struggles. These will be used to begin the assessment and intervention process.

The role of the SLP in CBLA is to assess how the student's language and communication abilities and disabilities influence performance within the selected tasks, and how things might be improved. This is accomplished by moving through four steps, each with its own organizing question (Nelson, 1989, 1998):

1. What language and communication skills are required for a typical student to experience success in the targeted curricular task?
2. What language and communication skills and strategies does this student currently bring to the task?
3. What new skills or strategies should the student learn to improve functioning on the task?
4. What modifications in the task make it possible for the student to do better?

To answer these four questions, the SLP uses broad knowledge of language and communication as reviewed throughout this book and in other sources (e.g., Calculator & Jorgensen, 1994; Merritt & Culatta, 1998; Nelson, 1998; Paul, 2000). Although professional knowledge is required, the process is not as complex as it might sound. Additionally, although it is not as quick and simple as some of the CBM tasks

TABLE 7.4	A Summary of Six Curricula Students Must Master to Succeed in School
Official Curriculum	The outline produced by curriculum committees in many school districts. May or may not have major influence in a particular classroom. To find out, ask the teacher to show you a copy.
Cultural Curriculum	The unpoken expectations for students to know enough about the mainstream culture to use it as background context in understanding various aspects of the official curriculum.
De facto Curriculum	The use of textbook selections rather than an official outline to determine the curriculum. Classrooms in the same district often vary in the degree to which "teacher manual teaching" occurs.
School Culture Curriculum	The set of spoken and unspoken rules about communication and behavior in classroom interactions. Includes expectations for metapragmatic awareness of rules about such things as when to talk, when not to talk, and how to request a turn.
Hidden Curriculum	The subtle expectations that teachers have for determining who the "good students" are in their classrooms. They vary with the value systems of individual teachers. Even students who are insensitive to the rules of the school culture curriculum usually know where they fall on a classroom continuum of "good" and "problem" students.
Underground Curriculum	The rules for social interaction among peers that determine who will be accepted and who not. Includes expectations for using the latest slang and pragmatic rules of social interaction discourse as diverse as bragging and peer tutoring.

Source: From Nelson, N. W. (1998), p. 404. Copyright 1992, 2000 by N. W. Nelson. Shared by permission of the author.

described previously, CBLA has advantages in yielding information about the best objectives and strategies for intervention.

Consider the example of a second-grade boy, Tyler, with language and learning disabilities for whom reading is identified as the curricular area of greatest concern. In contemplating **the first question,** the SLP or other specialist based her observations on the "simple view" of reading as decoding plus comprehension (Gough & Tunmer, 1986; Hoover & Gough, 1990). She knew that this view was favored by many practitioners and researchers (Kamhi, 1999) and was the one used by the American Speech-Language-Hearing Association (2001) in developing its position statement and guidelines for the roles of SLPs in reading and writing. Further, she knew that decoding occurs through word recognition processes for transforming print to words through both: (1) direct visual-orthographic routes, and (2) indirect sound-symbol correspondence ones, and that (3) comprehension occurs through construction of meaning at the word, sentence, and discourse levels.

When the SLP observed Tyler attempting to read aloud (addressing **the second question,** about what the child does currently), it was clear that he had limited ability to decode words using either sound–symbol or visual–orthographic strategies. Yet when the SLP read aloud to him from second-grade reading passages and asked comprehension questions (Leslie & Caldwell, 1995), Tyler seemed to understand with little difficulty. This was consistent with what other team members had reported. Analyzing Tyler's decoding performance further, the SLP observed that he rarely attempted to form even the first sound of most words unless prompted to do so. Neither did he use his relatively better sentence comprehension and formulation skills to predict what word might come next and narrow down the possibilities. Instead, he made erratic guesses or said, "I don't know." Because sound–symbol associations seemed wobbly, the SLP did a quick inventory by writing letter symbols and asking Tyler to tell the associated sound; then producing individual sounds and asking him to print the corresponding symbol. Although not a strength, Tyler was found to have sound–symbol association knowledge that he was not using.

Moving to **the third question,** about what the student might learn to do differently, the SLP used dynamic assessment techniques to instruct Tyler about new strategies and observe the effects. For example, the next time he came to an unknown word and said, "I don't know," the SLP framed the first letter or letter combination, such as "ch" or "sh," and asked, "What do these letters tell you about how the word starts? You know these sounds." After a response, the SLP encouraged, "See, your brain knows more than you think. If you get your mouth ready, and think about the sentence so far, it may be easier to figure out that tricky vowel sound that comes next." The SLP then scaffolded other strategies, such as, "Look at the end of the word too. You know that sound." Later, she encouraged greater independence, "Great! Let's try some more. I'll help if you need it, but you're doing a wonderful job." The result of this step-by-step dynamic assessment process was the formation of therapy goals aimed at strengthening sound–symbol associations and the phonological awareness skills that were weak for Tyler. For a second grader, the team decided to address the goals simultaneously because reading decoding could not wait for the remediation of phonological awareness problems.

Addressing **the fourth question,** about how the task might be modified, the team decided that Tyler's independent reading skills were not yet sufficiently developed for him to benefit from the half-hour silent reading periods the teacher conducted daily. What he needed, they decided, was intensive word decoding practice with adult support. The SLP assumed responsibility to assist with the process of firming up phonemic awareness and sound–symbol associations in pull-out sessions. The SLP, teacher, and learning disabilities teacher consultant conferred regarding the scaffolding strategies that seemed to help Tyler the most, and together they showed the paraprofessional how to use those strategies to support him while reading aloud in a quiet space outside the classroom during silent reading time. When the curriculum goal was to read stories for comprehension, the paraprofessional read aloud to Tyler, pointing to each word while reading, and stopping occasionally at direct-route "sight words" Tyler knew, or to encourage him to use developing decoding skills on regularly spelled words. The whole team, including Tyler and his parents, established a goal for this accommodation to be faded as he became a more independent reader by the end of the school year.

Other students might have more difficulty with direction following (part of the school culture curriculum) or social communication (part of the underground curriculum) than with the official curriculum. If a teacher identifies direction following as a problem, the SLP might offer to sit in during a lesson where directions are an important feature. Then CBLA procedures can involve writing down what the teacher says, what a typical student does (the first step), and what the target student does (the second step). The teacher and SLP can confer later to analyze what might be happening when the student does not respond correctly. For example, it might be necessary for the SLP to probe the student's understanding of directional vocabulary in a pull-out session to identify the need for specific instruction at the word level (the third step). Working collaboratively with the SLP, the teacher might observe that the student does better when directions are presented in fewer steps, and that it is important to check the student's comprehension by asking strategic question—not to catch the student in an error, but to support, confirm, and solidify understanding (the fourth step).

Similar procedures would be used for assessing problems of social communication across grade levels or for assessing comprehension of complex texts or note-taking problems in the upper grades (Merritt & Culatta, 1998). The advantage of CBLA is that the process relates smoothly to the design and implementation of intervention strategies that will make a difference for students. In intervention, language skills across all systems—phonology, morphology, syntax, semantics, pragmatics—and levels—sound, syllable, word, sentence, discourse—can be targeted in any curricular context, spoken or written. The curriculum-based language assessment and intervention process is recursive and flexible. It works across grade levels and situations, and for students with severe disabilities (Calculator & Jorgensen, 1994) as well as for students who are closer to their peers in ability.

Participation

The regulatory language of IDEA requires that children with disabilities be educated in the "least restrictive environment" (LRE). Strategies for meeting this requirement were discussed previously, along with the requirements for students' IEPs to be implemented for the child—"to be involved and progress in the general curriculum" in accordance with the child's needs, "to participate in extracurricular and other nonacademic activities," and "to be educated and participate with other children with disabilities and nondisabled children" [Sec. 614(d)(1)(A)(iii)].

Focusing on students' needs to participate in the general education curriculum and with general education peers is more than a requirement. It is essential for making changes relevant to students' needs. Meeting this standard requires a participatory attitude and values as much as a set of procedural steps. As in any aspect of school practice that is governed by policy, a real danger exists that valuable practices will be overshadowed by the demands of paperwork. It is possible for teams to go through the motions of considering LRE concerns for a particular child without taking the steps that would actually enhance participation. It is also possible for a student to be "included" full time in a general education classroom in body, but to participate only minimally in actuality.

Academic and social communication both are essential to successful participation in classrooms (Brinton, Fukiki, Montague, & Hanton, 2000; Merritt & Culatta,

1998), and SLPs have knowledge about how to foster such participation, but they are not necessarily in the best position to do so. General education teachers have greater opportunities in role, place, and time to foster the participation of students in natural environments with their peers, but they may not be sure how much to expect from their students with disabilities or how to draw the best from them.

Collaboration among professionals is clearly needed. Regardless of service delivery model, focusing assessment and intervention on issues of concern to teachers will enhance the likelihood of students learning the school culture and hidden curriculum necessary for classroom acceptance and participation. This process starts by asking the student's teachers, "If you could change just one thing for this student, what would that be?" Even this question may be premature, however, when students have the status more of "visitor" than true members of the class (Van Meter, 1999).

Some students are included in the general education classroom but are not expected to participate in any of the general education activities or even to meet the teacher's usual behavioral expectations. This was the case for Shannon, a third-grade student with significant cognitive, speech, and language difficulties. Shannon was included part time in a general education third-grade classroom. Her teacher had a rule that no student could leave his or her seat during formal lessons, yet the teacher ignored the infraction when Shannon left her seat, distanced herself by rummaging in her desk with the lid up, and generally ignored what the rest of the class was doing. When asked about the difference in rule enforcement, the teacher commented that the student in question was "special." In fact, the teacher said, "She's not one of my students."

Uncertainty about what to do with a special needs student, fear of doing the wrong thing, and worry about taking time away from other students makes many general education teachers reluctant to play a major role in facilitating participation for students with more severe disabilities. In Shannon's case, the teacher was not sure what to expect, but reported that she could not do any of the things that the other students did, saying "She can't even write." The SLP acknowledged that Shannon was especially challenging to teach. Her reading and writing were at emergent levels, her speech was difficult for her peers and teacher to understand, her language was marked by disordered sentence structure and limited vocabulary, and her pragmatic skills often left her listeners with inadequate information. In addition, her avoidance skills were well developed, not only hiding behind her raised desk lid and making frequent trips to the bathroom, but when she did finally sit down to write, with intensive scaffolding, she often would erase her work before her frustrated teachers could stop her. Shannon rarely made any communicative overtures to her peers, and they mostly ignored her.

The SLP was in the third-grade classroom two days per week and in the school's computer lab with the class one day per week to implement a writing lab approach (Nelson, Van Meter, Chamberlain, & Bahr, in press). This approach was an inclusive intervention program for fostering the language and communication skills of students with special education needs along with those of their classrooms, many of whom had educational risks of their own. The students had been diagnosed with a variety of disabilities (speech-language impairment, hearing impairment, learning disability, educational mental impairment, and emotional impairment), but all had communication needs and all had IEP goals in the area of written language. The teacher wondered how Shannon could fit into the writing lab activities when she could not write, but as the SLP and teacher looked at Shannon's initial attempts, they did find some strengths. She could make most letters, although she tended to string them together vertically and intersperse them with numbers in early spelling attempts. She also could copy text and generate some initial letters for invented spellings, skills learned in her special education classroom. She could even spell a few high-frequency words (see Figure 7.3). Although Shannon's spoken language was disordered, she was able to tell a kernel of a narrative about her cat (named Snowball) with extensive step-by-step questioning, but "It was like pulling teeth."

Collaborating, the SLP and teacher developed a set of goals and objectives (see Figure 7.4) and strategies to support Shannon in participating in writing lab activities with her peers. For example, when a more competent peer was asked to form a pair with Shannon to work on a project, the peer rolled her eyes and expressed reluctance. The SLP's intervention focused on helping the peer see that she could use her skills to help Shannon express her ideas before writing, that she would be making an important contribution, and that the SLP would help the student know what to say and do to help Shannon. When the peer began to show interest in Shannon's ideas and help her get them on paper, Shannon dropped some of her avoidance strategies and communicated more directly, meeting her planning objectives.

With scaffolding in this and other interactions, Shannon learned to tell a more complete story with less scaffolding and to apply some of her developing sound–symbol associations to write more words with less assistance. She also learned to read

FIGURE 7.3

Shannon's Initial Story-Writing Attempt

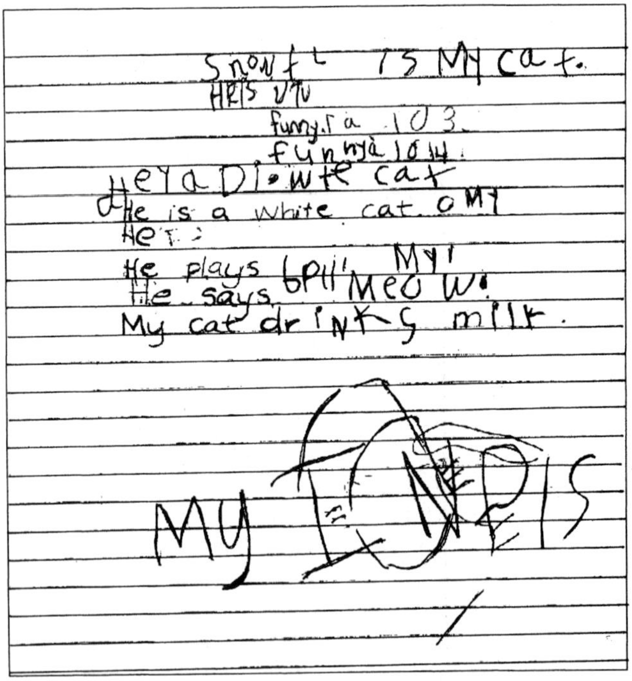

Shannon will

1. Increase independent planning
   a. Brainstorm 3 topic ideas
   b. Set daily writing goals and record progress with adult support
   c. Participate in a peer conference to plan
   d. Guide self with written or computer supported prompts (rather than intensive teacher scaffolding)

2. Improve spelling and word knowledge by
   a. Using association strategies taught in the special education room to generate initial and final sounds and letters
   b. Using word chunking strategies
   c. Referring to personal supports (personal dictionary, software supported word bank, word wall)

3. Improve reading by using strategies, such as
   a. Look for chunks
   b. Get your mouth ready
   c. Think about what makes sense
   d. Check accuracy with computer synthesizer reading

FIGURE 7.4

Shannon's Writing Lab Goals and Objectives

her story aloud with support from her peers. As Shannon began to participate in classroom activities to work on planning and drafting her own stories, her classmates began to accept her as a member of the class. The avoidance behaviors faded and the improved communication and participation outcomes became apparent when Shannon's story of how Snowball died held the attention of her peers. Her participation in the class became even clearer when she brought in pictures of her new baby sister, and the girls in the class gathered around asking questions and remarking about the baby. If Shannon had maintained only her special education student identity, it is unlikely that such scenes ever would have occurred.

MAKING IT ALL WORK

SLPs who provide services in school settings have unique opportunities, but also face unique challenges. Primary among these is the challenge to fit all of the many school-related roles and responsibilities into the confines of a school day and week. Maximum caseload size is codified in policy in most states. Such policies often indicate that caseload size should be determined by the collective IEPs and IFSPs of the children being served, allowing time for any of the other roles summarized in Table 7.1. The American Speech-Language-Hearing Association (1993, 1999b) also has published guidelines for determining caseload size:

> Caseload size must reflect a balance between how many hours are available in the school day for services to students, and how many hours are needed to complete paperwork, staffing, and other required activities. The recommended maximum caseload for appropriate services is 40 students, regardless of the type or number of service delivery models selected. Special populations may dictate fewer

students on the caseload. A recommended maximum caseload composed entirely of preschoolers is 25. Other populations that may require additional time, and therefore fewer students on the caseload, include students who are technologically dependent, medically fragile, multilingual or limited English proficient. Some states limit the number of students in self-contained classrooms. Eight students without a support person, or 12 students with a support person, are the recommendation for this type of setting. [ASHA, 1999b, p. 38]

When establishing a schedule, the SLP needs to plan time for conducting the specific activities associated with managing a caseload. A partial list includes:

- Conducting speech-language-hearing screenings
- Writing reports
- Participating as a member of multidisciplinary teams and conferences
- Completing required documentation
- Participating in continuing education
- Coordinating assistive technology services
- Planning curricular/instructional changes
- Serving on teacher assistance teams
- Carrying out comprehensive diagnostic evaluations
- Developing IEPs
- Participating in ongoing teacher/parent conferences
- Providing in-service documentation
- Participating in annual review conferences
- Participating/leading child study committees
- Supervising support personnel/Clinical Fellowship Years
- Serving as a mentor teacher
- Meeting other school responsibilities (ASHA, 1993, p. III-106)

Not all of these activities need to be built into a single workweek. Some are spread out over longer periods of time. Creating a balance also may vary with a particular caseload and career stage. More responsibilities can be handled after an SLP gains experience in a particular position, but at any point, it is important to keep supervisors informed when a workload gets out of control in order to avoid professional burn out. Bringing the supervisor into the problem-solving process may make it easier to find creative solutions, and it is part of the advocacy and leadership role mentioned in Table 7.1.

SUMMARY

This chapter has provided information about several key pieces of legislation that govern school-based service delivery, including Section 504 of the Rehabilitation Act, Parts B and C of the Individuals with Disabilities Education Act, and the Americans with Disabilities Act. Roles for school-based SLPs were described as including prevention, prereferral study, identification, assessment, evaluation, eligibility determination, IEP/IFSP development, caseload management, intervention for communication disorders and for communication variations (when appropriate), provision of technological supports, consulting regarding students both on the caseload and not, reevaluating, assisting with transitions, supervising, documenting, and serving as advocates and leaders.

Regulations and strategies were described for providing comprehensive services to infants/toddlers and their families under Part C, to preschoolers under Part C or B, and to school-age students under Part B of IDEA. A continuum of services was listed from less to more restrictive: consultation, home- or community-based, classroom-based, pull-out, self-contained classrooms, and separate school or facility. The point was made that although a continuum may be described, the determination of what is "least restrictive" must be determined for individual children by their IEP teams.

Special opportunities of working in school settings were presented. These include collaborative consultation with key participants across the age span, curriculum-based language assessment, and strategies for fostering students' participation with peers and in the general education curriculum. The chapter ended with suggestions for managing a full caseload.

STUDY QUESTIONS

1. Describe at least two ways that Section 504 of the Rehabilitation Act influences children with disabilities in school settings and differentiate it from IDEA.
2. Compare and contrast IEPS and IFSPs.
3. Differentiate multidisciplinary, interdisciplinary, and transdisciplinary team models; describe a situation in which each might be most likely used.
4. Describe collaborative roles that SLPs might play and how they differ for children with special needs as infants or toddlers, preschoolers, school-age children and adolescents, and young adults.
5. What are the four questions of curriculum-based language assessment and intervention, and how are they used?
6. What does it mean for a student with disabilities to participate in school contexts? How could an SLP support this participation?

REFERENCES

American Speech-Language-Hearing Association. (1985, June). Clinical management of communicatively handicapped minority language populations. *ASHA, 27,* 29–32.

American Speech-Language-Hearing Association. (1989a). Communication-based services for infants, toddlers, and their families. *ASHA, 31,* 32–34, 94.

American Speech-Language-Hearing Association. (1989b). Issues in determining eligibility for language intervention. *ASHA, 31,* 113–118.

American Speech-Language-Hearing Association. (1990). The roles of speech-language pathologists in service delivery to infants, toddlers, and their families (Position Statement). *ASHA, 32(Suppl. 2),* 4.

American Speech-Language-Hearing Association. (1991, March). Guidelines for speech-language pathologists serving persons with language, socio-communicative, and/or cognitive/communication impairments. *ASHA, 33,* 21–28.

American Speech-Language-Hearing Association. (1993). Guidelines for caseload size and speech-language service delivery in the schools. *ASHA, 35* (Suppl. 10), 33–39.

American Speech-Language-Hearing Association. (1996). Inclusive practices for children and youths with communication disorders. Position statement and technical report. *ASHA, 38* (Suppl. 16), 35–44.

American Speech-Language-Hearing Association. (1998a). *Bilingualism, LEP (limited English proficiency), and ESL (English as a second language).* Rockville, MD: ASHA, Office of Multicultural Affairs.

American Speech-Language-Hearing Association. (1998b). *Maximizing the provision of appropriate technology services and devices for students in schools: Technical report.* Rockville, MD: ASHA.

American Speech-Language-Hearing Association. (1999a). *Guidelines for the roles and responsibilities of the school-based speech-language pathologist.* Rockville, MD: ASHA.

American Speech-Language-Hearing Association. (1999b). *IDEA and your caseload: A template for eligibility and dismissal criteria for students ages 3 to 21.* Rockville, MD: ASHA.

American Speech-Language-Hearing Association. (2001). *Roles and responsibilities of the speech-language pathologist with respect to reading and writing in children and adolescents.* Rockville, MD: ASHA.

Anderson, G. M., & Nelson, N. W. (1988). Integrating language intervention and education in an alternate adolescent language classroom. *Seminars in Speech and Language, 9*(4), 341–353.

Arvedson, J. C. (2000). Evaluation of children with feeding and swallowing problems. *Language, Speech, and Hearing Services in Schools, 31,* 28–41.

Bashir, A., Conte, B. M., & Heerde, S. M. (1998) Language and school success: Collaborative challenges and choices. In D. Merritt & B. Culatta (Eds.), *Language intervention in the classroom* (pp. 1–36). San Diego, CA: Singular.

Battle, D. E. (Ed.). (1993). *Communication disorders in multicultural populations.* Boston: Andover Medical Publishers.

Beck, A. R., & Dennis, M. (1997). Speech-Language pathologists' and teachers' perceptions of classroom-based interventions. *Language, Speech, and Hearing Services in Schools, 28,* 146–153.

Brinton, B., Fujiki, M., Montague, E. C., & Hanton, J. (2000). Children with language impairment in cooperative work groups. *Language, Speech, and Hearing Services in Schools, 31,* 252–264.

Buttrill J., Niizawa, J., Biemer, C., Takahashi, C., & Hearn, S. (1989). Servicing the language disabled adolescent: A strategies-based model. *Language, Speech, and Hearing Services in Schools, 20,* 185–204.

Calculator, S. N., & Jorgensen, C. M. (1994). *Including students with severe disabilities in schools: Fostering communication, interaction, and participation.* San Diego, CA: Singular.

Casby, M. W. (1992). The cognitive hypothesis and its influence on speech-language services in schools. *Language, Speech, and Hearing Services in Schools, 23,* 198–202.

Cole, K. N., Dale, P. S., & Mills, P. E. (1990). Defining language delay in young children by cognitive referencing: Are we saying more than we know? *Applied Psycholinguistics, 11,* 291–302.

Cole, K. N., Dale, P. S., & Mills, P. E. (1992). Stability of the intelligence quotient–language quotient relation: Is discrepancy modeling based on a myth? *American Journal on Mental Retardation, 97,* 131–143.

Cole, K. N., & Harris, S. R. (1992). Instability of the intelligence quotient–motor quotient relationship. *Developmental Medicine and Child Neurology, 34,* 633–641.

Cole, K. N., Mills, P. E., & Kelley, D. (1994). Agreement of assessment profiles used in cognitive referencing. *Language, Speech, and Hearing Services in Schools, 25,* 25–31.

Coufal, K. (Ed.). (1993). Collaborative consultation for speech-language pathologists. *Topics in Language Disorders, 14*(1), 1–14.

Crandell, C. C., & Smaldino, J. J. (2000). Classroom acoustics for children with normal hearing and with hearing impairment. *Language, Speech, and Hearing Services in Schools, 31,* 362–370.

Deno, S. L., Martston, D., & Mirkin, P. L. (1982). Valid measurement procedures for continuous evaluation of written expression. *Exceptional Children, 48,* 368–371.

Deno, S. L., Mirkin, P. K., & Chiang, B. (1982). Valid measurement procedures for continuous evaluation of written expression. *Exceptional Children, 48,* 368–371.

DiMeo, J., Merritt, D., & Culatta, B. (1998). Collaborative partnerships and decision making. In D. Merritt & B. Culatta (Eds.), *Language intervention in the classroom* (pp. 37–97). San Diego, CA: Singular.

Ebert, K. A., & Prelock, P. A. (1994). Teachers' perception of their students with communication disorders. *Language, Speech, and Hearing Services in Schools, 25,* 211–214.

Ehren, B. (2000). Maintaining a therapeutic focus and sharing responsibility for student success: Keys to in-class speech-language services. *Language, Speech, and Hearing Services in Schools, 31,* 219–229.

Elksnin, L. K., & Capilouto, G. (1994). Speech-language pathologists' perceptions of integrated service delivery in school settings. *Language, Speech, and Hearing Services in Schools, 25,* 258–267.

Espin, C., Shin, J., Deno, S. L., Skare, S., Robinson, S., & Benner, B. (2000). Identifying indicators of written expression proficiency for middle school students. *The Journal of Special Education, 34*(3), 140–153.

Ferguson, M. L. (1991). Collaborative/consultative service delivery: An introduction. *Language, Speech, and Hearing Services in Schools, 22,* 147.

Fey, M. E., Long, S. H., & Cleave, P. L. (1994). Reconsideration of IQ criteria in the definition of specific language impairment. In R. V. Watkins & M. Rice (Eds.), Specific language impairments in children. Baltimore: Paul H. Brookes.

Francis, D. J., Fletcher, J. M., Shaywitz, B. A., Shaywitz, S. E., & Rourke, B. P. (1996). Defining learning and language disabilities: Conceptual and psychometric issues with the use of IQ tests. *Language, Speech, and Hearing Services in Schools, 27,* 132–143.

Fuchs, L. S., Fuchs, D., & Maxwell, L. (1988). The validity of informal reading comprehension measures. *Remedial and Special Education, 9*(2), 20–28.

Gough, P., & Tunmer, W. (1986). Decoding, reading and reading disability. *Remedial and Special Education, 7,* 6–10.

Hoover, W., & Gough, P. (1990). The simple view of reading. *Reading and Writing: An Interdisciplinary Journal, 2,* 127–160.

Idol, L., Paolucci-Whitcomb, P., & Nevin, A. (1986). *Models of curriculum-based assessment.* Rockville, MD: Aspen.

Jenkins, J. R., & Jewell, M. (1993). Examining the validity of two measures for formative teaching: Reading aloud and maze. *Exceptional children, 59,* 421–432.

Johnson, D. W., & Johnson, R. (1975). *Learning together and alone.* Englewood Cliffs, NJ: Prentice-Hall.

Kamhi, A. (1999). Language and reading: Convergences and divergences. In H. Catts & A. Kamhi (Eds.), *Language and reading disabilities* (pp. 1–24). Boston: Allyn & Bacon.

Leslie, L., & Caldwell, J. (1995). *Qualitative reading inventory-II (QRI-II).* New York: Longman.

Linder, T. (1993). *Transdisciplinary play-based assessment* (rev. ed.). Baltimore: Paul H. Brookes.

Lyon, S., & Lyon, G. (1980). Team functioning and staff development: A role release approach to providing integrated educational services for severely handicapped students. *Journal of the Association for the Severely Handicapped, 5*(3), 59–61.

McCormick, L. (1990). Extracurricular roles and relationships. In L. McCormick & R. L. Schiefelbusch (Eds.), *Early language intervention: An introduction* (2d ed.). (pp. 216–260). Columbus, OH: Merrill.

Merritt, D. D., & Culatta, B. (1998). *Language intervention in the classroom.* San Diego, CA: Singular.

Nelson, N. W. (1989). Curriculum-based language assessment and intervention. *Language, Speech, and Hearing Services in Schools, 20,* 170–184.

Nelson, N. W. (1998). *Childhood language disorders in context: Infancy through adolescence* (2d ed.). Boston: Allyn & Bacon.

Nelson, N. W., & Staskowski, M. (2000). Service delivery issues for schools. In R. Lubinske & C. Fratalli (Eds.), *Professional issues in speech-language pathology and audiology* (2d ed.). (pp. 277–300). San Diego, CA: Singular.

Nelson, N. W., Van Meter, A. M., Chamberlain, D. M., & Bahr, C. M. (In press). Roles of speech-language pathologists in a writing lab approach. *Seminars in Speech and Language.*

Nelson, P. B., & Soli, S. (2000). Acoustical barriers to learning: Children at risk in every classroom. *Language, Speech, and Hearing Services in Schools, 31,* 356–361.

Paul, R. (2000). *Language disorders from infancy through adolescence: Assessment and intervention* (2d ed.). St. Louis: Mosby.

Polmanteer, K., & Turbiville, V. (2000). Family-responsive Individualized Family Service Plans for speech-language pathologists. *Language, Speech, and Hearing Services in Schools, 31,* 4–14.

Prelock, P. A. (1997). Language-based curriculum analysis: A collaborative assessment and intervention process. *Journal of Childhood Communication Disorders, 19,* 35–42.

Prelock, P. A. (2000). Prologue: Multiple perspectives for determining the roles of speech-language pathologists in inclusionary classrooms. *Language, Speech, and Hearing Services in Schools, 31,* 213–218.

Prelock, P. A., Beatson, J., Contompasis, S. H., & Bishop, K. K. (1999). A model for family-centered interdisciplinary practice in the community. *Topics in Language Disorders, 19*(3), 36–51.

Prelock, P. A., Miller, B. L., & Reed, N. L. (1995). Collaborative partnerships in a language in the classroom program. *Language, Speech, and Hearing Services in Schools, 26,* 286–292.

Public Law 105-17. (1997, June). Individuals with Disabilities Education Act Amendments of 1997 (IDEA97). *Federal Register.*

Secord, W., & Wiig, E. (Eds.). (1990). *Best practices in school speech-language pathology: Collaborative programs in the schools—Concepts, models, and procedures.* San Antonio, TX: The Psychological Corporation.

Shackelford, J. (2000). State and jurisdictional eligibility definitions for infants and toddlers with disabilities under IDEA. *NECTAS Notes, Issue No. 5.* Chapel Hill, NC: National Early Childhood Technical Assistance System (www.nectas.unc.edu).

Sieben, G. W., Gold, M. A., Sieben, G. W., & Ermann, M. G. (2000). Ten ways to provide a high-quality acoustical environment in schools. *Language, Speech, and Hearing Services in Schools, 31,* 376–384.

Simon, C., & Myrold-Gunyuz, M. (1990). *Into the classroom: The SLP in the collaborative role.* San Antonio, TX: Communication Skill Builders.

Smaldino, J. J., & Crandell, C. C. (2000). Classroom amplification technology: Theory and practice. *Language, Speech, and Hearing Services in Schools, 31,* 371–375.

Sorkin, D. L. (2000). The classroom acoustical environment and the Americans with Disabilities Act. *Language, Speech, and Hearing Services in Schools, 31,* 385–388.

Taylor, O. L., & Payne, K. T. (1983). Culturally valid testing: A proactive approach. *Topics in Language Disorders, 3*(3), 8–20.

Tucker, J. A. (1985). Curriculum-based assessment: An introduction. *Exceptional Children, 52,* 199–204.

Van Meter, A. M. (1999, February). *Strategies for fostering inclusion in a computer supported writing lab.* Presentation at the Symposium on Literacy and Disabilities, Chapel Hill, NC.

Warner, C., & Nelson, N. W. (2000). Assessment of communication, language, and speech: Questions of "What to do next?" In B. Bracken (Ed.), *The psychoeducational assessment of preschool children* (3d ed.) (pp. 145–185). Boston: Allyn & Bacon.

Zhang, X., & Tomblin, J. B. (2000). The association of intervention receipt with speech-language profiles and social-demographic variables. *American Journal of Speech-Language Pathology, 9,* 345–357.

CHAPTER 8

Language Development and Disorders in Culturally and Linguistically Diverse Children

Dolores E. Battle
Buffalo State College

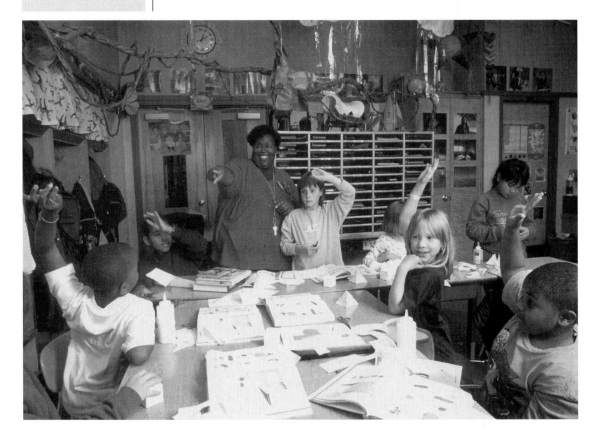

LINGUISTIC DIVERSITY IN THE UNITED STATES

From its beginning, the United States has been a nation of immigrants. The original immigrants came from European countries that shared a common European cultural background. Although they came from different parts of Europe, they shared common religious beliefs and learned to use English as the common language of the land. The country became a melting pot of persons of European heritage, who adopted the culture and language of their new country in order to share economic success and prosperity. The prosperity of the nation brought nonvoluntary immigration in the form of slavery from the countries of Africa. It also brought people from Asia to develop the western gold mines and build railroads linking the eastern and western parts of the nation. These groups added to the diversity of the Native Americans who had occupied the land before the European immigration. The resultant nation had a diversity unlike any found in other parts of the world. In order to maintain their economic power, the European majority adopted policies to restrict the immigration of persons from countries other than European ones. Political policies were established to maintain social and economic control over others such as Asians, Native Americans, and African Americans (Vecoli, 1995).

As the political and economic climate of the country changed at the beginning of the twentieth century, so did the patterns of immigration. The industrial revolution brought 18 million immigrants to the country from Europe and a large group of persons from Asia, primarily China and Japan. Concerns about the differences between Asians and Europeans led to the Immigration Acts of 1921 and 1924, which restricted the immigration of persons who were considered nonwhite. The United States, however, still became a nation of persons from many different cultures, speaking many different languages, and holding many different cultural values. The economic value of cultural and linguistic assimilation was not always strong, and immigrants sought to maintain their cultural and linguistic connections with their home country. Later, immigrations added to the cultural diversity. The Great Depression and World War II brought a hiatus in immigration. However, beginning in 1965, a new wave of immigration began with persons coming primarily from Central and South America, Asia and the Pacific Islands, as well as from the Middle East and Africa. This third wave of immigration was different from the previous two because the great majority of immigrants came from non-European countries. The result has been a change in the diversity of the country that has affected the understanding of language development and language disorders. No longer is the United States a nation of European immigrants with European cultural values speaking English as the primary language. Unlike the initial immigrants, the new immigrants were interested in maintaining their cultural identity and their native language while they learned the language and culture necessary to achieve success in this country.

The population of the country has changed dramatically in the past twenty years. There has been a significant increase in the number of persons immigrating to the United States from Central and South America, the Caribbean, and the Asian and Pacific Islands, as well as from the Middle East and Africa. Current population projections are that by the year 2050, persons of white European heritage will be in the minority in this country.

As shown in Table 8.1, of the more than 270 million people in this country, nearly 30 percent identify themselves as being nonwhite. This represents a nearly 5 percent increase from the number of nonwhites in 1990. African Americans make up the largest group at 12.1 percent, followed by Hispanic Americans at 11.1 percent, Asian Americans at 3.65 percent, and Native Americans at 0.8 percent.

The most significant changes have come from increases in the Hispanic and Asian populations. In 1996 alone, nearly 800,000 persons were legal immigrants from Mexico, the Philippines, India, Vietnam, China, the Dominican Republic, and Cuba. That same year, 128,565 persons were admitted as permanent residents under refugee acts from Europe, the former Soviet Union, Asia, and Africa, and an estimated 5 million persons were undocumented immigrants, including nearly 2.7 million from Mexico (U.S. Bureau of the Census, 1999). The immigrants can be found in nearly every state of the country, with differences in the populations that have settled in different regions. For example, nearly 30 percent of immigrants to Washington state came from Vietnam and the Philippines. Immigrants from Cuba settled in Florida, whereas immigrants from other Caribbean countries such as Puerto Rico, Jamaica, the Dominican Republic, and Haiti settled in the mid-Atlantic states of New York, New Jersey, and Pennsylvania. The projections are that by the year 2020, the population of the United States will be more than 35 percent racial and ethnic "minorities," and by 2050 what is now the "majority" will be the "minority" (U.S. Bureau of the Census, 1999).

It is important not to simplify the diversity of residents in this country by looking solely at the broad categories used in the Census. Each of the groups identified by the Census has tremendous heterogeneity. To say that 0.8 percent of the population is Native American ignores the fact that each of the more than 500 tribal groups in the country has its own beliefs and values. Although most tribal groups are declining in number, there are twenty-three tribes with 10,000 or more members living throughout the United States (U.S. Bureau of the Census, 1999). The largest tribal groups in the United States are the Cherokee and the Navajo, followed by the Chippewa and Sioux. There are Native Americans in every state, either living on reservations or in urban and rural communities. To classify Asians as one group is also to

TABLE 8.1	Resident Population of the United States by Race, 1990 and 1998		
		1990	**1998**
All races		248,765,000	270,299,000
American Indian, Eskimo, Aleut		2,065,000	2,360,000
Asian/Pacific Islander		7,462,000	10,507,000
Black		30,511,000	34,431,000
Hispanic origin		22,122,000	29,707,000
White		208,727,000	223,001,000

Source: U.S. Bureau of the Census. Current population reports, 1125–1130. In U.S. Bureau of the Census, *Statistical Abstract of the United States No. 20 and 21.*

ignore the diversity among those classified as Asian, which includes persons from Afghanistan, Cambodia, China, Hong Kong, Japan, Laos, Philippines, Thailand, and Vietnam, to name a few. The same can be said for the various cultures included under the classification of Hispanic or Latino, which includes people from Mexico, Puerto Rico, Cuba, Jamaica, Haiti, Columbia, Venezuela, and the many other countries of Central and South America and the Caribbean. Each country has its own culture and its own language or dialect. Although most Hispanic or Latin countries speak Spanish as their primary language, the primary language of Brazil is Portuguese. Any understanding of cultural diversity in American must include the full scope of diversity, with its many cultures and many languages beyond those classified by the Census data.

As a result of its traditional history and new immigration, the nation has become culturally diverse. Currently, one in ten U.S. citizens was born in a country other than the United States. Immigrants from various parts of the world bring with them cultural values that are often different from the cultural foundation of the original European settlers who forged what came to be understood as American culture. The country includes a diversity of cultures, beliefs, and values that shape the language and the language development of young children. Each culture has its own traditions and history, length of residence in the United States, immigration patterns to and from the country, and migration patterns within the country. Other factors, such as socioeconomic status, formal education, and degree of language proficiency in the home language as well as in English, add to the complexity of culture in America (Langdon, 1996).

As a second result of the increases in immigration, the linguistic diversity of children in the schools has increased dramatically. Many children in the public schools speak little or no English or use a language other than English at home. This presents a tremendous challenge for those charged with their education. In 1996, 5.1 percent of children aged five to seventeen spoke English less than very well. According to the U.S. Bureau of the Census, in 1995 there were 36.5 million children aged five to seventeen who spoke a language other than English at home. Although Spanish is by far the most commonly used language besides English (Spanish is used by 17,339,172 children), other languages used at home include French, German, Italian, Chinese, and Tagalog, each of which is used by more than 1 million children. Other languages used at home vary with the population, with some school districts reporting as many as 100 different languages being used by children and their families.

Language Disorders and Diversity

The American Speech-Language-Hearing Association (ASHA, 1991) and the National Institution for Deafness and Other Communication Disorders (1991) estimate that between 10 and 15 percent of the U.S. population has a speech-language or hearing disorder. The prevalence of speech-language disorders among culturally and linguistically diverse populations is difficult to determine. Using current population figures and estimates of prevalence, it would be expected that 27 million persons in the country have a communication disorder. This would indicate that nearly 7.56 million persons from culturally and linguistically diverse groups have a disorder of speech, language, or hearing, including 6 million children under the age of 18 years. These estimates are low because there is believed to be a greater risk for disorders among persons from socially and economically disadvantaged groups, including low-income persons from diverse populations. Socially and economically disadvantaged groups, including recent immigrants, are more likely to have disorders related to trauma, poor prenatal care, poor health care, poor access to preventive care, high lead levels, drug and alcohol abuse, and a higher incidence of medical conditions associated with stroke, such as high blood pressure.

To understand the factors associated with language and language disorders in culturally and linguistically diverse populations, it is necessary to understand (1) the relationship between culture and language, (2) the meaning of language dialects, (3) the nature of language development in monolingual and bilingual populations, (4) the issues related to the identification of language disorders, and (5) appropriate interventions to foster language development.

LANGUAGE AND CULTURE

The values, beliefs, attitudes, folkways, behavioral styles, and traditions of a people define culture. Culture encompasses a set of behaviors, institutions, and worldviews passed on and maintained by an identifiable group, and linked to form an integrated whole that functions to identify a society (Terrell & Terrell, 1993). Language is the primary mode of communication used by members of a cultural group to express their fundamental thoughts, principles, and attitudes. It is developed within a cultural group and is defined by the rules governing language form, content, and use. It is the fabric that serves to both bind and unify members of a society and to separate the group from others. Language helps to shape a culture, and a culture is shaped by its language. Cultural values influencing speech-language behavior include ethnic origin, race, place of birth, immigration pattern, age, gender, socioeconomic status, educational level, language or dialects spoken, religious beliefs, health-care practices and beliefs, and family and community networks.

Culture, Family, and Language

The family is a major variable in the culture of a people. The structure of the family, the roles of individual members within the family, and the expectations of the members of the family are important variables in the development of language. Children acquire language in the context of the family. The language system used by the family is passed to the child.

The structure of the family and the roles of individual members in the family in the development of language vary across cultural groups (Anderson & Battle, 1998). Many families are structured as nuclear families. Nuclear families are usually defined as parents and their children. The increase in the number of single-parent homes and blended families, in which the child has both parents and step-parents, siblings and step-siblings, has changed the perception of the nuclear family and the roles that individual family members play in language development. In traditional nuclear families, the parents are the primary caretakers participating in providing a language environment for the child.

Other families are known as extended families. Extended families include parents, children, and other relatives or close friends living in the same household or very nearby and who play a role in the development and rearing of the child. In extended families, the persons responsible for the development of language may be other persons in addition to the parents, such as grandparents, aunts, or older siblings

Children learn language as a social function within the context of the family. Each culture has its own communication rules and accepted ways of communicating within the group and with others who are not part of the group. Children learn the importance of language in their culture as a medium for interacting with others and for transmitting information to others. Cultural information is transmitted to the child through daily interaction with primary caretakers and significant others in a variety of situations. These daily interactions, including preferred language patterns and modes of interaction, influence the number and type of communication functions that the child will develop.

In some white middle-class homes, mothers or primary caretakers structure their children's language learning environment. The children are encouraged to engage in two-way conversations and exchanges with other individuals, especially the primary caretaker. The interchange begins in infancy during daily caretaking routines and continues throughout childhood. Caretakers see the teaching of language as one of their primary responsibilities. In other cultures and socioeconomic groups, however, children are often passive observers of the conversations of others. They are indirect participants in conversations and are encouraged to speak only when spoken to. Children learn through observation or gradual participation in adult tasks rather than involvement in child-centered activities (Heath, 1983b; Owens, 1992; Kayser, 1998; Harris, 1998).

It is difficult to make specific comparisons of the role of the family in language development by cultural group because of the pattern of intercultural and interethnic marriage, by which there may be various cultural backgrounds within a single family. The 1998 Census tallied more than 1.3 million racially mixed marriages in the United States. Intergroup marriages in 1998 included white/black (9 percent), White/Native American (12 percent), White/Asian (19 percent), and White/Hispanic (52 percent). The number of interethnic marriages is also increasing, such that nearly one in six Asian Americans is married to an Asian of a different ethnic background, such as Chinese/Japanese. Interethnic and interracial marriages are shaping what had been understood as descriptors of the values of families by cultural group (U.S. Bureau of the Census, 1999).

As stated by Schieffelin and Ochs (1986), "little is known about how caretakers and children speak and act toward one another and how that is linked to cultural patterns that extend and have consequences beyond specific interactions observed" (p. 116). According to recent work by Hammer & Weiss (2000), African American mothers from low and middle socioeconomic groups believed that children learn to talk by experiencing (watching, listening, imitating, and participating in communicative interactions). The mothers varied, however, in the extent to which they expected their children to participate in the interactions in order to learn how to communicate. Hammer and Weiss also found that, in general, the views of the African American mothers did not differ from the views of white middle-class mothers with respect to their role in their child's language development. They support the view of Crago (1992) that particular language socializing practices "are not the unique holding of any one culture" (p. 30). What can be said is that in most cultures, children learn language and cultural rules by watching the interactions among family members, receiving verbal stimulation from the members of the extended family through story telling, rhyming, poetry, and the encouragement of communication from early ages (Lynch & Hanson, 1993). Some, but not all, families' cultural and linguistic behaviors are transmitted by the primary caretaker in two-way conversations in which the child is encouraged to be an active participant. The child is expected to engage in social communication, and the role of the caretakers is to encourage and facilitate that engagement. In some families, children learn language through the efforts of extended family caretakers and language is learned through nonverbal instructions rather than direct conversations (Owens, 1992; Kayser, 1998). Children are not expected to engage in social conversation with parents, but rather are expected to observe or engage in conversation with age peers until they are competent to engage in interactions with adults. However, differences that may have been observed in the past seem to have been eradicated by increased contact between the cultural groups and exposure to effective child-rearing practices through the media. In addition, previously perceived differences related to race may not be as strong as those related to socioeconomic status (Hammer & Weiss, 2000).

Hall, Nagy, and Linn (1984) audiotaped middle-class and working-class parents talking to their preschool children. The middle-class parents used nearly 30 percent more words while talking to their children than the working-class parents. The middle-class children used more words per hour in their conversations than did the working-class children. Hart and Risley (1995), who compared the language experiences of infants and toddlers in professional, working-class, and welfare families, obtained similar results. The children from working-class and professional homes had significantly more language experiences than the children from welfare families. In addition, the types of language and feedback to the children were different across the socioeconomic groups. When the socioeconomic factors are added to the variation in cultures within and between families, the exact role of language development in an individual family must be examined or considered on an individual basis.

LANGUAGE DEVELOPMENT, DIALECTS, AND LANGUAGE DISORDERS

Dialects and Languages

A **dialect** is a variety of a language that is shared by a particular speech community for the purposes of interaction (Taylor, 1986). A dialect is a rule-governed variation in a language used by a racial, ethnic, geographic, or socioeconomic group. Although dialects of a language are generally intelligible to individuals outside the speech community, they reflect variations in almost every aspect of language, including phonology, semantics, syntax, and pragmatics. Dialects reflect basic behavioral difference between groups within a society and are a cultural manifestation of the group. Dialects of the same language may differ in form, pronunciation, vocabulary, and/or grammar from each other; however, they are enough alike to be mutually understood by speakers of different dialects of the same language.

Linguists consider any variety of language a dialect, including those that are considered "standard." The dialects of American English are commonly identified as Standard American English (SAE), African American English (AAE), Appalachian English, Southern White English, and numerous other regional dialects. They are spoken by groups of people who came together by geography and/or social history and serve as primary identifiers of the particular group. Because of the relationship between social history and the development of a dialect, certain dialects carry with them social stigma. African American dialects, for example, are often associated with persons of lower social class because of the history of slavery in this country. Spanish dialects are often associated with poverty and illegal immigration because of the large number of undocumented immigrants from Central and South America. However, New England dialects, especially Boston dialects, are considered prestigious because of their association with European culture, literature, and education (Taylor, 1999).

The dialects of Spanish are spoken by persons with historical roots in as many as twenty different countries. The vocabulary and pronunciations of certain words may vary, but the underlying principles of the language allow the dialects to be understood by most Spanish speakers. They are considered to be mutually intelligible. For example, although there may be vocabulary and pronunciation differences between the dialect of Spanish spoken in Cuba and the dialect spoken in Mexico, the people in these countries are able to communicate with each other and be understood while each uses his own dialect.

Some dialects of a language are not understood by speakers of the same language. They are considered mutually unintelligible. For example, there are 87 mutually unintelligible languages and dialects spoken in the 7,107 islands that make up the Philippines. Asian Indians in the United States mostly speak a dialect of Hindu or Kananadi (Cheng, 1995). Arabic, the sixth most common language spoken in the world and the primary language in eighteen countries of the Middle East, has so many dialects that are so different as to preclude communication unless Standard Arabic is used. The 500 Native American tribal entities in the United States speak as many as 200 distinct languages and dialects, some of which are mutually intelligible, but most of which are mutually unintelligible to other Native American speakers (Harris, 1998).

Most speakers of a dialect are able to speak the standard language, such as Standard English. They may chose to use the dialect to identify themselves as a member of a cultural group, but are able to switch to the use of the standard depending on the context, the message, or the communication partner. This is known as **code switching.** For example, children who use African American dialect have been shown to use fewer features of the dialect when talking to their teachers than when talking to their age peers. They have been shown to use fewer features of the dialect when retelling a story than when reporting an event (Wyatt, 1991). It is important to recognize the use of a dialect as a social, linguistic, and cultural bond between people and not to form a judgment of the value of the people or their ability to use language based on their use of a dialect. This is particularly important in making judgments about the language proficiency of children who use language dialects.

Dialects and Language Disorders

The American Speech-Language-Hearing Association (ASHA, 1993) defines a language disorder as "impaired comprehension and/or use of spoken, written, and/or other symbol systems. The disorder may involve (1) the form of language (phonology, morphology, or syntax), (2) the content of language (semantics), and/or (3) the function of language in communication (pragmatics in any combination)." Since language is embedded in culture, any definition of a language disorder must be defined by the parameters established by the community of which the child is a member. As culturally defined, a language disorder is impaired comprehension and/or use of a spoken, written, and/or other symbol system used by the child's indigenous culture and language group (Taylor, 1986).

According to the 1983 ASHA Position Paper on Social Dialects, "No dialectal variety of English (or any other language) is a disorder or pathological form of speech or language. Each social dialect is adequate as a functional and effective variety of English. Each serves a communication function as well as a social solidarity function. It maintains the communication network and the social construct of the community of speakers who use it" (pp. 23–24).

The identification of language disorders among children who are in the process of developing language is difficult. Distinctions have to be made between what is expected of the child at a particular age. When considering a child from a culturally and linguistically different background, the task is more challenging. Distinction must be made between what is expected of the child in his language, in his culture, and at his stage of language development. Much is known about the development of language by children developing Standard American English (Brown, 1973; Bloom & Lahey, 1978). Less is known about the development of language by children learning African American English, Spanish-influenced English, or English being developed by children who speak other languages.

Language Development, Dialects, and Disorders in AAE Children

African American English (AAE) is the dialect of English spoken by many, but not all, persons in working-class African American families. It reflects the complex social history of persons of African heritage in the United States and patterns of migration from the rural South to the urban North (Dillard, 1972). Because of its historical roots, the use of African American English carries a negative social stigma to persons in economic power in the country. Many attempts have been made to eradicate or eliminate the use of the dialect by school children, spurred by the feeling that its use will delay the development of literacy in Standard American English. However, members of the African American community continue to use the dialect in certain social situations, particularly when they are among their social and cultural peers.

Most are able to code switch to the use of Standard American English forms when educational, social, and economic mobility are required.

The major contrasts between Standard American English and African American English occur in phonology, morphology, syntax, and in the pragmatic and nonlinguistic features of language.

Development of Phonology in AAE Speakers

All of the phonetic sounds of English are used by speakers of AAE. The early development of phonology in infants and toddlers from homes where SAE and AAE is used is similar. At 36 months, the conversational speech of children exposed to African American English includes the same sounds as those used by speakers of Standard American English (e.g., /n/, /m/, /b/, /d/, /t/, /g/, /k/, /f/, /h/, and /w/) (Seymour & Ralabate, 1985; Seymour & Seymour, 1981; Steffersen, 1974; Stockman, 1998).

Some differences in the use of sounds occur among those sounds that develop after age 5 years. Differences occur in the use of /f/ for /è/ in words such as *thumb*, and the use of /b/ for /v/ in words such as *valentine*. Although there are other differences that become evident among later-developing phonological forms, the consonants that distinguish between AAE and SAE are not usually evident until after the age of 5 years. According to Bleile and Wallach (1992), the features that do not contrast between AAE and SAE are useful in distinguishing between AAE that is developing normally and that which may be delayed. These features include the following: the use of more than one or two stop errors (e.g., /p/, /t/, /k/, /g/); initial-word position errors; errors in /r/ or /l/ in children over the age of 4 years; more than a few cluster errors (e.g., /t/ for /st/); and fricative errors other than /è/ (e.g., /f/).

Development of Semantics and Pragmatics in AAE Speakers

Infants and toddlers in homes where AAE is spoken develop communication intent and semantic meanings in the same manner as has been described for children in homes where SAE is spoken (see Chapter 1) (Bridgeforth, 1984; Stockman, 1998; Davis, Williams, & Vaughn-Cooke, 1992–1993; Vaughn-Cooke & Wright-Harp, 1992). The number of language functions used increases with age through the preschool years. Young children from homes where AAE is spoken imitate, ask questions, express their needs both verbally and nonverbally, answer questions, and are interested in both telling and listening to stories in the same manner as children in other homes (Stockman, 1996).

The development of oral language skills and literacy are important in both African American and European American children. Differences in narrative production are a by-product of sociocultural differences, individual differences and preferences, and individual experiences. Consequently, cultural expectations and patterns influence the manner in which narrative style and literacy are developed. The expectations for the involvement of the children may be different in different families, depending on the culture and the family members' understanding of their role in the development of language. For example, in some working-class homes, storybooks and other forms of children's literature are not prominent. Although stories are often told, comprehension is not negotiated through questions and expectation of feedback. In some families, the children may be expected to engage in conversations with peers and give recounts of the day. However, recall and discussion of past experiences may be rare among children in other families. For example, talking about events of the day begins early in Asian and European American families, but is less likely to occur in Hispanic and African American families. The differences observed and frequently reported across cultural groups may be more related to social class and the education and expectations of family members than racial or ethnic identity.

There has been much discussion about the differences in narrative styles across cultural groups. For example, the narratives of some Japanese speakers are considered succinct and unelaborated. The narratives of children from Latin or Hispanic families do not appear to pay attention to sequencing of events. The narratives of working-class African American speakers are characterized by accounts that allow the speaker to share information with the listener. The children use more descriptions and have a complex organization and structure (Champion, Seymour, & Camarata, 1995). Speakers from European American families frequently use descriptions or explanation of events and past experiences (Heath, 1986). Selection of narrative style reflects cultural values as well as individual preferences, task demands, and linguistic experiences (Hester, 1996). It is important to distinguish between a narrative that reflects a speaker's cultural style and personal preferences and one that reflects disordered communication (McCabe, 1995).

Preferences for narrative style and for organization of discourse had been thought to be related to cultural and racial differences. There are generally two types of narrative styles, topic associative and topic centered. In **topic-associative style** the narrative moves from one topic to another linked by covert semantic or thematic associations related to the main topic. Frequent shifts in temporal, locative, and character references, and multiple experiences, are told in one story (Gee, 1989; Hyon & Sulzby, 1992). In **topic-centered narratives,** component events are linked in explicit chronological or sequential order. There is consistent use of temporal, locational, and character references; beginnings and ends are clearly marked (Hyon & Sulzby, 1992; Michaels, 1998). The narrative styles are evident in both oral language and in writing in school children.

Early research in the cultural differences in the use of narratives indicated that speakers of SAE were more likely to use topic-centered narratives and that speakers of AAE used the topic-associative style (Campbell, 1994; Gutierrez-Clellan & Quinn, 1993). More recent research has shown that children who use AAE use both topic-centered and topic-associative narrative styles, depending on the communicative context. Hester (1996) found that children switch narrative styles according to the discourse task, such as a conversation, story retelling, and fictional story telling. The narratives produced by African American children from low-income families aged 6 to 10 years have a complex organization and structure (Champion et al., 1995). It is therefore necessary to distinguish between narratives that reflect a speaker's cultural style or preference in a given communication event from those that reflect disordered communication.

Narrative ability depends on the cultural background and experiences of speakers and listeners. Differences in cultural background may influence the interpretation of the narrative produced by the child. Differences in narrative style between the speaker and the listener may result in communication breakdown. When listening to a child who uses a topic-associative style, the listener may interrupt with questions and comments to seek clarification. The interruptions may result in a communication breakdown and frustrate the child's further attempts to communicate (Bliss, Covington, & McCabe, 1999).

Development of Morphology in AAE speakers

The morphological development of children who speak AAE is similar to that of children who use SAE up to the age of 3 years (Blake, 1984; Stockman, 1986). By the age of 18 months, children in homes where AAE is used make one- and two-word utterances similar to those of children from homes where SAE is used (Steffersen, 1974; Stockman & Vaughn-Cooke, 1992; Blake, 1984). The morphological features of plural -s, possessive -s, past-tense -ed, and third-person singular -s are acquired in the same pattern as in children using SAE. (See Chapter 1 for information on normal language development.) Similarly, the features marking tense, mood, aspect markers of the verb phrase, and negation develop in the later preschool years. At the age of 3 years, children from homes where AAE is used produce well-formed, multiword constructions, simple declaratives, questions, and a few complex sentences. As the children develop through the preschool years, a variety of complex sentences including coordinated, subordinate, and relative clause sentences are used (Craig & Washington, 1994, 1995). Thus, in the preschool years, the morphological development of children in homes where AAE is used is similar to that of children in homes where SAE is used.

The features that differ between AAE and SAE involve the later-developing morphological forms. Forms used by speakers of AAE after the age of 5 years include the use of *at* in questions (e.g., "Where my shoes at?"); *go* as a copula (e.g., "There go my shoes."); deletion of *be* (e.g., "He working."). The use of other forms such as habitual *be* (e.g., "She be working."), and the use of *what* in embedded clauses (e.g., "He the one what ate it.") also develop later in the preschool years.

Speakers who use African American English do not use all of the features of the dialect in all contexts. Some children use only a few features, whereas others use more. The patterns of variability for particular features have important implications for understanding the use of AAE. For example, a child may omit the copula in some contexts ("He a boy."), but use it in others ("John is a boy."). Wyatt (1995) reported that school-age children used more features of the dialect when talking to their age peers and when excited about the topic than when retelling a story or talking to their teacher. Failure to use the copula or any form when it is expected in both SAE and AAE may be an indicator of a communication disorder. It is important to consider the content and the context of the communication event to distinguish between morphology that is developing normally and that which may be disordered.

Language Disorders in Speakers of AAE

The linguistic features of AAE can appear to be identical to symptoms that are found in children with language disorders. Differences in phonology and morphology as described above between AAE and SAE can be identified as a disorder when used by a child who does not use AAE. They can be identified as normal features of AAE when the child is actually exposed to AAE at home. For example, an eight-year-old child who uses /f/ for /è/ may be thought to be using AAE when his home language is actually SAE. He might be considered to be developing normally, although he actually has a disorder (Seymour, Bland-Stewart, & Green, 1998). The same can be said for a child who appears to omit copula verb forms as used in AAE. The omission of the copula is frequently cited as a feature of AAE. However, research has shown that the omission of the copula by AAE speakers decreases between the ages of 5 and 7 years, and its use in younger children is dependent on the linguistic context (Wyatt, 1991). An older speaker of AAE who omits the copula may be considered to be developing normally when in actuality he may have a disorder. These differences can extend to pragmatics and semantic areas as well.

Differentiating between normal language development, the development of linguistic features of a dialect, and a language disorder requires considerable expertise. It may be more beneficial to focus on the features that are shared between SAE and AAE than to make distinctions between them in determining the presence of a disorder. Regardless of the use of a dialect, children with language disorders use fewer prepositions, articles, conjunctions, locatives *(here, there)*, complex sentences, and modals *(want, will, could, can)* than do children without disorders. However, there do not appear to be significant differences between SAE and AAE in the use of pronouns, present progressive verbs *(-ing)*, or demonstratives *(this, that, these, those)*. Determination of a language disorder in children who are thought to use AAE should focus on those forms that are shared between the two dialects, rather than on those that are different (Seymour, Bland-Stewart, & Green, 1998).

Language Development and Disorders in Hispanic/Latino Children

Development of Phonology

Spanish phonology has 18 consonants, 4 semivowels, and 5 vowels, compared to 24 consonants, 3 semivowels, and 12 to 14 vowels in SAE. There are thus several English consonants that are not present in Spanish, including /v/, /w/, and /sh/. There are consonants in Spanish that are not present in English, such as the trilled /r/, the flap /rr/, and /ñ/. In addition, some Spanish consonants are not aspirated, giving the perception of a near-voiced sound for an unvoiced sound, such as *baber* for *paper* or *pad* for *pat*. In spite of the differences in the sounds of the language, the course of normal development of phonology in children learning Spanish parallels that of children learning English. Most researchers agree that by the age of 4–4.5 years children learning Spanish have mastered all consonant sounds except the liquids /j/, /l/, /ch/, /s/, /rr/, and sometimes /ñ/. By the age of 6 years, all of the later-developing sounds are learned (Acevedo, 1989; Eblen, 1982; Linares, 1982; Jimenez, 1987). According to Ambert (1986) and Hodson, Becker, Diamond, and Meza (1989), unintelligible 4-year-old children who use Spanish make the same types of errors in Spanish as unintelligible 4-year-old children using English, namely, omitting, distorting, reversing the order of sounds in words, and shortening the length of words (i.e., *nana* for *banana*), and making sound errors primarily involving /s/, /r/, /l/, and /rr/. They also show reduction of consonant sequences (e.g., *epexo* for *espejo*), liquid deviation (e.g., *ádbol* for *árbol*), and stridency deletion (e.g., *lápi* for *lápiz*). These patterns are similar to those reported by Bleile and Wallach (1992) for children who use AAE.

Morphological Development and Disorders in Spanish Speakers

The development of Spanish morphology has been studied by several researchers (Merino, 1982, 1992; Gudemar, 1981; Echeverria, 1975; Keller, 1976). Although they used different methods of investigation and different criteria for acceptance of the form being acquired, the age of acquisition of the various morphological forms differed by one or two years at the most. The studies indicated that children learning to use Spanish morphology acquire morphological forms at ages similar to those of children learning English. Similar to children learning English, children learning Spanish learn specific morphological forms in Spanish earlier than others. Present progressive verb form (*-ing*), plural (*-s*), and past-tense verbs (*-ed*) are mastered before passives, subjunctives, and indirect objects. Children learning Spanish learn plural forms and first- and second-person pronouns before the age of 2.5 years. Before the age of 3 years, they have learned present progressive, present indicative, simple preterit, present indicative, direct imperative, singular object nouns, third-person subject pronouns, and plural clitic pronouns. Before entry to school they have mastered complex forms involving tense and mood, similar to children learning English. Because of several differences between Spanish and English, it is challenging to make comparisons between all aspects of morphological development. For example, gender of nouns and noun adjectives is marked in Spanish, but not in English (e.g., "un niño cortés" versus "una niña cortés"—a polite boy versus a polite girl). Children learning English do not have to learn the gender of nouns except when a pronoun is used (e.g., *She* is used for ships and *it* is used for other gender-neutral nouns).

There are several differences in the development of Spanish morphology that affect the perception of a language disorder. The differences occur in noun and gender agreement, and in linguistic complexity. The use of articles in Spanish is different from that in English. Spanish speakers must use the correct gender of the article for the noun that is to be expressed. For example, in English the article *the* is used to modify all nouns. In Spanish, the language learner must distinguish between masculine nouns and feminine nouns so that the proper article can be used. For example, in the phrase, "the red car," the child must learn that *car* is masculine and therefore takes a masculine article: "el carro rojo." If the noun is plural, the child must mark the plural on the article, the adjective, and the noun (e.g., "los carros rojos"). Children learning Spanish have difficulty with gender and number agreement as late as 6 years of age (Garcia, Maez, & Gonzalez, 1984).

Because of the morphological contrasts between Standard American English and Spanish, children learning English as a second language may be perceived as having a language disorder. As seen in Table 8.2, differences in the order of morphological markers may be mistaken for language disorder. The differences involve, for example, the placement of noun modifiers, absence of plural noun markers, and placement of negation markers. These difficulties become even greater challenges when the child is learning English as a second language.

TABLE 8.2	Morphological Contrasts between Standard American English (SAE) and Spanish-English	
	Spanish-English	**SAE**
Possession	"hat of my brother"	"my brother's hat"
Plural	"The boy are here."	"The boys are here."
Regular past	"I walk yesterday."	"I walked yesterday."
Third-person regular	"He run fast."	"He runs fast."
Negation	"He no eat."	"He does not eat."
Question inversion	"Carlos is coming?"	"Is Carlos coming?"

Second Language Acquisition: Bilingualism or Multilingualism

The term *bilingual* or *multilingual* is defined by the level of competence a speaker has in two or more languages. A bilingual or multilingual speaker is one who has native or near-native language proficiency in two or more different languages. When a child is in an environment where two languages are used, the child is expected to develop two linguistic systems. While the child is in the process of developing language, the two systems interact with each other and affect the acquisition of each language. The age of exposure to the languages affects the way the child will develop the languages.

Baetens-Bearsmore (1986) identified two types of bilinguals: natural bilinguals and academic bilinguals. A natural bilingual is one who has learned the second language without any formal training. An academic bilingual is one who learns the second or third language through formal instruction, such as in an academic program. Natural bilinguals may be either simultaneous or successive second language learners. The acquisition of two or more languages can occur either simultaneously or in succession. Simultaneous bilingualism occurs when a child is exposed to two or more languages from the onset of the development of language, usually before the age of 3 years. Children learning two or more languages at the same time acquire both languages at the same rate, usually at the normally expected rate (Dulay, Hernandez-Chavez, & Burt, 1978; Doyle, Champagne, & Segalowitz, 1978). Although there may be some initial interference with syntactic organization, choice of lexical forms, or phonology, simultaneous bilingual learners are able to use both languages with equal proficiency (Ambert, 1986). They are able to code-switch (switch between the languages) depending on the language of their communication partner or the situation. Code switching may also occur when a concept is more accurately expressed in one language than the other.

Successive or sequential bilingualism occurs when a child learns the second language after the acquisition of the first language. The forms learned in the second language are learned in an order similar to the forms learned in the first language. There is usually interference of the first language when the new language is being learned.

Common influences include omission and overextension of morphological markers, double marking, and changes in the ordering of words or sentence components. In addition to the interference of one language with the other, the development and use of a second language may result in the loss of the first language or a slowing of development of the second language, particularly when the first language is not used at home. This may give the perception of language disorder or delay, since the child may not be using either language at the level expected. Clinicians may believe that the child has a disorder of delay because the first language is not well developed. It is thus very important to understand fully the history of the child with both languages in order to distinguish whether the difference from the expected in either language is a result of the normal course of bilingual language development.

Bilingual children become proficient in the language that they use the most. Children may become more proficient in the second language as they progress through the school years. Since much of academic education and new concepts are presented in the second language the child may develop advanced proficiency in the second language while either not using the first language or using it only for social rather than academic purposes. Vocabulary, morphology, and syntax may become more advanced in the language used in the school than in the language used at home for social communication. This is particularly the case when the child decides not to use the home language at all in order to advance more rapidly in the language of the school. Any testing in the home language in these cases may not provide an accurate assessment of the child's true language ability.

Bilingualism and Language Disorders

When a child uses the school language as his primary language, development of proficiency in the first language, which may be the language of the home, may be slowed or stopped. The child may be misidentified as having a disorder in the first language because the first language has not continued to develop because of nonuse or use for only social purposes. The child may be perceived as having a disorder in both the first and the second languages. The first language may not have developed beyond the basic communication skills and may not be at the level expected for chronological age. The child may not have developed the language proficiency in the second language to be able to use the language for complex academic tasks. As children enter school and are expected to use language for literacy such as reading and writing, it is critical that they have a firm foundation in the ability to use complex language skills in a language. This is usually the language of the home.

Language proficiency for academic tasks must consider the cognitive level of the material being presented and the amount of contextual support available to the child to assist in understanding the material or activity (Cummins, 1984). Contextual support may be in the form of pictures and interactive, multimodal exposure to presentations to assist the child in putting the material into a frame of reference. A child learning a second language may require two to three years to achieve social proficiency in basic interpersonal communicative skills (BICS) in the second language. This includes learning the vocabulary, morphology, and syntax, and pragmatic rules necessary to express his ideas and thoughts and to understand the ideas and thoughts of others, to share information. It may take five to seven years to develop the language skills necessary for the cognitive tasks expected in the academic environment. Cognitive academic language proficiency (CALP) requires the child to use language to analyze, synthesize, and evaluate information in the academic curriculum in oral communication and in reading and writing. In the lower grades, textbooks and classroom activity provide support through extensive use of pictures and hands-on activities. As the child advances in the academic program, the amount of contextualized support is reduced. In upper grades the textbooks may not include pictures to support the text material. The material may refer to events in the past that are not subject to observation or hands-on activities. The child may be expected to be able to generate the concept from verbally presented material in written format. Students may have the basic communication skills necessary for conversation or for understanding highly contextualized material, but they may not have the cognitive academic language skills to perform more complex abstract academic tasks expected in upper elementary and middle school grades. This may contribute to the very high failure rate of Hispanic youth in middle and secondary school (Langdon & Cheng, 1992).

The development of complex language skills in the first language is necessary while the child learns the basic forms in the second language. Failure to provide early academic instruction in reading and writing in the first language may result in language deficits throughout the academic program.

Mercer (1987) and Damico, Oller, and Storey (1983) have suggested that certain indicators of learning disabilities may also be characteristics of students in the process of learning a second language. The indicators are given as the following:

- A discrepancy between verbal and nonverbal performance measures on intelligence tests
- Academic learning difficulty, particularly with the abstract concepts required in upper elementary and secondary grades
- Inability to perceive and organize and remember information when such information is based on different experiences, different cultural values, or different linguistic backgrounds
- Social and emotional difficulties related to difficulty in ability to communicate or to problems related to adjustment to a new culture and cultural expectations in a new academic environment
- The appearance of attention-deficit problems because of difficulty comprehending information presented
- Delays in responding to questions, or silence or not responding, may be the result of difficulty understanding the second language rather than a word-finding or expression problem.

Nonlinguistic behaviors of second language learners or children from different cultures may also contribute to the identification of language disorders. Eye-contact behavior is culturally determined. Use of averted or indirect eye contact, while expected in some cultures, may give the appearance that the child is not paying attention in others. In some cultures it is considered disrespectful for a child or person in a subordinate position to establish or maintain eye contact with a superior or elder.

In other cultures a more sustained direct eye contact may be perceived as defiance or disrespect. For example, looking a person in the eyes while talking or listening is considered to be very aggressive in Japan, where it is appropriate to look at a person's cheek, not at the eyes while in conversation.

Second language–second culture children are sometimes perceived as being disorganized, lacking responsibility, arriving late or not using time wisely, or having difficulty changing activities. These behaviors can often be explained by cultural differences in the perception of time across cultures, difficulty adapting to a new culture, or failure to understand the directions, especially those given indirectly or using advanced syntactic structures.

A child learning a second language is often also learning a second culture. This is even more important if the child arrives in the new culture at an age when she is expected to enter the academic environment. Both the neighborhood culture and the school culture may be different from the environment of her first culture. In addition to learning the new language, the child must learn new rules for communicating, interacting, and learning in the new culture. The adjustment to the new culture may be further complicated by frequent trips back to the home country, when the child must shift again to the home culture and then shift back to the new culture, often in yet another new neighborhood and a new school. This may also lead to a perception of slower language development or a disorder. It thus becomes critical to obtain a full history of the child's opportunity to learn the new language before a diagnosis of language disorder can be made.

There are sociocultural factors that must be considered when determining that a second language learner has a language disorder or learning disability. Children in a new and different language environment frequently do not respond when spoken to or prefer to be alone. The child may be hesitant to speak with less than adequate language skills. When learning a second language and placed in a strange learning environment, the child may go through a silent period of three to six months during which he listens to the language and observes the behavior of others. This may be particularly true of children from cultures where they are encouraged to observe until they are competent to participate. Care must be taken to understand the social history, the cultural history, and the language history of the child, so that all factors affecting language development can be considered.

When the child is determined to have a language disorder, the clinical decisions for intervention are challenging. Most questions revolve around decisions about the appropriate language of instruction for a child whose primary language is not English. Should instruction be in the language of the home or in the language of the school? Current literature stresses the need to develop a firm language base in the child's first language before teaching a second language (Hamayan, 1992; Wong-Fillmore, 1991a, 1991b). Teaching the language of the home allows the family to continue to be involved in the development of language. Once the language base is established in the first language, the child will more readily learn the second language. If the second language is begun before a firm base in language is established, the child may forever be delayed in the ability to develop the higher-level cognitive skills required for academic work and literacy.

ASSESSMENT OF LANGUAGE IN CULTURALLY AND LINGUISTICALLY DIVERSE CHILDREN

Norm-Referenced Assessment

Because language is a sociocultural phenomenon, the assessment of language abilities must occur in a sociocultural context. The language skills of children from culturally and linguistically diverse backgrounds are often assessed using tests and procedures that are not culturally relevant to their needs. There are few tests of language abilities that are not inherently biased against culturally and linguistically diverse backgrounds. Test taking itself is a cultural phenomenon, thus by its very nature is biased against children who do not have family backgrounds that frequently ask the child to perform or respond to an item out of context. For example, if a child does not have experience naming pictures in books, the child will not do well on a picture-naming task on a test. Likewise, if the child has little experience telling stories or describing pictures, the child will not do well on tests in those formats. These problems in assessment are in addition to the obvious ones of expecting the child to identify pictures, places, and events with which he has had limited experience.

Formal standardized norm-referenced language tests are biased against children from culturally and linguistically diverse backgrounds because they are not included in the normative sample. Although some tests may indicate that the test was standardized on a representative sample of the population of the United States, there is no assurance that the child being tested is "representative" of children in the United States. The child has unique cultural and language experiences different from any other child and cannot be assumed to be represented in the sample in sufficient manner for the data to serve as a comparative baseline of normal behavior for the child. Every formal standardized test score obtained on a child from a culturally and linguistically diverse background must be considered suspect. The question must be asked whether the child had the opportunity to develop the skills being tested.

Weddington (1987) has made suggestions for using standardized tests with culturally and linguistically diverse children. They include alteration in the time limits for the test, rewording instructions, providing practice items, and ignoring ceiling and baseline scores. The primary consideration, before any of these alterations, must consider the appropriateness of the test format, test content, and mode of responding of the test. If these factors are not considered, then no alteration in test administration can render the test valid. When any alteration in the test format is used, the test scores cannot be used in interpretation. If scoring was based on standard administration, any alteration renders the scores invalid and they should not be represented or interpreted as valid indicators of the child's language ability.

Culturally and linguistically diverse children are often assessed using nonverbal assessments (Hamayan & Damico, 1991). Although nonverbal tests do not require verbal ability, there are cultural variables that may affect the child's performance on these tests as well. Nonverbal aspects of assessment including perception and use of time, display learning, competitiveness, and sociolinguistic dimensions such as cross-racial relationships between the child and the adult may also affect the child's ability to perform on nonverbal tests. Vaughn-Cooke (1983) and Musselwhite (1983) present several questions that may be useful in evaluating whether norm-referenced assessment instruments are appropriate for children from culturally and linguistically diverse families.

1. Has the child had the opportunity to become familiar with the underlying assumptions in the format of the test?
2. Is the child represented in the normative sample in a meaningful way?
3. Has the child had experience with the content of the test?
4. Has the child had an opportunity to learn the content of the test?
5. Does the test allow a reliable determination of whether the child is developing normally in the child's own linguistic and cultural community?
6. Can the test distinguish between normal development, dialectal differences, and disorders?
7. Does the test provide an opportunity for the child to express ideas without structural constraints on form?
8. Does the test allow the child to demonstrate understanding of an idea or concept in alternative ways with alternative linguistic formats?
9. Does the format of the test include an opportunity to obtain a sample of the child's spontaneous language?
10. Can the test provide an adequate description of the child's language ability as an integrated whole?

If the answer to any of these questions is "no," the test should not be used as a valid indicator of the child's ability to understand and use language. It should not be used to make educational judgments about the presence of a disorder or the need for special education or related services. If the test is used, the report of the results should carry a disclaimer about the interpretation of the validity of results.

Criterion-Referenced Assessment

Criterion-referenced assessment is usually more appropriate than norm-referenced assessment for determining the presence of a language disorder in culturally and linguistically diverse children. Criterion-referenced assessment allows a description of the child's performance on specific, independently defined criteria rather than comparison against an artificially established and culturally irrelevant group. The assessment results are interpreted by comparison against predetermined criteria rather than against norm-based scores (Scriven, 1991). Criterion-referenced assessment has limitations in defining the specific criteria that should be used; however, it is far superior to norm-referenced testing because it allows for full consideration of the child's cultural and linguistic background.

Criterion-referenced assessment should include a family-centered ethnographic interview and an analysis of the child's speech and communication skills in natural contexts. It involves the triangulation of cultural, linguistic, and experiential factors of communication. It considers the social context in which communication occurs and how language is used in a particular culture to share knowledge and establish order (Crago & Cole, 1991; Cheng, 1990). The family-centered ethnographic interview allows the evaluator to consider the environmental influences on the development of language in the home and the perception of the child's communication competence by the family (Westby, 1990). The family centered interview allows investigation of the child's communication with age peers, siblings, and adult communication partners against the background of the familiar social context. Items addressed in a family-centered ethnographic interview include the following:

1. What language(s) do the parents use in speaking to the child?
2. What language(s) do the parents use in speaking to each other?
3. What language does the child use in speaking to age peers? Adults?
4. How does the child express needs to the primary caretakers at home?
5. Does the child initiate conversations at home? With whom?
6. How does the child interact with the caretakers? With age peers? With siblings?
7. What is the parent's perception of the child's language ability?
8. Do members of the family understand the child?
9. Do other children use language with the child in the same manner that they do with his age peers?
10. Does the child understand language and instructions at home as expected for her age?
11. Does the family communicate to the child with gestures or simplified speech as compared to the child's age peers?
12. Is the child interested in objects and toys at the level expected in his home and by his cultural age peers?

A language sample should be a part of any assessment of language and communication of a child. The sample of normal communication should be collected through observation of the child in multiple contexts and with multiple communication partners. The sample should be collected in environments that are familiar to the child, with objects that are culturally relevant and familiar to the child. Cheng (1991) suggests collecting the language sample using several different tasks, including relating past events, describing objects, describing pictures, retelling culturally familiar stories, asking for assistance, or other tasks that are appropriate for the child's age and level of language development. The sample should be analyzed using criteria established for the phonology, syntax, morphology, and pragmatics of the child's language and dialect. Analysis should consider normal development in the child's language and the child's language history. Because normative data is often not available, the report should be descriptive rather than normative.

The following guidelines can be used to conduct a criterion-referenced ethnographic assessment.

- Interview members of the family to collect information on the child's language skills in the home environment and the family's perception of his or her overall development.
- Observe and describe the child's use of language in conversation with familiar partners, with familiar objects, and in familiar situations.
- Observe the child over time in different contexts with different communication partners.

- Interact with the child, considering the child's frame of reference, life experiences, and familiarity with unfamiliar communication partners.
- Collect narrative samples using books, pictures, toys, and objects that are familiar to the child and that have low cognitive demand.

The following criteria can be used as a guide in determining the existence of a language disorder within the parameters established for the culture and linguistic environment of the child:

- Rarely initiates verbal interactions or activities with peers or family members.
- Does not respond verbally when verbal interactions are initiated by peers or family members.
- Has difficulty using language at the level used by her age peers.
- Has a smaller vocabulary than expected for her age, regardless of the language used.
- Uses shorter, less complex sentences than would be expected by her age.
- Has difficulty communicating verbally with parents or cultural and linguistic age peers.
- Relies heavily on gestures and nonverbal means to communicate.
- Parents and language peers frequently repeat and rephrase instructions for the child.
- Is inordinately slow in responding to questions or instructions.
- Has difficulty with the noncontrastive elements of language form.
- Peers rarely initiate verbal exchanges with the child or use a notably lower level of verbal communication with the child than with age peers.
- Peers have difficulty understanding the child.
- Does not attempt to repair her communication failures.
- Does not comment on the action of others or express feelings verbally.
- Does not take turns or maintain conversations with peers.
- Does not ask for clarification or assistance verbally.
- Uses false starts, self-interruptions, or revisions.
- Makes frequent use of *it, thing, this,* or *that.*
- Does not learn new concepts or vocabulary or forgets material assumed to be learned. (Mattes & Omark, 1991; Kayser, 1990).

Using a combination of a comprehensive review of the child's language history and life experiences, observation of the child using language, interview with the family, and criterion-referenced assessment, the speech-language pathologist can make a judgment about the presence or absence of a speech-language disorder. Once that decision is made, decisions can be made about the need for intervention.

Using Interpreters in Assessment

When the clinical service provider does not have native or near-native proficiency in the language of the child or the family, it is difficult to make judgments about the language proficiency of the child. In these cases the service provider should seek the services of an interpreter to assist in assessment and possible intervention. According to

ASHA (1985), the interpreter must be trained in speech-language development and must be trained to work with families and children. The interpreter should be familiar with the language, dialect, and culture of the child and family, and should be able to assist the service provider in selecting the appropriate assessment techniques and materials considering the culture of the child and family. The interpreter should be not only able to interpret the speech and language of the child and parents, he or she should also be a cultural informant who is able to provide guidance on other cultural phenomena affecting the situation.

The clinician should discuss with the interpreter the items and questions to be used in the assessment, in advance of the session, to determine their cultural appropriateness. The interpreter should be instructed in advance to provide a translation and an interpretation of the meanings and feelings expressed by the client. During the session the interpreter should also be able to alert the clinician to any verbal and nonverbal cues that may be misunderstood and thus affect the interaction. After the session, the interpreter and the service provider should debrief to determine whether there were any verbal or nonverbal issues that were particularly relevant to the session.

LANGUAGE INTERVENTION IN CULTURALLY AND LINGUISTICALLY DIVERSE CHILDREN

Providing appropriate intervention for culturally and linguistically diverse children with language disorders is challenging. Intervention should focus on developing the language that the child will need in the primary environment in which he or she will function. Emphasis should be placed on teaching function and the use of language and semantics before emphasis on form. Stress should be given to helping the child develop a means of communicating from the level where he is and building according to individual need.

In creating a culturally appropriate intervention process, the clinician should establish a collaborative relationship with the family within their cultural boundaries. There are cultural differences in the extent of the families' perception of their role in intervention. Some families expect the clinician to be the teacher and they just observers. Others welcome the opportunity to be fully involved in the intervention program. In developing an intervention plan, it is critical to incorporate those practices that are culturally comfortable for the family. Intervention goals, objectives, and anticipated outcomes should be consistent with the concerns, priorities, and expectations of the family. Intervention materials should be based on experiences and situations that are familiar to the child and family and that will be functional in the child's life. Familiar concepts of family, housing, foods, art, music, dress, religious experiences, and cultural holidays and celebration should be appropriate to the child and family. When the familiar base is established and coded in the language of the child, new experiences can be added to enrich the language used.

The following suggestions are useful in guiding clinical intervention with children with communication disorders from culturally and linguistically diverse populations.

1. View each clinical interaction as a socially situated communicative event that is influenced by the rules of culture and language of both the clinician and the client.
2. Present clear explanations of objectives, goals, and expected outcomes using language, concepts, and cultural values that are appropriate and understood by the family.
3. Adapt materials and experiences to the client's individual needs and the life experiences of the child.
4. Preview materials and strategies to be used to determine whether they are culturally relevant and appropriate.
5. Review the lessons to determine whether the child's inability to acquire the concepts could be explained by cultural or linguistic factors.
6. Incorporate content from the child's culture while helping the child learn new concepts; review and expand familiar structures and concepts with new experiences.
7. Present materials and information using timing, pacing, and manner of communication appropriate for the culture. Expect responses according to those expected in the child's culture and language.
8. Use speech and language appropriate for the child's level of comprehension. Repeat and rephrase instructions to increase the likelihood that the instruction or concept is understood.
9. Use multiple modes to support the language being developed.
10. Use small group sessions of age peers to encourage supportive, cooperative interactions along with individual sessions to teach particular skills and functions.

CONCLUSION

The outcome of more than three decades of research on the acquisition of language and language disorders in culturally and linguistically diverse children has resulted in increased understanding of the complexity of the issue. The more we come to understand about the great diversity among and between children and groups of people, the more we realize what we do not know. While we have learned much about the language development of children from European American middle-class homes, we have yet to understand all we need to know about differential diagnosis of children from other cultures, other socioeconomic groups, those who speak another language or dialect, and those who live in different cultures. As we learn, the diversity in the country continues to increase at remarkable rates, such that soon there will be no minority or majority culture. The clinical skills necessary to provide appropriate clinical service and education to children with disorders and to assist them in the development of language will provide challenges and opportunities for new discoveries for years to come.

STUDY QUESTIONS

1. What is the responsibility of the monolingual English-speaking speech-language pathologist in providing clinical service to a monolingual Spanish-speaking child

and family? How can the speech-language pathologist work with other members of the educational team to assist the child in learning language?

2. What resources can the speech-language pathologist use to assist with providing culturally and linguistically relevant clinical services to a culturally and linguistically different child with a speech-language disorder?

3. What resources are available in your area to help you understand the culture and language of the children and families likely to require clinical services?

4. What opportunities are there for continuing education to prepare speech-language pathologists for serving culturally and linguistically diverse children and families?

5. What is the ethical responsibility of the speech-language pathologist in providing clinical services for a culturally and linguistically diverse child and family with a language disorder?

SUGGESTED READING

American Speech-Language-Hearing Association. (1983). Position paper on social dialects. *ASHA, 25*(9), 23–24.

American Speech-Language-Hearing Association. (1985). Clinical management of communicatively handicapped minority language populations. *ASHA, 27*(6), 29–32.

Battle, D. E. (Ed.). (in press). *Communication disorders in multicultural populations* (4th ed.). Newton, MA: Butterworth-Heinemann.

Taylor, O. L., & Leonard, L. B. (1999). *Language development across America: Cross cultural and cross-linguistic perspectives.* San Diego, CA: Singular.

Kamhi, A. G., Pollock, K. E., & Harris, J. L. (1996). *Communication development and disorders in African American children: Research, assessment, and intervention.* Baltimore: Paul H. Brookes.

REFERENCES

Acevedo, M. (1989, November). Typical speech misarticulations of Mexican-American preschoolers. Paper presented at the annual meeting *of* the American-Speech-Language-Hearing Association, St. Louis.

Ambert, A. (1986). Identifying language disorders in Spanish speakers. In A. C. Willig & H. F. Greenberg (Eds.), *Bilingualism and learning disabilities* (pp. 15–33). New York: American Library.

American Speech-Language-Hearing-Association. (1983). Position paper on social dialects. *ASHA, 25*(9), 23–24.

American Speech-Language-Hearing-Association. (1985). Clinical management of communicatively handicapped minority language populations. *ASHA, 27*(6), 29–32.

American Speech-Language-Hearing-Association. (1991). Did you know? *Perspectives, 12*(2), 11.

American Speech-Language-Hearing-Association. (1993). Definitions of communication disorders and variations. *ASHA, 35*(Suppl. 10), 40–41.

Anderson, N., & Battle, D. (1998). Culturally diverse families and the development of language. In D. Battle (Ed.), *Communication disorders in multicultural populations* (pp. 213–246). Newton, MA: Butterworth-Heinemann.

Baetens-Beardsmore, H. (1986). *Bilingualism: Basic principles* (2nd ed.). San Diego: College Hill.

Blake, I. (1984). Language development in working class black children: An examination of form, content and use. Doctoral dissertation, Columbia University, New York.

Bleile, K., & Wallach, H. (1992). A sociolinguistic investigation of the speech of African American preschoolers. *American Journal of Speech Language Pathology 1*(2), 54–62.

Bliss, L. S., Covington, Z., & McCabe, A. (1999). Assessing the narratives of African American children. *Contemporary Issues in Communication Sciences and Disorders, 26,* 160–167.

Bloom, M., & Lahey, M. (1978). *Language development and disorders.* New York: Wiley.

Bridgeforth, C. (1984). The development of language functions among black children from working class families. Paper presented at the presession of the 35th Annual Georgetown University Round Table on Language and Linguistics, Washington, DC.

Brown, R. (1973). *A first language, the early stages.* Cambridge, MA: Harvard University Press.

Campbell, L. (1994). Discourse diversity and Black English vernacular. In D. Ripich & N. Creaghead (Eds.), *School discourse problems* (pp. 93–131). San Diego, CA: Singular.

Champion, T., Seymour, H., & Camarata, S. (1995). Narrative discourse in African American children. Journal of *Narrative and Life History, 5,* 333–352.

Cheng, L. L. (1990). Identification of communicative disorders in Asian-Pacific students. *Journal of Childhood Communication Disorders, 13*(1), 113–119.

Cheng, L. L. (1991). *Assessing Asian language performance* (2d ed). Oceanside, CA: Academic Communication Associates.

Cheng, L. L. (1995). *Integrating language and learning for inclusion: An Asian-Pacific focus.* San Diego, CA: Singular.

Cheng, L. L. (1998). Asian and Pacific Island cultures. In D. Battle (Ed.), *Communication disorders in multicultural populations* (pp. 73–116). Newton, MA: Butterworth-Heinemann.

Cole, L. (1980). A development analysis of social dialect features in the spontaneous language of preschool black children. Doctoral dissertation, Northwestern University, Evanston, IL.

Cole, R., & Taylor, O. (1990). Performance of working-class African-American children on three tests of articulation. *Language, Speech, and Hearing Services in Schools, 24,* 161–166.

Crago, M. B. (1992). Ethnography and language socialization: A cross-cultural perspective. *Topics in Language Disorders 12*(3), 28–39.

Crago, M. B., & Cole, E. (1991). Using ethnography to bring children's communicative and cultural words into focus. In T. M. Gallagher (Ed.), *Pragmatics of language: Clinical practice issues* (pp. 99–132). San Diego, CA: Singular.

Craig, H., & Washington, J. A. (1994). The complex syntax skills of poor, urban, African-American preschoolers at school entry. *Language, Speech, and Hearing Services in Schools, 25*(2), 181–190.

Craig, H., & Washington, J. A. (1995). African-American English and linguistic complexity in preschool discourse: A second look. *Language, Speech, and Hearing Services in Schools, 26*(1), 87–93.

Cummins, J. (1984). *Bilingualism and special education.* San Diego, CA: College-Hill.

Damico, J. (1991). Descriptive assessment of communicative ability. In E. V. Hamayan & J. S. Damico (Eds.), *Limiting bias in the assessments of bilingual students.* Austin, TX: Pro-Ed.

Damico, J. S., Oller, J. W., & Storey, M. E. (1983). The diagnosis of language disorders in bilingual children: Surface-oriented and pragmatic criteria. *Journal of Speech and Hearing Disorders, 46,* 385–394.

Davis, P., Williams, J., & Vaughn-Cooke, F. (1992–1993). A comparison of lexical development in a child with normal language development and in a child with language delay. *National Student Speech-Language-Hearing Association Journal, 20,* 63–77.

Dillard, J. (1972). *Black English: Its history and usage.* New York: Random House.

Doyle, A., Champagne, M., & Segalowitz, N. (1978). Some issues in the assessment of linguistic consequences of early bilingualism. In M. Paradis (Ed.), *Aspects of bilingualism.* Columbia, SC: Hornbeam.

Dulay, H., & Burt, M. K. (1974). Natural sequences in second language acquisition. *Language Learning, 24,* 37–53.

Dulay, H., Hernandez-Chavez, E., & Burt, M. K. (1978). The process of becoming bilingual. In S. Singh & L. Lynch (Eds.), *Diagnostic procedures in hearing, language and speech* (pp. 305–326). Baltimore: University Park.

Eblen, R. E. (1982). A study of the acquisition of fricatives by 3 year old children learning Mexican Spanish. *Language and Speech, 25,* 201–220.

Echeverria, M. (1975). Late stages in the acquisition of Spanish syntax. Doctoral dissertation, University of Washington, Seattle.

Farran, D. (1982). Mother–child interaction, language development and the school performance of poverty children. In L. Feagans & D. Farran, (Eds.), *The language of children reared in poverty: Implications for evaluation and intervention.* New York: Academic.

Fasold, R. W., & Wolfram, W. (1978). Some linguistic features of Negro dialect. In P. Stoller (Ed.), *Black American English* (pp. 49–83). New York: Delta.

Garcia, E. E., Maez, L. F., & Gonzalez, G. (1984). *A national study of Spanish/English bilingualism in young Hispanic children of the United States.* Los Angeles: California State University, National Dissemination and Assessment Center.

Gee, J. P. (1989). Two styles of narrative construction and their linguistic and educational implications. *Discourse Processes, 12,* 287–307.

Gomperz, J. (1982). *Discourse strategies.* New York: Cambridge University Press.

Gonzales, G. (1983). Expressing time through verb tenses and temporal expression in Spanish: Age 2.0–4.6. *NABE Journal, 7,* 69–82.

Gudeman, R. H. (1981). Learning Spanish: A cross-sectional study of imitation, comprehension and production of Spanish grammatical forms by rural Panamanians. Doctoral dissertation, University of Minnesota, Minneapolis.

Gutiérrez-Clellen, V., Peña, E., & Quinn, R. (1995). Accommodating cultural differences in narrative style: A multicultural perspective. *Topics in Language Disorders, 15*(4), 54–67.

Gutiérrez-Clellen, V., & Quinn, R. (1993). Assessing narratives of children from diverse cultural/linguistic groups. *Language, Speech, and Hearing Services in Schools, 24*(1), 2–9.

Hall, W., Nagy, W., & Linn, R. (1984). *Spoken words: Effects of stimulation and social group on oral word usage and frequency.* Hillsdale, NJ: Erlbaum.

Hamayan, E. (1992, September). Meeting the challenge of cultural and linguistic diversity in the schools: Best practices in language intervention. Paper presented at the Broward County Exceptional Student Education In-Service, Ft. Lauderdale, FL.

Hamayan, E. V., & Damico, J. S. (1991). *Limiting bias in the assessment of bilingual students.* Austin, TX: Pro-Ed.

Hammer, C. S., & Weiss, A. L. (2000). African American mothers' views of their infants' language development and language-learning environment. *American Journal of Speech-Language Pathology, 9,* 126–140.

Harris, G. (1998). American Indian culture: A lesson in diversity. In D. Battle (Ed.), *Communication disorders in multicultural populations* (pp. 78–113). Newton, MA: Butterworth-Heinemann.

Hart, B., & Risley, T. (1995). *Meaningful differences in the everyday experiences of young American children.* Baltimore: Paul H. Brookes.

Haynes, W. O., & Moran, M. (1989). A cross-sectional development study of final consonant production in Southern Black children from preschool to third grade. *Language, Speech, and Hearing Services in Schools, 21*(4), 400–406.

Haynes, W. O., & Shulman, B. B. (1994). *Communication development: Foundations, processes, and clinical applications.* Englewood Cliffs, NJ: Prentice Hall.

Heath, S. B. (1982). What no bedtime story means: Narrative skills at home and school. *Language and Society, 11,* 49–76.

Heath, S. B. (1983a). *Ways with words: Language, life, and work in communities and classrooms.* New York: Cambridge University Press.

Heath, S. B. (1983b). Sociocultural contexts of language development. In *Beyond Language.* Los Angeles: Evaluation, Dissemination and Assessment Center.

Heath, S. B. (1986). Taking a cross cultural look at narratives. *Topics in Language Disorders, 7*(1), 84–89.

Heath, S. B. (1989, February). Oral and literate traditions among Black Americans living in poverty. *American Psychologist,* 367–373.

Hester, E. J. (1996). Using oral narratives to assess communicative competence. In A. G. Kamhi, K. E. Pollock, & J. L. Harris (Eds.), *Communication development and disorders in African American children* (pp. 227–246). Baltimore: Paul H. Brookes.

Hodson, B., Becker, M., Diamond, F., & Meza, P. (1989). Phonological analysis of unintelligible children's utterances: English and Spanish. In *Occasional papers on linguistics: The uses of phonology.* Carbondale: Southern Illinois University Press.

Hoover, J. J., & Collier, C. (1985). Referring culturally different children: Sociocultural considerations. *Academic Therapy, 20*(4), 503–509.

Hyon, S., & Sulzby, L. (1992, April). Black kindergarteners' spoken narratives: Style, structure and task. Paper presented at the annual meeting of the American Educational Research Association, San Francisco, CA.

Jimenez, B. C. (1987). Acquisition of Spanish consonants in children aged 3–5 years. *Language, Speech, and Hearing Services in Schools, 18*(4), 357–363.

Kayser, H. (1989). Speech and language assessment of Spanish-English speaking children. *Language, Speech, and Hearing Services in Schools, 20*, 226–244.

Kayser, H. (1990). Social communicative behaviors of language-disordered Mexican-American students. *Child Language Teaching Therapy, 6*(3), 255–269.

Kayser, H. (1993). Hispanic cultures. In D. Battle (Ed.), *Communication disorders in multicultural populations* (pp. 114–157). Newton, MA: Butterworth-Heinemann.

Kayser, H. (1998). Hispanic cultures and language. In Battle, D. E. (Ed.), *Communication disorders in multicultural populations* (2nd ed.) (pp. 157–196). Boston: Butterworth-Heinemann.

Keller, G. (1976). Acquisition of the English and Spanish passive voices among bilingual children. In G. D. Keller, R. V. Teschner, & S. Viera (Eds.), *Bilingualism in the bicentennial and beyond* (pp. 161–168). New York: Bilingual Press.

Kovac, C. (1980). Children's acquisition of variable features. Doctoral dissertation, Georgetown University, Washington, DC.

Labov, W. (1972). *Language in the inner city.* Philadelphia: University of Pennsylvania Press.

Langdon, H. W. (1996). English language learning by immigrant Spanish speakers: A United States perspective. *Topics in Language Disorders, 16*, 38–53.

Langdon, H. W., & Cheng, L. (Eds.). (1992). *Hispanic children and adults with communication disorders: Assessments and intervention.* Gaithersburg, MD: Aspen.

Linares, T. A. (1982). Articulation skills of Spanish-speaking children. *Ethnoperspectives in bilingual education, series vol III: Bilingual education technology* (pp. 363–387), Ypsilanti, MI.

Lynch, E. W., & Hanson, M. J. (1993). *Developing cross-cultural competence: A guide for working with young children and their families.* Baltimore: Paul H. Brookes.

Marge, M. (1993). Disability prevention: Are we ready for this challenge? *ASHA 35,* 42–44.

Mattes, L. J., & Omark, D. R. (1991). *Speech and language assessment for the bilingual handicapped* (2d ed.) San Diego, CA: College Hill.

McCabe, A. (1995). Evaluation of narrative discourse skills. In K. N. Cole, P. S. Dale, & D. J. Thal (Eds.), *Assessment of communication and language* (pp. 121–142). Baltimore, MD: Paul Brookes.

Median, V. (1982). *Interpretation and translation in bilingual B. A. S. A.* San Diego, CA: Superintendent of Schools, Department of Education, San Diego County.

Mercer, C. D. (1987). *Students with learning disabilities* (3d ed.). New York: Merrill.

Merino, B. J. (1982, October–November). Language development in Spanish as a first language: Implications of assessment. Paper presented at the National Conference on the Exceptional Bilingual Child, Phoenix, AZ.

Merino, B. J. (1992). Acquisition of syntactic and phonological features in Spanish. In H. W. Langdon & L. L. Cheng (Eds.), *Hispanic children and adults with communication disorders* (pp. 57–98). Gaithersburg, MD: Aspen.

Michaels, S. (1981). "Sharing time": Children's narrative styles and differential access to literacy. *Language in Society, 10,* 423–442.

Moran, M. (1993). Final consonant deletion in African American children speaking Black English: A closer look. *Language, Speech, and Hearing Services in Schools, 24,* 161–166.

Musselwhite, C. (1983). Pluralistic assessment in speech-language pathology: Use of dual norms in the placement process. *Language, Speech and Hearing Services in Schools, 14,* 29–37.

National Deafness and Other Communication Disorders Advisory Board. (1991). *Research in human communication,* Annual report (NIH Publication No. 92–3317). Bethesda, MD: National Institutes of Health.

Ochs, E., & Schieffelin, B. (1984). Language acquisition and socialization. In R. Shwedder & R. Levine (Eds.), *Culture theory: Essays on mind, self, and emotion* (pp. 246–322). New York: Cambridge University Press.

Office of Scientific and Health Reports. (1988). *Developmental speech and language disorders: Hope through research* (NIH Publication No. 88–2757). Bethesda, MD: National Institutes of Neurological and Communicative Disorders and Stroke.

Owens, R. (1992). *Language disorders: A functional approach to assessment and intervention.* New York: Merrill.

Ratusnik, D., & Koenigsknecht, R. (1975). Influence of certain clinical variables on Black preschoolers' nonstandard phonological and grammatical performance. *Journal of Communication Disorders, 8,* 281–297.

Reveron, W. (1978). The acquisition of variable features. Doctoral dissertation, Ohio State University, Columbus.

Rickford, J. R. (In press). Regional and social variation. In S. L. McKay & N. H. Hornberger (Eds.), *Sociolinguistics and language teaching.* Oxford, UK: Oxford University Press.

Ripich, D., & Creaghead, N. (1995). *School discourse problems* (2d ed.). San Diego, CA: Singular.

Saville-Troike, M. (1986). Anthropological considerations in the study of communication. In O. Taylor (Ed.), *Nature of communication disorders in culturally and linguistically diverse populations* (pp. 47–72). San Diego, CA: College Hill.

Schieffelin, B., & Ochs, E. (1986). Language socialization. *Annual Review of Anthropology, 15,* 163–191.

Scriven, M. (1991). *Evaluation thesaurus* (4th ed.). New York: Sage.

Seymour, H. (1995, November). *Theory and practice in evaluating child African-American English.* Paper presented to meeting of the American Speech-Language-Hearing Association, Orlando, FL.

Seymour, H., Bland-Stewart, L., & Green, L. J. (1998). Difference versus deficit in child African American English. *Language, Speech, and Hearing Services in Schools, 29,* 96–108.

Seymour, H., & Ralabate, P. (1985). The acquisition of a phonological feature of Black English. *Journal of Communication Disorders, 18,* 139–148.

Seymour, H., & Seymour, C. (1981). Black English and Standard English contrasts in consonantal development of four- and five-year old children. *Journal of Speech and Hearing Disorders, 46,* 274–280.

Shipley, K. G., & McAfee, J. G. (1992). *Assessment in speech-language pathology: A resource manual.* San Diego, CA: Singular.

Steffersen, M. (1974). The acquisition of Black English. Doctoral dissertation, University of Illinois, Evanston.

Stockman, I. (1986). Language acquisition in culturally diverse populations: The black child as a case study. In O. Taylor (Ed.), *Nature of communication disorders in culturally and linguistically diverse populations* (pp. 117–155). San Diego, CA: College Hill.

Stockman, I. (1991, November). *Constraints on final consonant deletion in Black English.* Paper presented to meeting of the American Speech-Language-Hearing Association, Atlanta, GA.

Stockman, I. (1993). Variable word initial and medial consonants relationships in children's speech sound articulation. *Perceptual and Motor Skills, 76,* 675–689.

Stockman, I. (1995, November). Early morphosyntactic patterns of African-American children. Paper presented to the meeting of the American Speech-Language-Hearing Association, Orlando, FL.

Stockman, I. (1996). The promise and pitfalls of language sample analysis as an assessment tool for linguistic minority children. *Language, Speech, and Hearing Services in Schools, 27,* 355–366.

Stockman, I. (1998). The promises and pitfalls of language sample analysis as an assessment tool for linguistic minority children. *Language Speech and Hearing Services in Schools, 27*(4), 355–365.

Stockman, I., & Settle, M. S. (1991, November). Initial consonants in young Black children's conversational speech. Paper presented to the meeting of the American Speech-Language-Hearing Association.

Stockman, I., & Vaughn-Cooke, F. (1992). Lexical elaboration in children's locative action expressions. *Child Development, 63,* 1104–1125.

Taylor, O. (1986). *Nature of communication disorders in culturally and linguistically diverse populations.* San Diego, CA: College Hill.

Taylor, O. (In press). Clinical practice as a social occasion. In L. Cole & V. Deal (Eds.), *Communication disorders in multicultural populations.* Rockville, MD: American Speech-Language-Hearing Association.

Taylor, O., & Clarke, M. G. (1994). Culture and communication disorders: A theoretical framework. *Seminars in Speech and Language, 15*(2), 103–113.

Taylor, O. T. (1999). Cultural Issues and Language Acquisition. In O. T. Taylor & L. B. Leonard (Eds.), *Language acquisition across North America: Cross-cultural and cross linguistic perspectives.* San Diego, CA: Singular.

Terrell, S., & Terrell, F. (1993). African-American cultures. In D. E. Battle (Ed.), *Communication disorders in multicultural populations* (pp. 3–37). Newton, MA: Butterworth-Heinemann.

Thal, D., Jackson-Maldonado, D., & Acosta, D. (2000). Validity of a parent report measure of vocabulary and grammar for Spanish-Speaking toddlers. *Journal of Speech, Language, and Hearing Research, 43,* 1087–1100.

U.S. Bureau of the Census. (1990). *Statistical Abstract of the United States: 1990* (110th ed.). Washington, DC: U.S. Department of Commerce.

U.S. Bureau of the Census. (1993). *Household and family characteristics:* March 1993. *Current population report series P-20.* Washington, DC: U.S. Government Printing Office.

U.S. Bureau of the Census. (1999). *Statistical Abstract of the United States: 1999* (119th ed.). Washington, DC: U.S. Department of Commerce.

U.S. Department of Education. (1994). To assure the free appropriate public education of all Americans: Sixteenth annual report to Congress on the implementation of The Individuals with Disabilities Education Act (ED/OSERS Publication No. 065 000 00700–2). Washington, DC: U.S. Government Printing Office.

Vaughn-Cooke, F. (1983). Improving language assessment in minority children. *ASHA, 9,* 29–34.

Vaughn-Cooke, F. (1986). Lexical diffusion: Evidence from a decreolizing variety of Black English. In M. Montgomery & G. Bailey (Eds.), *Language variety in the South* (pp. 111–130). Tuscaloosa: University of Alabama Press.

Vaughn-Cooke, F., & Wright-Harp, W. (1992). *Lexical development in working-class Black children.* National Institutes of Health grant #RR08005–23.

Vecoli, R. J. (1995). Introduction. In J. Galens, A. Sheets, & R. V. Young (Eds.), *Gale encyclopedia of multicultural America.* New York: Gale Research.

Washington, J., & Craig, H. (1992). Articulation test performance of low-income, African-American preschoolers with communication impairments. *Language, Speech, and Hearing Services in Schools, 23,* 245–252.

Wayman, K. I., Lynch, E. W., & Hanson, M. J. (1990). Home-based early childhood services: Cultural sensitivity in a family systems approach. *Topics in Early Childhood Special Education, 10,* 65–66.

Weddington, G. T. (1987). *The assessment and treatment of communication disorders in culturally diverse populations.* Unpublished manuscript. San Jose State University.

Westby, C. (1990). Ethnographic interviewing. *Journal of Childhood Communication Disorders, 13*(1), 110–118.

Westby, C. (1994). Multicultural issues. In J. B. Tomblin, H. L. Morris, & D. C. Spriestersbach (Eds.), *Diagnosis in speech-language pathology.* San Diego, CA: Singular.

Wolfram, W., & Fasold, R. (1974). *The study of social dialects in American English.* Englewood Cliffs, NJ: Prentice Hall.

Wong-Fillmore, L. (1991a). Second language learning in children: A model of language learning in social context. In E. Bialystok (Ed.), *Language processing in bilingual children* (pp. 49–69). Cambridge, UK: Cambridge University Press.

Wong-Fillmore, L., (1991b). When learning a second language means losing the first. *Early Childhood Research Quarterly, 6,* 323–346.

Wyatt, T. (1991). Linguistic constraints on copula production in Black English child speech. *Dissertation Abstracts International, 523*(2), 781B (University Microfilms No. DA9120958).

Wyatt, T. (1995). Language development in African American child speech. *Linguistsics and Education, 7,* 7–22.

Language Disorders and Special Populations

CHAPTER 9

Pearl L. Seidenberg

*Long Island
University,
C. W. Post Campus*

Understanding Learning Disabilities

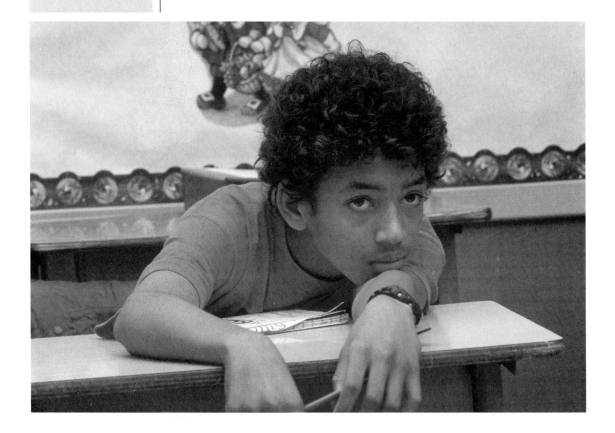

THE CONCEPT OF LEARNING DISABILITIES

Historical Origins

Learning disabilities is the most recent classification to be included as a category of disability. Since the term was introduced, its use has become widespread in education, but many educators still remain unsure about the nature of this category. The struggle to understand and define learning disabilities has characterized the field since its inception.

Lerner (1981) and Wiederholt (1974) divided the history of learning disabilities into four distinct phases:

1. *Foundation phase* (about 1800–1930), a period devoted to scientific investigation of brain function
2. *Transition phase* (about 1930–1960), during which it was assumed that children who were not learning possessed brain function deficits resulting in disordered behaviors; professionals (Cruickshank, Bentzen, Razburg, & Tannhauser, 1961; Orton, 1937; Strauss & Lehtinen, 1947) began to develop assessment and treatment methods for these children
3. *Integration phase* (about 1960–1980), a period characterized by increased interest in learning disabilities with a subsequent increase in school programs for the learning disabled and research into assessment practices and teaching methods
4. *Contemporary phase* (1980 to the present), in which the direction is toward widening the definition of individuals served and the integration of services provided across school programs

One of the first to propose the term *learning disability* was Samuel Kirk (1963), who used it to describe a group of children with specific learning deficits. He stated that a learning disability refers to a retardation, disorder, or delayed development in one or more of the processes of speech, language, reading, spelling, writing, or arithmetic. The learning disability results from a possible cerebral dysfunction and/or emotional or behavioral disturbance, not from mental retardation, sensory deprivation, or cultural or instructional factors. Kirk explained that these disabilities refer to a discrepancy between the child's achievement and apparent capacity to learn as indicated by aptitude tests, verbal understanding, and arithmetic computational skills.

Although the concept covered diverse learning deficits, the term established a frame of reference for thinking about a child with specific learning disorders. The term avoided placing the blame for failure to learn solely on dysfunctions within the child, who was assumed to have more intellectual ability than the child who is mentally retarded. Because the term did not specify a cause, it focused attention on the educational problems that the child faces and laid the framework for educational decision making and special education services.

In 1963, when the Association for Children with Learning Disabilities (ACLD) was formed, the term *learning disability* was adopted. In 1969, the following definition was presented to Congress by the National Advisory Committee on Handicapped Children:

> The term "children with specific learning disabilities" means those children who
> have a disorder in one or more of the basic psychological processes involved in
> understanding or in using language, spoken or written, which disorder may man-
> ifest itself in an imperfect ability to listen, think, speak, read, write, spell or do
> mathematical calculations. Such disorders include such conditions as perceptual
> handicaps, brain injury, minimal brain dysfunction, dyslexia and developmental
> aphasia. The term does not include children who have learning problems which
> are primarily the result of visual, hearing or motor handicaps, of mental retar-
> dation, of emotional disturbance, or of environmental, cultural or economic dis-
> advantage. (U.S. Office of Education, 1977)

In 1975, this definition was included in the Education for All Handicapped Children
Act, Public Law 94-142.

In 1981, the National Joint Committee on Learning Disabilities revised the definition (Hammill, Leiger, McNutt, & Larsen, 1981) and agreed on the following:

> Learning disability is a generic term that refers to a heterogeneous group of dis-
> orders manifested by significant difficulties in the acquisition and use of listen-
> ing, speaking, reading, writing, reasoning, or mathematical abilities. These
> disorders are intrinsic to the individual and are presumed to be due to central
> nervous system dysfunction. Even though a learning disability may occur con-
> comitantly with other handicapping conditions or environmental influences, it
> is not the direct result of those conditions or influences. (p. 336)

This definition has been accepted by the Council for Learning Disabilities, the International Reading Association, the Division for Children with Communication Disorders, the Orton Society, and the American Speech-Language-Hearing Association.

The most basic and important difference from the definition included in Public
Law 94–142 is the elimination of the phrase "basic psychological processes." The
joint committee agreed that the original purpose of the statement, which was to emphasize the *intrinsic* nature of learning disabilities, had been confounded by the controversy that resulted from the association of the term with the perceptual-motor and
specific abilities training models that were in use at the time the original definition
was adopted. Currently, explanations of the kinds of *cognitive, metacognitive,* and
ability deficits that characterize the nature of the intrinsic disorders of the learning-
disabled population are based on linguistic science and information-processing theory.

Defining Learning Disabilities

Because human behavior and learning are complex, learning disabilities may be difficult to define, but they are usually readily identifiable and distinguishable from other
disabilities. Although professionals may be unable to agree on a single definition, in
practice most do not deny the validity of the condition.

The term is used to describe children and adolescents who are not learning at an
expected rate despite the fact that they have experienced traditionally adequate instructional programs. The term *learning disability* does not identify a specific dysfunction or a syndrome of dysfunctions. The decision to describe a child as learning disabled
is made by eliminating other causes of school failure such as emotional disturbance,
mental retardation, or environmental or cultural disadvantage. The label encompasses
a heterogeneous group of learners with diverse characteristics, who have common prob-

lems with learning, and who do not present a clearly identifiable reason for their learning deficits. Although the label is descriptive rather than diagnostic and does not denote a specific etiology or a specific cluster of characteristics, there are a number of behavioral characteristics that are often attributed to children with learning disabilities.

Characteristics of Children with Learning Disabilities

Although the characteristics associated with learning disability are not likely to be present in all or even many learning-disabled children, the behavioral characteristics are useful for helping us to understand the category. The following nine characteristics are mentioned most frequently:

1. *Hyperactivity*—inappropriate excessive motor activity such as tapping of finger or foot, jumping out of seat, or skipping from task to task
2. *Attention deficits*—distracted by irrelevant stimuli or perseveration, or attention becomes fixed on a single task or behavior that is repeated over and over
3. *Motor deficits*—general coordination problems resulting in awkward or clumsy movements
4. *Perceptual-motor deficits*—difficulty in integrating a visual or auditory stimulus with a motor response
5. *Language deficits*—delays in speech and difficulty in understanding and/or formulating spoken language
6. *Impulsivity*—lack of reflective behavior
7. *Cognitive deficits*—deficits in memory and concept formation
8. *Orientation deficits*—poorly developed spatial or temporal concepts
9. *Specific learning deficits*—problems in acquiring reading, writing, or arithmetic skills

These behavioral characteristics, for the most part, are *process* oriented, as opposed to *effect* oriented. That is, they focus on deficit behaviors exhibited by children with learning problems. In contrast, the identification of the effects of the learning deficits (e.g., deficits in verbal or written language development) directs attention to the child's deficiencies in level of performance or skill acquisition in academic areas. These effect-oriented characteristics are the only performance indicators that are useful in helping to develop appropriate educational interventions.

Attention Deficit Hyperactivity Disorder (ADHD) and Learning Disabilities

Controversy continues to surround the relationship between the diagnostic classification of attention deficit hyperactivity disorder (ADHD) and learning disabilities. Historically, there have been significant changes in the diagnostic criteria that were intended to separate ADHD and learning disabilities. The current Diagnostic and Statistical Manual (DSM-IV) of the American Psychiatric Association (1994) continues to categorize learning disabilities as *specific developmental disabilities*, while attention deficit disorders are categorized as *disruptive disorders of children*. At the same time, clarification of the status of ADHD as a handicapping condition by the U.S. Department of Education (DOE) recognized that ADHD could co-occur with other handicapping conditions and result in learning problems. However, the DOE did not believe that ADHD needed to be added as a separate disability category, indicating that children with ADHD are eligible for services under the category of learning disabled or emotionally disturbed if they satisfy the specific category criteria (Davila, Williams, & MacDonald, 1991).

Research has consistently demonstrated that learning disabilities involve a number of components, such as cognitive, attentional, and behavioral deficits and including hyperactivity and impulsivity among some students (Hiebert, Wong, & Hunter, 1982; Kavale & Nye, 1985; McKinney & Reagans, 1983, 1984; Walker, 1985; Williams, Gridley, & Fitzhugh-Bell, 1992).

At the same time, a number of studies have shown that children diagnosed as ADHD experience significant academic achievement problems (August & Garfinkel, 1990; Barkley, Fischer, Edelbrock, & Smallish, 1990; McGee, Williams, Moffett, & Anderson, 1989). However, it is still not clear whether academic failure in children with ADHD is related to attention/impulsivity, cognitive deficits (learning disabilities), or a combination of both (Biederman, Newcorn, & Sprich, 1991).

Although the results of a large number of studies suggest a relationship between LD and ADHD, the underlying nature of the relationship has not as yet been clearly defined (Cantwell & Baker, 1991; Epstein, Shaywitz, Shaywitz, & Woolston, 1991; Shaywitz & Shaywitz, 1991). It has been suggested that the co-occurrence of learning disabilities (LD) and ADHD in subgroups of each of these populations is likely to be the result of differences in underlying neurological functioning that result in common cognitive deficits (Epstein et al., 1991; Shaywitz & Shaywitz, 1991). Based on evidence of underlying neurological dysfunction, it has been suggested that subgroups of both LD and ADHD children may present with attentional problems (August & Garfinkel, 1990; Fleisher, Soodak, & Jelin, 1984; Levine, Busch, & Aufsieser, 1982). In addition, the presence of a language disorder appears to characterize both LD and ADHD children. For children with learning disabilities, language deficits appear to be a major underlying problem (Catts, 1991; Gibbs & Cooper, 1989; Newhoff, 1990; Paul, 1992). Similarly, many children diagnosed with attention deficit disorders demonstrate some type of language disorder (Baker & Cantwell, 1990; Cohen, Devine, & Meloche-Kelly, 1989). Because of these findings, it has been suggested that linguistic development may represent the key element that underlies the relationships between some LD and ADHD children at a cognitive level and the resultant academic achievement problems demonstrated by these children (August & Garfinkel, 1990).

At the same time, because of the paucity of evidence that specifies the educational characteristics or needs of students with ADHD without the complications imposed by other co-existing conditions such as learning disabilities, educational interventions for this population should address the co-occurring learning disabilities and/or language deficits before any other accommodations are provided (Zentall, 1993).

AN INFORMATION-PROCESSING PERSPECTIVE

Current characterizations of the intrinsic disorders manifested in the ability deficits of students with learning disabilities are based on information-processing theory.

Attention has shifted from an interest in identifying and remediating discrete underlying processing ability deficits to a focus on the inefficient or maladaptive information-processing skills of children with learning disabilities. An information-processing orientation provides a way to understand performance in more complex, higher-order cognitive and linguistic tasks such as reading and writing. This perspective provides for useful conceptualizations of the cognitive processes (such as coding, comparing, storing, and retrieving) that underlie observable performance. Learning failure is viewed in terms of deficiencies in underlying cognitive processes (Torgesen, 1986; Swanson, 1989).

Psychological Processes

For some time, learning disabilities were considered to be the result of various types of specific underlying ability deficits. Historically, the research in learning disabilities centered on various psychological processing tasks involving attention, perception, and memory. Comparisons were made between learning-disabled and non-learning-disabled students. These tasks were considered to be measures of underlying cognitive abilities and were used to assess separate discrete functions (visual closure, visual and/or auditory figure–ground differentiation, auditory discrimination, visual and/or auditory memory, etc.). Because early theorists contended that these factors had to be adequately developed before learning could occur, training programs and materials were designed to remediate specific processing deficits (Frostig, 1968; Kephart, 1971; Kirk & Kirk, 1972).

An assumption underlying the specific abilities deficit model was that the areas were distinct from each other and that their component parts could be identified and assessed. Therefore, each system could be measured independently. The interactive nature of the processes of perception, attention, and memory was not considered. Also, the role of the learner in cognitive processing was not viewed as an active one, and thus confounding variables such as meaningfulness of material or organizational abilities were not taken into consideration. The passive view of the child led to the belief that what was to be attended to, perceived, or memorized was "out there." Modification of the demands of tasks rather than attempts to influence the child's approach to a problem was emphasized.

From an information-processing perspective, perception, attention, and memory are considered interactive cognitive processes whose functioning reflects the influence and control of higher-order, integrated, goal-directed cognitive structures (Anderson, 1975). We develop control mechanisms, "a plan to execute a plan" (Miller, Galanter, & Pribam, 1960), which organize and direct the lower-order processes. Therefore, the learning difficulties experienced by some otherwise normally developing children have come to be recognized as related to the higher-order cognitive controls, or strategies, that regulate attention, perception, and memory. This strategy-oriented view of learning disabilities focuses on cognitive processes that are modifiable by instruction rather than on separate, more elementary processing differences or deficits (Swanson, 1991).

The most important and useful feature of information-processing theory is that it enhances our understanding of the problems of children with learning disabilities.

A much more complex picture of the learning process is emerging that focuses attention on the strategies a child uses in approaching learning tasks and suggests very different educational interventions.

The Information-Processing Model

In 1969, Chalfont and Scheffelin described learning disabilities as problems involving deviation in the ability to process information and as an inefficiency in the reception, analysis, synthesis, and symbolic use of information. Since then, information-processing concepts have provided a useful framework for understanding learning disabilities.

The conceptual model arising from information-processing theory enables us to describe systematically the way students who exhibit learning deficits process information. Cognitive psychology, or information-processing psychology, deals with the study of mental processes and begins with the idea that we have the innate capacity to make sense of our experiences. We pick up information, organize it, retain it, and retrieve it. We can call on previously stored information to help us in managing new information. The fact that we make sense of our experience, even though nothing ever happens to us in exactly the same way twice, must mean that we are organized in some systematic way (Farnham-Diggory, 1980). Figure 9.1 is an example of an information-processing model.

Auditory, visual, and tactile stimuli (sensory data) are transmitted to the central processing mechanism (the brain), where they are analyzed, integrated, and stored. The behavioral responses of the individual serve as an additional input source (feedback) for correcting or further modifying the responses. The input is always into a dynamic, organized, interactive system. Behavioral responses are determined not only by the actual stimulus but also by the ongoing programs, the result of past experiences that are already stored in the system.

Modern information-processing theory suggests that individuals may differ from one another cognitively in two broad areas. First, they may differ in the basic structure of their information-processing systems. These structural, or architectural (Cam-

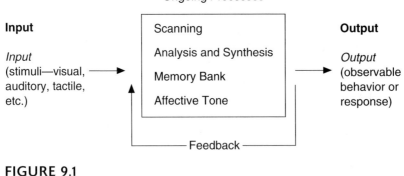

FIGURE 9.1

Information-Processing Model

pione & Brown, 1978), features are the elements of the system that operate outside the conscious control of the individual. Such things as capacity of short-term memory, duration of memory traces, and speed of operations of various processes are all part of the structure of the system.

Second, individual differences can be the result of differences in information and skills that are *learned* as a result of experience. These are the content of long-term memory (i.e., programs already in the system) and are made up of general organized knowledge of the world (i.e., hierarchical semantic structures), habitual ways of thinking (i.e., concrete versus abstract), and rules and strategies that guide performance and adaptation to tasks. The content of long-term memory and the functional features of the system are modifiable by instruction and are under our conscious control (Torgesen, 1982).

The distinction between structural and functional areas of cognitive performance made by information-processing theorists has led to new ways of thinking about the cognitive system of individuals with learning disabilities. Traditionally, learning-disabled children's academic problems and poor performance on experimental tasks were explained in terms of specific ability deficits necessary for normal processing of information. A large number of disabilities, such as perceptual-motor deficits, inter-model integration deficits, and psycholinguistic processing problems, were considered to be relatively enduring cognitive deficits that restricted information processing. In information-processing terms, these earlier explanations claimed that all problems with learning were due to differences in the structural features of the system.

Concepts derived from information-processing theory have greater explanatory power. They provide a framework for analyzing learning deficits that differentiates between the structural and the functional elements of the system, that is, between the system and the programs that use the system. In the child who is learning disabled, some information-processing components are not operating effectively for certain tasks. Therefore, the primary problem appears to be one of programming, and although there may also be some system defects, we can search for ways to develop programs that will compensate for them. A major assumption that underlies the information-processing view is that the rules and specific strategies used by children with learning disabilities do not appear to be appropriate to their intellectual ability. They appear to have knowledge that they are unable to access under certain conditions, to have strategies that they fail to use, or to have not learned when to select particular strategies.

To account for the poor task performance of students with learning disabilities, researchers have generated a number of information-processing models that focus on isolating specific processing deficits involving metacognitive and metalinguistic variables, such as a verbal processing deficit (Vellutino, 1977), a phonological recoding deficit (Shankweiler, Liberman, Mark, Fowler, & Fischer, 1979), a rehearsal deficiency (Bauer, 1977), a selective attention deficit (Hallahan & Reeves, 1980), or a memory deficit (Mastropieri, Scruggs, & Levin, 1987; Scruggs, Mastropieri, & Levin, 1987).

In addition, more general metacognitive models have been proposed that focus on higher-order cognitive processing problems involving mechanisms such as the regulation or coordination of mental activities (e.g., general control processes involved in the planful consideration, selection, execution, and evaluation of strategies) as well as the relation of affective belief systems (e.g., appropriate attributions of performance outcomes) to strategic processing (Borkowski, Johnston, & Reid, 1987; Borkowski & Kurtz, 1987; Swanson, 1988, 1989).

Based on these more global metacognitive models, a number of studies support the notion that students with learning disabilities have difficulty modifying or transforming simple strategies into the more complex, efficient procedures needed to meet the requirements of many academic tasks (Swanson, 1988; Swanson & Cooney, 1985; Swanson & Rhine, 1985). The higher-order cognitive processing problems are undoubtedly influenced by specific strategic processing deficits and dysfunctional belief systems (outlined earlier), which probably become more pervasive over time in their influence on academic performance. At the same time, a considerable body of evidence shows that training students with learning disabilities to use more efficient task-specific cognitive strategies improves their performance on many school-related tasks (Deshler, Schumaker, & Lenz, 1984; Ellis & Lenz, 1987; Ryan, Weed, & Short, 1986; Schunk & Cox, 1986; Wong, 1985).

The metacognitive and metalinguistic variables generated by these diverse information-processing models have important implications for our understanding of the three major areas of learning disabilities: (1) deficiencies in oral language, (2) deficiencies in cognitive abilities, and (3) deficiencies in written language.

MAJOR AREAS OF LEARNING DISABILITIES

Deficits in Oral Language

Failure to develop adequate verbal language skills results in subsequent failure in many other areas of learning. It is important to understand the interdependencies of language disorders and learning disabilities. For many decades, the field of learning disabilities generally did not emphasize the role of language processes. Because of the origins of the field, an interest in perceptual-motor functioning and other nonverbal tasks dominated both the literature and educational programs. It was not until the 1970s that researchers began to investigate the relationship between deficits in oral language and learning disabilities. Currently, many researchers believe that language deficits are implicated in learning disabilities (Catts & Kamhi, 1999; Dillon & Dodd, 1994; Leong, 1999; Vellutino, 1979). They propose that these deficits have an impact on reading ability and academic success. Following is a brief overview of the language problems presented by students with learning disabilities.

Preschool Language Deficits

Preschool children who exhibit language deficits or delays are generally at risk for later school failure. Early language disorders are demonstrated in a number of areas. At-risk children frequently show no interest in verbal activities, are unable to follow a story line, and do not enjoy being read to. Although nouns, verbs, and most prepositions are understood, these children may have word-retrieval difficulties or difficulty in following a series of oral directions. There is often a sustained delay in speech and language development, and syntax may be primitive, with incidence of inadequate morphological pattern acquisition. Overall verbal concept development may be slow, and the children are often still unable to name colors, letters, or days of the week when they enter school.

In a comprehensive review of the research regarding young children with language impairments, Leonard (1979) presented a description of at-risk children's linguistic problems. In general, the language skills of preschoolers with language delays are similar to those of younger, normally developing children. Syntactically, the structures used by both groups of children seem to be the same, although at-risk children appear to use them less frequently and in more limited contexts. The size of their vocabulary and the length of their utterances (MLU) also resemble those of younger children. Similar findings relate to the areas of pragmatics and phonology. There is evidence of greater delays in the language-impaired child's use of the pragmatic and phonological features of language.

Because inadequate language development is often the precursor to learning problems during the school years, there is an urgent need for early identification of children who show developmental language delays. As discussed in earlier chapters, recognition of the importance of early identification and intervention programs for infants and toddlers at risk for developmental delays and preschoolers with disabilities spurred passage of the Education of Handicapped Children Act Amendments of 1986 (PL 99–457). It is well established that early intervention can prevent later learning problems from developing and can offset the negative emotional consequences of school failure (Majsterek & Ellenwood, 1990).

Language Deficits of the School-Age Child

Many children with learning disabilities exhibit a number of language deficits that affect both language comprehension and production. The linguistic demands of a classroom require a level of abstractness and complexity much greater than that needed for ordinary social communicative competence. The mismatch between the linguistic demands of instructional language and the poor linguistic abilities of many children with learning disabilities may account in part for the hyperactive, impulsive behaviors and attentional deficits often attributed to these children.

Generally, language-impaired, learning-disabled children have difficulty in understanding *wh-* questions and in processing and using pronouns and possessives. Other aspects of syntax that often cause difficulty are the passive construction, negative constructions, relative clauses, negations, contractions, and adjective transformations (Vogel, 1975; Wiig & Semel, 1973, 1974, 1975). There is evidence of reduced mastery of the grammatical inflections for adjectives, verb tense markers, and possession (Vogel, 1975; Wiig, Semel, & Crouse, 1973). Specific difficulty with verb tense markers was found primarily in irregular past-tense forms (Moran & Bryne, 1977) and with more complex grammatical structures (Edwards & Kallail, 1977).

Linguistic concepts expressing comparative, spatial, and temporal relationships are also problems for children with learning disabilities. Wiig and Semel (1976) have demonstrated that the ability to process these structures follows a developmental course, with comparative relations being easiest, followed in difficulty by temporal and spatial relationships. It is important to note that not all children who have learning disabilities will have the same difficulties with the same linguistic concepts.

An extensive description of areas of possible difficulty with different form classes, including nouns, verbs, adjectives, adverbs, and prepositions, was provided by Wiig and Semel (1984). The authors related many of the linguistic problems to more primary cognitive difficulties. They suggested that if relationships are not accurately perceived by children in their interactions with their environment, they will not be able to comprehend these relationships when they are coded linguistically. In addition, they believed that a child who has difficulty in generalizing and has a tendency toward concreteness will maintain narrower word meanings and have problems processing sentences containing multiple-meaning words and figurative language. It has been shown that elementary-age students with learning disabilities do have difficulty understanding metaphoric language when compared with their non-learning-disabled peers. It appears that, although many learning-disabled children have the requisite cognitive strategies for understanding metaphors (e.g., generating and comparing semantic attributes), they fail to spontaneously access and apply them when they should (Seidenberg & Bernstein, 1986, 1988).

In development of their semantic system, children with and without learning disabilities generally have been found to perform equally well in tasks of receptive vocabulary (Wiig & Semel, 1973; Vogel, 1975). However, children with learning disabilities exhibit word-finding difficulties (Denckla & Rudel, 1976; Johnson & Myklebust, 1967; Kail & Leonard, 1986) and semantic memory deficits (Baker, Ceci, & Hermann, 1987). They also demonstrate specific deficits in rapid naming tasks, naming pictures, naming opposites, and giving word definitions (Wiig & Semel, 1976).

The primary productive syntactic language problems evidenced by children with learning disabilities appear to be a delay in the acquisition of basic operations such as negative, interrogative, or passive transformations. In sentence repetition tasks, these children appear to maintain the basic meaning or semantic relations of a sentence without difficulty, but they repeat the sentence in a reduced fashion (Menyuk & Looney, 1972). In general, children with learning disabilities appear to be performing similarly to younger, normally developing children in this area.

Generally, the phonological problems of children with language impairments are more complex than the problems exhibited by children with only an articulation disorder. The problems appear to be related to morpho-syntactic delays as well as to the ability to carry out accurately the complex motor programs of speech (Berry, 1980). Often, the language learning disabled child evidences inconsistencies in sound production. Sounds may be produced accurately in a simple sentence, but when the sentences become longer and more complex, production difficulties become evident. The child with language delays appears more vulnerable to the syntactic demands of more complex structures, in which requirements of motor patterning and idea formulation appear to create organizational problems and subsequent problems in speech production (Lieberman, Meskill, Chatillon, & Schupack, 1985).

Finally, children with learning disabilities may have deficits in pragmatics, the understanding of the rules governing the use of language in social contexts. In a review of a series of studies dealing with pragmatic competence, Bryan (1981) presented an overview of these deficits. In general, the children with learning disabilities did *not* differ from nondisabled children in conversational turn taking or in referential communicative competence when a required response was unambiguous. However, when a situation was ambiguous or socially complex, the performance of the two groups differed. In these situations, children with learning disabilities had difficulty with such pragmatic skills as asking questions, responding to inadequate messages, disagreeing, supporting an argument, and sustaining or monitoring a conversation. The studies also indicated that the relationships among syntactic-semantic knowledge, social knowledge, and development of communicative competence are interactive and complex and may be dependent on the development of both linguistic skills and cognitive abilities.

Deficits in Cognitive Abilities

Any attempt to understand the performance of learning-disabled children in academic learning must consider the interaction of language and thought and the cognitive correlates of such an interaction. In processing written language, the learner is confronted with a combination of both abstract concepts and complex language. Without adequate development in both language and cognitive strategies for processing information, a serious mismatch between the child's ability and the academic task demands can result. The cognitive functions of perception, attention, and memory are related to each other, as well as to the acquisition of language. Understanding the nature of these interactions in the processing of verbally encoded information contributes to our understanding of the problems experienced by many children with learning disabilities.

According to current theory in cognitive psychology, perception, attention, and memory are interactive processes that reconstruct, organize, and internalize information. Cognitive development is continually emerging through stages of newly acquired strategies for actively processing environmental information. The child becomes increasingly able to attend selectively to critical attributes during perception and to hold more than one aspect of perceived information in memory simultaneously to perform cognitively on that information. As age increases, memory abilities are enhanced by the use of categorization and verbal rehearsal strategies (Ring, 1976). Similarly, with maturation, children develop increased ability to focus attention on the relevant aspects of learning tasks and to diminish attention to incidental stimuli (Hallahan & Sapona, 1984; Tarver, Hallahan, Kaufman, & Ball, 1976).

Memory, attention, and perception interact and are interdependent. The individual actively analyzes and processes information by developing strategies that tap previously stored information acquired through past experience and organizational structures. Also, there appears to be a reciprocal relationship between language development and the development of cognitive abilities. This interactive nature of the relationship is viewed within the broader framework of the child's overall ability to organize, plan, monitor, and integrate information. The view that is generally held is that the development of cognitive strategies complements linguistic development in a way that facilitates the processing of verbally encoded information. Also, increased linguistic abilities contribute to the development of a number of cognitive functions such as memory and attention.

For example, many children who have learning disabilities exhibit deficits in short-term memory of verbal information (Cohen, 1982; Jorm, 1983; Torgesen, 1985), resulting from difficulties in the use of such elaborative encoding strategies as verbal grouping and verbal rehearsal (e.g., repeating information to oneself to encourage recall). These difficulties appear to reduce the effectiveness of attention and memory in processing information. At the same time, children with learning disabilities exhibit inadequate use of the organizational structure of syntax and of category clustering of verbal material, and these deficits also appear to be related to problems in processing verbal material (Bauer, 1977; Gelheiser, 1984; Hallahan, Gajar, Cohen, & Tarver, 1978; Kamhi & Koenig, 1985; Pressley, Borkowski, & O'Sullivan, 1984; Torgesen, 1978).

In a number of previously reported studies, the performance of children with learning disabilities improved after they were taught to use selected processing strategies. These observed changes in behavior have led to the conclusion that children with learning disabilities have more ability than can be presumed from their performance. Some of their learning deficits are not due to an inability to acquire effective cognitive strategies, but to other factors that interfere with their development. One factor that appears to result in poor performance is that many children with learning disabilities tend to lack motivation and are thus characterized as inactive learners (Torgesen & Licht, 1983). It has been suggested that this passive approach to learning is the result of the children's tendency *not* to link performance outcomes to their own efforts or abilities; that is, they often regard what happens to them as unrelated to what they themselves do. It has been proposed that this view of themselves and the learning environment may prevent children with learning disabilities from actively using appropriate cognitive strategies (Butkowsky & Willows, 1980; Hallahan et al., 1978; Johnston & Winograd, 1985; Kurtz & Borkowski, 1984; Licht, 1984; Winograd & Niquette, 1988).

Some aspects of the relationship between cognition and language have yet to be examined; however, many of the behaviors reported in learning disabled children appear to support a hypothesis of a delay in cognitive development. Their cognitive development indicates deficits in the use of higher-order cognitive strategies such as (1) simultaneous processing of perceptual information, (2) development of organizational structures that encode larger amounts of information, and (3) use of verbal strategies to facilitate storage and retrieval of information. Because of the importance of these higher order cognitive and linguistic variables for academic learning (e.g., metacognitive and metalinguistic abilities), they are discussed in some detail in the following section.

Deficits in Reading and Writing

The largest subgroup among the learning disabled population are those children and adolescents identified as having deficits associated with learning to read and write (Stanovich, 1986). Children with disorders in the comprehension or formulation of written language appear to process information differently than non-learning-disabled children. Often they fail to use effective strategies in interacting with written material and show deficits in their performance of reading and writing tasks.

Reading Deficits

Although most children learn to read as effortlessly as they learn to speak, regardless of the method used to teach them, a small proportion of children with no clearly identifiable intellectual, physical, or social disabilities find it extremely difficult to learn to read or write. For these children, learning to read is a formidable task. Those who are responsible for teaching these children find the task equally difficult. However, current theoretical advances in the cognitive and linguistic sciences provide some new approaches to this problem. Insights derived from a developmental cognitive-linguistic perspective emphasize the complex, interactive nature of the reading process and provide an additional dimension for understanding the nature of reading disabilities.

This perspective assumes that there are critical age-related cognitive and linguistic characteristics that interact with reading instruction and result in an inability to acquire specific reading skills. It is believed that the learner's cognitive-linguistic abilities set the parameters for the child's information-processing capacities. These underlying information-processing capabilities are important for learning to read and are reflected in a student's specific reading behaviors. Because reading disability is *not* a unitary phenomenon, the actual causes of difficulties in learning to read vary. There can be various points of breakdown for different learners in the learning-to-read process. Deficits in the learner's underlying information-processing capacities relative to the skills being taught contribute to these breakdowns.

Efficient reading requires the acquisition and integration of different skills at different points in the process. The acquisition of these skills is dependent on the integrative functioning of cognitive abilities (i.e., perception, attention, and memory) and their interface with linguistic variables. Therefore, the concept of reading disability can be understood only within a developmental context that considers what learners bring to the task of learning to read and how it affects reading efficiency.

Defining the Reading Process

Reading may be broadly defined as a communication process in that it involves the ability to respond to written language. It is a process of obtaining meaning and is currently categorized not as a perceptual act, but as a language-based activity. Goodman (1973) described reading as a "psycholinguistic guessing game" in which the reader samples only a minimal amount of the visual information, relying heavily on the redundancy of language (i.e., phonology, semantics, and syntax) to predict structures. As the reader processes the subsequent language, these predictions are tested against the semantic content and are confirmed. Reading is viewed as a constructive process in which the reader's knowledge about the language and the world (i.e., past experience) interact with the textual information (Anderson, Spiro, & Montague, 1977).

To bridge the gap from print to meaning, the reader must engage a number of subprocesses that involve auditory and visual perceptual abilities, cognitive abilities (i.e., attention, memory, organization), language knowledge, and past experiences. Reading performance can be viewed as a product of the reader's cognitive and linguistic abilities, prior knowledge, and mastery of specific reading skills (see Figure 9.2). Reading performance reflects the interaction of these diverse factors, each of which contributes collectively to the reading process and, therefore, to observable reading behaviors.

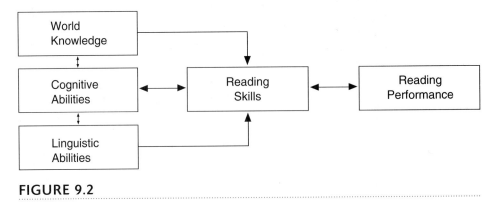

FIGURE 9.2

Interactive Model of Reading Performance

Although reading may start with print and the specific skills taught in reading instruction, the level of reading efficiency demonstrated at any given point in the learning-to-read process is linked to the reader's information-processing capabilities within the different components of the model. Reading performance reflects the knowledge and competencies available to the learner and how these are activated and coordinated during the reading process.

Deficits in Verbal Processing

The possibility of verbal deficiencies in poor readers is currently receiving greater attention than it has in past years. There is an emerging consensus about the importance of a variety of linguistic or language-based skills in explaining reading disabilities (Catts & Kamhi, 1986; Stanovich, 1986; Vellutino, 1979).

Because reading achievement necessitates the efficient use of all of the learner's cognitive and linguistic abilities, deficits in linguistic functioning have impacts on both initial reading skill acquisition and on the later stages of the learning-to-read process. One theory suggests that many children with reading disabilities have deficits in processing the phonological aspects of language (Catts & Kamhi, 1999; Liberman, 1983; Stackhouse & Wells, 1997; Torgesen, Wagner, & Rashotte, 1994).

Difficulty in acquiring beginning reading skills has been linked with deficits in phonological processing. For example, Vellutino (1979) maintained that the apparent visual-perceptual problems (i.e., word identification) encountered by beginning readers are, in fact, associated with problems in verbal mediation and/or phonological deficits. He contended that many of the errors implicated in reading disability can be understood as linguistic intrusion errors rather than as deficits in visual perception. Thus, when poor readers call a *b* a *d* or substitute *was* for *saw,* it is not because they are processing the visual information inaccurately, it is because they have difficulty in naming the letter or word correctly. Similarly, he suggested that awareness of the phonological structure of spoken language is important for the acquisition of word-decoding skills. Success in beginning reading, specifically in code acquisition (e.g., learning sound–symbol relationships), requires that learners have the ability to segment words at the phonemic level and to associate the separate phonemes with their counterparts in print. Poor readers appear to lack the phonological segmentation ability and, therefore, have difficulty in phonemic decoding and in developing phoneme–grapheme correspondences.

A number of other researchers support the idea that poor readers are less adequate than better readers in phonological segmentation ability and in both short- and long-term memory for verbal material. These difficulties have been linked to (1) a lack of phonological awareness, (2) problems in encoding verbal stimuli phonologically, and (3) deficits in retrieving phonological information from memory. In studies of phonological segmentation ability, poor readers performed less well on phoneme and syllable segmentation tasks and on tasks involving rhyming and alliteration than good readers (Bryant & Bradley, 1981; Fox & Routh, 1980; Lieberman et al., 1985; O'Connor & Jenkins, 1999; Williams, 1984b). Research indicating that poor readers exhibit deficits in short-term memory of verbal information has attributed the deficits to difficulties in using phonologically based codes to store verbal information (Perfetti & Lesgold, 1979; Ring, 1976; Torgesen, 1985; Torgesen, Rashotte, Greenstein, & Portes, 1991).

Another aspect of the phonological processing deficits of children with reading disabilities is inadequacy associated with deficits in the basic naming and labeling of verbal stimuli and in word retrieval (Blackman, 1984; Ceci, 1982; Denckla & Rudel, 1976; Perfetti & Hogaboam, 1975; Torgesen & Houck, 1980). It has been proposed that these naming and retrieval deficits are due to difficulties children have in accessing the phonological representations of words from their lexicons (Catts, 1986; Ellis, 1981).

A number of additional studies implicate other aspects of linguistic functioning in reader group differences in the development of reading comprehension abilities. These studies indicate that poor readers are not as proficient as better readers at understanding syntactically complex sentences (Brittain, 1970; Hook & Johnson, 1978; Vogel, 1975), at comprehending and using inflectional morphology (Berko, 1958; Bougere, 1969), at using syntactic constraints to assist in word identification (Samuels, Begg, & Chen, 1976; Steiner, Werner, & Cromer, 1971), in lexical development (Jansky & deHirsh, 1972; Vellutino, 1979), and at using knowledge of text or story structure (Englert & Raphael, 1988; Short & Ryan, 1984; Vallecorsa & Garriss, 1990; Williams, 1984a; Winograd, 1984, Wong, Wong, Perry, & Sawatsky, 1986).

Deficits in Metacognitive and Metalinguistic Abilities

In addition to linguistic competence, efficient reading requires a more comprehensive awareness of cognitive and linguistic functioning. Metacognition, for example, is the ability to deal abstractly with one's own thought processes in comprehension and reasoning tasks and to identify and regulate the use of appropriate strategies (Brown, 1978; Flavell, 1978). Similarly, metalinguistic skills involve linguistic awareness, which is the ability to reflect consciously on the nature and discrete properties of language. In general, metalinguistic abilities interact with and reflect general cognitive and metacognitive abilities at different points in development (van Kleeck, 1984). Deficits in metalinguistic and/or metacognitive knowledge appear to be important factors that affect the acquisition of effective reading skills among poor readers.

It has been proposed that the development of reading skills requires a level of linguistic awareness above that required for the development and use of spoken language (Seidenberg, 1982). Many children who have learning disabilities appear to have deficits not solely in their verbal language systems but also in their metalinguistic abilities. For example, the phonological processing abilities outlined earlier that are required for the acquisition of phonics skills in beginning reading involve metalinguistic awareness, and there are developmental differences in children's ability to analyze and differentiate the phonemes in words (Cazden, 1972). The ability to make explicit judgments about the properties of language—that is, to analyze words, blend word parts, and reconstruct words—requires metalinguistic skills (Kamhi & Koenig, 1985). Similarly, the ability to recognize the syntactic structures in written text, to understand the relatedness among sentences in connected discourse, and to consider pertinent contextual information—that is, the ability to resolve contextual ambiguities—involves metalinguistic skills that are related to problems in reading comprehension. Many poor readers appear to have deficits in the ability to grasp grammatical structure and abstract meaning from larger contexts (Denner, 1970). Some poor readers are unable to segment texts into meaningful units and are therefore unable to attend to the focal or propositional information (Fleisher, Jenkins, & Pany, 1979). Poor readers also appear to have deficits in the metalinguistic awareness and cognitive strategies needed for monitoring and repairing comprehension failures due to textual inadequacies or inconsistencies (e.g., analogies, absurdities, anaphoric usage, figurative language, and idioms; see Chan, Cole, & Barfett, 1987; Seidenberg & Bernstein, 1988).

Research on metacognitive differences between good and poor readers indicates that less skilled readers appear to be unaware of their own failures to comprehend (Bos & Filip, 1984; Garner & Reis, 1981; Markman, 1977; Wong et al., 1986; Wong & Jones, 1982) and do not access or use effective comprehension-monitoring or repair strategies. In general, poor readers appear to be less able to evaluate task difficulty and to identify appropriate reading or studying strategies (Bransford, Stein, Shelton, & Owings, 1980; McGee, 1982; Paris & Meyers, 1981; Rinehart, Stahl, & Erickson, 1986; Schumaker, Deshler, Alley, Warner, & Denton, 1984). They are also characterized as overreliant on ineffective or inappropriate reading comprehension strategies. Poor readers continue to use inappropriate bottom-up strategies (word-decoding strategies) that affect comprehension, or inappropriate top-down strategies (conceptual strategies based on prior knowledge) that interfere with accurate word recognition (Pearson & Spiro, 1980). Additionally, poor readers tend not to use effective strategies for integrating word and sentence meanings, for extracting important information from the text, for drawing inferences, and for integrating background knowledge with the text (Golinkoff, 1976; Jenkins, Heliotis, Stein, & Haynes, 1987; Williams, 1984a; Winograd, 1984; Wong, 1978).

Writing Deficits

Generally, the student with learning disabilities involving either verbal language skills or reading skills will also experience difficulties in the acquisition of writing skills. Research indicates that writing skills are among the best correlates of reading, and that a strong relationship exists among reading, the receptive aspect of written language, and almost all other aspects of written language (Hammill & McNutt, 1981). Writing is a highly complex, interactive process that builds on preexisting cognitive and linguistic structures. It is the final and most formal aspect of language that has to be learned. Writing disorders can be understood only within a multiple framework encompassing knowledge of what the writer must bring to the task (i.e., underlying cognitive and linguistic abilities) and knowledge of the nature of the writing task itself.

There are two major categories of problems associated with writing disorders: (1) those due to deficits in underlying cognitive or linguistic processes required for writing and (2) those due to the nature of the complex components inherent in writing activities and their interaction with underlying abilities. Written language facility involves a number of component skills, including handwriting, spelling, punctuation, capitalization, vocabulary, syntax, and the formulation and organization of ideas. Typically, students with learning disabilities have difficulty in more than one aspect of written language. Therefore, it is important to understand the development of these component skills and their relationship to proficiency in written language.

Acquisition of Written Language Skills

The abilities to read and write follow developmentally the abilities to listen and speak. Myklebust (1965, 1978) described the hierarchical process of language acquisition as developing through auditory receptive, auditory expressive, visual receptive, and visual expressive forms. He maintained that the development of abilities in the language hierarchy relies on the initial intactness of the oral language capacity. If there are significant verbal language problems, then all capacities above this level will be affected. The many cognitive and linguistic abilities outlined earlier underlie basic oral language capacities. Therefore, those aspects of functioning that affect the verbal language system will also affect writing performance.

However, the ability to write requires an additional kind of analysis beyond that required for verbal language. Writing is a form of representation that is further from the reality it represents than is spoken language. Vygotsky (1962) referred to writing as a "second-order symbol system." Writing does not represent experience directly, but rather represents a previously acquired linguistic code, a system of arbitrary signs, by means of a new system. Vygotsky concluded that writing is highly abstract compared with the immediacy of spoken language. Although written language is similar to verbal language in thought and imagery, its structure and mode of functioning differ.

Because of the complexity of writing, underlying processing capacities of attention and memory as well as higher levels of cognitive functioning need to be adapted and used in unique ways. For example, children must acquire the linguistic awareness that enables them to use effectively the syntactic and semantic aspects of language in writing. A writing task demands an awareness and control of linguistic processes that are different by nature and medium from speech. The conventions of writing have their own discourse rules that demand more formal use of complete syntactic conventions, such as connectives and embedded clauses, than those required for speech. There is also a demand for more cohesiveness, less redundancy, and fewer examples or illustrations.

Children need to develop metacognitive skills so that they are capable of monitoring their own production, evaluating what they are writing in light of their purpose, taking perspective into account, and using an expanded knowledge base. Finally, they need to develop a concept of text, an understanding of the way that coherence or unity is achieved in written language. Children need to acquire the concept of a story (as well as of other genres) that they will bring to the writing task. It is this concept of text structure that appears to support organization and memory during the writing activity (Applebee, 1978; Englert & Raphael, 1988; Thomas, Englert, & Gregg, 1987).

Before they can write, children must be able to perform the motor act of writing and must have attained a level of proficiency in spelling. Handwriting is a grapho-motor skill and is primarily dependent on visual-perceptual ability, visual memory, and eye–hand coordination. Johnson and Myklebust (1967) termed the inability to learn the appropriate motor behaviors for writing **dysgraphia.** Severe deficits in hand-writing may include the inability to maintain an appropriate pencil grasp. Less severe problems may result in handwriting that is poorly spaced, awkward, or immature. Handwriting difficulties may be only one manifestation of more generalized difficulties in the performance of motor activities (e.g., catching or throwing a ball, buttoning a coat, or following a pattern or sequence of movements).

Handwriting difficulties also may be affected by the rate of performance. In order for writing to be efficient, it must be performed at a rate appropriate for the task. Although a child's handwriting may appear adequate, it may have been produced slowly and with difficulty. Such problems result from a lack of automatic motor patterns for letter formation or from slowness in processing and organizing information for the writing task.

Another of the skills necessary for writing is the ability to recall the spelling of words. Cici (1980) outlined some of the underlying abilities necessary for children to learn to spell words. The abilities to articulate the word correctly, to recall the spoken pattern (i.e., the auditory sequence of the phonemes or syllables), and to recall the visual letter sequences are necessary for learning to spell. Also, children must be able to recall the motor pattern for writing a word and to execute the plan for the motor act. Because the complex nature of the writing task requires the simultaneous use of semantic, syntactic, and graphophonic information, trying to satisfy all of these constraints at one time makes writing difficult.

Disorders in Written Language

Because the complexity of the writing task involves the integration of linguistic, cognitive, and motoric activities, writing presents a major problem for many students with learning disabilities. Lerner (1981) suggested that poor facility in expressing thoughts through written language is the most prevalent disorder in the acquisition of communication skills. Students who have responded well to remediation in spoken language or reading instruction during the elementary grades often continue to have difficulties with written expressive language. Among the learning disabled population, written language disorders often persist into adolescence and adulthood (Blalock, 1981; Isaacson, 1987; Johnson, Blalock, & Nesbitt, 1978; Moran, Schumaker, & Vetter, 1981).

Children with learning disabilities often continue to have spelling difficulties even after they have learned to read. Some adolescents who exhibit severe spelling deficits may also show subtle verbal language deficits, including problems with word retrieval and phonological segmentation (Gerber, 1984, 1986).

Wiig and Semel (1976) reported that in writing tasks, students with learning disabilities frequently omit words, confuse word order, use incorrect verbs and pronouns, use incorrect word endings, and leave out punctuation. They also indicated that, at the syntactic level, children with learning disabilities frequently produce agrammatical sentences in which elements of several transformations are combined or reversed. Learning-disabled children have been found to score significantly lower on indices of syntax, vocabulary, and ideation when their writing samples are compared with those of nondisabled peers (Blair & Crump, 1984; Gregg, 1983; Myklebust, 1973; Norris & Crump, 1982). Research documents the organizational deficiencies of learning-disabled students in story narrative writing skills and in generating expository compositions (Nodine, Barenbaum, & Newcomer, 1985; Thomas et al., 1987). Typically, individuals with learning disabilities approach both narrative and informational writing as an associative or linear process in which any separate idea associatively stimulates subsequent unrelated ideas. These students show no awareness or use of an overall organizational plan that restricts the generation of ideas or that ties each idea back to a major proposition or theme (Englert & Thomas, 1987). Students with learning disabilities also show significant mechanical writing skills deficits on measures of spelling, grammatical correctness, capitalization, and punctuation. In addition, their written language performance on these factors becomes more discrepant as grade level increases (Gerber, 1984; Poplin, Gray, Larsen, Banikowski, & Mehring, 1980).

Although reading and writing make different demands on underlying linguistic and cognitive capabilities, the skills needed for conveying meaning in writing are clearly interrelated with the skills necessary for extracting meaning from reading. For example, as already indicated, the reading and writing performance of students with learning disabilities suggests that they approach both tasks without sensitivity to the overall organizational pattern of the text (e.g., story schema or expository text structure type). They therefore fail to recognize the organizational pattern in written materials and neglect to use it to construct meaning while reading or writing. Because these students do not link the ideas in text into groupings of related ideas, they recall or they generate only isolated pieces of information (Raphael & Englert, 1990; Seidenberg, 1989). The interrelated, reciprocal relationship inherent in reading and writing activities and the positive influence of this relationship on the development of both processes cannot be overemphasized. It assumes special significance in our understanding of the nature of the learning disabilities associated with written language.

ASSESSMENT OF LEARNING DISABILITIES

The measurement of a student's psychoeducational abilities and skills has historically been a major theme in the development and delivery of special education programs and services. Assessment, the collection and interpretation of relevant data, is a supporting activity for all subsequent decision-making activities. Before the need for a special education program or the instructional focus of the educational program can be determined for a student suspected of having a learning disability, a comprehensive functional assessment must be done.

Functional assessment and testing are not the same. Assessment involves far more than the administration of a group of tests. When we assess students, we have to consider the way they perform a variety of tasks in a variety of settings or contexts (e.g., the child with a short attention span for reading instruction but not for model plane building), the meaning of their performance in terms of their total functioning (e.g., the child's short attention span is related directly to the task demand—reading versus model plane building), and explanations for their performance (e.g., the nature of the reading instructional program may be inappropriate for the child's information-processing capacities). Assessment is always an evaluative, interpretive appraisal of performance that provides information to teachers and other school-based personnel, allowing them to make effective educational decisions for children.

Comprehensive Evaluation

A single set of indicators cannot be used to decide that a child is learning disabled because there are different causes for and, therefore, different types of learning disability. Therefore, a careful clinical description of the individual child is of primary importance in making an appropriate identification. Assessment of children suspected of having learning disabilities must be flexible and responsive to the individual differences exhibited by these children.

Because of the heterogeneity of the learning disabled population, the regulations of Public Law 94–142 mandate that a comprehensive evaluation be done by a multidisciplinary team. For the assessment of children suspected of having specific learning disabilities, the regulations (Section 12 la. 540) state explicitly that the team must be made up of

- A person knowledgeable in the area of the suspected disability
- The child's classroom teacher, or, if the child does not have a classroom teacher, a teacher qualified to teach the child
- At least one additional specialist such as a psychologist, a speech-language pathologist, or a remedial reading specialist, qualified to administer individual diagnostic assessments

Because of the interactive relationship between language disability and learning disability for many students, competent assessment requires a comprehensive evaluation that includes findings from both of these disciplines as well as from other disciplines (physician, psychologist, reading specialist, regular teacher, etc.). It is very important to the overall identification of specific learning disabilities that the team's assessment approach reflect a multidimensional model, taking into account factors ranging from the purposes of assessment to a broad-based conceptualization of the nature of learning.

The Assessment Model

Assessment is undertaken to determine if special education is warranted and, if so, to determine the nature of the student's special educational needs. To make these decisions, a systematic approach to the organization and interpretation of evaluation data must be used. Testing information must identify meaningful patterns of functioning and provide data that are relevant for learning.

An information-processing model is one of the most fruitful approaches to understanding learning disabilities. Such a model accommodates the major concerns and problems areas in learning, including the cognitive and linguistic processes necessary for the acquisition of academic skills. Also, aspects of information-processing theory serve as the foundation for an important component of intervention that must address and integrate both the process-oriented data (e.g., cognitive, linguistic) and the content-oriented data (e.g., component skills needed for acquisition of reading and writing).

There is always a potential for bias in assessment, and it can affect both the descriptive and programmatic phases of assessment. Diverse professionals involved in the assessment process are generally influenced by the knowledge base in their respective disciplines and look for what they understand to be important aspects of learning and behavior. The adoption of a comprehensive assessment model can clarify the interrelationships among disciplines and improve current practice in evaluating and developing programming for the student with a learning disability.

The translation of a comprehensive assessment model into strategies for obtaining information relevant for identification and educational planning places considerable demands on the multidisciplinary team. It requires that team members have a strong foundation of knowledge pertaining to both the process-oriented and the content-oriented aspects, and skills in translating these factors into specific assessment techniques. Team decision making requires that members have a sound knowledge base, the ability to recognize interactive patterns, and a firm understanding of how a particular testing paradigm affects the interpretation of test results. The assessment of learning disabilities, therefore, must have a sound theoretical base, and the team members must be informed specialists who have kept up with current research in their own and related fields.

Assessment for Identification

Until we refine our understanding of what constitutes a learning disability, the decision to classify a child as learning disabled is made on the basis of a discrepancy between expected and attained achievement and by the progressive exclusion of other causes for the learning deficits. The professional expertise of the multidisciplinary team is of critical importance, and the basis for making the decision must be carefully documented. Assessment to determine eligibility for special education obtains objective descriptions of a child's cognitive, linguistic, and social/emotional status as well as descriptions of educational performance.

In general, formal tests—tests that are norm referenced or standardized—are used extensively for screening and identification purposes. A child suspected of having learning disabilities should be measured in each of the domains (cognitive, linguistic, and social/emotional). Although the cognitive domain can be defined in many different ways, in practice it almost always refers to the measurement of intelligence, The Wechsler Intelligence Scale for Children—Revised (WISC—R) (Wechsler, 1974) is used most often and is related to and predictive of academic success. With the learning disabled child, the intelligence test is used to establish that the child is functioning intellectually within the normal range. Data from the test can also provide information on the underlying abilities that constitute intelligence. Extensive scatter or unevenness within the profile of cognitive abilities may provide insight into the child's information-processing abilities. Skilled clinical analysis of the data can provide information that can be useful in the development of an intervention program.

As is the case in cognitive assessment, formal measurement in the social/emotional domain is used to provide identification information and to rule out severe emotional disturbances as the primary cause of the learning deficits. A language assessment determines whether the child has difficulties in processing linguistically encoded information. Many children with learning disabilities have language problems that impact directly on their academic learning.

Formal measures of academic achievement are used to provide information on the difference between actual achievement and estimated potential in order to implement the identification procedures outlined in the federal rules and regulations. For the most part, the learning disabilities classification has not been operationally defined and still remains largely a matter of clinical judgment, underscoring the importance of team decision making.

Assessment for Instructional Programming

The Individualized Education Program

In order to ensure that a child with a disability receives appropriate services based on planned educational goals and activities determined by the child's parents and school-based personnel, an Individualized Education Program (IEP) is included as a key component of Public Law 94-142. The team decision-making process described earlier is an important component of the law and is also built into the IEP process.

The specific demands of the IEP require that collected data be organized and analyzed systematically. Therefore, it is important that information be collected methodically, organized in an interpretable way, and analyzed for instructional implications. The formal tests that are administered for identification represent only the starting point in the IEP process and generally will be useful only for the most basic aspects of instructional planning. Informal assessment procedures are often the necessary bridge between formal procedures and the instructional program. Data derived from informal measures can be readily used in the construction of the IEP.

Formal measures have serious limitations in terms of generating data to explain underlying systems or in providing directly relevant intervention alternatives. Informal measures are often more descriptive and relevant to the individual and are useful in educational planning for children with learning disabilities, where an understanding of individual differences is critical to effective intervention. Informal assessment approaches assess behavior in more natural contexts (i.e., classroom observations) and in the specific curriculum content of the classroom (criterion-referenced tests, teacher-made tests, etc.). Informal assessment, which generates both qualitative and quantitative data, corresponds more closely to actual behavior. The data and conclusions are specific, representative, and relevant. Informal assessment data can be directly translated into an intervention program more closely tied to meaningful goals, strategies, and activities based on the content of the regular curriculum, the context of the classroom, and the performance patterns of the child.

Quantitative and Qualitative Data

Although formal measures are used primarily to provide identification information rather than instructional programming information, both quantitative and qualitative data can result from the administration of a formal test. **Quantitative data** refers to the actual scores achieved on the test. Examples of quantitative data are statements such as "James scored at the 83rd percentile on the Comprehension subtest of the Stanford Diagnostic Reading Test" or "Robin earned a scaled score of 12 on the Picture Completion subtest of the Wechsler Intelligence Scale for Children—Revised."

Qualitative data consists of (1) observations made while a child is being tested (e.g., child's response characteristics such as frustration tolerance, self-directive behavior, and risk taking) and (2) systematic analysis of the child's performance in order to understand *how* the child achieved the score (e.g., item analysis). In assessment, the nature of the child's errors is often more important than knowing the child's score. For example, on the measure of reading comprehension ability, James may have performed best on factual questions while demonstrating a weakness in the ability to respond to questions requiring inferential reasoning. And, although Robin was able to score in the above-average range on the Picture Completion subtest of the WISC—R, some of her word choices indicated word-retrieval difficulties: she pointed to the "nostril" and said "ear," substituted "the things you pull on" for "knobs," and said, "the thing over here on the door" for "hinge." When tests are used in assessment, the score earned by a child is often the *least* relevant piece of information for instructional planning.

Capacity versus Strategy Deficits

In clinical assessment, a distinction should always be made between underlying abilities and performance. Performance on a task involves the availability of four aspects of cognitive functioning: (1) underlying abilities (i.e., perception, attention, memory), (2) acquired knowledge (i.e., language skills, knowledge of the world in general based on past experience), (3) strategies (i.e., activities undertaken to achieve specific objectives), and (4) metacognition (i.e., awareness of one's own thought processes and the executive functions necessary to regulate the use of basic abilities, knowledge, and strategies).

The purpose of assessment is to measure not only acquired knowledge and how it is used, but also what the child is capable of learning. A child may have the underlying abilities but not an appropriate strategy for effectively acquiring, accessing, or applying knowledge. For example, a child with a learning disability may have the underlying ability or capacity to store verbal information in short-term memory but may not have an effective verbal rehearsal or category clustering strategy for coding the information for storage and retrieval. On the other hand, word-retrieval difficulties may be implicated in short-term memory deficits, in that the child may not have readily accessible high-quality verbal memory codes to represent information in short-term memory. Some children who have learning disabilities appear to have poorer access to a phonetic code or access to a degraded phonetic representation on memory span tasks (Shankweiler et al., 1979). Similarly, reduced language performance does not always indicate that a child does not have adequate knowledge of the linguistic system. Knowledge of the language system may be intact, and reduced language the result of memory processing constraints or situational constraints (Ervin-Tripp, 1971; Slobin, 1971). Performance characteristics in response to specific tasks do not always clearly reflect specific underlying systems; therefore, data available from testing alone cannot always be taken as evidence of underlying ability and/or knowledge deficits.

Assessment that focuses on quantitative data deals only with the products of underlying systems (e.g., the observable responses). Such assessment is more restrictive in determining educational goals than assessment that also measures the patterns of functioning that reflect underlying systems. Patterns of performance that more fully describe the nature of the individual's difficulties are important aspects of a comprehensive assessment and guide the development of effective educational goals and strategies.

Planning Assessment for Intervention

For planning educational interventions, two levels of assessment must be considered and integrated: the content-oriented level and the process-oriented level. At the level of content, assessment must determine what academic abilities or skills the child has already learned and what aspects still remain to be learned. The second level of assessment relates to *how* academic skills are learned, the underlying cognitive or linguistic processes relevant to the acquisition of academic skills. Information obtained from such a broadened perspective may not indicate which specific areas require intervention, but it provides considerable insight into patterns of performance, the child's readiness for structured intervention in academic areas, and appropriate strategies for either intervention or compensatory techniques.

In order to integrate the content-oriented and process-oriented approaches, the assessment process must be based on identification of the component skills that underlie performance of a specific academic task (reading, writing, etc.) and the subsequent development of specific procedures to assess the prerequisite skills and underlying processes required to learn these component skills. For the assessment of specific reading disability, the reading battery should be based on knowledge of the reading acquisition process (knowledge of letter–sound correspondences, automatization of word recognition skills, comprehension skills, etc.); the cognitive battery should be based on an analysis of the cognitive and metacognitive processes relevant to learning to read (short-term verbal memory, phonemic segmentation ability, etc.); and the language battery should be based on an analysis of the language acquisition process relevant to the acquisition of reading skills (understanding sentences and paragraphs, morphophonemic processing, etc.). With these data, the team members can make relevant decisions concerning the *why, what,* and *how* of intervention. The summary of a case history included later in this chapter illustrates how members of an evaluation team can integrate assessment data to make relevant decisions about the educational needs of a student who is language learning disabled.

Because a more complex picture of learning problems has emerged based on linguistic science and information-processing models of learning, assessment of a learning-disabled child requires a multifaceted approach. An effective, interactive team approach to assessment provides the initial foundation for determining the need and nature of an intervention program.

THE INTERVENTION PROGRAM

Intervention, like assessment, requires a multidimensional approach. Decisions to intervene must be made jointly, and interventions must be well planned, integrated, and carefully monitored. The specialists and regular classroom teachers who work with children who have learning disabilities will, to a great extent, be faced with a series of individual problems, and the goal will be to capitalize on the strengths and minimize the limitations of the individual in the interactive learning environment. Learning disabilities are usually identified after children enter school and encounter academic failure. Intervention procedures must take into account the continuing educational demands on the child despite cognitive and/or linguistic deficits. In addition to providing specialized instruction, the specialists working with the child, in collaboration with the regular teacher, must develop procedures that will ameliorate some of the child's problems by modifying the failure-producing aspects of the regular classroom learning environments (e.g., language of the classroom and task demands of the curriculum).

Also, it is important to maximize intervention efforts by integrating planning and implementation across disciplines. Intervention should be an integrated, comprehensive set of activities involving systematic ongoing implementation and evaluation. Specialized content and procedures, including remedial techniques, should be reconceptualized to focus on intervention both within a specific discipline and across disciplines. A generic understanding of intervention planning and implementation across disciplines helps to clarify the interrelationships among disciplines, expands the range of options available, and improves current practice in the delivery of specialized instruction for the learning disabled.

Some of the factors basic to all interventions include the following:

- *Content match.* The information and tasks must not be too different from the child's current knowledge base and way of understanding and learning.
- *Sequence.* Instruction must be sequentially ordered to correspond to the sequence of information needed by the child.
- *Pace.* Instruction must provide for practice, repetition, and overlearning of information that needs to be accessed automatically.
- *Structure.* Intervention components should be taught within and across disciplines and should correspond with the demands of the regular curriculum content.
- *Motivation.* Interventions need to accommodate interests, attitudes, and learning style. Activities that are reinforced will be continued, and immediate feedback will support the maintenance of attention.

The Transdisciplinary Approach

Practitioners should have a comprehensive and generic understanding of intervention planning and implementation across disciplines. This understanding requires a sound grounding in the fundamentals and interrelationships of the diverse disciplines involved in the diagnostic-instructional process. Educational interventions undertaken on behalf of the learning disabled are often arbitrary and fragmented. We are only beginning to understand the developmental and behavioral characteristics of individuals with learning disabilities. Potential interventions based on linguistic science and information-processing models of learning are emerging. They strongly suggest the need for a holistic, integrated, transdisciplinary approach to educational planning. The complex interactive nature of cognitive and linguistic processes and academic learning indicates the need for a broad-based, multidimensional approach to the development of an educational program for the student with learning disabilities.

At the same time, the new requirements of the 1997 reauthorization of the Individuals with Disabilities Act (IDEA) mandate that Individualized Education Programs (IEPs) must be developed in the context of the general education curriculum in order to better support academic learning in the regular classroom. This new inclusionary model of service delivery has led to a redefinition of the roles and responsibilities of all school-based practitioners, who must now function as partners in educational teams in regular classrooms. Collaborative in-classroom intervention underscores the need for a transdisciplinary framework that focuses on a shared understanding of instructional purposes and the interrelatedness of instructional goals and objectives across diverse disciplines (Giangrico, Prelock, Reid, Dennis & Edelman, 2000; Landerholm, 1990; Whitmere, 2000).

With specific reference to the student who has a language learning disability, the interactive nature of underlying information-processing abilities and academic learning has specific implications for the development of interrelated educational goals, objectives, and activities. Integration of instruction across diverse disciplines can enhance both the compensatory and remedial aspects of instruction for the student with a language learning disability.

Compensatory aspects of instruction can be addressed by the language specialist, who can make recommendations for modifications in both the style and structure of the language of the classroom. There are aspects of language processing that are applicable to the educational management of the child whose processing abilities have not developed optimally. Instructional personnel could be guided to simplify the language of instruction by using shorter, less complex sentences and by making longer pauses and more frequent restatements of information. Knowledge of more specific aspects of language processing is also important. As an example, instructional personnel should be aware that formulating oral or written instructions or directions in the affirmative whenever possible, rather than in the negative, will reduce language processing difficulties. Also, because implicit negatives such as *different* (i.e., not the same), *absent* (i.e., not present), and *except* (i.e., not all) are processed in the same way as explicit negatives, these will be equally difficult for some children.

Similarly, the integration of remedial aspects of instruction can increase the impact of educational planning for the student with a language learning disability. An assessment model that identifies the interactive cognitive and/or linguistic correlates of reading skill acquisition at both the initial and transitional stages of reading instruction has implications for the integration of instruction. For example, at the initial stages of reading instruction, phonemic segmentation skills are critical in learning to use phonic cues (i.e., to make use of letter–sound correspondences) to help in identifying the words represented by a sequence of letters. Many children with learning disabilities have trouble learning to use phonic cues because they do not recognize that words can be segmented into syllables and syllables into distinct phonemes, and that phonemic segmentation is represented graphically by the use of specific letters placed in sequence. Assessment and subsequent remedial training of phonemic segmentation skills could be undertaken jointly by the language and learning disabilities specialists. Also, modifications in the method of teaching initial reading need to be made for the child with poor segmentation skills. An instructional procedure that places less initial emphasis on phonic skills (e.g., a word-family or structural analysis approach) should be used for the teaching of word recognition skills.

Also, many elements of whole-language instruction should be considered for use with students with learning disabilities. This instructional approach derives from the belief that children can acquire spoken literacy in much the same way that they acquire language and emphasizes the wholeness of reading and writing. Because whole-language practices include daily writing and the reading of authentic literature (e.g., trade books), this emphasis on the inherent reciprocity and interdependence of reading and writing maximizes learning of literacy skills for students. However, explicit instruction that promotes facility in word recognition is vitally important for efficient reading, especially for beginning readers who are likely to be at risk for reading failure (Mather, 1992; Pressley & Rankin, 1994; Stanovich, 1991; Vellutino & Scanlon, 1991). Therefore, current research appears to support a balanced approach to initial reading instruction (Dahl & Scharer, 2000; Pressley, Rankin, Gaskins, Brown, & El-Dinary, 1995; Sawyer, 1991).

For students who have difficulty in making progress primarily though immersion in a language-rich environment, explicit code-based instruction should be integrated with the reading of whole authentic texts and student journal writing. The assimilation of skill instruction into a meaningful context enables children to learn that the ultimate goal of all reading instruction is to enhance their ability to derive meaning from text.

Similar interrelated educational goals and activities can be identified at the transitional stage of reading acquisition. The syntactic language problems evidenced by a student with a language learning disability will also be reflected in various reading behaviors such as understanding syntactically complex sentences or using syntactic constraints to assist in word identification. Remedial training to intensify awareness of the syntactic structure of complex sentences by manipulating clausal units would be a valid transdisciplinary activity that could be integrated into language, reading, and writing instruction. For example, the learning disabled student's linguistic skills and linguistic awareness can be improved by training in sentence expansion and in sentence combining and/or sentence decombining exercises (Norris & Crump, 1982; Seidenberg, 1982; Wallach & Wallach, 1976).

Because the semantic processing problems of many students with language learning disabilities also affect reading comprehension and content learning, an integrated instructional approach focusing on the structure and process of semantic memory can ameliorate some of their learning problems. Transdisciplinary training in the use of more effective word elaboration strategies (e.g., classifying and categorizing) as well as in the use of strategies for analyzing semantic features of concepts, such as semantic mapping or webbing (e.g., explicating the relationships among superordinate, coordinate, and subordinate concepts), can enhance both content learning and text comprehension (Anders & Bos, 1986; Bos, Anders, Filip, & Jaffe, 1989; Mastropieri et al., 1987).

Additionally, it is important that practitioners develop comprehensive intervention programs that incorporate instructional sequences that explicitly teach critical metacognitive strategies to students with learning disabilities (Seidenberg, 1991). Currently, strategy deficit models of learning disabilities are the most prevalent theoretical orientation shaping both intervention research and practice for this population (Scruggs, 1991). As indicated earlier, a considerable body of literature supports the notion that many children with learning disabilities are inactive learners who fail spontaneously to access or use effective cognitive strategies for solving academic problems. These students tend not to believe in their own efforts or abilities and have an inadequate understanding of the cognitive strategies available for successful performance on academic tasks (Borkowski, Weyhing, & Carr, 1988; Torgesen, 1986). Therefore, students with learning disabilities frequently require direct instruction in those strategic processing skills that non-learning-disabled students acquire and apply automatically (Harris, 1990; Harris & Pressley, 1991).

Also, interventions derived from an information-processing perspective emphasize specific instruction and practice on component reading and writing skills in contrast to practice in general language or problem-solving skills in a context outside of reading and writing tasks. Information-processing research supports the context-bound nature of strategic processing skills for many academic tasks (Paris & Oka, 1989; Siegler, 1983; Stanovich, 1986; Vellutino, 1979). There is evidence that training students with learning disabilities to use task-specific cognitive strategies improves their performance particularly on complex reading and writing tasks that have high information-processing demands (Dye, 2000; Graham, Harris, & Troia, 2000; Swanson, 1991).

Students with learning disabilities who have been taught metacognitive strategies have shown improved performance in a variety of tasks, including the self-monitoring of on-task behavior (Kneedler & Hallahan, 1981), the detection of contextual inconsistencies (Capelli & Markman, 1982), comprehension monitoring (Wong & Jones, 1982; Palincsar & Brown, 1986), improvement of spelling ability (Gerber, 1986; Wong, 1986), and awareness and use of text organization for improved comprehension and composing skills (Englert, Raphael, Anderson, Gregg, & Anthony, 1989; Englert & Raphael, 1988; Welch, 1992; Wong & Wilson, 1984; Wong, Butler, Ficzere & Kuperis, 1996).

The instructional principles derived from the intervention research highlight the importance of interactive dialogues and the modeling of strategic activities as well as the scaffolding of instruction around domain-specific content knowledge and strategic knowledge (e.g., the associated task-specific cognitive strategies). Effective instructional interventions for complex academic tasks share a number of features, including:

1. Heightening the learner's awareness of the demands of a task
2. Instructing the learner in the appropriate strategies to facilitate successful task completion

3. Explicit modeling of the use of the strategies
4. Providing guided practice and feedback regarding the application of the strategies
5. Providing instruction for generalized use of the strategies

Table 9.1 provides an example of an instructional sequence for teaching the strategic processing skills needed for successful performance of a complex academic task. Interventions based on an information-processing perspective that address students' academic deficits directly and incorporate an instructional technology focusing on the interactive nature of the teaching–learning process appear to hold the most promise for enabling students with learning disabilities to become more successful learners.

Therefore, practitioners need to enlarge the scope of their instructional practices by gaining a better understanding of the role that metacognitive factors play in the learning needs of the learning-disabled population. At the same time, practitioners must integrate their efforts in order to maximize the impact of the instructional program for students with learning disabilities in inclusionary classroom settings.

TABLE 9.1 | **Teaching a Cognitive Strategy for a Complex Academic Task**

Step 1: *Introduction of Strategy and Performance Review*
The teacher explains the strategy, and students and teacher review the students' current level of performance (e.g., pretest outcomes).

Step 2: *Relevance of the Strategy*
The teacher explains why the strategy should be learned, and students and teacher generate examples of strategy application.

Step 3: *Strategy Description*
The teacher describes how to use the strategy and provides the students with a "help sheet" listing the steps.

Step 4: *Modeling the Strategy*
The teacher models the use of the strategy, demonstrating aloud the thinking process underlying the separate steps. As a group, the teacher and students model and rehearse the use of the strategy.

Step 5: *When to Use the Strategy*
The teacher explains the conditions for use of the strategy.

Step 6: *Practice in Controlled Material*
The students apply the strategy to controlled practice material while the teacher provides prompts and corrective feedback as necessary.

Step 7: *Evaluation of Strategy Use*
The teacher shows students a method for evaluating the use of the strategy.

Step 8: *Strategy Generalization*
The students apply the strategy to complete assignments required in regular content area classrooms.

Source: P. L. Seidenberg, Cognitive and academic instructional intervention for learning disabled adolescents, *Topics in Language Disorders, 8,* No. 3, p. 65, reprinted with permission of Aspen Publishers, Inc. © 1988.

Careful planning and identification of effective cognitive strategies that are most likely to facilitate a student's academic learning are essential for supporting accessibility to the regular education curriculum. Educators need to assume new collaborative roles and responsibilities to meet this challenge and to fulfill the promise of meeting the special educational needs of students with learning disabilities.

CASE STUDY

The following summary of a case history for Robert, a first grader, illustrates how members of a multidisciplinary team identify a child as learning disabled. The screening team, comprised of professionals from diverse disciplines, meets at the time of initial referral and, based on the nature of the referral information, develops a plan to guide the assessment process. Wherever possible, they see the child jointly in order to avoid miscommunication based on different disciplinary outlooks. The professionals (school psychologist, learning disability specialist, language specialist, etc.) involved in the evaluation process discuss their findings, and the final report reflects the conclusions of each team member.

Identification Information

Name: Robert G.	Birthdate: July 10, 1993
Age: 6 yrs. 6 mos.	School Placement: Windmere Elementary School
Grade: First	Date of Report: January 15, 2000

Reason for Referral

At the request of his classroom teacher and with the written consent of his parents, Robert was referred for a psychoeducational evaluation. Robert is reported to be having difficulty learning to read and write. The teacher reports that he exhibits written reversals, transposition of letters, and poor phonic decoding skills. The teacher also states that Robert's difficulties appear to be associated with distractibility, confusions in directionality and sequencing, and poor ability to process auditory information. An evaluation is being done to better understand Robert's current functional ability and to assist in educational planning.

Summary of Behavioral Observations

Robert is a sturdy, well-built youngster. He appears active and alert and was not overly apprehensive during the initial testing session. Robert speaks in well-organized sentences that are logical and easy to follow, and his vocabulary appears to be within normal limits. He exhibits some articulation difficulties. Robert was able to work steadily and persistently on many of the tasks presented. However, there were also tasks on which he performed poorly or was completely unable to perform, and restlessness and increased distractibility were observable at these times.

Summary of Background Information

Birth and developmental milestones for Robert are described as "normal." Robert's health history indicates hospitalization for a myringotomy just prior to school entrance. He also experiences an allergic reaction to milk and milk products. He still has a recurrent hearing problem, and his most recent audiological examination again detected fluid in the middle ear. This may account, in part, for his articulation problems.

Summary of Assessment Procedures

Tests administered include:

1. *Wechsler Intelligence Scale for Children—Revised* (WISC—III)

Verbal IQ	115
Performance IQ	105
Full Scale IQ	112

   Verbal Scaled Score

Information	10
Similarities	15
Arithmetic	11
Vocabulary	14
Comprehension	13
(Digit Span)	(9)

   Performance Scaled Score

Picture Completion	13
Picture Arrangement	9
Block Design	9
Object Assembly	15
Coding	8

2. *Bender Visual-Motor Gestalt Test* (Initial and Recall)
3. *Human Figure Drawing*
4. *Wepman Auditory Discrimination Test*
5. *Clinical Evaluation of Language Functions* (CELF—R)
   Recalling Sentences
   Formulating Sentences
   Semantic Relationships
   Oral Directions
6. *Key Math Diagnostic Arithmetic Test*
7. *Metropolitan Reading Test—Level II* (Form P)
   Beginning Consonants
   Sound–Letter Correspondence
   Visual Matching
   Listening

In addition to the formal tests, Robert was asked to copy numbers, letters, and words. He also completed a trial reading lesson using a language-experience approach. He dictated a brief story and then was asked to read his story to the examiner. Robert also identified a word in his own story that he wanted to learn to read and write. A multisensory approach was used successfully to teach word-recognition and spelling skills.

Summary of Test Results

Robert's scores on the WISC—III indicate that he is functioning intellectually in the high average range. However, there are variations in the subtest scores ranging from below average to superior.

Robert's fund of information was average, with failures on comparatively easy items and successes on more difficult ones. Verbal fluency appeared to interfere with performance on this task, and he would comment, "I know the name but I forget," or "I can't think of the name of it." At the same time, expressive vocabulary was in the superior range, and he was able to make excellent responses when he was not limited to retrieving a specific word from memory but could make semantic substitutions.

Abstract verbal reasoning (similarities) and judgment, common sense, and reality testing (comprehension) were all in the high average range. The quality of his responses indicated good ability to make abstractions and understand superordinate classification. His ability to do in-the-head arithmetic was above average, and his lowest score was on the Digit Span subtest, which was below average. He was able to repeat up to five digits forward but was unable to repeat more than two digits backward without reversing the order of presentation.

On the performance tasks, Robert's highest score (very superior on Object Assembly) reflected an ability to organize and work toward a concrete goal. His visual memory, necessary for recognition of essential details, was also above average. On the remaining tasks, such as replicating designs of blocks and sequencing a series of pictures in a logical order, he scored below average. His lowest score was for the transposition of symbols within a time limit (Coding) and was in the defective range. Robert appears to have visual-motor coordination difficulties. He is also experiencing problems with more integrative visual skills, such as sequencing, directionality, and perception of spatially defined complex stimuli (e.g., block designs). On the other hand, Robert's figure drawing was age appropriate and indicated the ability to integrate and organize the spatial details.

Robert's performance on the Bender-Gestalt, an assessment of his own response to his perceptual organization of visual information, also indicated difficulty in integration of details and organization of spatially defined stimuli. Problems with integrative skills were evidenced in his loss of angulation and difficulties in maintaining the overall structure of shapes. He has difficulty in reproducing details and in storing visual information. His visual memory for designs indicates that he was able to recall only two of the Bender designs after the initial copying task. Also, there is evidence of slowness of response to graphomotor tasks, not only on the Coding subtest of the WISC—R but also in his handwriting.

Robert's performance on a number of formal and informal language-processing measures showed an inconsistent response pattern similar to his intelligence test profile. Informal observation of his language skills indicated that he is able to understand everyday conversation and to express his ideas in age-appropriate syntax. On the Wepman Auditory Discrimination Test, Robert was able to differentiate the phonemic likenesses and differences in word pairs. However, he has articulation difficulties that appear to be persistent and systematic. Further assessment is indicated in this area. On the recalling sentences subtest of the Clinical Evaluation of Language Function (CELF—R), Robert performed well above age expectancy but at only the beginning first-grade level for a task requiring the formulation of sentences (e.g., "Make a sentence with the word *car*"). His performance was age appropriate for a task tapping his understanding of semantic relationships. However, he had difficulty in retaining a series of oral directions in short-term memory and executing them. Robert attempted to use verbal rehearsal strategy to facilitate recall, but because his phonological reproduction and verbal fluency are faulty, rehearsal is also impaired.

Robert's performance on the Metropolitan Readiness subtests was slightly better for a task requiring the matching of beginning sounds (60th percentile) than it was for the other subtests administered (50th percentile). In making sound–letter correspondences, both initial-consonant and consonant-blend inaccuracies were noted. He was not able to match the letters *c, g, d, pl, tr, gr,* and *cl* to their phonemic counterparts in words (*cat, goat,* etc.). However, on the visual matching subtest, Robert was able to match all of the letter sequences accurately and encountered difficulty only with the letterlike shapes or designs. His performance on the listening subtest indicates good ability to integrate and draw inferences when information is presented orally but poor comprehension of comparative relationships (*taller, bigger,* etc.).

On the Key Math Diagnostic Test, Robert scored at an overall grade equivalent of 1.5. His understanding of the number system was at a 2.5 grade level, and his numerical reasoning and ability to solve simple one-step story problems was at a 2.0 grade level. His ability to perform written, single-digit addition and subtraction computations was at a 1.6 grade level. He had difficulty with money problems (e.g., coin values), but he can recognize and apply common units of measurement (e.g., ruler, thermometer) and units of time (e.g., clock, calendar). Robert was able to write the numbers from 1 to 10, but there were still some directional confusions noted (e.g., 6, 9, and 10) that are not inappropriate for a beginning first-grader. Although his graphomotor responses are slow and labored, he can copy letters and numbers accurately.

Summary of Conclusions

Robert appears to be a child of above-average intelligence with indications for better potential. He would be expected to function in academic areas at or above his grade placement. At this time, he is impeded academically by specific learning deficits in oral language, reading, and writing. His uneven performance patterns indicate that he is experiencing difficulties in those areas involving expressive language abilities (e.g., speech production, verbal fluency, and sentence formulation), auditory and visual sequential memory, spatial concepts, and visual-motor integration. He also exhibits fatigue and distractibility, especially when tasks are hard or frustrating. His arithmetic concepts and ability to do in-the-head arithmetic are excellent, but he is not doing as well as most of the other children in his grade in the acquisition of reading and writing skills. The evaluation data indicate that Robert will not acquire reading and writing skills consistent with expectations without special education and related services, and, therefore, the classification of *learning disabled* is indicated.

Summary of Recommendations

Robert's oral expressive language deficits are implicated in his learning difficulties and indicate the need for further assessment by the speech-language pathologist. In-depth testing of Robert's receptive and expressive language skills is recommended, including a phonological, semantic, syntactic, and pragmatic analysis of a language sample. The content of an appropriate language intervention program for Robert will depend on the results of the language assessment.

A traditional synthetic phonics approach to initial reading instruction would not be appropriate for Robert at this time. Although he uses immediate rehearsal to re-create a discrete phoneme (sound), the phonological reproduction is inaccurate, resulting in impaired or inconsistent recall of phonemes and phonemic patterns. Robert would benefit from training in rhyming, phoneme segmentation, and recognition of syllable types in order to increase phonological awareness. He needs guided practice in parsing written words into the spelling units that correspond to phonemes and/or syllables. Also, instruction should proceed in both directions, that is, from spelling units to phonemes and from phonemes to spelling.

In order to utilize his cognitive and linguistic abilities, a language experience approach in which he dictates and then reads his own stories would be an effective component of initial reading instruction. A method for the teaching of word recognition and spelling should integrate the visual, tactile, and auditory modes (e.g., Fernold technique) and could be based, initially, on the words found in his own stories. Additionally, daily writing from dictation and many opportunities to read connected text for fluency and meaning could be used successfully with Robert at this time.

Robert has difficulty in attending to oral directions. He attempts to use verbal rehearsal to facilitate recall, but his reproductions are inconsistent and inaccurate, and interfere with his retrieval of the auditory information. It is important, therefore, that his teachers speak clearly, use short sentences with simple syntax, and check periodically on the accuracy of his recall of the information. Robert could be asked to repeat directions to be sure that he recalls them accurately

Robert uses a great deal of verbal mediation; that is, he talks himself through tasks. This is an excellent strategy for him and should be encouraged. For example, he could be taught to use verbal supports or associations to focus attention on relevant directional aspects of letters or numbers and, thus, guide his graphomotor responses.

Handwriting skills will need to be taught in carefully sequenced incremental steps, and particular attention will need to be paid to establishing the fine-motor patterns needed for writing. Initially, he will profit from handwriting automaticity training to improve fluency in retrieving and producing the one- and two-letter spelling units in written words that correspond to the phoneme–letter(s) associations that specifically underlie the alphabetic principle. Gradually, the training should be expanded to also include whole words and syllable structure types. Also, lengthy tasks requiring graphomotor responses (workbook exercises, copying from the chalkboard, etc.) should be adjusted for Robert's current level of functioning. He attempts to compensate cognitively for his visual-motor difficulties. He can be successful if given adequate structure and time.

As is typical of underachieving youngsters with excellent potential, Robert is beginning to experience confusion in reconciling the apparent conflict in feedback from the important adults in his life. That is, on the one hand, that he is a capable youngster; and, on the other, that he is having difficulties in learning. He is becoming extremely frustrated and unhappy because of his uneven functioning. Therefore, it is important that the educational program planned for Robert provide him with opportunities to use his cognitive and linguistic strengths and help him to compensate for his deficit areas.

SUMMARY

That deficits in learning are a major cause of school failure is currently well accepted, and new approaches to identification and educational planning have developed that are based on information-processing theory. Learning disabilities derive from innate disorders that alter cognitive processes. These alterations in cognitive functioning vary in type and degree of severity and, therefore, in behavioral consequences.

An understanding of the interactive nature of language and cognition contributes to our understanding of the problems in comprehension and formulation of written language experienced by many children who have learning disabilities. Both reading and writing performance reflect the knowledge and the linguistic and cognitive competencies available to the learner and how these are activated and integrated during the acquisition of reading and writing skills. In addition to disorders in verbal language, a fundamental deficit for many children with learning disabilities appears to be an inability to use effective cognitive strategies for the comprehension or production of written language.

Because of the heterogeneity of the learning-disabled population, the assessment process must be flexible and responsive to individual differences (see Chapter 5). Practitioners from diverse disciplines need to collaborate in decision-making activities. A multidisciplinary approach based on a comprehensive assessment model that provides for the systematic collection, organization, and analysis of assessment data needs to be adopted. The data must adequately describe the nature of an individual's difficulties and guide the development of an effective educational program. An interactive, collaborative, team approach to assessment and intervention also provides the foundation for the integration of learning experiences and educational services for children with learning disabilities.

STUDY QUESTIONS

1. Identify and discuss the major components of the information-processing model. Include in the discussion the implications for understanding the perceptual, attentional, and memory deficits of the student who is learning-disabled.
2. Briefly present six characteristics that may be exhibited by learning disabled students with language deficits.
3. How does the interaction of linguistic and cognitive variables affect the acquisition of reading and writing skills?
4. Outline the research findings pertaining to cognitive and/or metacognitive deficits in relation to how students with learning disabilities acquire reading skills.
5. Briefly discuss several factors that may be related to writing disabilities. Discuss some writing behaviors exhibited by students with learning disabilities.
6. Discuss the advantages and disadvantages of formal and informal assessment in the identification of students with learning disabilities.

7. What are the important characteristics of an effective intervention program for the student who is learning disabled?
8. Describe and discuss the key components of intervention programs that incorporate instruction in metacognitive strategies.

REFERENCES

American Psychiatric Association. (1994). *Diagnostic and statistical manual of mental disorders* (4th ed.). Washington, DC: APA.

Anders, P. L., & Bos, C. S. (1986). Semantic feature analysis: An interactive strategy for vocabulary development and text comprehension. *Journal of Reading, 29,* 610–616.

Anderson, B. R. (1975). *Cognitive psychology.* New York: Academic.

Anderson, R. C., Spiro, R. J., & Montague, W. D. (1977). *Schooling and the acquisition of knowledge.* Hillsdale, NJ: Lawrence Erlbaum Associates.

Applebee, A. (1978). *The child's concept of story.* Chicago: University of Chicago Press.

August, G. J. & Garfinkel, B. D. (1990). Comorbity of ADHD among clinic-referred children. *Journal of Abnormal Child Psychology, 18,* 29–45.

Baker, J. G., Ceci, S. J., & Hermann, D. (1987). Semantic structure and processing: Implications for the learning disabled child. In H. L. Swanson (Ed.), *Memory and learning disabilities: Advances in learning and behavioral disabilities.* Greenwich, CT: JAI Press.

Baker, L., & Cantwell, D. S. (1990). The association between emotional/behavior disorders and learning disorders with speech/language disorders. *Advances in Learning and Behavioral Disabilities, 6,* 26–46.

Barkley, R. A., Fischer, M., Edelbrock, C., & Smallish, L. (1990). The adolescent outcome of hyperactive children diagnosed by research criteria: An 8-year follow-up study. *Journal of the American Academy of Child and Adolescent Psychology, 29,* 546–557.

Bauer, R. H. (1977). Memory processes in children with learning disabilities. *Journal of Experimental Child Psychology, 18,* 283–296.

Berko, J. (1958). The child's learning of English morphology. *Word, 14,* 150–177.

Berry, M. F. (1980). *Teaching linguistically handicapped children.* Englewood Cliffs, NJ: Prentice Hall.

Biederman, J., Newcorn, J., & Sprich, S. (1991). Comorbidity of ADHD with conduct, depression, anxiety, and other disorders. *American Journal of Psychiatry, 148,* 564–577.

Blackman, B. (1984). Language analysis skills and early reading acquisition. In G. Wallach & K. Buder (Eds.), *Language learning disabilities in school-age children.* Baltimore: Williams & Wilkins.

Blair, T. K., & Crump, W. D. (1984). Effects of discourse made on the syntactic complexity of learning disabled students' written expression. *Learning Disability Quarterly, 17,* 19–29.

Blalock, J. (1981). Persistent problems and concerns of young adults with learning disabilities. In W. Cruickshank & A. Silvers (Eds.), *Bridges to tomorrow: The best of ACDL* (Vol. 2). Syracuse, NY: Syracuse University Press.

Borkowski, J. G., Johnston, M. D., & Reid, M. (1987). Metacognition, motivation and controlled performance. In S. Ceci (Ed.), *Handbook of cognitive, social and neurological aspects of learning disabilities.* Hillsdale, NJ: Lawrence Erlbaum Associates.

Borkowski, J. G., & Kurtz, B. E. (1987). Motivation and executive control. In J. G. Borkowski and J. D. Day (Eds.), *Cognition in special children.* Norwood, NJ: Ablex.

Borkowski, J. G., Weyhing, R. S., & Carr, M. (1988). Effects of attributional retraining on strategy-based reading comprehension in learning disabled students. *Journal of Educational Psychology, 75,* 544–552.

Bos, C., Anders, P. L., Filip, D., & Jaffe, L. E. (1989). The effects of an interactive instructional strategy for enhancing learning disabled students' reading comprehension and content area learning. *Journal of Learning Disabilities, 22,* 384–390.

Bos, C. S., & Filip, D. (1984). Comprehension monitoring in learning disabled and average students. *Journal of Learning Disabilities, 17,* 229–233.

Bougere, M. (1969). Selected factors in oral language related to first grade reading performance. *Reading Research Quarterly, 5,* 31–58.

Bransford, J. D., Stein, B. S., Shelton, T. S., & Owings, R. A. (1980). Cognition and adaptation: The importance of learning to learn. In J. Harvey (Ed.), *Cognition, social behavior and the environment.* Hillsdale, NJ: Lawrence Erlbaum Associates.

Brittain, M. A. (1970). Inflectional performance and early reading achievement. *Reading Research Quarterly, 6,* 34–48.

Brown, A. L. (1978). Knowing when, where and how to remember, a problem of metacognition. In R. Glaser (Ed.), *Advances in instructional psychology.* Hillsdale, NJ: Lawrence Erlbaum Associates.

Bryan, J. H. (1981). Social behaviors of learning disabled children. In J. Gottlieb & S. Strichart (Eds.), *Developmental theory and research in learning disabilities.* Baltimore: University Park Press.

Bryant, P., & Bradley, L. (1981). Visual memory and phonological skills in reading and spelling backwardness. *Psychological Research, 43,* 193–199.

Butkowsky, I. S., & Willows, D. M. (1980). Cognitive-motivational characteristics of children varying in reading ability: Evidence for learned helplessness in poor readers. *Journal of Educational Psychology, 72,* 408–422.

Campione, J. C., & Brown, A. L. (1978). Toward a theory of intelligence. *Intelligence, 2,* 279–304.

Cantwell, D. P., & Baker, L. (1991). Association between attention deficit hyperactivity disorders and learning disorders. *Journal of Learning Disabilities, 24,* 88–95.

Capelli, C. A., & Markman, E. M. (1982). Suggestions for training comprehension monitoring. *Topics in Learning and Learning Disorders, 2,* 87–96.

Catts, H., & Kamhi, A. (1999). Causes of reading disabilities. In H. Catts & A. Kamhi (Eds.), *Language and Reading Disabilities* (pp. 95–127). Boston: Allyn & Bacon.

Catts, H. W. (1991). Early identification of dyslexia: Evidence of a follow-up study of speech-language impaired children. *Annals of Dyslexia, 41,* 143–157.

Catts, H. W., & Kamhi, A. G. (1986). The linguistic basis of reading disorders: Implications for the speech-language pathologist. *Language, Speech and Hearing Services in Schools, 17,* 329–341.

Cazden, C. B. (1972). *Child language and education.* New York: Holt, Rinehart & Winston.

Ceci, S. J. (1982). Extracting meaning from stimuli: Automatic and purposive processing of the language-based learning disabled. *Topics in Learning and Learning Disabilities, 2,* 46–53.

Chalfont, J. C., & Scheffelin, M. A. (1969). *Central processing dysfunctions in children: A review of research* (NINDS Monograph No. 9). Bethesda, MD: U.S. Department of Health, Education and Welfare.

Chan, L. K. S., Cole, P. G., & Barfett, S. (1987). Comprehension monitoring: Detection and identification of text inconsistencies by LD and normal students. *Learning Disabilities Quarterly, 10,* 114–124.

Cici, R. (1980). Written language disorders. *Bulletin of the Orton Society, 30,* 240–251.

Cohen, N. J., Devine, M., & Meloche-Kelly, M. (1989). Prevalence of unsuspected language in child psychiatric population. *Journal of American Academy of Child and Adolescent Psychiatry, 28,* 107–111.

Cohen, R. (1982). Individual differences in short-term memory. *International Review of Research in Mental Retardation, 11,* 43–77.

Connolly, A., Nachtman, W., & Pritchett, E. (1971). *Key Math Diagnostic Arithmetic Test.* Circle Pines, MN: American Guidance Services.

Cruickshank, W., Bentzen, F., Razburg, F., & Tannhauser, M. (1961). *A teaching-method for brain-injured and hyperactive children.* Syracuse, NY: Syracuse University Press.

Dahl, K. L., & Scharer, P. L. (2000). Phonics teaching and learning in whole language classrooms: New evidence from research. *The Reading Teacher, 53,* 516–523.

Davila, R. R., Williams, M. L., & MacDonald, J. T. (1991). *Clarification of policy to address the needs of children with attention deficit disorders within general and special education.* Washington, DC: U.S. Department of Education.

Denckla, M. B., & Rudel, R. (1976). Naming of pictured objects by dyslexic and other learning-disabled children. *Brain and Language, 39,* 1–15.

Denner, F. (1970). Representational and syntactic competence of problem readers. *Child Development, 41,* 881–887.

Deshler, D. L., Schumaker, J. B., & Lenz, B. K. (1984). Academic and cognitive interventions for LD adolescents: Part I. *Journal of Learning Disabilities, 17,* 108–117.

Dillon, G., & Dodd, B. (1994). A prospective study of the relationship between phonological, semantic and syntactic skills and specific reading disability. *Reading and Writing, 6,* 321–345.

Dye, G. A. (2000). Graphic organizers to the rescue. Helping students link and remember information. *Exceptional Children, 66,* 72–76.

Edwards, H. T., & Kallail, K. J. (1977, November). Ability of learning disabled and regular classroom adolescents to close structure and content words. Paper presented at the national convention of the American Speech and Hearing Association, Chicago.

Ellis, E. S., & Lenz, B. K. (1987). A component analysis of effective learning strategies for LD students. *Learning Disabilities Focus, 2,* 94–107.

Ellis, N. (1981). Visual and name coding in dyslexic children. *Psychological Research, 43,* 201–219.

Englert, C. S., & Raphael, T. E. (1988). Constructing well-formed prose: Process, structure and metacognitive knowledge. *Exceptional Children, 54,* 513–520.

Englert, C. S., Raphael, T. E., Anderson, L. M., Gregg, S. L., & Anthony, H. M. (1989). Exposition: Reading, writing and metacognitive knowledge of learning disabled students. *Learning Disabilities Research, 5,* 5–24.

Englert, C. S., & Thomas, C. C. (1987). Sensitivity to text structure in reading and writing: A comparison of learning disabled and nonhandicapped students. *Learning Disability Quarterly, 10,* 93–105.

Epstein, M. A., Shaywitz, S. E., Shaywitz, B. A., & Woolston, J. L. (1991). The boundaries of attention deficit disorder. *Journal of Disabilities, 24,* 78–86.

Ervin-Tripp, S. (1971). Social backgrounds and verbal skills. In T. Moore (Ed.), *Language acquisition: Models and methods.* New York: Academic.

Farnham-Diggory, S. (1980). Learning disabilities: A view from cognitive science. *Journal of the American Academy of Child Psychiatry, 19,* 570–578.

Flavell, J. H. (1978). Metacognitive development. In J. M. Scandura & C. J. Brainerd (Eds.), *Structural process theories of human behavior.* Hillsdale, NJ: Lawrence Erlbaum Associates.

Fleisher, L. S., Jenkins, J. R., & Pany, D. (1979). Effects on poor readers' comprehension of training in rapid decoding. *Reading Research Quarterly, 15,* 30–48.

Fleisher, L. S., Soodak, L. C., & Jelin, M. A. (1984). Selective attention deficits in learning disabled children: Analysis of the database. *Exceptional Children, 51,* 136–141.

Fox, B., & Routh, D. K. (1980). Phonemic analysis and severe reading disability in children. *Journal of Psycholinguistic Research, 9,* 115–119.

Frostig, M. (1968). Education for children with hearing disabilities. In H. Myklebust (Ed.), *Progress in learning disabilities.* New York: Grune & Stratton.

Garner, R., & Reis, R. (1981). Monitoring and resolving comprehension obstacles. *Reading Research Quarterly, 16,* 569–582.

Gelheiser, L. M. (1984). Generalization from categorical memory tasks to prose by learning disabled adolescents. *Journal of Educational Psychology, 76,* 1128–1138.

Gerber, M. M. (1984). Investigations of the orthographic problem-solving ability in learning disabled and normally achieving students. *Learning Disability Quarterly, 7,* 157–164.

Gerber, M. M. (1986). Generalization of spelling strategies by LD students as a result of contingent imitation/modeling and mastery criteria. *Journal of Learning Disabilities, 19,* 530–537.

Giangrico, M. F., Prelock, P. A., Reid, R. R., Dennis, R. E., & Edelman, S. W. (2000). Role of related services personnel in inclusive schools. In R. A. Villa & J. S. Thousand (Eds.), *Restructuring for Caring and Effective Education: Piecing the Puzzle Together* (pp. 360–388). Baltimore: Paul H. Brookes.

Gibbs, D. P., & Cooper, E. B. (1989). Prevalence of communication disorders in students with learning disabilities. *Journal of Learning Disabilities, 22,* 60–63.

Golinkoff, R. M. (1976). A comparison of reading comprehension processes in good and poor comprehenders. *Reading Research Quarterly, 11,* 623–659.

Goodman, K. S. (1973). Psycholinguistic universals in the reading process. In F. Smith (Ed.), *Psycholinguistics and reading.* New York: Holt, Rinehart & Winston.

Graham, S., Harris, K. R., & Troia, G. A. (2000). Self-regulated strategy development revisited: Teaching writing strategies to struggling writers. *Topics in Language Disorders, 20,* 1–14.

Gregg, N. (1983). College learning disabled writer: Error patterns and instructional alternatives. *Journal of Learning Disabilities, 16,* 334–338.

Hallahan, D., Gajar, A., Cohen, S., & Tarver, S. (1978). Selective attention and locus of control in learning disabled and normal children. *Journal of Learning Disabilities, 4,* 47–52.

Hallahan, D., & Reeves, R. (1980). Selective attention and distractibility. In B. Keogh (Ed.), *Advances in special education.* Greenwich, CT: JAI Press.

Hallahan, D., & Sapona, R. (1984). Self-monitoring of attention with learning disabled children: Past practice and current issues. *Annual Review of Learning Disabilities, 2,* 97–101.

Hammill, D., Leiger, J., McNutt, G., & Larsen, T. (1981). A new definition of learning disabilities. *Learning Disability Quarterly, 4,* 336–342.

Hammill, D., & McNutt, B. (1981). *Correlates of reading: The consensus of thirty years of research.* Austin, TX: Pro-Ed.

Harris, K. (1990). Developing self-regulation learners: The role of private speech and self-instructions. *Educational Psychologist, 25,* 35–50.

Harris, K., Pressley, M. (1991). The nature of cognitive strategy instruction: Interactive strategy construction. *Exceptional Children, 57,* 392–404.

Hiebert, B., Wong, B. Y., & Hunter, M. (1982). Affective influence on learning disabled adolescence. *Learning Disability Quarterly, 5,* 334–343.

Hook, P. E., & Johnson, D. J. (1978). Metalinguistic awareness and reading strategies. *Bulletin of the Orton Society, 28,* 62–78.

Isaacson, S. (1987). Effective instruction in written language. *Focus on Exceptional Children, 19,* 1–12.

Jansky, J., & deHirsh, K. (1972). *Preventing reading failure: Prediction, diagnosis, intervention.* New York: Harper & Row.

Jenkins, J. J., Heliotis, J. D., Stein, M. L., & Haynes, M. C. (1987). Improving reading comprehension by using paragraph restatements. *Exceptional Children, 54,* 54–59.

Johnson, D., Blalock, J., & Nesbitt, J. (1978). Adolescents with learning disabilities: Perspectives from an educational clinic. *Learning Disability Quarterly, 1,* 24–36.

Johnson, D., & Myklebust, H. (1967). *Learning disabilities: Educational principles and practices.* New York: Grune & Stratton.

Johnston, P. H., & Winograd, P. (1985). Passive failure in reading. *Journal of Reading Behavior, 4,* 279–301.

Jorm, A. (1983). Specific reading retardation and working memory: A review. *British Journal of Psychology, 74,* 311–342.

Kail, R., & Leonard, L. B. (1986). Sources of word-finding problems in language-impaired children. In S. J. Ceci (Ed.), *Handbook of cognitive social and neuropsychological aspects of learning disabilities.* Hillsdale, NJ: Lawrence Erlbaum Associates.

Kamhi, A. G., & Koenig, L. A. (1985). Metalinguistic awareness in normal and language-disordered children. *Language, Speech, and Hearing Services in Schools, 16,* 199–210.

Kavale, K. A., & Nye, C. (1985). Parameters of LD in achievement, linguistic, neuro-psychological, and social/behavioral domains. *Journal of Special Education, 19,* 443–457.

Kephart, N. (1971). *The slow learner in the classroom.* Columbus, OH: Merrill/Macmillan.

Kirk, S. A. (1963). Behavioral diagnosis and remediation of learning disabilities. *Conference on Exploration into the Problems of the Perceptually Handicapped Child*. Evanston, IL: Fund for Perceptually Handicapped Children.

Kirk, S. A., & Kirk, W. P. (1972). *Psycholinguistic learning disabilities*. Urbana: University of Illinois Press.

Kneedler, R. D., & Hallahan, D. P. (1981). Self-monitoring of on-task behavior with learning-disabled children: Current studies and future directions. *Exceptional Education Quarterly, 2*, 73–82.

Kurtz, B. E., & Borkowski, J. G. (1984). Children's metacognition: Exploring relationships among knowledge, process and motivational variables. *Journal of Experimental Child Psychology, 37*, 335–354.

Landerholm, E. (1990). The trans-disciplinary team approach. *Teaching Exceptional Children, 21*, 66–70.

Leonard, L. B. (1979). Language impairment in children. *Merrill-Palmer Quarterly, 25*, 205–232.

Leong, C. K. (1999). Phonological and morphological processing in students with learning disabilities. *Journal of Learning Disabilities, 32*, 224–238.

Lerner, J. W. (1981). *Learning disabilities* (3d ed.). Boston: Houghton Mifflin.

Levine, M. D., Busch, B., & Aufseiser, C. (1982). The dimensions of inattention among children with school problems. *Pediatrics, 70*, 387–395.

Liberman, I. Y. (1983). A language-oriented view of reading and its disorders. In H. Myklebust (Ed.), *Progress in learning disabilities* (Vol. 5). New York: Grune & Stratton.

Licht, B. G. (1984). Cognitive-motivational factors that contribute to the achievement of learning-disabled children. *Annual Review of Learning Disabilities, 2*, 119–126.

Lieberman, P., Meskill, R. H., Chatillon, M., & Schupack, H. (1985). Phonetic speech perception deficits in dyslexia. *Journal of Speech and Hearing Research, 28*, 480–486.

Majsterek, D. J., & Ellenwood, A. (1990). Screening preschoolers for reading and learning disabilities: Promising procedures. *L. D. Forum, 16*, 6–14.

Markman, E. M. (1977). Realizing that you don't understand: A preliminary investigation. *Child Development, 48*, 989–992.

Mastropieri, M. A., Scruggs, T. E., & Levin, J. R. (1987). Facilitating LD students memory for expository prose. *American Educational Research Journal, 24*, 505–519.

Mather, R. E. (1992). Whole language reading instruction for students with learning disabilities: Caught in the crossfire. *Learning Disabilities Research and Practice, 7*, 87–95.

McGee, L. M. (1982). Awareness of text structure: Effects on children's recall of expository text. *Reading Research Quarterly, 17*, 581–590.

McGee, R., Williams, S., Moffett, T., & Anderson, J. (1989). A comparison of 13-year-old-boys with an attention deficit and/or reading disabilities on neuropsychological measures. *Journal of Abnormal Child Psychology, 17*, 37–53.

Menyuk, P., & Looney, P. (1972). A problem of language disorder: Length versus structure. *Journal of Speech and Hearing Research, 15*, 264–279.

Miller, G. A., Galanter, E., & Pribam, K. (1960). *Plans and the structure of behavior*. New York: Holt, Rinehart & Winston.

Moran, M. R., & Bryne, M. C. (1977). Mastery of verb tense markers by normal and learning disabled children. *Journal of Speech and Hearing Research, 20,* 529–542.

Moran, M. R., Schumaker, J. B., & Vetter, A. F. (1981). Teaching a paragraph organization strategy to learning disabled adolescents (Research Rep. No. 54). Lawrence: University of Kansas Institute for Research in Learning Disabilities.

Myklebust, H. R. (1965). *Development and disorders of written language, Vol. I: The Picture Story Language Test.* New York: Grune & Stratton.

Myklebust, H. R. (1973). *Development and disorders of written language, Vol. 2: Studies of normal and exceptional children.* New York: Grune & Stratton.

Myklebust, H. R. (1978). Toward a science of dyslexiology. In H. Myklebust (Ed.), *Progress in learning disabilities* (Vol. 4). New York: Grune & Stratton.

Newhoff, M. (1990). Oral language deficits as the basis of learning disabilities. *Clinical Connection, 4,* 16–17.

Nodine, B. F., Barenbaum, E., & Newcomer, P. (1985). Story composition by learning disabled, reading disabled and normal children. *Learning Disability Quarterly, 8,* 167–181.

Norris, N. T., & Crump, W. D. (1982). Syntactic and vocabulary development in the written language of learning disabled and non-learning disabled students at four age levels. *Learning Disability Quarterly, 5,* 167–181.

O'Connor, R. E., & Jenkins, J. R. (1999). Prediction of reading disabilities in kindergarten and first grade. *Scientific Studies of Reading, 3,* 159–197.

Orton, S. T. (1937). *Reading, writing and speech problems in children.* New York: Norton.

Palincsar, A. S., & Brown, A. L. (1986). Interactive teaching to promote independent learning from text. *The Reading Teacher, 39,* 771–777.

Paris, S. G., & Meyers, M. (1981). Comprehension monitoring, memory and study strategies of good and poor readers. *Journal of Reading Behavior, 13,* 7–22.

Paris, S. G., & Oka, E. R. (1989). Strategies for comprehending text and coping with reading difficulties. *Learning Disability Quarterly, 12,* 32–42.

Paul, R. (1992). Language and speech disorders. In S. R. Hooper, G. W. Hynd, & R. E. Mattison (Eds.). *Developmental disorders: Diagnostic criteria and clinical assessment* (pp. 209–238). Hillsdale, NJ: Lawrence Erlbaum Associates.

Pearson, P. D., & Spiro, R. J. (1980). Toward a theory of reading instruction. *Topics in Language Disorders, 1,* 71–88.

Perfetti, C. A., & Hogaboam, T. W. (1975). The relationship between single word decoding and reading comprehension skill. *Journal of Educational Psychology, 67,* 461–469.

Perfetti, C. A., & Lesgold, A. M. (1979). Coding and comprehension in skilled reading and implications for reading instruction. In L. B. Resnick & P. A. Weaver (Eds.), *Theory and practice of early reading* (Vol. 1). Hillsdale, NJ: Lawrence Erlbaum Associates.

Poplin, M., Gray, R., Larsen, S., Banikowski, A., & Mehring, T. (1980). A comparison of components of written expression abilities in learning disabled and non-learning disabled students at three grade-levels. *Learning Disability Quarterly, 3,* 46–53.

Pressley, M., Borkowski, J. G., & O'Sullivan, J. T. (1984). Memory strategy instruction is made of this: Metamemory and durable strategy use. *Educational Psychologist, 19,* 94–107.

Pressley, M., & Rankin, J. (1994). More about whole language methods of reading instruction for students at-risk for early reading failure. *Learning Disabilities Research and Practice, 9,* 157–168.

Pressley, M., Rankin, J., Gaskins, I., Brown, R., & El-Dinary, P. (1995). Mapping the cutting edge in primary level literacy for at-risk readers. In T. E. Scruggs and M. Mastropieri (Eds.). *Advances in learning and behavioral disabilities* (pp. 47–90). Greenwich, CT: JAI Press.

Raphael, T. S., & Englert, C. S. (1990). Reading and writing: Partners in constructing meaning. *The Reading Teacher, 43,* 388–400.

Rinehart, S. D., Stahl, S. A., & Erickson, L. G. (1986). Some effects of summarization training on reading and studying. *Reading Research Quarterly, 12,* 422–438.

Ring, B. C. (1976). Effects of input organization on auditory short-term memory. *Journal of Learning Disabilities, 9,* 59–63.

Ryan, E. B., Weed, K. A., & Short, E. J. (1986). Cognitive behavior modifications: Promoting active self-regulatory learning styles. In J. Torgesen & B. Wong (Eds.), *Psychological and educational perspectives on learning disabilities.* New York: Academic.

Samuels, S. J., Begg, G., & Chen, C. C. (1976). Comparison of word recognition speed and strategies of less skilled and more highly skilled readers. *Reading Research Quarterly, 1,* 73–86.

Sawyer, D. J. (1991). Whole language in context: Insights into the current great debate. *Topics in Language Disorders, 11,* 1–13.

Schumaker, J., Deshler, D., Alley, G., Warner, M., & Denton, P. (1984). Multipass: A learning strategy for improving reading comprehension. *Learning Disability Quarterly, 5,* 295–304.

Schunk, D. H., & Cox, P. D. (1986). Strategy training and attributional feedback with learning disabled students. *Journal of Educational Psychology, 78,* 201–209.

Scruggs, T. E. (1991). Commentary: Foundations of interaction research. In T. E. Scruggs and B. Y. L. Wong (Eds.), *Intervention research in learning disabilities.* New York: Springer-Verlag.

Scruggs, T. E., Mastropieri, M. A., & Levin, J. R. (1987). Transformational mnemonic strategies for learning disabled students. In H. L. Swanson (Ed.), *Memory and learning disabilities.* Greenwich, CT: JAI Press.

Seidenberg, P. L. (1982). Implications of schemata theory for learning disabled readers. *Journal of Learning Disabilities, 15,* 352–355.

Seidenberg, P. L. (1988). Cognitive and academic instructional intervention for learning disabled adolescents. *Topics in Language Disorders, 8,* 56–71.

Seidenberg, P. L. (1989). Relating text-processing research to reading and writing instruction for learning disabled students. *Learning Disabilities Focus, 5,* 4–12.

Seidenberg, P. L. (1991). *Reading, writing and studying strategies: An integrated curriculum.* Gaithersburg, MD: Aspen.

Seidenberg, P. L., & Bernstein, D. K. (1986). The comprehension of similies and metaphors by learning disabled and non-learning disabled children. *Language, Speech and Hearing Services in Schools, 17,* 219–229.

Seidenberg, P. L., & Bernstein, D. K. (1988). Metaphor comprehension and performance on metaphor-related language tasks: A comparison of good and poor readers. *Remedial and Special Education, 9,* 39–45.

Shankweiler, D., Liberman, I. Y., Mark, L. S., Fowler, C. A., & Fischer, F. W. (1979). The speech code and learning to read. *Journal of Experimental Psychology, 5,* 531–545.

Shaywitz, B. A., & Shaywitz, S. E. (1991). Comorbidity: A critical issue in attention deficit disorder. *Journal of Child Neurology, 6,* 13–22.

Short, E., & Ryan, E. (1984). Metacognitive differences between skilled and less skilled readers: Remediating deficits through story grammar and attribution training. *Journal of Educational Psychology, 76,* 225–235.

Siegler, R. S. (1983). Information processing approaches to development. In H. Mussen (Ed.), *Carmichael's manual of child psychology.* New York: Wiley.

Slobin, D. (1971). *Psycholinguistics.* Glenview, IL: Scott Foresman.

Stackhouse, J., & Wells, B. (1997). How do speech and language problems affect literacy development? In C. Hulme & M. Snowling (Eds.), *Dyslexia, biology, cognition, and intervention* (pp. 182–211). London: Whurr.

Stanovich, K. E. (1986). Cognitive processes and the reading problems of learning disabled children: Evaluating the assumption of specificity. In J. K. Torgesen & B. Y. L. Wong (Eds.), *Psychological and educational perspectives in learning disabilities.* New York: Academic.

Stanovich, K. E. (1991). Word recognition: Changing perspectives. In R. Barr, M. L. Kamil, P. Mosenthal, & P. E. Pearson (Eds.). *Handbook of reading research* (pp. 418–452). New York: Longman.

Steiner, R., Werner, M., & Cromer, W. (1971). Comprehension training and identification of poor and good readers. *Journal of Educational Psychology, 62,* 506–513.

Strauss, A., & Lehtinen, L. (1947). *Psychopathology and education of the brain-injured child.* New York: Grune & Stratton.

Swanson, H. L. (1988). Learning disabled children's problem-solving: Identifying mental processes underlying intelligent performance. *Intelligence, 12,* 261–278.

Swanson, H. L. (1989). Central processing strategy difference in gifted, normal achieving, learning disabled and mentally retarded children. *Journal of Experimental Child Psychology, 47,* 378–397.

Swanson, H. L. (1991). Instruction derived from the strategy deficit model: Overview of principles and procedures. In T. E. Scruggs & B. Y. L. Wong (Eds.), *Intervention research in learning disabilities.* New York: Springer-Verlag.

Swanson, H. L., & Cooney, J. (1985). Strategy transformations in learning disabled children. *Learning Disability Quarterly, 8,* 221–231.

Swanson, H. L., & Rhine, B. (1985). Strategy transformations in learning disabled children's math performance: Clues to the development of expertise. *Journal of Learning Disabilities, 18,* 596–603.

Tarver, S. G., Hallahan, D. P., Kaufman, J. M., & Ball, D. W. (1976). Verbal rehearsal and selective attention in children with learning disabilities: A developmental lag. *Journal of Experimental Child Psychology, 22,* 375–385.

Thomas, C. C., Englert, C. S., & Gregg, S. (1987). An analysis of errors and strategies in the expository writing of learning disabled students. *Remedial and Special Education, 8,* 21–30.

Torgesen, J. K. (1978). Performance of reading disabled children on serial memory tasks: A review. *Reading Research Quarterly, 19*, 57–87.

Torgesen, J. K. (1982). The study of short-term memory in learning disabled children. In K. Gadow & I. Bialer (Eds.), *Advances in learning and behavioral disabilities* (Vol. 1). Greenwich, CT: JAI Press.

Torgesen, J. K. (1985). Memory processes in reading disabled children. *Journal of Learning Disabilities, 18*, 350–357.

Torgesen, J. K. (1986). Learning disabilities theory: Its current state and future prospects. *Journal of Learning Disabilities, 19*, 399–407.

Torgesen, J. K., & Houck, G. (1980). Processing deficiencies in learning disabled children who perform poorly on the digit span task. *Journal of Educational Psychology, 72*, 141–160.

Torgesen, J. K., & Licht, B. G. (1983). The learning disabled child as an inactive learner: Retrospect and prospects. In J. D. McKinney & L. Feagan (Eds.), *Current topics in learning disabilities* (Vol. 1). Normand, NJ: Ablex.

Torgesen, J. K., Rashotte, C. A., Greenstein, J., & Portes, P. (1991). Further studies of learning disabled children with severe performance problems on the digit span test. *Learning Disabilities Research and Practice, 6*, 134–144.

Torgesen, J., Wagner, R., & Rashotte, C. (1994). Longitudinal studies of phonological processing and reading. *Journal of Educational Psychology, 84*, 364–370.

U.S. Office of Education. (1977, December). Education of handicapped children: Assistance to states: Procedures for evaluating specific learning disabilities. *Federal Register, Part III*. Washington, DC: Department of Health, Education and Welfare.

U.S. Department of Education. (1986, October). Education of handicapped children act: Amendments of 1986. *Federal Register.* Washington, DC: Department of Education.

Vallecorsa, A. L., & Garriss, E. (1990). Story composition skills of middle-grade students with learning disabilities. *Exceptional Children, 57*, 48–55.

van Kleeck, A. (1984). Metalinguistic skills: Cutting across spoken and written language and problem solving abilities. In G. P. Wallach & K. G. Butler (Eds.), *Language learning disabilities in school-age children.* Baltimore: Williams & Wilkins.

Vellutino, F. R. (1977). Alternative conceptualizations of dyslexia: Evidence in support of a verbal-deficit hypothesis. *Harvard Educational Review, 47*, 334–354.

Vellutino, F. R. (1979). *Dyslexia: Theory and research.* Cambridge, MA: MIT Press.

Vellutino, F. R. (1991). Has basic research in reading increased our understanding of developmental reading and how to teach reading? *Psychological Science, 2*, 81–83.

Vellutino, F. R., & Scanlon, D. M. (1979, April). The effect of phonemic segmentation training and response acquisition on coding ability in poor and normal readers. Paper presented at the American Education Research Association annual meeting, San Francisco.

Vellutino, F. R., & Scanlon, D. M. (1991). The preeminence of phonologically based skills in learning to read. In S. Brady & D. Shankweiler (Eds.), *Phonological processes in literacy* (pp. 237–252). Hillsdale, NJ: Erlbaum.

Vogel, S. A. (1975). *Syntactic abilities in normal and dyslexic children.* Baltimore: University Park Press.

Vygotsky, L. S. (1962). *Thought and language.* Cambridge, MA: MIT Press.

Walker, N. W. (1985). Impulsivity in learning disabled children, past research findings and methodological inconsistencies. *Learning Disabilities Quarterly, 8,* 85–94.

Wallach, G. P., & Butler, K. G. (1984). *Language learning disabilities in school-age children.* Baltimore: Williams & Wilkins.

Wallach, M. A., & Wallach, L. (1976). *Teaching all children to read.* Chicago: University of Chicago Press.

Wechsler, D. (1974). *Wechsler Intelligence Scale for Children—Revised* (manual). Austin, TX: Psychological Corp.

Welch, M. (1992). The PLEASE strategy: A metacognitive learning strategy for improving the paragraph writing of students with mild learning disabilities. *Learning Disability Quarterly, 15,* 119–128.

Wepman, J. M. (1973). *Wepman Auditory Discrimination Test.* Chicago: Language Research Associates.

Whitmere, K. (2000). Action: School services. *Language, Speech and Hearing Services in Schools, 31,* 194–199.

Wiederholt, J. L. (1974). Historical perspectives in the education of the learning disabled. In L. Mann & D. Sabatino (Eds.), *The second review of special education.* Philadelphia: Journal of Special Education Press.

Wiig, E. H., & Semel, E. M. (1973). Comprehension of linguistic concepts requiring logical operations by learning disabled children. *Journal of Speech and Hearing Research, 16,* 627–636.

Wiig, E. H., & Semel, E. M. (1974). Logico-grammatical sentence comprehension by learning disabled adolescents. *Perceptual Motor Skills, 38,* 1331–1334.

Wiig, E. H., & Semel, E. M. (1975). Productive language abilities in learning disabled adolescents. *Journal of Learning Disabilities, 8,* 578–586.

Wiig, E. H., & Semel, E. M. (1976). *Language disabilities in children and adolescents.* Columbus, OH: Merrill/Macmillan.

Wiig, E. H., & Semel, E. M. (1984). *Language assessment and intervention for the learning disabled* (2d ed.). Columbus, OH: Merrill/Macmillan.

Wiig, E. H., Semel, E. M., & Crouse, M. A. (1973). The use of English morphology by high risk and learning disabled children. *Journal of Learning Disabilities, 6,* 457–465.

Williams, D. L., Gridley, B. E., & Fitzhugh-Bell, K. (1992). Cluster analysis of children and adolescents with brain damage and learning disabilities using neuropsychological, psychoeducational, sacrobehavioral variables. *Journal of Learning Disabilities, 25,* 290–299.

Williams, J. P. (1984a). Categorization, macrostructure, and finding the main idea. *Journal of Educational Psychology, 76,* 874–879.

Williams, J. P. (1984b). Phonemic analysis and how it relates to reading. *Journal of Learning Disabilities, 17,* 240–245.

Winograd, P. (1984). Strategic difficulties in summarizing texts. *Reading Research Quarterly, 21,* 404–425.

Winograd, P., & Niquette, G. (1988). Assessing learned helplessness in poor readers. *Topics in Language Disorders, 8,* 38–55.

Wong, B. Y. L. (1978). The effects of directive cues on the organization of memory and recall in good and poor readers. *Journal of Education Research, 72,* 32–38.

Wong, B. Y. L. (1985). Metacognition and learning disabilities. In T. G. Weller, D. Forrest, & E. MacKinnon (Eds.), *Metacognition, cognition and human performance.* New York: Academic.

Wong, B. Y. L. (1986). A cognitive approach to teaching spelling. *Exceptional Children, 53,* 169–173.

Wong, B. Y. L., Butler, D. L., Ficzere, S. A., & Kuperis, S. (1996). Teaching adolescents with learning disabilities to plan, write, and revise opinion essays. *Journal of Learning Disabilities, 29,* 197–212.

Wong, B. Y. L., & Jones, W. (1982). Increasing metacomprehension in learning disabled and normally achieving students through self-questioning training. *Learning Disability Quarterly, 5,* 228–246.

Wong, B. Y. L., & Wilson, M. (1984). Investigating awareness of and teaching passage organization in learning disabled children. *Journal of Learning Disabilities, 17,* 477–482.

Wong, B. Y. L., Wong, R., Perry, N., & Sawatsky, D. (1986). The efficacy of a self-questioning summarization strategy for use by underachievers and learning disabled adolescents in social studies. *Learning Disabilities Focus, 2,* 20–35.

Zentall, S. (1993). Research on the educational implications of attention deficit hyperactivity disorder. *Exceptional Children, 60,* 143–153.

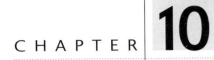

Mental Retardation

Difference and Delay

Robert E. Owens, Jr.

*State University
of New York
at Geneseo*

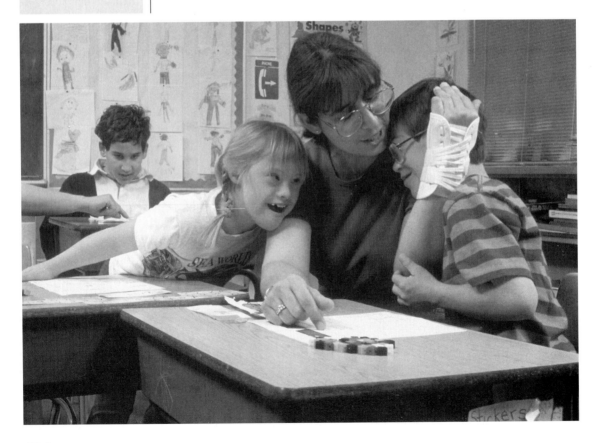

- Discuss how we characterize or define the mentally retarded population
- List the cognitive and linguistic characteristics of the mentally retarded population
- Discuss intervention techniques that are suggested by the learning characteristics of the mentally retarded population
- Describe the developmental intervention approach, and how it is used
- Describe behaviors that should be targeted, and techniques that should be used in intervention by the speech-language pathologist

> I wanted to make this book all about pop music, but my Dad says people will be more interested in my adventures. But I must write a bit about pop. (Hunt, 1967, p. 89)

In *The World of Nigel Hunt,* the author expresses the interests of many other teenagers. This particular adolescent has mental retardation. He was born with Down syndrome, a genetic disorder that is one of hundreds of identifiable causes of or factors related to mental retardation. Yet Nigel is more like his nonretarded peers than he is unlike them.

It is difficult to characterize the mentally retarded population because of its diversity. This heterogeneous population includes individuals who are totally dependent and those who are nearly independent in their daily living. We can say, however, that they develop more slowly or at a more retarded rate than the non-mentally retarded population. In addition, they are different in some ways from the nonretarded population. This characteristic can be seen in several aspects of the development of individuals with mental retardation, including language.

In this chapter, I will explore a definition of mental retardation and discuss the implications for communication and language development. I will characterize the special language problems of this population and suggest intervention techniques and programs that might be helpful for the speech-language pathologist.

A DEFINITION OF MENTAL RETARDATION

The American Association on Mental Deficiency (AAMD), the primary organization for professionals working with the mentally retarded population, defines mental retardation as a "significantly subaverage general intellectual functioning, existing concurrently with related limitations in two or more . . . adaptive skill areas[, and] . . . manifest[ed] before age 18" (American Association on Mental Retardation, 1992). To understand this definition fully, we must look at its various components.

Significantly subaverage is generally defined as an IQ of 70 or lower, but this upper limit is not inflexible and may be extended upward, depending on the reliability of the testing that helped to establish the IQ. In the entire population, the mean or average IQ is 100, but the range of normality extends from 85 to 115. This range contains two-thirds of the population. An IQ of 70 is significantly below average.

Intellectual functioning refers to the results of a culture-free standardized general intelligence test. The generally accepted measurement of intelligence is IQ, a ratio of mental age to chronological age. If the mental age is 10 years and the chronological age is 10 years, the relationship is 10/10 or 1, which is interpreted as an IQ of 100. In contrast, a mental age of 5 and a chronological age of 10 yields 5/10 or 0.5, which is an IQ of 50.

Testing should be pluralistic and culture free. A test based solely on language abilities would be unfair to many second-language learners and to many children with learning disabilities. Intelligence testing should also include nonlinguistic abilities, such as problem solving, sensorimotor development, and social skills. Likewise, culturally biased tests would be prejudicial to many minorities. The author knows of one recent Southeast Asian immigrant classified as mentally retarded based on an English receptive vocabulary test.

Adaptive skills vary for different ages. During infancy and the preschool years, adaptive skills include sensorimotor, speech and language, self-help, and interactional development. In middle childhood and early adolescence, the emphasis shifts to academic and reasoning skill development and to group and interpersonal relationships. Late adolescent and adult adaptive skill development relates to vocational and social responsibility. Adaptive behavior frequently correlates very positively with intelligence but not always, especially for very low IQs (Grossman, 1983).

The period *prior to age 18* is considered by many to be the **developmental period.** For those with mental retardation, development may be slow, arrested, or incomplete. The developmental rate decreases as all humans reach the late teens. Thus, young adults who are profoundly retarded may experience only moderate developmental change after age 18, although they function at a mental age of only 3 years.

The AAMD definition includes only those individuals who meet all the criteria. Children who have learning disabilities are not included because they possess normal intelligence; and elderly patients who have aphasia do not qualify because their disorder did not manifest itself during the developmental period. Although individuals with both types of disorders might function within the retarded range on some tasks, they cannot be classified as mentally retarded. Figure 10.1 illustrates the AAMD definition.

The definition does not specify causes or etiologies but emphasizes the current functioning level of the individual. In other words, it is not assumed that Down syndrome is synonymous with mental retardation. In part, the definition reflects a belief that functioning levels can be modified or changed, that the individual with mental retardation is a developmental being.

PREVALENCE AND LEVELS OF FUNCTIONING

The exact number of individuals with mental retardation in the United States is unknown. Estimates vary from 1 to 3 percent of the population, or approximately 2.5

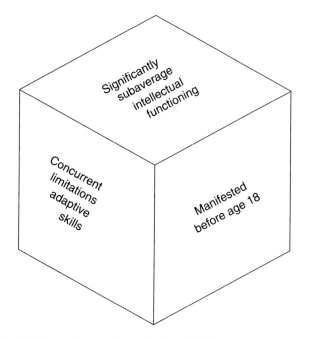

All criteria must be met in order to establish mental retardation

FIGURE 10.1

AAMD Definition of Mental Retardation

(Adapted from American Association on Mental Retardation, 1992.)

to 7 million individuals. Upper figures are based solely on IQ score data. Mental retardation is approximately fifteen times more prevalent than blindness. Most of the approximately 125,000 individuals with retardation born in the United States each year are only mildly retarded.

There are four categories of mental retardation, based on IQ—mild, moderate, severe, and profound. The characteristics of each category are listed in Table 10.1.

The distribution of mental retardation within the population is not uniform. The distribution of individuals with severe and profound retardation reflects the general population. However, among the mildly and moderately retarded, there is a greater percentage of poor and minority individuals as well as a greater percentage of individuals with a family history of retardation. The disproportionately higher percentage among the poor and minority populations may reflect the environmental effects of poverty. In American culture, many minorities are found in the lower socioeconomic levels because of discriminatory practices. Also, middle-class professionals are more likely to classify lower-class or minority children as retarded. Lack of proper nutrition or poor health may contribute to delayed development among the poor. In addition, because parents with mild mental retardation are most likely to find themselves among the poor, genetic influences may play a role. These adults are more likely than nonretarded adults to produce offspring with depressed cognitive functioning. This factor does not occur with the severely and profoundly retarded, because very few of these individuals produce offspring.

| TABLE 10.1 | | Categories of Mental Retardation | | |

Category	IQ Range	% of MR Population	Characteristics
Mild	52–68	89	Usually absorbed into the community, where they work and live independently
Moderate	36–51	6	Capable of learning self-care skills and working within a sheltered environment; live semi-independently, with relatives or in a community residence
Severe	20–35	$3\frac{1}{2}$	Capable of learning some self-care skills and are not totally dependent; often exhibit physical disabilities and deficits in speech and language
Profound	Below 20	$1\frac{1}{2}$	Capable of learning some basic living skills but require continual care and supervision; often exhibit severe physical and/or sensory problems

Source: Adapted from American Association on Mental Retardation (1992).

CAUSES OF MENTAL RETARDATION

Biological causes may be a factor for more than half of the individuals within the mentally retarded population. Many individuals whose mental retardation was previously believed to have resulted from social-environmental factors may actually exhibit a relatively recently discovered syndrome called Fragile X (Nussvaum & Ledbetter, 1986; Wolff, Gardner, Lappen, Paccia, & Meryash, 1988). Fragile X syndrome is the most common cause of mental retardation after Down syndrome (Caron, 1994). A weakness in the female, or X, chromosome found in all humans is related to mental retardation and possibly to other learning disorders. Fragile X, a recessive trait more prevalent in males because they carry only one X chromosome, is found in 1 of every 1,350 live male births and 1 of every 2,033 live female births (Love & Webb, 1986). Most males with the Fragile X trait are mentally retarded, whereas only about a third of females with the trait are so affected (Caron, 1994). Language problems affect all males with Fragile X, even those whose IQs are within normal limits (Caron, 1994). Females are more likely to exhibit characteristics of a learning disability (Wolff et al., 1988).

Other biological causes may be genetic, such as Down syndrome; congenital, such as metabolic disorders or malformations of the skull and brain; or illness or toxin related, such as maternal rubella or lead poisoning. The correlation between severity of retardation and biological factors is very strong.

Social-environmental factors are not as easy to identify as biological factors and involve many interactive variables. Poor housing and hygiene, as well as inadequate medical care and nutrition, may contribute. Lack of prenatal care and of infant stimulation may affect the developing child more directly.

Certainly any discussion of causality offers only the grossest of estimates and must be taken cautiously for several reasons. First, certain conditions may be related to mental retardation but not be a direct causal agent. Second, individuals may have several identifiable causes or related factors. Third, the specific etiology is unknown for a significant portion of the retarded population. Known causes of mental retardation are listed in Table 10.2.

ASSOCIATED NEUROLOGICAL DISORDERS

There is a higher incidence of neurological disorders among the mentally retarded population, especially that segment that is severely and profoundly involved. Cerebral palsy and/or epilepsy are found in a greater percentage of the mentally retarded population than in the nonretarded population. This difference is especially evident among the severely and profoundly retarded. These individuals frequently exhibit neuromuscular disorders as part of a complex of multiple disabilities.

Among the cerebral palsied population, approximately 50 percent demonstrate IQs lower than 70. Such scores may reflect a lack of sophistication by the tester or by the test. In other words, individuals with cerebral palsy may be difficult to test using standard procedures because of neuromuscular interference. Nonetheless, it seems safe to conclude that a substantial proportion of the cerebral palsied population also exhibits mental retardation.

Epilepsy affects less than 1 percent of the general population. The percentage increases with decreased intelligence, and as high as 65 percent of the profoundly retarded population may exhibit seizure activity. Frequent causes of epilepsy in young children are central nervous system (CNS) malformation, CNS injury from infection or accident, and CNS malfunction caused by a metabolic error.

Related neurological disorders further complicate learning tasks for persons with mental retardation. The increased occurrence with decreased intelligence may also indicate an underlying organic cause for the more severe forms of retardation.

COGNITIVE FUNCTIONING

Volumes of research have been published on the cognitive abilities of individuals with mental retardation. Still, for a number of reasons, we do not fully understand the cognitive and learning processes of this population (Cegelka & Prehm, 1982). First, the complex nature of the cognitive process necessitates research that targets very limited aspects. Therefore, there are no definitive studies of the entire process of cognitive functioning among either the retarded or the nonretarded population. Second, the cognitive functioning level of subjects with mental retardation in many studies is poorly defined. This factor can be extremely important because there seems to be a very strong link between IQ and cognitive abilities. It is difficult to draw conclusions across studies when the functioning levels of the subjects differ greatly. Finally,

TABLE 10.2 Known Causes of Mental Retardation

Type	Examples	Characteristics
Biological		
Genetic and chromosomal	Down syndrome (Trisomy 21)	Broad head and characteristic facial features, small stature, mental retardation
	Klinefelter syndrome (sex-linked, XXY)	Feminine roundness to body, small testes, possible mental retardation
	Cri-du-chat syndrome	Catlike cry, microcephaly, mental retardation
Infectious processes	Maternal rubella	Cardiac defects, cataracts, hearing loss, microcephaly, possible mental retardation
	Congenital syphilis	Deafness, vision problems, possible epilepsy or cerebral palsy, mental retardation
Toxins and chemical agents	Fetal alcohol syndrome	Persistently deficient growth, low brain weight, facial abnormalities, cardiac defects, mental retardation
	Lead poisoning	Central nervous system and kidney damage, hyperactivity
Nutrition and metabolism	Phenylketonuria (PKU)	Reduced pigmentation, motor coordination problems, convulsions, microcephaly, mental retardation
	Tay-Sachs disease	Progressive deterioration of nervous system and vision, mental retardation, death in preschool years
	Inadequate diet	Small stature, possible mental retardation
Gestational disorders	Hydrocephalus	Enlarged head caused by increased volume of cerebro-spinal fluid, visual defects, epilepsy, mental retardation
	Cerebral malformation	Absence or underdevelopment of cerebral cortex and resultant mental retardation
	Craniofacial anomalies	Malformed skull and associated mental retardation
Complications of pregnancy and delivery	Extreme immaturity or preterm infant	Low birth weight, higher prevalence of central nervous system disorders
	Exceptionally large baby	Possible birth injury to central nervous system
	Maternal nutritional disorders	Low birth weight, higher prevalence of central nervous system disorders
Gross brain diseases	Tumors and tuberous sclerosis	Tumors in heart, seizures, tuberous "bumps" on nose and cheeks, mental retardation
	Huntington disease	Degenerative neurological functioning evidenced in progressive dementia and cerebral palsy
Social-Environmental		
Psychosocial disadvantage	Subnormal intellectual functioning in immediate family and/or impoverished environment	Functional retardation
Sensory deprivation	Maternal deprivation Prolonged isolation	Functional retardation and failure to thrive

Adapted from Grossman (1983).

it is difficult to extrapolate from a limited experimental setting to the daily environments of individuals.

Researchers have interpreted their data in two general ways. One interpretation holds that there are discrepancies or differences in the cognitive processing abilities of the mentally retarded population that cannot be accounted for by mental age alone. Individuals with mental retardation do not perform in the same manner as nonretarded peers of the same mental age. Pointing to methodological problems in many of these studies, a second group of researchers considers the mentally retarded population to develop cognitively in the same manner as the nonretarded population, but at a slower rate (Kamhi, 1981).

In general, individuals in the mentally retarded population develop many cognitive skills in a developmental sequence similar to that of the nonmentally retarded population. There are differences, however, that indicate fundamental processing differences. Some of these similarities and differences can be identified in learning processes and in memory. **Learning** is a change in behavior that results from rehearsal of the behavior to be learned. Cognitive abilities important for learning include attention, organization, transfer, and memory. The variables to which an individual attends and the organization of these variables are important for memory, which in turn affects transfer or generalization to novel situations or problems. Figure 10.2 demonstrates this process schematically.

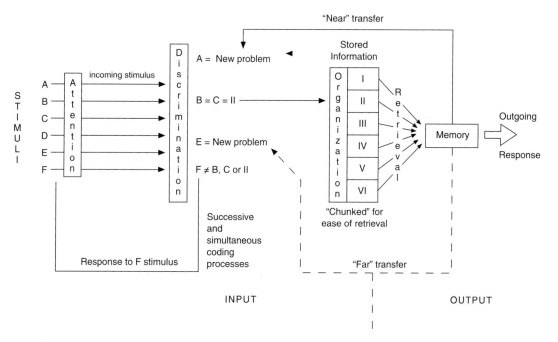

FIGURE 10.2

Schematic of Major Cognitive Functions

Attention

Attention includes awareness of a learning situation and active cognitive processing. As noted in Figure 10.2, we do not attend to all stimuli. Research on attention has examined the orienting, reacting, and discriminating abilities of individuals with mental retardation. **Orientation** is the ability to sustain attention over time. In general, individuals with mild retardation exhibit equal or slightly greater ability to sustain attention and to orient when compared to their mental age-matched (MA-matched) nonretarded peers.

Reaction time refers to the amount of time required for an individual to respond to a stimulus. In Figure 10.2, the subject responds to stimulus F immediately. Individuals with mild mental retardation react similarly to MA-matched nonretarded peers, but their performance is very individualistic. In part, reaction time is a function of the individual's ability to select the relevant dimensions of a task before responding. Individuals with mental retardation appear to be deficient in their abilities to scan and attend selectively.

Discrimination is the ability to identify differing stimuli from a field of similar stimuli. For example, a discrimination task might involve picking a different pitch tone from a series of pitch tones. In a more complicated task, a subject might be required to attend to several dimensions of a sample, such as color, shape, and size, at the same time. For example, in Figure 10.2, stimuli B and C are found to be similar to each other and to information already stored. In contrast, A and E are new information. In general, individuals with mental retardation exhibit difficulties identifying and maintaining attention to the relevant stimulus dimensions. As a group, persons with mild and moderate retardation attend to fewer dimensions of a task than do the nonretarded, and these dimensions are not necessarily the salient or important ones. This deficiency reduces an individual's ability to compare new information with stored information from previous learning. In addition, it takes a longer time and more practice for persons with mental retardation to understand the dimensions of a task. Once a task is understood or learned, however, individuals with mental retardation can perform as well as their MA-matched nonretarded peers. In general, individuals with mental retardation who have higher functioning abilities can learn discrimination tasks more rapidly than those who have lower functioning abilities (Ellis et al., 1982). There are substantial individual differences among persons with severe and profound retardation, however, and some subjects learn tasks as well as those with mild retardation, although they may have more limited attentional capacity and may be less efficient at attention allocation (Nugent & Mosley, 1987).

In general, persons with mental retardation seem able to attend as well as their MA-matched nonretarded peers. They may be less able, however, to select the relevant information from a field. Therefore, new or relevant features of a task need to be highlighted in order to call attention to them (Meador, 1984).

Organization of Input Material

The organization of incoming sensory information is very important for later retrieval. This organization can be demonstrated when we try to recall the name of an object.

Frequently, the names of related objects will also come to mind. Therefore, we may name the washing machine *dryer* or *refrigerator,* but rarely *spoon* or *window.* As shown in Figure 10.2, information is organized or "chunked" by category for easy retrieval. Nonretarded persons and those with mild retardation exhibit similar developmental trends in the grouping of information. In general, individuals with mental retardation exhibit difficulty developing categorizing strategies for organizing new material into more easily remembered "chunks." Because it is much more difficult to remember unrelated bits of information, any organizational deficit will hinder later recall and quickly overload memory capacity. Every reader can recognize that it is easier to recall a ten-word sentence than ten unrelated words. If, as some propose, memory capacity is fixed, more efficient processing will require increasingly better organization. In turn, better organization leaves more room for new input.

Individuals with mild and moderate mental retardation do not seem to rely on mediation or associative learning strategies nor to use them as efficiently as do the nonretarded. In mediating strategies, a word or symbol forms a link between two inputs. For example, a person's name might relate past experiences with feelings, lifestyles, or opinions. In associative strategies, one word or symbol aids in recall of another. Common examples are "salt and _____," "black and _____," and so on. Mildly retarded individuals can use associative strategies if the two symbols are easily associated and nonabstract.

Four components of information integration may be input, sensory register, central processor, and output. The three processes of the central processor are simultaneous synthesis, sequential or successive synthesis, and regulatory activities. Simultaneous synthesis, or coding, which takes place in the occipital-parietal region of the brain, is related to higher thought. Separate elements are synthesized into groups so that all members of the group can be retrieved simultaneously. For example, various examples of dogs are coded for the *dog* category. In sentence coding, the overall meaning, rather than the individual syntactic and phonological units, is processed. Sequential, or successive, coding is related to language form and takes place in the frontal-temporal region of the brain. Linguistic information is coded in linear fashion. Both processes are used for coding input and for planning behavior. Obviously, these coding processes are influenced by sensory input, memory, and other intellectual processes.

Both nonretarded persons and those with mild retardation exhibit simultaneous and successive coding. There appears to be some difference in the use of this coding for the planning function, however, and the two groups may *employ* the coding process differently. Individuals with Down syndrome may even possess different coding functions. As a group, persons with Down syndrome perform more poorly than either brain-damaged individuals or other MA-matched individuals with retardation on successive processing tasks. This deficiency may be an underlying cause for auditory memory and expressive language problems of the Down syndrome population. The poor auditory processing and memory behavior of individuals with Down syndrome may indicate a structural difference in the processing portions of the brain (Ellis, Deacon, & Wooldridge, 1985; Lincoln, Courchesne, Kilman, & Galambos, 1985). Persons with more severe retardation may sustain some organic problems and, therefore, have qualitatively different neurological functioning also (Snart, O'Grady, & Das, 1982).

In general, individuals with mental retardation demonstrate some organizing difficulties and thus benefit from preorganized input. Organizational deficits can hinder recall and generalization, both essential for learning.

Transfer

Transfer, or generalization, is the ability to apply previously learned material in the solving of similar but novel problems. Although persons with mild retardation can be taught cognitive processing strategies, attempts to generalize these strategies have been less successful. The learning of individuals with more severe retardation is characterized by even weaker transfer (Ellis et al., 1982; Reid, 1980). Learning enhances performance but not generalization.

Near transfer involves only minimal changes between the training and novel, testing situations, whereas **far transfer** involves substantial changes. In Figure 10.2, Stimulus A is considered to be similar enough to stored information to qualify for near transfer. Stimulus E is less similar and thus represents far transfer. Persons with mental retardation have difficulties with both near and far transfer, which appear to be a function not of the similarity of the old and new tasks but of the level of awareness required to detect such similarities.

Understanding the task is essential for transfer. Individuals with mental retardation can benefit from training in all components of a task and in applying these components to new task settings (Burger, Blackman, Clark, & Reis, 1982). However, explicit training does not appear to be necessary for all retarded individuals. Persons with mild retardation can gain knowledge to increase transfer solely through observation of the task (Burger, Blackman, & Clark, 1981).

The generalization deficits of individuals with mental retardation may reflect the selection and organization problems noted previously. Generalization can be facilitated, however, if the client is helped in analyzing the similarities between old and new tasks.

Memory

The ability to retrieve needed information that was previously learned is necessary for recall or memory. Individuals with mild and moderate retardation seem to be able to retain information within long-term memory as well as nonretarded individuals, although overall recall is slower (Merrill, 1985). Organizational deficits, however, may result in an overreliance on rote memory by persons with mild retardation. In contrast, individuals with profound mental retardation exhibit significant forgetting of learned behavior within only a short interval.

Short-term memory deficiencies are more evident in the retarded population (Gutowski & Chechile, 1987). In turn, such deficiencies may affect discrimination abilities. In general, short-term memory is very limited—nonretarded individuals can hold fewer than ten entities only briefly. Individuals with mental retardation may experience difficulty with short-term storage due to a lack of associational strategies (Gutowski & Chechile, 1987). They retain pictures better than printed words or letters (as compared with nonretarded adolescents and adults, for whom the reverse is true). Short-term memory is particularly affected by the rapid rate of forgetting found in the retarded population, especially within the first ten seconds (Ellis et al., 1985). Increased encoding time does not normalize the rate of forgetting, indicating encoding and storage deficits (Ellis et al., 1985).

Information is retained and/or transferred to long-term memory through rehearsal or repetition. It has been reported that persons with mental retardation do not rehearse information spontaneously (Reid, 1980). Rehearsal does occur when the individual is given increased time (Turner & Bray, 1985).

The type of information and the stimulus mode greatly affect memory. For example, there appears to be little difference in spatial location memory for non-mentally retarded children and adults and adults with mental retardation, even those with IQs as low as 30 (Ellis, Woodley-Zanthos, & Dulaney, 1989). In contrast, adults with mental retardation perform much less well on free-recall tasks of auditory information.

Each auditory stimulus event has a sensory, or sign, impression inherent in the event and an abstract, or symbol, representation for that event. The sign is meaningful but nonlinguistic. For example, the sound of a horn may signal an automobile. In contrast, the abstract representation, or word, is linguistic in nature. Memory should be better for signs because internal representation is based originally on perception. In other words, our early meaning of *doggie* is based on the perceptual attributes of the examples of *doggie* that we have encountered. The name or word *doggie* is superimposed later. Our ability to infer an entity from an auditory sign is part of our early linguistic knowledge base. Children with mental retardation and MA-matched nonretarded preschoolers have similar recall for signal information, but children with mental retardation have significantly poorer recognition and recall of symbolic representations (Lamberts, 1981). There may be a link, therefore, between the reported language deficits and auditory memory deficits of the mentally retarded population.

Sentence recall probably involves reproduction of the memory episode and then editing of the text. Because individuals with mental retardation make frequent word-substitution errors, performance may break down in the second stage (Bilsky, Walker, & Sakales, 1983). Poor sentence recall by individuals in the retarded population may reflect poor editing skills or a breakdown in syntactic-semantic analysis, although phonological processing may be unaffected (Merrill & Mar, 1987).

Poor reading recall, on the other hand, may be related to failure to use important textual information for organization. Selective attention to important portions of reading passages can be taught, however, with resultant recall improvement (Luftig & Johnson, 1982).

Auditory memory deficits are particularly evident in the Down syndrome population (Marcell & Armstrong, 1982; Marcell & Weeks, 1988). This difficulty may be related to **echoic memory,** "the ability to hear a sound for some time after physical stimulation has ceased" (Watkins & Watkins, 1980, p. 252). In other words, echoic memory is the ability to remember what has been heard even when it is no longer present. Echoic memory is a passive retention strategy related to immediate recall of linguistic stimuli and seems to be most efficient with the fast rates found in conversation. Among individuals with Down syndrome, however, this echo may decay more rapidly than in the nonretarded population, or at a rate at which the slower processing of the retarded cannot access it. Individuals with Down syndrome may not realize how to use such passive strategies effectively (Marcell & Armstrong, 1982). Other studies have demonstrated the generally inefficient use of memory strategies by the retarded population. As reported previously, individuals with Down syndrome have poorer successive cognitive processing than do other retarded individuals and, thus, poorer auditory sequential memory (Snart et al., 1982). Individuals with Down syndrome also exhibit difficulties in vocabulary storage and retrieval (Varnhagen, Das, & Varnhagen, 1987). These data support the reportedly low language performance of those with Down syndrome in comparison to other retarded individuals.

In general, persons with mental retardation demonstrate poorer recall than MA-matched nonretarded peers. Not all areas are affected equally, and there is some indication that memory for spatial location is a strength that can be used to enhance learning (Nigro & Roak, 1987).

Conclusion

The mentally retarded population seems to develop cognitively in a manner similar to the nonretarded but at a slower rate. Overall, mental development of adults, as measured in Down syndrome individuals, continues well into midlife (Berry, Groeneweg, Gibson, & Brown, 1984). Some cognitive processing differences exist, however, especially in organization and memory. It is important to remember, too, that information processing differences do not explain mental retardation and may represent the cause or result, or a concurrent problem (Leonard, 1987).

Reported differences in personality and motivational functioning may reflect experiential differences (Leahy, Balla, & Zigler, 1982). In general, as the level of severity increases, wide individual differences become more apparent. With more severe retardation, cognitive functioning may be complicated by accompanying organic disorders. For persons with mild retardation, however, IQ alone is not a particularly powerful predictor of life adjustment. It is important to recall that individuals with mental retardation, especially those who are noninstitutionalized, exhibit integrated problem-solving abilities daily. For example, they must make decisions regarding their daily schedule, personal hygiene, nutrition, and employment. The individuals who are independent or challenged early are even more flexible problem solvers, because they have developed internal models of the mechanics of addressing problems (Levine & Langness, 1985).

LANGUAGE AND COMMUNICATION SKILLS: DIFFERENCE AND DELAY

The language behavior of the mentally retarded population is frequently one of the most problematic areas of adaptive behavior and may be the single most important characteristic of this population. Ultimately, language behavior will determine an individual's ability to function independently in the outside world. Although MA-matched nonretarded individuals and those with mental retardation may be similar in many cognitive functions, individuals with mental retardation often exhibit difficulty with symbolic functions, including language (Kamhi, 1981).

The exact relationship of cognition and language for all humans is unknown. The relationship may be inconsistent—cognition might influence language at some phases of development and language influence cognition during other phases (Miller, Chapman, & MacKenzie, 1981). Among individuals with mental retardation, several patterns emerge and may vary with age, severity of retardation, and task. The most frequent patterns are as follows (Miller et al., 1981):

1. Comprehension and cognition are at similar levels, but production is below that of cognition.
2. Both comprehension and production are below the level of cognition.
3. Both comprehension and production are at the level of cognition.

As much as 50 percent of the mentally retarded population may be within the third group. It is important to note that the relationship of cognition and language is not stable over time for any individual (Cole, Dale, & Mills, 1992).

Questions of difference versus delay and quality versus quantity of language and communication behaviors have been debated for decades (Kamhi & Masterson, 1989). In general, before a mental age of 10 years, the language development of the retarded population seems to follow that of the nonretarded and to differ only in the speed or in the quantity of language or the length of utterances produced (Weiss, Weisz, & Bromfield, 1986). After a mental age of 10 years, the developmental paths seem to deviate, and the language of the two groups shows qualitative differences as well.

Such debates may turn on nonissues, given that language and cognition are not the same (Kamhi & Masterson, 1989). Nor can we assume that all aspects of language differ in a similar manner. Some areas of language and cognition overlap; others are distinct.

Studies of the language development of the retarded population suffer from a number of limitations (Kamhi & Masterson, 1989). First, the retarded population is not homogeneous and it is difficult to make generalizations. Second, results may vary with the assessment instruments used. Third, attempts to match subjects by mental age may be inappropriate given the lack of knowledge of the relationship between cognition and language.

I will attempt to describe the results of a number of studies of language in the retarded population, threading through the mix of severity of retardation, subject matching, and level of development. The major characteristics of the language of the retarded population are listed in Table 10.3. This table is based on summarized data and on group data. Individuals or specific subgroups, especially those with more severe impairment, may exhibit different behavior. Some individuals with profound retardation will not use expressive language beyond single symbols, if at all.

Parameters of Language

Five parameters of language are generally recognized—syntax, morphology, phonology, semantics, and pragmatics. All five parameters have been examined in research studies of the language of persons with mental retardation.

TABLE 10.3	**Language Characteristics of Children with Mental Retardation**
Pragmatics	Gestural and intentional developmental patterns similar to those of children developing normally. Delayed gestural requesting. May take less dominant conversational role. No difference in clarification skills from mental age-matched peers developing typically.
Semantics	More concrete word meanings. Slow vocabulary growth. More limited use of a variety of semantic units. Children with Down syndrome able to learn word meanings from exposure in context as well as mental age-matched peers developing typically.
Syntax/ morphology	Length–complexity relationship similar to that of preschoolers developing typically. Same sequence of general sentence development as children developing typically. Shorter, less-complex sentences, with fewer subject elaborations or relative clauses than mental age-matched peers developing typically. Sentence word order takes precedence over word relationships. Reliance on less mature forms, though capable of more advanced. Same order of morpheme development as preschoolers developing typically.
Phonology	Phonological rules similar to those of preschoolers developing typically, but reliance on less mature forms, though capable of more advanced ones.
Comprehension	Poorer receptive language skills, especially children with Down syndrome, than mental age-matched peers developing typically. Poorer sentence recall than mental age-matched peers. More reliance on context to extract meaning.

Sources: Based on Abbeduto, Davies, Solesby, & Furman (1991); Abbeduto, Short-Meyerson, Benson, & Dolish (1997); Bender & Carlson (1982); Chapman, Kay-Raining Bird, & Schwartz (1990); Chapman, Schwartz, & Kay-Raining Bird (1988); Kernan (1990); Klink, Gerstman, Raphael, Schlanger, & Newsome (1986); Lobato, Barrera, & Feldman (1981); McLeavey, Toomey, & Dempsey (1982); Merrill & Bilsky (1990); Mervis (1988); Moran, Money, & Leonard (1984); Mundy, Kasari, Sigman, & Ruskin, (1995); Owens & MacDonald (1982); Prater (1982); Rondal, Ghiotto, Bredart, & Bachelet (1988); Rosin, Swift, Bless, & Vetter (1988); Shriberg & Widder (1990).

Pragmatics

Many individuals with mental retardation "are seriously and basically deficient in this area of social . . . functions" (McLean & Snyder-McLean, 1978, p. 190). Research studies have reached varying conclusions, but there is little doubt that those individuals residing in developmental centers demonstrate greater deficiencies in language use.

Pragmatic functions first become evident with the development of gestures. At this point, children begin to express primitive intentions, such as signaling notice, attracting attention, or making demands. Both nonretarded children and those with mild and moderate retardation accompanying Down syndrome exhibit gestures at the same level of cognitive development (Greenwald & Leonard, 1979). Both groups of children use gestures to enlist help or to gain an object and use declarative gestures to gain attention. These gestures develop in Piaget's sensorimotor substage 4 (age 8–12 months for the nonretarded infant).

Gestures may be classified as contact, such as touching an object or a person, or as distal, such as pointing. More mature distal gestures are associated with a wider range and a greater frequency of communication functions across individuals with mental retardation (McLean, Brady, McLean, & Behrens, 1999).

For children with severe retardation, gestures do not appear until substage 5 (Lobato, Barrera, & Feldman, 1981). The gestures of individuals with profound mental retardation primarily function to regulate behavior of others (Ogletree, Wetherby, & Westling, 1992). Initiated by the individual rather than by the conversational partner, these gestures are often performed in isolation with little vocalization.

Among children with Down syndrome, grammatical production lags well behind comprehension. Word comprehension and gestural production appear to be closely correlated among these children, suggesting that a strong gestural repertoire influences their comprehension (Caselli, Vicari, Longobardi, Lami, Pizzoli, & Stella, 1998).

For both the retarded and nonretarded populations, the appearance of language is strongly correlated with the cognitive functions of substage 4 (Lobato et al., 1981). In general, the language of retarded and nonretarded children fulfills the functions earlier expressed in gestures. The distribution of most functions is similar for both groups of children when matched for language development level (Owens & MacDonald, 1982). Both groups of children are able to answer and to ask questions spontaneously, to reply to the comments of others, to make spontaneous declarations and demands, to name or label entities, and to imitate and practice language spontaneously.

Imitation of others and self-repetition may develop differently for individuals with Down syndrome (Owens & MacDonald, 1982; Sokolov, 1992). In general, imitation decreases for children developing normally as they begin to learn syntax. The rate of decrease is significantly less for children with Down syndrome. This difference may indicate a continued reliance on outmoded learning strategies by children with mental retardation. The typically developing child may discard inefficient strategies more readily.

At the single-word or early multiword stage, typically developing children begin to demonstrate presuppositional skills. They presuppose that their communication partners are aware of redundant or old information in a situation, and therefore label only aspects of a situation that are undergoing change or are new information. For example, the child may not name the cup on the high chair each morning, but may label with the word *cup* a new cup recently received from Grandma. Toddlers with mild retardation also exhibit this behavior.

Presuppositional skills may be a forerunner of several perspective-taking behaviors used in everyday communication, such as the ability to assume the communication partner's perceptual viewpoint in interpretation of terms such as *here* and *there* and to assess a partner's knowledge or emotional state. Children with mild and moderate retardation and younger, nonretarded second graders matched for cognitive abilities exhibit similar perspective-taking behaviors (Bender & Carlson, 1982).

Although individuals with mental retardation reportedly are delayed in role taking and in referential communication, these differences are not found when subjects are matched for social maturity (Blacher, 1982). Referential communication refers to a target referent by distinguishing it from others, such as "the girl with the white dress" or "big doggie." Children with mental retardation are less able to distinguish referents for their listeners than are their MA-matched peers who are nonretarded (Brownell & Whitely, 1992). These referential skills can be taught.

Although individuals who are mentally retarded seem as adept as their MA-matched nonretarded peers in selecting the appropriate referent or subject of discussion within context, they are less skilled in requesting clarification of information when the context is uninformative (Abbeduto, Davies, Solesby, & Furman, 1991). This conclusion seems odd given the abilities of individuals with mental retardation to request clarification (Abbeduto & Rosenberg, 1980) and to use the context and linguistic memory for referent identification (Abbeduto & Rosenberg, 1980; Abbeduto, Short-Meyerson, Benson, Dolish, & Weissman, 1998). Possibly the requirements of conversation are such that the individual with mental retardation cannot integrate these skills when needed. An inability to seek such clarification may be critical, given a report that individuals with Down syndrome have difficulty understanding sentences without a supporting extralinguistic context (Kernan, 1990).

The requirements of the conversational context may also account for the amount of verbal perseveratives found in the speech of adults with mental retardation (Rein & Kernan, 1989). Verbal perseveration is excessive talking on a topic even when inappropriate or previously addressed in the conversation. Such behavior may be used by individuals with mental retardation to maintain the interaction or to "buy time" until they can produce a more appropriate response. The use of verbal perseveratives varies within the retarded population. Males with Fragile X syndrome have been shown to produce more perseverative, repetitive, inappropriate, and off-topic utterances than males with Down syndrome (Sudhalter, Cohen, Silverman, & Wolf-Schein, 1990; Wolf-Schein et al., 1987).

All of the preceding skills are interrelated in the conversational context. In a conversation, roles and topics change, and each partner must try to assess how much information his partner needs. In general, individuals with mental retardation are less able to judge the nonverbal emotions of their communication partners than are MA-matched nonretarded peers, and thus are less able to respond appropriately (Marcell & Jett, 1985). The conversational role of persons with mental retardation seems to be one of nondominance. Children with mental retardation are more likely to keep greater interpersonal distance, a possible reflection of the child's perception of little personal control. Likewise, adults with mental retardation rarely exert dominance in a conversation even when the communication partner is a child, although these adults possess the communication skills to do so. This subservient conversational behavior is more pronounced in institutionalized populations and can be noted in the case study at the end of the chapter.

Semantics

As a group, individuals with mental retardation exhibit poorer receptive language skills than their MA-matched peers, although there are many variations among individuals (Abbeduto, Furman, & Davies, 1989). These two facts may relate to the type and severity of mental retardation, to cognitive processing, and/or to environment.

Word meanings of the retarded population seem more concrete than those of the nonretarded. For example, *cold* may be defined in relation to temperature but not to the psychological aspects, such as in a *cold personality*. There appears to be no difference in the quality of definition, however, as measured by the Stanford-Binet intelligence test.

Word meanings are established in a two-step process that includes a quick, general determination of meaning from the context, a process called fast mapping, and a slower evolution of meaning from use. Children with Down syndrome are as skilled as MA-matched peers who are nonretarded in inferring novel word meanings. They are also equally skilled at producing words correctly thereafter (Chapman, Kay-Raining Bird, & Schwartz, 1990).

As might be expected, figurative language such as idioms poses particular difficulties. Context is very important in aiding comprehension for individuals with Down syndrome (Ezell & Goldstein, 1991).

Finally, both individuals with mild retardation accompanying Down syndrome and MA-matched nonretarded individuals display all features of verbs and noun inflections. Individuals with Down syndrome use these features less frequently.

Syntax

In general, the overall sequence of development of syntactic structures is similar for the mildly retarded and the nonretarded populations; however, the rate of development is slower among those with mental retardation. Both sentence length and complexity increase with development. In addition, the same sentence types appear and in the same order for both groups. There is a general trend from simple declarative to negative sentences, and then interrogative to negative interrogative sentences. Within interrogatives, the order of development is also similar. For example, *what* and *where* types develop initially, and *when, why,* and *how* appear last.

Even at equivalent mental age levels, however, individuals with retardation appear to use shorter, less complex sentences than their nonretarded peers (McLeavey, Toomey, & Dempsey, 1982). These characteristics are evident in the case study at the end of this chapter. Individuals with mild retardation use fewer complex structures, such as subject elaborations and relative clauses. These deficiencies may reflect poorer linguistic rule generalization. Poor rule generalization does not imply an inability to learn language rules, although persons with mental retardation seem to rely more on sequential placement than on grammatical rules. In other words, sentence word order takes precedence over the relationships between different word classes. The result is less flexible linguistic structure although still a rule-oriented approach to language (McLeavey et al., 1982). Even individuals with severe retardation are capable of using linguistic rules. Taken together, these findings suggest that persons with retardation learn and use linguistic rules but also rely more on primitive word-order rules than do their nonretarded language peers.

One measure of sentence complexity for initial sentence development is mean length of utterance (MLU). For children both with Down syndrome and those who are nonretarded, MLU correlates strongly with chronological age and predicts complexity and diversity of sentence development (Rondal, Ghiotto, Bredart, & Bachelet, 1988). MLU appears to be a good measure of complexity to an average of 3.5 morphemes for both groups.

Any syntactic lag noted among persons with retardation may represent a dependence on older syntactic forms for a longer time during development (McLeavey et al., 1982). Advanced syntactic forms are learned but used less frequently.

Finally, individuals with mental retardation exhibit poorer recall of sentences than their MA-matched peers (Merrill & Bilsky, 1990). Within the mentally retarded population, males with Fragile X syndrome appear to have more difficulty with auditory sequential memory and auditory reception than males with Down syndrome (Hagerman, Kemper, & Hudson, 1985). This poorer performance may reflect poorer quality mental representations of the sentences to be recalled or an inability to encode the significant semantic information for a holistic, integrated memory (Merrill & Mar, 1987). Although individuals with Down syndrome seem to have recall patterns similar to those of nonretarded individuals, they have greater difficulty when there is no supporting extralinguistic context (Kernan, 1990).

Sentence recall and context utilization for individuals with mental retardation can be enhanced when the semantic relatedness of the words in a sentence is increased (Merrill & Jackson, 1992). For example, the sentence, "The hunter shot the rabbit," has more relatedness across the words than "The photographer chased the rabbit" and is thus easier to recall.

Morphology

In developmental studies, the same order of morphological acquisition has been reported for both the retarded and the nonretarded populations. The pattern of development seems to be delayed, even beyond what one might expect for mental age, but not significantly different.

Phonology

Individuals with profound retardation vocalize less when gesturing than do individuals developing typically. These vocalizations often lack consonants (Ogletree et al., 1992). Infants with Down syndrome and less severe retardation babble in a fashion similar to that of chronologically age-matched peers who are developing typically (Steffens, Oller, Lynch, & Urbano, 1992). Over time, both groups of children produce more mature vowels and more well-formed syllables, and fewer quasi-vowel sounds and fewer marginal syllables.

The articulation and phonologic characteristics of the mentally retarded population can be summarized as follows (Shriberg & Widder, 1990):

1. Articulation errors are more common than in the nonretarded population.
2. Most frequent error is deletion of consonants.
3. Errors are likely to be inconsistent.
4. Patterns are similar to those of nonretarded children or children with a functional delay.
5. Individuals with Down syndrome have perceptually and acoustically distinct prosody.

The types of errors and the level of mental retardation do not seem to be related, although a majority of institutionalized and/or severely retarded persons exhibit articulation disorders.

In general, individuals with mental retardation use the same phonological processes as nonretarded children but with greater frequency (Klink, Gerstman, Raphael, Schlanger, & Newsome, 1986; Moran, Money, & Leonard, 1984). The most common phonological processes exhibited by the mentally retarded population are reduction of consonant clusters and final-consonant deletion (Klink et al., 1986; Bleile & Schwartz, 1984; Oller & Seibert, 1988; Sommers, Patterson, & Wildgren, 1988; Van Borsel, 1988). When a nonretarded child cannot produce two consonants together (e.g., *stop*), the child deletes one consonant to produce a simpler version (e.g., *top*). Final-consonant deletion is usually the result of consonant–vowel (CV) syllable learning. In this process, words consist of CV or CVCV constructions. Because final consonants, such as a CVC construction, violate this process, the child may delete the final consonant. Individuals with mental retardation may exhibit much variability in their use of these processes.

Other processes are the same as those of younger, nonretarded children (Prater, 1982). Individuals with mental retardation may use these processes even when they are capable of producing the deleted or modified sound. It is possible, therefore, that these processes serve a different purpose for the retarded population than for the nonretarded. For example, consonant deletions may reflect cognitive processing constraints in the motor assembly stage of speech production (Shriberg & Widder, 1990).

Oral language skills correlate closely with reading skills. Phonological awareness—rhyming, syllabication, phoneme recognition and identification—is a prerequisite of reading. Children with Down syndrome have similar phonological awareness skills to non-Down syndrome peers relative to reading ability (Cupples & Iacono, 2000).

Summary

Studies of the language of the mentally retarded population offer varying, sometimes conflicting, results. In general, however, the language abilities of persons with retardation are similar to those of mental age-matched nonretarded peers, although some differences do exist.

Several studies have indicated that language abilities among individuals with mental retardation are delayed beyond expectations based on mental age alone, although the course of development is similar to that for nonretarded persons. This language delay, particularly evident among individuals with Down syndrome (Mahoney, Glover, & Finger, 1981), becomes evident soon after language acquisition begins, as the level of vocabulary development begins to lag behind cognitive development (Cardosa-Martins, Mervis, & Mervis, 1985).

Individuals with Down syndrome continue to develop language well into adolescence and early adulthood. In general, these individuals produce shorter utterances with fewer words and fewer different words in an overall language sample than MA-matched non-Down syndrome peers (Chapman, Seung, Schwartz, & Kay-Raining Bird, 1998). Down syndrome is only one of hundreds of possible conditions related to mental retardation. Others may exhibit distinct patterns of speech, language, and communication (Alvares & Downing, 1998).

Differences in mental age and language may reflect symbol processing deficiencies within the retarded population. Therefore, in language therapy, "it seems more defensible to teach individuals how to learn, and this implies the training of underlying processes" (Ashman, 1982, p. 636).

Environmental Influences on the Language of Individuals with Mental Retardation

Individuals with mental retardation are generally found in two types of environments: home centered or residential. The different environmental influences on learning have been well documented (Conroy, Efthimiou, & Lemanowicz, 1982). In general, individuals who live in institutions have fewer adaptive skills and are more dependent. Both language and communication are adaptive behaviors. Some aspects of language may be affected differently by institutionalization, especially pragmatics and semantics. In general, there is a deterioration of language abilities with extended institutionalization. The adult described at the end of this chapter exhibits few conversational initiations. Her verbal behavior is mostly responsive.

Parent–Child Interaction

Is there some special feature of the language-learning home environment of children with mental retardation that can account for the mental age–language age gap? One theory contends that if infants with mental retardation behave differently from nonretarded infants, the mothers of each group must respond to their infants differently. According to this notion, mother–child interaction patterns can adversely affect a child's language development.

The importance of early mother–child interaction has been increasingly recognized. Typically developing children have an established repertoire of communication skills before they speak their first words. These words usually fulfill the communicative functions already in place. The infant's communication skills develop within the interaction of mother and child (Owens, 2001).

The stress that accompanies the birth of an infant with a handicapping condition may alter the dynamics of family relations. There is an initial period of grief before a more normal relationship evolves. The sense of grief may be compounded by feelings of estrangement from an infant whose communication skills do not fulfill parental expectations.

Because the interactional process is one of mutual adaptation by the two partners, some researchers assume that a child with retardation will alter the mother's behavior differently than will a nonretarded infant. In addition, infants with Down syndrome may allow less time for maternal turn taking and use less referential eye contact. Consequently, "this reduction in the quality of the dialogue of emotional expression may result in parents being less effective with such children" (Trotter, 1983, p. 20). Mothers of children with mental retardation must contend with ambiguous parent–child social norms and with inconsistent child behaviors (Eheart, 1982). The situation is made more acute by a lack of information on and assistance with development, by possible feelings of grief and guilt, and by fear of an unknown future.

Among children who are language delayed but who exhibit no other disability, some professionals have assumed that maternal or family language patterns are a contributing factor. For example, mothers of language-delayed children reportedly use more directives (Cardosa-Martins et al., 1985; Hanzlik & Stevenson, 1986), provide fewer opportunities for their children to use language, use less referential or object-directed speech (Cardosa-Martins et al., 1985), and are less verbally responsive (Hanzlik & Stevenson, 1986). Although this maternal behavior is found in some language-delay cases, it cannot be assumed that this pattern represents general maternal interaction with language-delayed children with mental retardation.

Mothers of preschool children with Down syndrome and MA-matched nonretarded children both use control to support and encourage their children's play (Tannock, 1988). As a group, mothers of children with Down syndrome have been found to exert more verbal control, whereas mothers of nonretarded children are more likely to watch quietly (Tannock, 1988). The mothers of children with Down syndrome talk to their children more (Berger & Cunningham, 1983). They initiate more topics, repeat more utterances, and take more turns (Maurer & Sherrod, 1987). In general, the children with Down syndrome are more passive and do not respond in turn as frequently. Both groups of mothers are equally responsive to their children's verbalizations.

In teaching situations, both groups of mothers have been found to be equally directive. Possibly the mothers of children with Down syndrome perceive their role as instructional, aware of their children's language learning difficulties (Davis, Stroud, & Green, 1988).

The patterns of directives used by mothers of retarded and nonretarded children are similar in their hierarchy of change over time, although the mothers of children with Down syndrome demonstrate more reluctance to change to more mature patterns such as indirect requests (Maurer & Sherrod, 1987).

Mothers act according to their expectations of the infants' behavior and attempt to keep their infants within these expectations. In general, more active and less irritable infants receive optimum maternal responsiveness. Infants with Down syndrome or early medical disorders exhibit rather inactive behavior. Infants in intensive-care nurseries are reported to have high irritability. It might be expected, therefore, that mothers of these children would be less responsive than mothers of nondisordered infants and that lack of maternal responsiveness might result in the infant's withdrawal. Further research is needed in this area.

Predictable and responsive infants participate more in the parent–infant interactional environment. At-risk infants are less predictable and less responsive (Affleck, Allen, McGrade, & McQueeney, 1982). Nevertheless, research does not support the conclusion that mothers of infants with mental retardation are more restrictive of the infants' activities and less responsive. In fact, these mothers interpret more of their children's behaviors as communicative than do mothers of nonretarded children (Yoder & Feagans, 1988). It is the mothers' attribution of meaning to the child's behavior, not just the behavior itself, that affects the mothers' responses (Harding, 1984).

In studies of the mothers of children with mental retardation and chronological age-matched (CA-matched) nonretarded peers, the mothers of the former have been found to use more "primitive" forms of speech. The unwarranted conclusion has been that these mothers are inhibiting their children's growth. We expect children with retardation to function at a lower cognitive and language level than chronological peers. Of more concern is the appropriateness of this maternal input for the linguistic competence of the child.

Mothers of children with Down syndrome alter their linguistic input appropriately for the language level of their children. Research has shown no significant difference between the mothers of children with Down syndrome and mothers of nonretarded children in both verbal and nonverbal behaviors (Buckhalt, Rutherford, & Goldberg, 1978; Cardosa-Martins & Mervis, 1990). Mothers use "Motherese," a style of speaking that is characterized by short sentences, redundancy, long pauses, gesturing, and exaggerated intonation and stress patterns.

In addition, mothers of Down syndrome and nonretarded children have been found to use similar response classes, with a few exceptions. Mothers of nonretarded children use more whole and partial repetitions, as do their children. In contrast, children with mental retardation and their mothers have been reported to use more comments and replies. In both groups, repetitions decrease and comments and replies increase with the children's increasing language abilities. In part, the more conversational style of the mothers with their retarded children may reflect the older age of these children compared to the nonretarded mental age-matched subjects.

Maternal changes accompany children's changing abilities (Petersen & Sherrod, 1982). With retarded and nonretarded children, and those with language delayed, mothers use language more prominently in interactions as their children's language progresses. Requests for nonverbal behavior decrease, and language-seeking utterances and verbal feedback increase. Language-seeking utterances consist of questions, requests for elaboration, labeling, and imitation. Both negative and positive feedback increase with children's increasing language abilities as mothers become more discriminating and more demanding (Petersen & Sherrod, 1982).

There are differences among these groups of mothers, however. Some researchers report a lack of rapport on the part of mothers of children with language delays and mothers of children with Down syndrome (Petersen & Sherrod, 1982). In addition, mothers of children with mental retardation dominate the parent–child interaction more than mothers of CA-matched nonretarded children (Eheart, 1982). Mothers of children with mental retardation are more directive and initiate interactions more frequently. For example, mothers of children with Down syndrome require their children to imitate more. The continued use of verbal imitation by children with Down syndrome long after such a language learning strategy has ceased to be a viable learning technique has been noted (Owens & MacDonald, 1982). If mothers foster imitation beyond a language age of approximately 30 months, it could negatively affect language development (Petersen & Sherrod, 1982). In addition, the utterances of mothers of children with mental retardation may be more noncontingent or more off-topic than those of mothers of nonretarded children (Mahoney, Fors, & Wood, 1990). These mothers incorporate fewer of their children's topics than do mothers of nonretarded children (Miller & Newhoff, 1978). Thus, the child may lack the vital extralinguistic and linguistic context needed for interpretation.

Children with mental retardation respond less frequently to their mothers' initiations (Eheart, 1982). In addition, the children initiate communication only half as often as nonretarded children. In part, this behavior may reflect a larger ratio of adult-to-child utterances.

Staff–Client Interaction

In general, a lack of appropriate verbal interactions seems to exist within large residential settings. A large percentage of directives are used by the institutional staff. Such behavior is unlikely to elicit much verbal interchange. Clients are least responsive following staff directives, the most frequent staff verbal behavior. In contrast, the least frequent behavior, staff-initiated conversation, elicits the most verbal client responses. When clients do verbalize, staff personnel are as likely to ignore the behavior as to respond with a verbal comment or reply. The most frequent staff behavior is a nonverbal agreement in the form of a head nod. Even though clients respond very little to staff instructions, such communication does provide language input. Yet, for most of the day, clients are left alone in unstructured settings. These features mitigate against the development of verbal communicative competence. Residence in a developmental center is likely to have its greatest effect on pragmatics. Individuals who reside in community residences are more likely to use their pragmatic skills (McLean et al., 1999; Van Der Gagg, 1989).

Professionals must shoulder some of the blame for the less dominant role that individuals with mental retardation take in conversations (Peter, 2000). The language used by professionals tends to objectify these individuals. Many aspects of the lives of individuals with mental retardation are defined by others. In short, they are treated as defective. Professional staff exert control in part through their use of directives and questions, two speech acts found infrequently among individuals with mental retardation (Domingo, Barrow, & Amato, 1998). Persons with mental retardation are often treated as category members rather than individuals, and are labeled with terms that demean or note their abnormality (Danforth & Navarro, 1998).

Summary

Individuals who are mentally retarded receive better linguistic input and more conversational opportunities within a home environment. The mother–child data are mixed, however, suggesting that although mothers adapt form and content to the linguistic competence of their children, these same mothers provide primarily a responsive verbal environment. Thus, children with mental retardation initiate less communication than their nonretarded peers. We cannot assume, however, that differences indicate a cause for language delay. The differences in speech and language of the mother may be in response to the children's language problems rather than their cause. Even if mothers of children with mental retardation did provide linguistic form, content, and use styles similar to those of mothers of nonretarded children, it might not be appropriate for the special language learning needs of their retarded children.

LANGUAGE AND COMMUNICATION INTERVENTION

Many of the language and communication intervention techniques discussed in this text for use with other language-disordered populations can also be used with individuals with mental retardation. Some intervention methods, however, seem particularly germane for this population.

Our knowledge of the cognitive functioning and language processes of the mentally retarded population, although limited, suggests some principles and techniques for intervention. I will discuss these globally and then specifically address various aspects of language assessment and intervention. The breadth of this topic and the discussion of and intervention in other chapters will allow for only general discussion of the topic.

Principles of Assessment and Intervention

The characteristics of the mentally retarded population suggest some guiding principles for speech-language pathologists. Of necessity, these principles will be general. The speech-language pathologist must remember that each person with mental retardation is an individual and that individual differences such as age, level of cognitive functioning, previous training, residential environment, and learning style will alter the methods actually used. The principles are summarized in Table 10.4.

Language and Communication Intervention Methodologies

In general, training goals should be explicit, with the information organized for easy learning and recall. For example, direct teaching of vocabulary words seems to be superior to more indirect training (Hanley-Maxwell, Wilcox, & Heal, 1982).

The clinician should consider the skills that the client brings to the task and those skills required for successful learning. To require too much in the form of new learning or transfer often hinders the client's ability to be successful. A question-probe technique can foster comprehension and help individuals with mental retardation to assess the learning that they bring to a new situation (Zetlin & Gallimore, 1983). In this technique, newly learned skills are questioned and probed continually as they are learned to ensure understanding by the client.

TABLE 10.4	Principles for Intervention with Clients Who Are Mentally Retarded

1. Highlight new or relevant material.
2. Preorganize information.
3. Train rehearsal strategies.
4. Use overlearning and repetition.
5. Train in the natural environment.
6. Begin as early as possible.
7. Follow developmental guidelines.

Some structured training is usually necessary for initial learning, and repetition of initial procedures may aid further learning of the targeted skill. It may even facilitate learning if the material is presented in the same order until a certain criterion of performance is reached.

Transfer can be facilitated by keeping the training situation as close to the everyday environment as possible. The clever clinician will use objects, persons, and events from this environment for training or, better still, train in the use environment.

The developmental model of language intervention also works well with individuals with mental retardation. Theoretically, the easiest structures are learned first by nonretarded children and therefore are targeted first for training.

Highlight New or Relevant Material

Individuals with mental retardation are capable of attending well when they understand to what they should attend. New information, materials, or methods should be highlighted so that the client does not miss them or assume that they are unimportant. For example, new pictures on a communication board might be drawn in a different color or placed in a special area of the board. Stimuli that require certain responses or language features that govern language use should also be highlighted. For example, words such as *yesterday* and *last week* signal use of past tense. The waiter's utterance, "What may I get for you?," signals a requesting response.

Attending need not be targeted directly for intervention. Improved attending has been reported as a result of augmentative communication training for institutionalized children and adults with severe retardation (Abrahamsen, Romski, & Sevcik, 1989).

Generalization is enhanced by a related principle: *Train scanning of a task for relevant or similar stimuli.* Generalization is often difficult for individuals with mental retardation because they are unsure of which stimuli are relevant.

Preorganize Information

Speech-language pathologists can aid learning by pregrouping information to facilitate organization and later recall. Organization strategies such as physical conceptual arrangement, grouping, and consistent ordering can also be taught. In general, persons with mental retardation are able to retain information better if it is organized first, and if the learning task is explained by the teacher. Individuals with mild retardation have better recall if material is grouped spatially rather than presented singly (Harris, 1982). For example, an adult who is experiencing difficulty recalling four digits, such as 6–3–8–5, may do better if the digits are grouped in pairs to form 63 and 85. Such grouping does not seem to aid the recall of nonretarded individuals, possibly because they already employ this strategy. In conclusion, instructions and procedures should be clear, logically sequenced, and involve as many senses as possible (Pruess, Vadasy, & Fewell, 1987).

Train Rehearsal Strategies

Individuals with mild and moderate mental retardation can improve their memory abilities through the training of rehearsal strategies (Burger, Blackman, & Tan, 1980; Reid, 1980). Rehearsal aids the transfer of learned material to long-term storage. This may be especially true for visual information such as communicative signs or gestures, the learning of which enhances associated word recall (Bowler, 1991).

Use Overlearning and Repetition

Although rehearsal or extra training facilitates learning and recall, it does not seem to directly enhance transfer (Day & Hall, 1988). Those who receive extra training, however, subsequently need less assistance with transfer.

Train in the Natural Environment

Individuals with mental retardation have great difficulty generalizing training to novel contexts. Although highly structured training may increase the rate of learning, especially for individuals with severe retardation, such training may be limited to the training context" (Salzberg & Villani, 1983). In other words, it is difficult to teach the spontaneous use of skills in untrained situations. Highly structured settings offer a limited variety of communication situations. Accordingly, "the problem is how to incorporate procedures into the initial training that will actively induce generalization" (Spradlin & Siegel, 1982, p. 3).

Although "many teachers view language as a 45-minute period or lesson . . . [it] is an integral part of any interpersonal communication and is best learned in the natural context of those daily interactions" (Looney, 1980, p. 31). We can expect little generalization with pictures or with objects not within the natural environment (Simic & Bucher, 1980). The typically limited stimuli used in the classroom or clinic often have little relation to the natural environment. In other words, difficulties in generalization can be minimized if training occurs using familiar materials within daily activities occurring in everyday locations of the client (Gullo & Gullo, 1984; McCormick, 1986; Stowitschek, McConaughy, Peatross, Salzberg, & Lignngaris/ Kraft, 1988). Most communication training approaches for individuals with moderate to severe mental retardation advocate use of the natural environment (Caro & Snell, 1989).

Language training is more functional if taught in the situations where there is actually a need for language to be used. The general result is more spontaneous usage, which in turn motivates the individual to learn more language. "One of the reasons so little spontaneity has been observed with this population is that the training has not been functional" (Wulz, Hall, & Klein, 1983, p. 3). Natural stimuli present in the training environment become "signals" associated with the behavior trained.

Everyday routines also provide an excellent vehicle for training and facilitate generalization. Routines provide a familiar script or scaffolding that enables the client to participate more fully by freeing cognitive energy that might otherwise be used to aid participation. Children with mental retardation seem to produce more speech and more diverse vocabulary in routine situations than in other less familiar situations (Yoder & Davies, 1992).

People within the natural environment, such as parents, teachers, and aides, should be included in the training as language trainers and as clients themselves (Owens, 1982d, 1999). In short, greater involvement by caregivers yields greater results for generalization to the home and other settings.

The effective use of parents as behavior change agents is well established (Heifetz, 1980). Infant stimulation programs conducted in the home by trained parents can significantly improve the functioning of children with mental retardation (Sharav & Shlomo, 1986). Several parent variables can affect the outcome. Parent socioeconomic status, pretraining skills, and experience positively correlate with the short-term learning outcomes (Clark, Baker, & Heifetz, 1982). Working-class mothers also can make positive strides with their children, because prior to training, these mothers often overlook natural teaching situations used by middle- and upper-class mothers. The successful use of higher-functioning individuals with mental retardation as language trainers for clients with more severe involvement has also been documented. The key to success with language trainers is consideration of individual trainer differences and learning styles, and individualization of the techniques that these trainers use (Reese & Serna, 1986).

In general, mothers of children with Down syndrome assume a manager or teacher role more often and are more responsive than fathers (Stoneman, Brody, & Abbott, 1983). Parents with some instruction were able to modify their speech to their children in order to improve the children's expressive skills. Apparently, knowledge of the direction in which training should proceed is sufficient information to allow some parents spontaneously to adopt suitable teaching strategies.

The variables that control transfer of parental skills to natural settings are not fully understood. Transfer increases with the similarity of the tasks and of training structure to the natural environment (Salzberg & Villani, 1983). Feedback from the speech-language pathologist regarding the application of newly acquired training skills is also important.

Successful use of parents as language facilitators seems to depend on three components (Salzberg & Villani, 1983).

- Parents must use their training skills at home.
- Parents must be specifically taught to adapt training techniques to these more informal situations.
- Parents need to receive professional feedback.

Interactive models that train parents in general interactive strategies may result in parents becoming more responsive, less directive, and better able to model language, but may have little effect on their children's development (Tannock, Girolametto, & Siegel, 1992). General strategies may result in achievement of general goals such as increased vocal turn taking, but specific skills training is needed by parents if more specific learning is expected.

Preintervention child–parent or client–caregiver interactional patterns may be nurturing but insufficient to effect real change. These interactions can be systematically modified. Thus, "a major task in parent training is to demonstrate to parents that, since they are the children's major language teachers, they can become more effective by incorporating language training principles in their natural interactions with their children" (MacDonald et al., 1974, p. 411). There is still no assurance that the new interactional patterns will be used in the home. Several suggestions are offered in Table 10.5 for facilitating language development in both clinical and more natural settings. Effective parent training requires that parental skills be used in the home.

TABLE 10.5	**Suggestions for Facilitating Language Generalization**

In the natural environment:
1. Arrange environment to accomplish with language what cannot be accomplished easily in other ways.
2. Delay reinforcement and provide cues when appropriate verbal response is obvious.
3. Be responsive to communication attempts.
4. Restructure environment to create opportunities for a particular response to occur.

In the language training environment:
1. Teach language skills generalizable outside of the clinic.
2. Vary the contexts, trainers, and training materials.
3. Use the consequences that are varied and related to language use being taught.
4. Reduce density of reinforcement as performance improves.

Source: Adapted from Spradlin and Siegel (1982).

There is often little or no generalization from the structured training mode to free-play situations in the home.

Generalization does not just happen. The environment must be modified systematically to increase the likelihood of generalization. The skilled speech-language pathologist can train other language facilitators to work with the child in various settings.

Initial Communication and Language Training

For many individuals with mental retardation, training begins at a presymbolic or early symbolic level. Many young children participate in infant stimulation or preschool programs. Nonspeaking adults with profound mental retardation may also be trained at this level.

Begin as Early as Possible

Training should begin as soon as it is recognized that the child may be at risk (Mahoney & Snow, 1983). Speech-language pathologists can work with caregivers to help them fine-tune the infant–caregiver interaction to better facilitate language learning.

Follow Developmental Guidelines

Behaviors observed in typical development can serve as a basis for training with disordered populations, especially individuals with mental retardation. Development or change follows a developmental hierarchy. Children use single-word verbalizations, then short, multiword utterances. In addition, behavioral change goes from simple to complex. Short word-order rules appear before complex syntactic systems. Complex behavior results from coordination or modification of simpler responses. Thus, localization to sound is presumed to result from a coordination of less complex visual and auditory skills.

Professional caregivers or parents cannot teach all of the complex behaviors found among humans and must determine which behaviors to target. Because development is rarely linear, educators must also determine the sequence of trained skills. In addition, intervention must consider the individual needs of the client.

Selection of appropriate training targets is critical. It cannot be assumed that all behaviors of the nonretarded child will be appropriate for the retarded child. Selection of content and training should reflect the expected functioning level and future use environment of the client.

Overall Model

In communication intervention with nonspeaking clients, clinicians often use a dual approach, with major emphasis on establishing an initial communication system and secondary emphasis on training presymbolic skills (Figure 10.3). These two paths merge when the client begins to use symbols. Clients who do not reach this point still

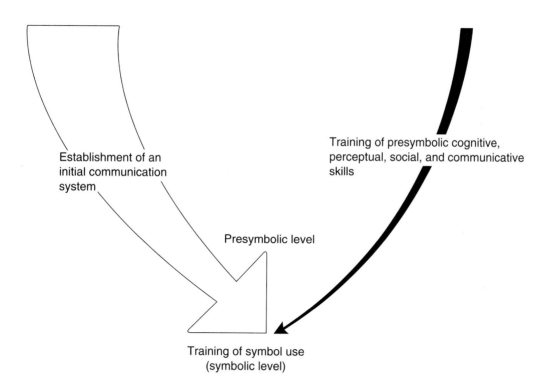

The primary presymbolic approach establishes an initial communication system, whereas the secondary approach teaches skills believed essential to symbol use. These two approaches join at the symbolic level in which the child is taught to use symbols within the context of the previously established communication system.

FIGURE 10.3

Dual-Intervention Approach with Presymbolic Children

(From R. Owens, *Language Disorders, a Functional Approach to Assessment and Intervention*. Reprinted with permission of Merrill, an imprint of Macmillan Publishing Company. Copyright © 1999 by Allyn & Bacon.)

have a communication system, even if it is limited to gestures or a generalized "request" signal.

Assessment

The goal of assessment is to identify the client's communication behaviors and to identify the contexts, times, and individuals that affect the client's communication (Mahoney & Weller, 1980). It is assumed that all individuals communicate, that each communication occurrence offers an opportunity for reciprocity, and that the behaviors of each communication partner affect the other (MacDonald, 1985). In addition, the speech-language pathologist is interested in the level of presymbolic functioning and the content of communication.

For presymbolic clients, it is essential that background data be integrated with observational and testing data to form an overall image of communication characteristics. Initial information can be gathered by observation and then supplemented through interviews with the client's caregivers. The speech-language pathologist should attempt to obtain information about the following (Calculator, 1988; Owens & Rogerson, 1988):

1. How does the client communicate primarily?
2. Does the client demonstrate any turn-taking behaviors?
3. What situations seem to be high-communication contexts?
4. What high-interest items does the client have?
5. Do caregivers provide enough time for the client to respond? How do caregivers cue the client to respond? How do they evaluate responses?
6. Which caregivers seem to elicit the most client responses? Why?
7. Does the client seem to enjoy making sounds? Give examples. How often does the client vocalize? Which situations elicit maximum vocalization? Imitated vocalizations?
8. Which daily situations result in the most client–caregiver interaction? Describe these interactions. When do these occur daily? Are the client's responses consistent?
9. Does the client ever initiate communication? How? In what situations?
10. Does the client—
    Make wants known? How?
    Request help? How?
    Point to things, name them, or both? Does the client look at the object and/or partner while pointing or naming?
    Ask questions or seek information? How?
    Indicate emotions (pain, happiness, like/dislike)? How?
    Seek attention? How? What happens if attention doesn't follow?

This general information can be supplemented by specific questions related to the functioning level of the client. Several language assessment tools are available for this purpose, as listed in Table 10.6. It is inappropriate to use an assessment tool design for infants with adults, even when these adults are functioning at a presymbolic level. Infants and adults are very different, and their presymbolic behaviors are manifested in very different ways. In addition, individuals with developmental delays may not exhibit stages found in children developing typically (Kangas & Lloyd, 1988).

TABLE 10.6   Assessment Protocols for Clients Functioning below Three Years

Assessment Tool	Infant–Preschool	School Age–Adult
Ages and Stages Questionnaires (ASQ): A Parent-Completed Child-Monitoring System. Bricker, D., Squires, J., & Mounts, L. (1995).	X	
Assessing Linguistic Behavior (ALB). Olswang, L., Stoel-Gammon, C., Coggins, T., & Carpenter, R. (1987a).	X	
Assessment, Evaluation, and Programming Systems: AEPS Measurement for Birth to Three Years (Volume 1). Bricker, D. (1993).	X	
Birth to Three Developmental Scales. Bangs, T., & Dodson, S. (1979).	X	
Callier-Azusa Scale. Stillman, R. (1978).	X	X
Caregiver Interview and Environmental Observation. Owens, R. (1982a).	X	X
Carolina Curriculum for Infants and Toddlers with Special Needs. Johnson-Martin, N., Jens, K, Attermeier, S., & Hacker, B. (1991).	X	
A Clinical and Educational Manual for Use With the Uzgris and Hunt Scales of Infant Psychological Development. Dunst, C. (1980).	X	X
Communication and Symbolic Behavior Scales. Wetherby, A., & Prizant, B. (1993).	X	X
Comprehension of Social-Action Games in Prelinguistic Children: Levels of Participation and Effect of Adult Structure. Platt, J., & Coggins, T. (1990).	X	
Developmental Activities Screening Inventory. Fewell, R., & Langley, M. (1984).	X	
Developmental Assessment Tool. Owens, R. (1982b).	X	X
Developmental Communication Curriculum Inventory. Hanna, R., Lippert, E., & Harris, A. (1982).	X	
Diagnostic Interactional Survey. Owens, R. (1982c).	X	
Early Language Milestone Scale. Coplan, J. (1987).	X	
Environmental Communication System (ECO). MacDonald, J., and Gillette, Y. (1978).	X	
Environmental Language Inventory. MacDonald, J. (1978a).	X	X
Environmental Prelanguage Battery. Horstmeier, D., & MacDonald, J. (1978).	X	X
Evaluating Acquired Skills In Communication. Riley, A. (1984).	X	X
Family Administered Neonatal Activities. Cardone, I., & Gilkerson, L. (1989).	X	
Infant-Toddler Language Scale. Rossetti, L. (1990).	X	
Language Development Survey. Rescorla, L. (1989).	X	X
MacArthur Communicative Development Inventories. Fenson, L., Dale, P., Reznick, S., Thal, D., Bates, E., Hartung, J., Pethnick, S., & Reilly, J. (1993).	X	X
Observation of Communicative Interactions. Klein, M., & Briggs, M. (1987).	X	
Parent/Professional Preschool Performance Profile (5Ps). Variety Pre-Schooler's Workshop. (1987).	X	
Preverbal Assessment Intervention Profile. Connard, P. (1984).	X	X
Receptive Expressive Emergent Language Test. Bzock, K., & League, R. (1978).	X	

The Ages and Stages Questionnaires (ASQ) (Bricker, Squires, & Mounts, 1995), Caregiver Interview and Environmental Observation (Owens, 1982a), Infant Scale of Communication Intent (Sacks & Young, 1982), MacArthur Communicative Development Inventories (Fenson et al., 1993), the Oliver (MacDonald, 1978), and Receptive Expressive Emergent Language Scale (REEL) (Bzock & League, 1978) are primarily questionnaire or interview format. The REEL, designed for children functioning between ages 0 and 36 months, and Infant Scale, 0–18 months, attempt to establish an approximate functional developmental age from a range of questions about communicative behaviors. Ages and Stages goes beyond communication to ask questions about motor, social, and problem-solving behaviors as well. The MacArthur Infant and Toddler scales ask caregivers to check gestures, words, and phrases comprehended and produced by the child. Data from such parental reports compares favorably to clinical data (Miller, Sedey, & Miolo, 1995). The Oliver uses a questionnaire format complemented by caregiver recall and actual eliciting of specific presymbolic behaviors. The Caregiver Interview and Environmental Observation also includes observation by the speech-language pathologist of specific communicative behavior.

The speech-language pathologist's goal is to obtain an estimate of client functioning in order to provide a more thorough assessment. In addition, such probing familiarizes the caregiver with the behaviors to be tested and taught. This familiarization is vital if caregivers are to become fully participating members in the intervention process. These tools are best used as guides for describing the client's behavior; the goal should not be to fix a developmental age.

Clients should also be observed by the caregiver and/or speech-pathologist to verify information from questionnaires and interviews and to enhance the validity of the overall assessment. Of interest are the methods used by the client to communicate and the contexts in which these behaviors occur, The Birth to Three Developmental Scales (Bangs & Dodson, 1979), Caregiver Interview and Environmental Observation, Diagnostic Interactional Survey (Owens, 1982a, 1982c), Ecological Communication System (ECO) (MacDonald & Gillette, 1988), Observation of Communicative Interactions (Klein & Briggs, 1987), and Parent/Professional Preschool Performance Profile (5Ps) (Variety Pre-Schooler's Workshop, 1987) offer formats for structured collection of observational data.

Clients who communicate in a nonstandard manner should be observed carefully to determine the intent of such communication (Houghton, Bronicki, & Guess, 1987). For example, a client who bashes her head with her fist might be attempting to communicate. By observing the times and circumstances of this behavior, the speech-language pathologist can form hypotheses about the child's intended meaning (Robinson & Owens, 1995). Not all such behaviors contain communicative content, although consistent, predictable behaviors are likely to be meaningful. Hypotheses on the intent of such behaviors can be tested by carefully manipulating the events that precede and follow the behavior and carefully recording the effect on the behavior. For example, it might be hypothesized that head bashing before meals indicates a request for help. If aid given before or after the behavior results in nonperformance or cessation of the behavior, respectively, this may confirm the hypothesis. The speech-language pathologist is interested in the range of communication needs expressed and in the modes of communication (visual, manual, vocal, tactile) used receptively and expressively (Owens, 1999; Caro & Snell, 1989).

Formal assessment of presymbolic skills might include the content listed in Table 10.7. Skills essential to language acquisition can be grouped as cognitive, perceptual, social, and communicative (McLean & Snyder-McLean, 1978; Owens,

TABLE 10.7 | **Possible Presymbolic Targets**

Behavior	Cognitive	Perceptual	Social	Communicative
Physical imitation—imitating behaviors of others	X		X	
Imitation with objects—using extension of self for imitation	X			
Deferred imitation—retrieving a behavior for imitation	X			
Repetitive and sequential imitation—retrieving patterns	X	X		
Object permanence—retrieving object form from memory	X			
Turn taking—using motor imitation or eye contact in turn				X
Functional use—using objects for intended purpose in order to gain functional knowledge of meaning	X			
Means–ends—using one object or person to attain another	X		X	
Communicative gestures—displaying early intentions				X
Auditory memory—remembering sound patterns	X	X		
Word recognition—pairing names with entities				X
Vocal response—vocalizing in response to another person			X	X
Vocal turn taking—vocalizing turns			X	X
Vocal imitation—shaping vocalizations to resemble a model		X		X
Sequencing vocal imitation—imitating vocal sequences		X		X

Source: Program for the Acquisition of Language with the Severely Impaired (PALS), by R. Owens, 1982, San Antonio: The Psychological Corporation. Copyright 1982 by The Psychological Corporation. Adapted by permission.

2001). Clients using symbols, such as words, signs, pictures, or pictographs, should be evaluated for the range of semantic and illocutionary functions expressed by these symbols (Table 10.8). This can be done using both formal testing and sampling, although the latter is more valuable as a source of information on typical performance.

Several formal assessment tools are available for use with presymbolic and minimally symbolic clients. These include Assessing Linguistic Behavior (Olswang, Stoel-Gammon, Coggins, & Carpenter, 1987b), Carolina Curriculum for Infants and Toddlers with Special Needs (Johnson-Martin, Jens, Attermeier, & Hacker, 1991), Communication and Symbolic Behavior Scales (Wetherby & Prizant, 1993), Developmental Activities Screening Inventory (Fewell & Langley, 1984), Developmental Assessment Tool (DAT) (Owens, 1982b), Developmental Communication Curriculum Inventory (Hanna, Lippert, & Harris, 1982), Environmental Prelanguage Battery (EPB) (Horstmeier & MacDonald, 1978), Environmental Language Inventory (ELI) (MacDonald, 1978a), and Infant-Toddler Language Scale (Rossetti, 1990). Many, such as the DAT and the Rossetti scale, use data collected by a variety of methods including direct testing, observation, and parental report.

Sampling may occur in a free-play situation or in a combination of free-play and structured sampling plus imitation (MacDonald, 1978b). Fifty utterances, either spoken, signed, or picture-indicated, should be an adequate sample unless the client repeats frequently. The clinician should be interested in both the breadth and depth of semantic and illocutionary functions. Of particular interest are the nonexistence of certain functions, the low incidence of others, and the length of each function. This can be accomplished by a short, rated sample (Owens, 1982d) or by a more descriptive analysis (Wilcox & Campbell, 1983).

Early single-word and early multiword utterances are organized following word-order rules based on semantics (Brown, 1973), and early prelinguistic and single-word semantic functions do exist (Table 10.8). These semantic functions can be expanded or combined into two-, three-, and four-word utterances.

Likewise, specific illocutionary acts or communicative intentions can be found in early vocalizations or single-word utterances. A language sample can be analyzed to determine the range of such functions. The speech-language pathologist should be cautioned that although these semantic and illocutionary categories represent what linguists believe children mean and intend by their early verbalizations, there is no way of knowing a child's actual meaning or intention. In addition, these categories are predetermined and may not accurately reflect the behavior of communicators with mental retardation (Leonard, Steckol, & Panther, 1983). More valid results may be attained if caregivers participate with the client, and if the client uses familiar objects, possibly in a play format (Westby, 1980).

Because caregivers act as language facilitators, the client–caregiver interaction is of importance in an assessment. A sample might range from a ten-minute rated play sample (Owens, 1982d) to a more descriptive, lengthier analysis (Wilcox & Campbell, 1983). Analysis might involve the physical distance of the communicators; the use of reinforcement, responses, and cues by the caregiver; appropriate language by the caregiver for the perceived language skills of the client; turn taking, body posture, and movement, and the termination and reengagement of the interaction (MacDonald & Gillette, 1982; Owens, 1982d; Wilcox & Campbell, 1983).

TABLE 10.8 Semantic and Illocutionary Targets of Early Childhood

Functions	Examples
Semantic	
Nomination—naming a person or object using a single- or multiword name or a demonstrative-plus as a name.	Doggie, Choo-choo This horsie
Location—marking spatial relationships. Utterances may contain single location words or two-word utterances containing an agent, action, or object plus a location word. The function can be demonstrated in response to *where* questions.	PARTNER: Where's doggie? CLIENT: Chair. Ball table, Doggie chair, Throw me, Throw here (X + locative)
Negation—marking of nonexistence, rejection, and denial using single negative words or a negative followed by another word (negative + *X*).	All gone (count as a single word), Away, No milk (client drank it), All gone car (the ride is over), No
Nonexistence generally develops first and marks the absence of a once-present object.	PARTNER: Time for bed. CLIENT: No (or No bed).
Rejection marks an attempt to prevent or to stop an event.	Stop it. No milk (pushes glass away).
Denial marks rejection of a proposition.	PARTNER: See the bear? CLIENT: No bear.
Modification	
Possession—appreciating that an object belongs to or is frequently associated with someone. Single-word utterances signal the owner's name. In two-word utterances, stress is usually on the initial word, the possessor.	Mine, My dollie, Johnnie bike (modifier + head) Dollie (client clutches doll)
Attribution—using descriptors for properties not inherently part of the object.	Yukky, Big doggie, Little baby (modifier + head)
Recurrence—understanding that an object can reappear or an event can be reenacted.	More, More milk, 'Nuther cookie (modifier + head)
Notice—signaling that an object has appeared, an event has happened, or an attempt to gain attention.	Hi Mommy, Bye-bye, Look Jim
Action—marking an activity.	
Action—single action words.	Jump, Eat
Agent + action—two-word signal that an animate initiated an activity.	Mommy throw, Doggie eat, Baby sleep
Action + object—two-word signal that an animate or inanimate object was the recipient of action.	Eat cookie, Throw ball
Illocutionary	
Answer—client responds to questions. The questioner's behaviors are a cue for the client's response; the response probably would not be produced without this cue. The client's responses are cognitively related to the question, although they may be incorrect.	PARTNER: (*holding doll*) What's this? CLIENT: Baby. PARTNER: Is this a mirror? CLIENT: No.
Question—client asks for information or verification by addressing the other person verbally. The client's behavior is a stimulus or cue and indicates that she expects an answer. The client can ask herself questions when engaged in egocentric play.	CLIENT: (*picks up toy telephone*) Phone? CLIENT: What this?

(continued)

TABLE 10.8 (Continued)

Functions	Examples
Reply—client makes meaningful response to the content of the other speaker's previous utterance, a verbal cue external to the client. The client may continue to build on the content and ignore the form of the utterance, such as responding to a word or thought in a question without answering the question. In many cases, the client will build on the content *and* respond with an appropriate form. This category does not include mere repetition.	PARTNER: Johnny, bring me the scissors. (command) CLIENT: No. PARTNER: May I have the keys? (request) CLIENT: In a minute. PARTNER: This is a cute dog. (declaration) CLIENT: My doggie.
Elicitation—client self-repeats in response to a request for repetition or clarification or in response to "Say X."	CLIENT: Kitty go. (declaration) PARTNER: What? CLIENT: Kitty go. PARTNER: Mary, say "ball." CLIENT: Ball.
Continuant—client signals that she is listening and wants to continue the interchange, or that she missed what was said.	Uh-huh, Okay, I see, Yes, What? Huh?
Declaration—client makes a statement that is situationally related and for communication but is not in response to another speaker. The utterance is more like a commentary. Cues are internal or situational but not verbal. This category also includes situationally related phonemic exclamations.	CLIENT: *(playing game with mother and glances out)* It raining out. CLIENT: *(playing with car)* Car go up. PARTNER: This is a cute doggie. CLIENT: My doggie. (reply) He lives in a house. (declaration) PARTNER: This is a cute doggie. CLIENT: My doggie. (reply) I have kitty, too. (declaration)
Practice—client repeats or imitates in whole or part what she or another person says with no change in intonation that would indicate a change of intent. In addition, internal replay without added new information is considered practice. This category also includes counting, singing, babbling, or rhyming behaviors in which the client seems to be experimenting or rehearsing.	PARTNER: Ball. CLIENT: Ball. PARTNER: See the red ball. CLIENT: Red ball. PARTNER: See the red ball. CLIENT: See ball. (practice) Ball, ball, ball. (practice)
Perseverative responses, even if the other person interjects an utterance between them, are considered practice as long as they do not mark discrete events or objects.	
Name—client labels an object or event that is present, but the label is not in response to a question. This verbal behavior is usually accomplished by pointing or nodding.	CLIENT: *(picks up ball)* Ball. CLIENT: *(points to ball)* That ball.
Suggestion, command, demand, request—The primary function of the client's utterance is to influence another person's behavior by getting that person to do something or to give the client permission. The form may be imperative, declarative, or interrogative.	CLIENT: Gimmie cookie. CLIENT: Stop that. CLIENT: Mommy. CLIENT: Throw ball. *(parent throws ball)* Throw ball. *(parent throws ball)* Throw ball.

Source: Program for the Acquisition of Language with the Severely Impaired (PALS), by R. Owens, 1982, San Antonio: The Psychological Corporation. Copyright 1982 by The Psychological Corporation. Adapted by permission.

Once the initial evaluation is complete, the speech-language pathologist should know the client's interactional strategies, most frequent topics, communication partners, functioning level, and the quality of the client–caregiver interaction. Throughout the clinical intervention phase, the speech-language pathologist should test and probe in order to fine-tune training techniques.

Intervention

The first step in training is to decide what to teach, who will teach it, and under what circumstances. In the previous section, I suggested a number of training targets for early intervention. The participants and the circumstances are related and will significantly shape the intervention program.

It is essential in initial language programming that the natural environment of the client be included. In establishing early communication, the speech-language pathologist must enlist the aid of the client's caregivers in the intervention process. Typically, the professional trains client responses, and the parents train and elicit these responses within the home (Wulz et al., 1983). The components are environmental manipulation and teaching interaction. In environmental manipulation, parents restructure needs-meeting situations so that their children's needs are not anticipated but are dependent on the children's communication behavior. Within the teaching phase, children are taught to respond to "need-to-communicate" situations. The purpose of the training is to expand the children's communication repertoire and to stimulate responding.

Home-based training should not be disruptive. The goal is not to give parents added responsibilities but rather to help them make use of teaching opportunities in daily routines by restructuring these ongoing activities (Wulz et al., 1983). Called **incidental teaching,** this type of training should be given primacy as an early communication training strategy (Owens, 1982d). If, for example, the parent is training object permanence—the knowledge that unseen entities still exist—nonfloating soap and toys can be incorporated into the bathing routine. Because almost any routine can be adapted for language training, there is no need to rely solely on formal, out-of-context training modes. With children, the modality for training may be play. Play is child centered, and the child's activity can provide the focus of training.

Training should occur in short, repetitive, daily activities in which the reinforcer is part of the activity, such as requesting another cookie at snack time (Halle, Alpert, & Anderson, 1984). The content should be meaningful in the situation and result in real consequences.

Environmental rules can also be used to restructure client–caregiver interactions (MacDonald, 1978b). Once clients have learned a skill, they are required to perform that skill in order to obtain desired entities or privileges. For example, if the client can sign *cookie,* the sign is required in order to get a cookie. Previously accepted pointing or whining is unacceptable. Environmental rules affect both client and caregiver behaviors.

Language stimulation techniques can also be used in the natural environment (Owens, 1982d). Ideally, such stimulation would precede slightly the client's actual level of functioning. Stimulation can take the form of "Motherese," discussed earlier. It is important that language trainers maintain an interactive style in order to preclude solitary nonlanguage activities common among children with mental retardation (Smith & Hagen, 1984).

The importance of formal or structured training cannot be overlooked but should be minimized when possible (MacDonald, 1985; Owens, 1982d). Often this training can be adapted to a play modality (Manolson, 1983). Two trainers can facilitate client responding (Richmond & Lewallen, 1983). One trainer cues the client while the second trainer models or prompts the appropriate response.

It is not always possible to train within the home. An alternative is the classroom (Brightman, Ambrose, & Baker, 1980). Within residential settings, aides, direct-care staff, or foster grandparents may serve as language facilitators (Owens, McNerney, Bigler-Burke, & Lepre-Clark, 1987). The behaviors of direct-care staff can be modified by simple praise or by feedback plus praise (Realon, Lewallen, & Wheeler, 1983).

Early communication in the form of basic signal systems can be established using **behavior chain interruption** techniques (Goetz, Gee, & Sailor, 1985; Hunt, Goetz, Alwell, & Sailor, 1986; Romer & Schoenberg, 1991; Sternberg, Pegnatore, & Hill, 1983). There are two basic elements to behavior chain interruption. First, the client engages in a pleasurable activity that the trainer interrupts. Second, the client is prompted to give a communicative response, such as a touch, in order to have the activity begin again. The communicative response or signal can be modified or expanded into a more conventional gesture or sign.

Communication systems can also be initiated through the use of pictures or signs to signal a generalized or nonspecific request (Reichle, 1990). This procedure will be discussed in more detail under augmentative communication.

Several programs target presymbolic and early symbolic skills (Guess, Sailor, & Baer, 1976; Hanna et al., 1982; MacDonald, 1978b; MacDonald & Gillette, 1982; Miller & Yoder, 1974; Musselwhite & St. Louis, 1982; Owens, 1982d). Programs designed for less severely delayed clients, such as the Environmental Language Intervention Program (MacDonald, 1978b), may contain fewer presymbolic skills than those presented in Table 10.7. Others, such as the Program for the Acquisition of Language with the Severely Impaired (PALS) (Owens, 1982d), target more. Decisions on the direction of therapy should be based on the client's social interactional skills, comprehension, and imitative and spontaneous expression (Crais & Roberts, 1991).

In general, the younger the client, the more important is such presymbolic training. With older children and adults, programming emphasizes establishing an initial communication system with less stress on presymbolic targets. Natural behaviors, such as reaching, can be modified into a requesting gesture or a point to a printed symbol (Reichle & Sigafoos, 1991).

All spontaneous vocalizations and other attempts to communicate should be encouraged and reinforced. The amount of vocalizing can be increased through reinforcement and modified into meaningful communication (Drash, Raver, Murrin, & Tudor, 1989; Poulson, 1988).

Once trained in imitation, a single word or sign can be trained in a variety of semantic and illocutionary functions. Thus, "a single form may be used to express several functions and several forms can express a single function" (Miller & Yoder, 1974, p. 523). Single words are typically trained in response to "What's this?," but this question-naming paradigm has only limited application. Possible semantic and illocutionary training targets appear in Table 10.8. Using this table, the clinician may pair each semantic category with each of the illocutionary acts. For example, a "location answer" response might follow the cue, "Where is baby?" A "nomination question" might consist of "Cup?" or "What?" A "location question" might also consist of "Cup?" if the client is trying to guess the location of some small object. Within these category combinations, longer utterances may also be learned. It has been demonstrated that children continue to use combinations of the semantic rules in utterances of up to four words. After this point, learning focuses on internal sentence reorganization, and new structures are learned.

Some developmental guidelines exist for the semantic functions. In general, the order of appearance is nomination, negation, action, objects, state or attribution, change in state or attribution, possession and location, experiencer of action, and agent (Menyuk, 1974). Initial two-word functions include nomination ("that _____"), recurrence ("more _____"), and nonexistence ("no _____"). Next, separate semantic classes are combined to produce utterances to indicate agent + action ("Mommy eat"), possession ("Baby cookie"), and location ("Doggie bed").

Augmentative and Alternative Communication

Some individuals with mental retardation, particularly those with more severe impairment, experience great difficulty with speech and with the use of symbols. For these nonspeaking clients, an augmentative and alternative form of communication may be necessary. Augmentative and alternative forms increase or expand the symbolic communication capabilities of these nonspeaking individuals. Common forms of augmentative and alternative communication include manual communication, communication boards, and electronic or computer-based communication. These forms will be discussed along with assessment and programming considerations.

Contrary to common misconception, use of augmentative and alternative communication systems does not deter further development of speech. Augmentative communication facilitates symbol learning; increases verbalization of trained symbols; increases attention, intentional communication, and sociability; facilitates spontaneous verbal communication; increases communication initiations; and increases the range of meanings and communication partners. Augmentative communication, however, "will not, in itself, assure effective communication" (Calculator & Luchko. 1983, p. 185). "It does not solve all of the communication problems of the non-speaking person" (Shane, Lipschultz, & Shane, 1982, p. 83).

Types of Augmentative and Alternative Communication

Augmentative and alternative communication systems can be divided into two types, aided and unaided. Aided augmentative communication uses a device such as a communication board or an electronic means of communication. Unaided systems consist of manual communication, such as gestures, signs, and finger spelling.

Communication boards come in many different shapes and varieties. In general, boards are easy to make, portable, and very adaptable. The visual symbols used may include, from least to most symbolic, models or miniatures, pictures, drawings, Rebus symbols, Blissymbols, or letters and words. Examples are presented in Figure 10.4.

FIGURE 10.4

Transparency of Graphic Augmentative Communication Systems

Sources: Bloomberg, Karlan, & Lloyd (1990); Burroughs, Albritton, Eaton, & Montague (1990); Mirenda & Locke (1989)

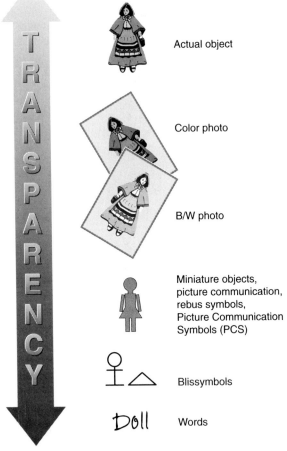

More transparent

Actual object

Color photo

B/W photo

Miniature objects, picture communication, rebus symbols, Picture Communication Symbols (PCS)

Blissymbols

Words

Less transparent

More transparent or more guessable visual systems are easier to learn than are less transparent ones.

Rebus symbols are pictographic representations of concepts. Blissymbols are generally less iconic than Rebus symbols but allow for more generative language use. For example, the Rebus symbol for the word *book* is a pictograph showing simplistic details of an open book; the Blissymbol is a square with a vertical line through its center that represents an open book schematically. These encoding forms are not exclusive and may be used in combination. In general, the more iconic or "guessable" the encoding system, the easier it is to learn (Clark, 1981). In turn, the less iconic systems are more flexible and generative, allowing more adultlike representation.

The tremendous growth of computer technology is opening many new possibilities for the nonspeaking (Vanderheiden, 1982). Input systems may be similar to those used on communication boards, and output may include print, graphics, and/or pre-recorded or synthesized speech. In general, three types of indicating methods are used by clients: scanning, encoding, and direct selection. In the scanning method, the device continually scans the display of symbols. The client stops the scan on the desired symbol. With encoding, a code such as numbers or digits is used to access the computer's memory. Finally, in direct selection, the client moves a cursor or pointer to the desired symbol or may, if possible, type the message.

Accessing computers may be the most difficult problem, particularly for individuals with severe motoric involvement. The interface switch between the client and the microcomputer must often be modified or custom designed to the motoric abilities of an individual client. The slowness of use of an interface device may actually negate some of the speed advantages associated with microcomputers.

There are several types of unaided sign systems, from American Sign Language (ASL), which is a language of its own, to Seeing Essential English (SEE$_1$) or Signing Exact English (SEE$_2$), which closely approximate English syntax. Signed English uses signs from other systems but does not adhere as closely to English morphological rules as SEE$_1$. American Indian sign language (Amer-Ind) has also been used successfully with persons with mental retardation. One reason for these results may be the transparency of Amer-Ind. Transparency is the ease of understanding a sign once its origin is explained. Amer-Ind is significantly more transparent than ASL (Daniloff, Lloyd, & Fristoe, 1983).

It may be advantageous for some clients to have more than one type of augmentative system. Different systems may have application in different environments.

Evaluation

Evaluative decisions on client use of an augmentative communication system are made by a team of professionals, usually consisting of a speech-language pathologist, psychologist, physical therapist, occupational therapist, special education teacher, a client advocate such as a parent, and the client. Assessment is a continuing process which, in this case, is essential to adapt the augmentative system to the client's changing needs and abilities.

The American Speech-Language-Hearing Association (ASHA) Ad Hoc Committee on Communication Processes and Non-Speaking Persons (1980) identified three components of the assessment for augmentative communication. First, the team must assess the appropriateness of an augmentative system. Not all nonspeaking individuals are candidates for augmentative communication. For example, the cognitive abilities needed for spontaneous symbol use apply to augmentative communication as well as to verbal language (Bryen, Goldman, & Quinlisk-Gill, 1988; Goossens, 1984; Owens & House, 1984; Shane & Bashir, 1980; Silverman, 1980). The environment also must be supportive of augmentative system use (Owens & House, 1984; Shane et al., 1982).

The second component of an evaluation is selection of the appropriate communication mode. The team must decide which type or types of augmentative systems will be appropriate for the nonspeaking individual. Of particular importance are the motoric abilities of the client in the context of the body's total movement patterns (Bottorf & DePape, 1982; Shane & Wilbur, 1980; Silverman, 1980). The evaluative team is interested in the range, speed, strength, and consistency of movement. Clients with good motor skills may be candidates for manual systems, whereas those with less ability may use communication boards or electronic systems. For electronic devices, decisions should be based on a task analysis that includes the client's present skills and those behaviors needed to operate the communication aid (Coleman, Cook, & Myers, 1980).

Finally, the team must select the appropriate symbol system or systems. Questions of appropriateness relate to cognitive ability, visual acuity, and environmental receptivity (Chapman & Miller, 1980). For example, greater cognitive skills and visual discrimination abilities are needed for word use than for picture use. Pictures are generally easier to discriminate than lexigrams (picture–letter combinations), which are, in turn, easier than printed words (Romski, Sevcik, Pate, & Rumbaugh, 1985). In addition, the use of a symbol system such as Blissymbols might hinder communication in a nonreceptive environment.

Intervention

The focus of intervention should be increasing successful interactions (Bottorf & De-Pape, 1982). In general, communication interactions can be fostered by adapting the augmentative system to the individual client and to the communication environment.

The speech-language pathologist should establish an augmentative environment around the client. The augmentative or alternative system is available at all times, and others are encouraged to use the system. Signs are always available, but others may not use them when talking to the client. Their use by others may facilitate client comprehension and help establish an atmosphere of sign. In addition, the unique daily routine of each client can foster augmentative and alternative communication use. Lack of generalization of augmentative systems may be related to lack of knowledge and infrequent use by caregivers (Bryen & McGinley, 1991).

Selection of individualized content should reflect client routines, interests, and needs. The vocabulary selected will affect the types of interactions in which it is used (Bottorf & DePape, 1982). Initial vocabularies should be based on each client's individual interests, routines, and basic needs, and on the recommendations of others within the environment. In addition, signs may be chosen on the basis of symmetry, taction, and iconicity. Individuals with severe retardation can learn signs more rapidly if the signs are symmetrical or contain identical hand movements, have some contact with the body (taction), and are iconic or highly representational (Kohl, 1981).

Augmentative and alternative communication is not a panacea, and the results are not always favorable. The average client with severe or profound mental retardation may learn to produce only a few signs spontaneously after years of training (Bryen, Goldman, & Quinlisk-Gill, 1988). Lack of progress seems to be related to overuse of imitative training with little thought toward spontaneous use, nonmeaningful training situations, inappropriate vocabulary or augmentative system, and little environmental support by caregivers.

Successful intervention builds on the client's current communication base and employs a multimodality strategy that uses all the client's means of communication (Paul, 2000). Thus, some clients may rely on a communication board supplemented by a few signs and vocalizations. The speech-language pathologist attempts to open new avenues of communication while strengthening and building existing ones.

The environment should be modified systematically to encourage augmentative communication. Nonspeaking clients must be given an opportunity to use their augmentative systems. Teachers and caregivers need to be cautioned not to dominate communication. Communication partners must be patient and await client responses. Clients should also be given a choice in their daily routine and among alternative activities in order to foster active system use. Even individuals with severe retardation can retain symbol vocabularies well over long periods of time if these symbols are used by them to control their daily environment (Romski, Sevcik, & Rumbaugh, 1985).

Summary

Augmentative communication systems can be part of a nonspeaking individual's effective interaction system if continually evaluated and adapted to that client's communication needs. These systems "can be used to express a variety of communication functions, but only if the environment provides opportunities for meaningful use" (Shane et al., 1982, p. 83).

Language Rule Training

Once the client begins to use symbols meaningfully, training targets become the rule systems used with these symbols. The speech-language pathologist should be knowledgeable in the rules used within the five generally recognized areas of language: syntax, morphology, phonology, semantics, and pragmatics.

Children with language delays differ in their comprehension of sentences according to linguistic stage (Page & Horn, 1987). For example, children using four-word sentences or less use semantic comprehension strategies, not syntactic ones. Therefore, clinicians must be concerned with selecting the appropriate level of linguistic input in order to facilitate both comprehension and production. It is best to present examples of the language code that slightly exceed the child's expressive language skills.

Professionals sometimes assume that only the adult forms of these rules are acceptable training targets. A typical two-year-old who says "What Mommy eating?" is not considered to be language disordered but to be following an age-appropriate rule. Likewise, individuals with mental retardation follow rules that generally reflect their level of cognitive functioning.

Evaluation

Initial evaluation should attempt to determine which rule systems the client uses expressively and which ones she comprehends. Assessment ideally should include both formal testing and informal evaluation.

Very few formal tests were designed for and normed on the retarded population. Most commercially available tests were developed and normed on nonretarded children. Careful consideration must be given to the appropriateness of such tests and materials with older retarded clients, particularly adults. The speech-language pathologist must consider the child's motor and cognitive abilities before choosing a language test or tests. The means of responding may need to be modified for those with oral motor difficulties or those who use augmentative communication. These individuals may need more time to complete timed tests.

Test norms may also be inappropriate for clients with mental retardation. It is of little value for intervention planning to demonstrate that a retarded client is in fact delayed in language. Testing can be of more value when used to help describe the client's language features and behavior.

Existing materials can be modified and new assessment tools developed (Owings & Guvette, 1982). Many speech-language pathologists supplement formal tests with their own locally prepared instruments (Pickett & Flynn, 1983).

Formal testing situations are artificial and generally lacking in the natural cues available in a conversation. Additional sources of information are needed. Informally collected language samples can provide valuable information. Samples can be analyzed in a number of ways. Initially, the speech-language pathologist should determine the MLU. Increasing MLU correlates with increasing complexity up to an MLU of 4.0 morphemes. Table 10.9 contains MLU values and equivalent ages.

Of the commercially available analysis methods, Miller's Assigning Structural Stage (1980), or its computer version, SALT, seems to be the most functional. Others, such as Developmental Sentence Scoring (Lee, 1974), result in a normative score but provide little direction for intervention. Using Miller's approach, the speech-language pathologist determines the correct percentage of use of Brown's (1973) fourteen morphemes. This data, plus the MLU, suggest a developmental stage. Internal sentence analysis of noun phrase, verb phrase, and sentence type development results in assignment of the client to a stage or stages of language development. Similar analysis can be performed semantically and phonologically.

Language samples may also be analyzed using less formal, more descriptive methods (Owens, 1999). The speech-language pathologist should attempt to describe all aspects of language. Pragmatic concerns, such as inappropriate communication, are difficult to measure directly but are very important for overall communication effectiveness.

TABLE 10.9 | **MLU and Approximate Age**

MLU	Predicted Chronological Age in Months	Predicted Age in Months ± 1 S. D.
1.5	23.0	18.5–27.5
2.0	26.9	21.5–32.3
2.5	30.8	23.9–37.7
3.0	34.8	28.0–41.6
3.5	38.7	30.8–46.6
4.0	42.6	36.7–48.5
4.5	46.6	40.3–52.9
5.0	50.5	42.1–58.9
5.5	54.4	46.0–62.8
6.0	58.3	49.9–66.7

Source: Adapted from Miller (1980).

Intervention

Again, generalization is best ensured by use of the natural environment for language training. Caregivers can be instructed in the use of evaluative feedback and in expansion techniques. For example, caregivers can provide corrective feedback in the form of modeling of the correct production. Incomplete or primitive responses can be expanded into a more adultlike form. The conversational context should not be overlooked for the training opportunity that it provides. As noted previously, generalization to spontaneous conversational use does not happen automatically for many clients with mental retardation. Training within structured conversations familiarize the client with the situations and the contexts that govern language feature use.

The primary criterion for selecting training targets should be the usefulness to the client of the language features targeted. Targets should include those language features or behaviors that facilitate communication, such as asking questions, or that offer more communication options to the client, such as using the telephone.

It is best if the trainer does not introduce too many new items into the training task. Training cues, prompts, and materials should change gradually. Previously trained information should be used to aid new learning. For example, knowledge of the semantic categories and rules previously discussed can be used to train syntax. Agent words (*mommy, doggie*), because of their position in the utterance and their use, can become subjects. Possession, previously expressed by word order, can be expanded through the training of the possessive marker ('s).

Miniature linguistic systems may be helpful in training word order (Bunce, Ruder, & Ruder, 1985). Table 10.10 demonstrates a miniature system matrix in which one language feature occupies each axis. The child can learn a word-order rule by combining words from each grouping. Good generalization has been reported with miniature systems from training of some but not all possible combinations. The Xs in Table 10.10 identify the combinations most effective in training.

New language features can be introduced using focused stimulation in which examples of the feature are given frequently in context. For example, when introducing the present progressive verb form (verb + *-ing*), the trainer might use self-talk to describe what he is doing or parallel talk to describe what the child is doing. Repeated use in context will highlight the feature for the child and help to focus attention.

When attempting to elicit full sentences, the speech-language pathologist should be very careful to use cues that make sense pragmatically and reflect general language use. For example, the cue "What do you want?" is most likely to elicit a single-word or short-phrase response, such as "Cookie." Demanding "I want cookie" as a response is inappropriate pragmatically.

Vocabulary, often a deficit area, can also be trained within the context of daily events in which the symbols have some relevance. The use of key words or pictures can facilitate learning and ensure memory better than direct instruction (Scruggs, Mastropieri, & Levin, 1985). For example, the word *popover* contains the key word *pop;* pictures that show the word *popover* or a toaster pastry "popping" out of a toaster may aid word recall. Stories can also be used to facilitate recall of single words or series of words (Glidden & Warner, 1985).

| TABLE 10.10 | Miniature Linguistic Systems |

	Cookie	Cake	Pudding	Pie	Bread
Eat	X	X	X	X	X
Bake	X				
Mix	X				
Want	X				
Give	X				

	Pet	Dog	Cat	Horse	Ferret
Feed	X	X			
Bathe		X	X		
Groom			X	X	
Walk				X	X
Brush	X				X

Verbs on one axis are combined with nouns on the other to form short phrases. Each combination taught is marked with an X. Rule learning will generalize to the untrained combinations.

Source: R. Owens, *Language Disorders, a Functional Approach to Assessment and Intervention.* Reprinted with permission of Merrill, an imprint of Macmillan. Copyright © 1991 by Allyn & Bacon.

In addition, speech-language pathologists should be aware of the special learning needs of the retarded population. Cognitive operations should be trained before linguistic skills that express those operations. For example, the client should understand reversibility of processes and time relationships before learning linguistic concepts such as *before, after,* and *because.*

Clients such as those with Down syndrome may need help with successive processing skills. Simultaneous skills related to overall meaning may be employed to facilitate sequential operations.

Finally, some individuals, such as those with Down syndrome, will require additional input beyond auditory symbols. Visual and tactile input can enhance learning for these persons. The use of pictures or experiential activities might facilitate concept learning and elicit more client responses. Involvement in activity by the client results in more verbal responsiveness than involvement by the clinician or use of pictures (Cook & Seymour, 1980). Likewise, active participation by the severely retarded client becomes a cue for verbal behavior that was situationally appropriate (Spiegel, 1983).

Language Use

With higher-functioning adults or teenagers with mental retardation in prevocational or vocational training programs, the focus of training should be language use.

Although a minimum of language structure is required, language forms are not as critical to life success.

The main difference between occupationally and socially successful and nonsuccessful adults with retardation seems to be integration at work and in society (Reiter & Levi, 1980). Further, there is great need among individuals in the retarded population for attaining regular employment and for having nonretarded friends. One difference between the successful and unsuccessful person is found in the area of social skills, including language. Therefore, more appropriate language use is a desirable training target.

Some language factors, such as following directions or asking questions, may be more important than others, particularly in the work setting. Adults with mental retardation are less likely to be employed if their language use is inappropriate, such as being abusive, argumentative, vulgar, bossy, loud, interruptive, or irrelevant. Additional skills for training might also include conversational abilities and direction following.

These vocational-interpersonal skills can be modified through a combination of modeling, coaching, and behavior rehearsal (LaGreca, Stone, & Bell, 1983). Appropriate verbal behavior can be modeled while clients are trained in appropriate use. Rehearsal and role playing in situations close to those of actual use can be beneficial. Social feedback in the form of praise, instruction, and reprimands has been more effective than reprimands and instruction in reducing inappropriate verbalizations.

Other conversational skills may also be taught. Teenagers who are mentally retarded may have particular difficulties communicating with their parents and expressing their feelings. As conversational partners, adults, including those with mental retardation, are expected to observe the rules of turn taking and to be able to introduce, sustain, and contribute to the topic of conversation. In addition, they should be able to take their communication partner's perspective and to vary their own role and informational contribution accordingly. Pragmatic abilities of those functioning at school-age or adult levels may also be assessed and trained for a range of intentions and forms of expression (Prutting & Kirchner, 1983). Normally developing peers can serve effectively as models and can elicit appropriate conversational responses (Wilkinson & Romski, 1995).

Critical social and communication skills can be taught within the classroom, home, or workplace (Stowitschek et al., 1988). Even adolescents and adults with severe retardation can be taught successfully to answer the telephone and to respond to a variety of messages and callers (Karen, Astin-Smith, & Creasy, 1985). Even individuals with mental retardation recognize the need for these conversational skills. In a "social" room in a day training program, the clients established the following rules:

- Stay on topic.
- Be quiet when others are talking.
- Listen to what you hear.
- Don't interrupt others.
- Take turns—give everyone a chance.
- Speak so others can hear you.
- Don't talk to yourself.

CASE STUDY

Catherine is a 33-year-old with severe mental retardation residing in a developmental center but attending a day training program in the community. She has been institutionalized since early childhood. The cause of her retardation is unknown. Her mental age measured on the Wechsler Intelligence Scale for Children—Revised is slightly above age 6, although her language performance is lower. She experiences seizures, primarily of the petit mal type. During seizure activity, Catherine usually stares and her expression is blank. Such episodes are usually a few seconds in duration, although on a few occasions she has lost consciousness. Currently, her seizures are controlled through medication. At times, Catherine will become violent and strike other clients for no apparent reason. Her placement in a community residence is dependent on control of this behavior. She has good self-help skills, such as dressing and feeding, but poor language, money, and time skills.

Catherine's receptive vocabulary age is approximately 5 years, as measured on the Peabody Picture Vocabulary Test. Although she can point to pictures named, she has difficulty explaining word meanings. Her equivalent receptive language age as measured by the Test for Auditory Comprehension of Language—Revised (TACL—R) is 4 years 2 months. This score is corroborated for her expressive language by the Carrow Elicited Language Inventory. In this sentence imitation test, she received an age equivalent of 46 months. Her performance was characterized by sentence simplification, omission of articles, and difficulties with verb tensing and pronouns. On the TACL—R she also made several errors in verb tensing and pronouns. A free sample analyzed using Miller's Assigning Structural Stage indicated that her language skills are primarily those found in Brown's Stage IV. Her MLU is approximately 3.67. Language is primarily responsive and characterized by short sentences, a scarcity of complex or compound sentences, little use of pronouns beyond *you, me, he, she,* and *him,* and absence of tensing markers. Some auxiliary verbs and modals are present, but there is some confusion with the verb *to be.* Most sentences are simple declaratives or negatives.

In the vocational training program, Catherine's communication behavior is mostly responsive, although staff report that she also exhibits perseverative verbal behavior. While in vocational training, she will continually repeat instructions she has been given or statements made to her. This behavior is whispered but still annoys others around her. Staff report that it is difficult to stop this behavior.

Catherine is seen by the speech-language pathologist twice weekly for individual programming and once a week for group training. Within the individual sessions, the speech-language pathologist works primarily on verb tensing, focusing on the regular and irregular past and the future tense. Once a correct response is given, the speech-language pathologist attempts to gain a longer verbalization. Group work attempts to encourage initiation of conversation and use of longer utterances. In her vocational training program, Catherine is expected by the staff to provide longer responses in conversation. A questioning technique is used to elicit expansions of previous utterances. In addition, she is reinforced for short periods without perseverative whispering.

SUMMARY

Within this chapter, I have explored a definition of mental retardation that considers cognitive functioning and adaptive behavior. Overall, this definition reflects empirical findings that individuals with mental retardation are developmental beings whose behavior is characterized by both delay and difference. This finding is also true for the language development of the retarded population, with special modification.

These characteristics suggest a developmental language intervention approach. The wise clinician will use nonretarded development as a guide for creative programming.

The language intervention targets will differ with the language skills of the client. Initial training should focus on cognitive, perceptual, social, and communicative skills and on the establishment of early communication. Early building blocks will be semantic and pragmatic. Once short multiword utterances are trained, the speech-language pathologist should target language rule systems. As the client becomes more capable in using language rules, language use becomes a tool for normalization training. Such training is particularly true of clients in vocational training programs.

We began this chapter with a quote from Nigel Hunt and will end with one as well:

Thank you ever so much for letting me write this book. I am most delightful. (p. 124)

STUDY QUESTIONS

1. What is the AAMD definition of mental retardation? Explain each portion of this definition.
2. How does cognitive functioning of the retarded population differ from that of the nonretarded population? How might these differences relate to overall intervention considerations?
3. Compare all aspects of the language abilities of the retarded and nonretarded populations.
4. Explain the developmental model of intervention and its relation to language training with persons with mental retardation.
5. What are some of the targets for language intervention with persons with mental retardation?

REFERENCES

Abbeduto, L., Davies, B., & Furman, L. (1988). The development of speech act comprehension in mentally retarded individuals and nonretarded children. *Child Development, 59*, 1460–1472.

Abbeduto, L., Davies, B., Solesby, S., & Furman, L. (1991). Identifying the referents of spoken messages: Use of context and clarification requests by children with and without mental retardation. *American Journal on Mental Retardation, 95*, 551–562.

Abbeduto, L., Furman, L., & Davies, B. (1989). Relation between the receptive language and mental age of persons with mental retardation. *American Journal on Mental Retardation, 93,* 535–543.

Abbeduto, L., & Rosenberg, S. (1980). The communicative competence of mildly retarded adults. *Applied Psycholinguistics, 1,* 405–426.

Abbeduto, L., Short-Meyerson, K., Benson, G., & Dolish, J. (1997). Signaling of noncomprehension by children and adolescents with mental retardation: Effects of problem type and speaker identity. *Journal of Speech, Language, and Hearing Research, 40,* 20–32.

Abbeduto, L., Short-Meyerson, K., Benson, G., Dolish, J., & Weissman, M. (1998). Understanding referential expressions in context: Use of common ground by children and adolescents with mental retardation. *Journal of Speech, Language, and Hearing Research, 41,* 1348–1362.

Abrahamsen, A., Romski, M., & Sevcik, R. (1989). Concomitants of success in acquiring an augmentative communication system: Changes in attention, communication, and sociability. *American Journal on Mental Retardation, 93,* 475–496.

Affleck, G. (1976). Role-taking ability and the interpersonal tactics of retarded children. *American Journal of Mental Deficiency, 80,* 667–670.

Affleck, G., Allen, D., McGrade, B., & McQueeney, M. (1982). Home environments of developmentally disabled infants as a function of parent and infant characteristics. *American Journal of Mental Deficiency, 86,* 445–452.

Alvares, R. L., & Downing, S. F. (1998). A survey of expressive communication skills in children with Angelman syndrome. *American Journal of Speech-Language Pathology.* 7(2), 14–24.

Ambron, S., & Irwin, D. (1975). Role-taking and moral judgment in 5- and 7-year olds. *Developmental Psychology, 11,* 102.

American Association on Mental Retardation. (1992). *Mental retardation: Definition, classification, and systems of support* (9th ed.). Washington, DC: American Association on Mental Retardation.

ASHA Ad Hoc Committee on Communication Processes and Nonspeaking Persons. (1980). Nonspeech communication: A position paper. *ASHA, 22,* 267–272.

Ashman, A. (1982). Coding, strategic behavior, and language performance of institutionalized mentally retarded young adults. *American Journal of Mental Deficiency, 86,* 627–636.

Baker, B. (1976). Parent involvement in programming for the developmentally disabled child. In L. Lloyd (Ed.), *Communication assessment and intervention.* Baltimore: University Park Press.

Balla, D., & Zigler, E. (1971). Luria's verbal deficiency theory of mental retardation and performance on sameness, symmetry and opposition tasks: A critique. *American Journal of Mental Deficiency, 75,* 400–413.

Balthazar, E., & Stevens, H. (1974). *The emotionally disturbed, mentally retarded: A historical and contemporary perspective.* Englewood Cliffs, NJ: Prentice Hall.

Bangs, T. (1961). Evaluating children with language delay. *Journal of Speech and Hearing Disorders, 26,* 6–18.

Bangs, T., & Dodson, S. (1979). *Birth to Three Developmental Scales.* Seattle: University of Washington Press.

Bates, E., Benigni, L., Bretherton, I., Camaioni, L., & Volterra, V. (1979). *The emergence of symbols: Cognition and communication in infancy.* New York: Academic.

Bedrosian, J., & Prutting, C. (1978). Communicative performance of mentally retarded adults in four conversational settings. *Journal of Speech and Hearing Research, 21,* 79–95.

Bee, H., Van Egeren, L., Streissguth, A., Nyman, B., & Leckie, M. (1969). Social class differences in maternal teaching strategies and speech patterns. *Developmental Psychology, 1,* 726–734.

Bellinger, D. (1980). Consistency in the pattern of change in mothers' speech: Some discriminant analysis. *Journal of Child Language, 7,* 469–487.

Belmont, J. (1967). Long-term memory in mental retardation. In N. Ellis (Ed.), *International review of research in mental retardation* (Vol. 1). New York: Academic.

Bender, N., & Carlson, J. (1982). Prosocial behavior and perspective-taking of mentally retarded and nonretarded children. *American Journal of Mental Deficiency, 86,* 361–366.

Berger, J., & Cunningham, C. (1983). The development of early vocal behaviors and interactions in Down syndrome and non-handicapped infant-mother pairs. *Developmental Psychology, 19,* 322–331.

Berko, J. (1958). The child's learning of English morphology. *Word, 14,* 150–177.

Berry, P., Groeneweg, G., Gibson, D., & Brown, R. (1984). Mental development of adults with Down's syndrome. *American Journal of Mental Deficiency, 89,* 252–256.

Bilsky, L., Walker, N., & Sakales, S. (1983). Comprehension and recall of sentences by mentally retarded and nonretarded individuals. *American Journal of Mental Deficiency, 87,* 558–565.

Birch, H., Richardson, S., Baird, D., Horobin, G., & Illsley, R. (1970). *Mental subnormality in the community: A clinical and epidemiological study.* Baltimore: Williams & Wilkins.

Blacher, J. (1982). Assessing social cognition of young mentally retarded and nonretarded children. *American Journal of Mental Deficiency, 86,* 473–484.

Bleile, K., & Schwartz, I. (1984). Three perspectives on the speech of children with Down's syndrome. *Journal of Communication Disorders, 17,* 87–94.

Blodgett, E., & Miller, V. (1981). The facilitative language model. Paper presented at the American Speech-Language-Hearing Association Annual Convention, Los Angeles.

Bloom, L. (1973). *One word at a time: The use of single-word utterances before syntax.* The Hague: Mouton.

Bloomberg, K., Karlan, G., & Lloyd, L. (1990). The comparative translucency of initial lexical items represented in five graphic symbol systems and sets. *Journal of Speech and Hearing Research, 33,* 717–725.

Borkowski, J., & Cavanaugh, J. (1979). Maintenance and generalization of skills and strategies by the retarded. In N. Ellis (Ed.), *Handbook of mental deficiency: Psychological theory and research.* Hillsdale, NJ: Lawrence Erlbaum Associates.

Borkowski, J., & Wanschura, P. (1974). Mediational processes in the retarded. In N. R. Ellis (Ed.), *International review of research in mental retardation* (Vol. 7). New York: Academic.

Bottorf, L., & DePape, D. (1982). Initiating communication systems for severely speech-impaired persons. *Topics in Language Disorders, 2,* 55–72.

Bowler, D. (1991). Rehearsal training and short-term free-recall of sign and word labels by severely handicapped children. *Journal of Mental Deficiency Research, 35,* 113–124.

Bradbury, B., & Lunzer, E. (1972). The learning of grammatical inflections in normal and subnormal children. *Journal of Child Psychology and Psychiatry, 13,* 239–248.

Bray, N. (1979). Strategy production in the retarded. In N. Ellis (Ed.), *Handbook of mental deficiency: Psychological theory and research.* Hillsdale, NJ: Lawrence Erlbaum Associates.

Bricker, D. (1972). Imitative sign training as a facilitator of word-object association with low-functioning children. *American Journal of Mental Deficiency, 76,* 509–516.

Bricker, D. (1993). *Assessment, Evaluation, and Programming Systems: AEPS Measurement for Birth to Three Years* (Vol. 1). Baltimore: Paul H. Brookes.

Bricker, D., Squires, J., & Mounts, L. (1995). *Ages and Stages Questionnaire (ASQ): A parent-completed child-monitoring system.* Baltimore: Paul H. Brookes.

Bricker, W., Heal, L., Bricker, D., Hayes, W., & Larsen, L. (1969). Discrimination learning and learning set with institutionalized retarded children. *American Journal of Mental Deficiency, 74,* 242–248.

Brightman, R., Ambrose, S., & Baker, B. (1980). Parent training: A school-based model for enhancing teaching performance. *Child Behavior Therapy, 2,* 35–47.

Brooks, P., & Baumeister, A. (1977). A plea for consideration of ecological validity in the experimental psychology of mental retardation: A guest editorial. *American Journal of Mental Deficiency, 81,* 407–416.

Brophy, J. (1970). Mothers as teachers of their own preschool children: The influence of socioeconomic status and task structure on teaching specificity. *Child Development, 41,* 79–94.

Brown, A. (1974). The role of strategic behavior in retardate memory. In N. Ellis (Ed.), *International review of research in mental retardation* (Vol. 7). New York: Academic.

Brown, A. (1978). Knowing when, where, and how to remember: A problem in meta cognition. In R. Glaser (Ed.), *Advances in instructional psychology.* Hillsdale, NJ: Lawrence Erlbaum Associates.

Brown, A., Campione, J., & Murphy, M. (1974). Keeping track of changing variables: Long-term retention of a trained rehearsal strategy by retarded adolescents. *American Journal of Mental Deficiency, 78,* 446–453.

Brown, R. (1973). *First language: The early stages.* Cambridge, MA: Harvard University Press.

Brownell, M. D., & Whiteley, J. H. (1992). Development and training of referential communication in children with mental retardation. *American Journal on Mental Retardation, 97,* 161–172.

Bruner, J. (1974–1975). From communication to language—A psychological perspective. *Cognition, 3,* 255–287.

Bruner, J. (1977). Early social interaction and language acquisition. In R. Schaffer (Ed.), *Studies in mother-infant interaction.* New York: Academic.

Bryen, D., Goldman, A., & Quinlisk-Gill, S. (1988). Sign language with students with severe/profound mental retardation: How effective is it? *Education and Training in Mental Retardation, 23,* 129–137.

Bryen, D., & McGinley, V. (1991). Sign language input to community residents with mental retardation. *Education and Training in Mental Retardation, 26,* 207–214.

Buckhalt, J., Rutherford, R., & Goldberg, K. (1978). Verbal and nonverbal interaction of mothers with their Down's syndrome and nonretarded infants. *American Journal of Mental Deficiency, 82,* 337–343.

Buium, N., Rynders, J., & Turnure, J. (1974). Early maternal linguistic environment of normal and Down's syndrome language-learning children. *American Journal of Mental Deficiency, 79,* 52–58.

Bullowa, M. (Ed.). (1979). *Before speech: The beginning of interpersonal communication.* New York: Cambridge University Press.

Bunce, B., Ruder, K., & Ruder, C. (1985). Using the miniature linguistic system in teaching syntax: Two case studies. *Journal of Speech and Hearing Disorders, 50,* 247–253.

Burger, A., Blackman, L., & Clark, H. (1981). Generalization of verbal abstraction strategies by EMR children and adolescents. *American Journal of Mental Deficiency, 85,* 611–618.

Burger, A., Blackman, L., Clark, H., & Reis, E. (1982). Effects of hypothesis testing and variable format training on generalization of a verbal abstraction strategy by EMR learners. *American Journal of Mental Deficiency, 86,* 405–413.

Burger, A., Blackman, L., Holmes, M., & Zetlin, A. (1978). Use of active sorting and retrieval strategies as a facilitator of recall, clustering, and sorting by EMR and nonretarded children. *American Journal of Mental Deficiency, 83,* 253–261.

Burger, A., Blackman, L., & Tan, N. (1980). Maintenance and generalization of a sorting and retrieval strategy by EMR and nonretarded individuals. *American Journal of Mental Deficiency, 84,* 373–380.

Burggraf, A. (1972). Sign language as a verbal-facilitator with mentally retarded children. Master's thesis, Ohio State University, Columbus.

Burr, D., & Rohr, A. (1978). Patterns of psycholinguistic development in the severely mentally retarded: A hypothesis. *Social Biology, 25,* 15–22.

Burroughs, J., Albritton, E., Eaton, B., & Montagne, J. (1990). A comparative study of language delayed preschool children's ability to recall symbols from two symbol systems. *Augmentative and Alternative Communication, 6,* 202–206.

Butterfield, E., & Belmont, J. (1978). Assessing and improving the cognitive functions of mentally retarded people. In I. Bialer & M. Sternlicht (Eds.), *The psychology of mental retardation: Issues and approaches.* New York: Psychological Dimensions.

Butterfield, E., Wambold, C., & Belmont, J. (1973). On the theory and practice of improving short-term memory. *American Journal of Mental Deficiency, 77,* 654–669.

Bzock, K., & League, R. (1978). *Receptive Expressive Emergent Language Scale.* Austin, TX: Pro-Ed.

Calculator, S. N. (1988). Exploring the language of adults with mental retardation. In S. Calculator & J. Bedrosian (Eds.), *Communication assessment and intervention for adults with mental retardation* (pp. 95–106). San Diego, CA: College-Hill.

Calculator, S., & Luchko, C. (1983). Evaluating the effectiveness of a communication board training program. *Journal of Speech and Hearing Disorders, 48,* 185–191.

Campione, J., & Brown, A. (1977). Memory and metamemory development in educable retarded children. In R. Kail & J. Hagen (Eds.), *Perspectives on the development of memory and cognition.* Hillsdale, NJ: Lawrence Erlbaum Associates.

Cardone, I., & Gilkerson, L. (1989). *Family administered neonatal activities.* Washington, DC: Bulletin of the National Center for Clinical Infant Programs.

Cardosa-Martins, C., & Mervis, C. (1990). Mothers' use of substantive deixis and nouns with their children with Down syndrome: Some discrepant findings. *American Journal on Mental Retardation, 94,* 633–637.

Cardosa-Martins, C., Mervis, C., & Mervis, C. (1985). Early vocabulary acquisition by children with Down's syndrome. *American Journal of Mental Deficiency, 90,* 177–184.

Caro, P., & Snell, M. (1989). Characteristics of teaching communication to people with moderate and severe disabilities. *Education and Training in Mental Retardation, 24,* 63–77.

Caron, J. (1994). Male-female characteristics of Fragile X syndrome. Typescript.

Case, R. (1978). Intellectual development from birth to adulthood: A neo-Piagetian interpretation. In R. Siegler (Ed.), *Children's thinking: What develops?* Hillsdale, NJ: Lawrence Erlbaum Associates.

Caselli, M. C., Vicari, S., Longobardi, E., Lami, L., Pizzoli, C., & Stella, G. (1998). Gestures and words in early development of children with Down syndrome. *Journal of Speech, Language, and Hearing Research, 41,*1125–1135.

Cegelka, P., & Prehm, H. (1982). *Mental retardation: From categories to people.* Columbus, OH: Merrill/Macmillan.

Chandler, M., Greenspan, S., & Barenboim, C. (1974). Assessment and training of role-taking and referential communication skills in institutionalized emotionally disturbed children. *Developmental Psychology, 10,* 546–553.

Chaney, R., Eyman, R., & Miller, C. (1979). Comparison of respiratory mortality in the profoundly mentally retarded and the less retarded. *Journal of Mental Deficiency Research, 23,* 107.

Chapman, R. S., Kay-Raining Bird, E., & Schwartz, S. E. (1990). Fast mapping of words in event contexts by children with Down syndrome. *Journal of Speech and Hearing Disorders, 55,* 761–770.

Chapman, R. S., & Miller, J. (1980). Analyzing language and communication in the child. In R. Schiefelbusch (Ed.), *Nonspeech language and communication: Analysis and intervention.* Baltimore: University Park Press.

Chapman, R. S., Schwartz, S. E., & Kay-Raining Bird, E. (1988, November). *Predicting comprehension of children with Down syndrome.* Paper presented at the Annual Convention of the American Speech-Language-Hearing Association, Boston.

Chapman, R. S., Seung, H.-K., Schwartz, S. E., & Kay-Raining Bird, E. (1998). Language skills of children and adolescents with Down syndrome: II. Production deficits. *Journal of Speech, Language, and Hearing Research, 41,* 861–873.

Cheseldine, S., & McConkey, R. (1979). Parental speech to young Down's syndrome children: An intervention study. *American Journal of Mental Deficiency, 83,* 612–620.

Clark, C. (1981). Learning words using traditional orthography and the symbols of Rebus, Bliss, and Carrier. *Journal of Speech and Hearing Disorders, 46,* 191–196.

Clark, D., Baker, B., & Heifetz, L. (1982). Behavioral training for parents of mentally retarded children: Prediction of outcome. *American Journal of Mental Deficiency, 87,* 14–19.

Cole, K. N., Dale, P. S., & Mills, P. E. (1992). Stability of intelligence quotient-language relation: Is discrepancy modeling based on a myth? *American Journal on Mental Retardation, 97,* 131–144.

Coleman, C., Cook, A., & Myers, L. (1980). Assessing non-oral clients for assistive communication devices. *Journal of Speech and Hearing Disorders, 45,* 515–526.

Connard, P. (1984). *Preverbal Assessment Intervention Profile,* Austin, TX: Pro-Ed.

Connor, F., Williamson, G., & Siepp, J. (1978). *Program guide for infants and toddlers with neuromotor and other developmental disabilities.* New York: Teachers College Press.

Conroy, J., Efthimiou, J., & Lemanowicz, J. (1982). A matched comparison of the developmental growth of institutionalized and deinstitutionalized mentally retarded clients. *American Journal of Mental Deficiency, 86,* 581–587.

Cook, D., & Seymour, H. (1980). A comparison among three language elicitation procedures. Paper presented at the American Speech-Language-Hearing Association Convention, Detroit.

Coplan, J. (1987). *Early Language Milestone Scale.* Tulsa, OK: Modern Education Corporation.

Crais, E., & Roberts, J. (1991). Decision making in assessment and early intervention planning. *Language, Speech and Hearing Services in Schools, 22,* 19–30.

Cummins, J. (1979). Language functions and cognitive processing. In J. Das, J. Kirby, & R. Jarman (Eds.), *Simultaneous and successive cognitive processes.* New York: Academic.

Cummins, J., & Das, J. (1978). Simultaneous and successive synthesis and linguistic processes. *International Journal of Psychology, 13,* 129–138.

Cupples, L., & Iacono, T. (2000). Phonological awareness and oral reading skills in children with Down syndrome. *Journal of Speech, Language, and Hearing Research, 43,* 595–608.

Dance, F. (1967). Toward a theory of human communication. In F. Dance (Ed.), *Human communication theory: Original essays.* New York: Holt, Rinehart & Winston.

Danforth, S., & Navarro, V. (1998). Speech acts: Sampling the social construction of mental retardation in everyday life. *Mental Retardation, 36,* 31–43.

Daniloff, J., Lloyd, L., & Fristoe, M. (1983). Amer-Ind transparency. *Journal of Speech and Hearing Disorders, 48,* 103–110.

Das, J. (1972). Patterns of cognitive ability in nonretarded and retarded children. *American Journal of Mental Deficiency, 77,* 6–12.

Das, J., Kirby, J., & Jarman, R. (1975). Simultaneous and successive synthesis: An alternative model for cognitive abilities. *Psychological Bulletin, 80,* 97–113.

Das, J., Kirby, J., & Jarman, R. (1979). *Simultaneous and successive cognitive processes.* New York: Academic.

Davis, H., Stroud, A., & Green, L. (1988). Maternal language environment of children with mental retardation. *American Journal on Mental Retardation, 93,* 144–153.

Day, J., & Hall, L. (1988). Intelligence-related differences in learning and transfer and enhancement of transfer among mentally retarded persons. *American Journal on Mental Retardation, 93,* 125–137.

Detterman, D. (1979). Memory in the mentally retarded. In N. Ellis (Ed.), *Handbook of mental deficiency: Psychological theory and research.* Hillsdale, NJ: Lawrence Erlbaum Associates.

Dever, R. (1978). *TALK—Teaching the American language to kids.* Columbus, OH: Merrill/Macmillan.

Dever, R., & Gardner, W. (1970). Performance of normal and retarded boys on Berko's test of morphology. *Language and Speech, 13,* 162–181.

Domingo, R. A., Barrow, M. B., & Amato, J. (1998). Exercise of linguistic control by speakers in an adult day treatment program. *Mental Retardation, 36,* 293–302.

Dore, J. (1974). A pragmatic description of early language development. *Journal of Psycholinguistic Research, 3,* 343–350.

Drash, P., Raver, S., Murrin, M., & Tudor, R. (1989). Three procedures for increasing vocal response to therapist prompt in infants and children with Down syndrome. *American Journal on Mental Retardation, 94,* 64–73.

Duhammel, T., Lin, S., Skelton, A., & Hantke, L. (1974). Early parental perceptions and the high risk neonate. *Clinical Pediatrics, 13,* 1052–1056.

Dunst, C. (1980). *A clinical and educational manual for use with the Uzgris and Hunt scales of infant psychological development.* Austin, TX: Pro-Ed.

Dwinell, M., & Connis, R. (1979). Reducing inappropriate verbalizations of a retarded adult. *American Journal of Mental Deficiency, 84,* 87–92.

Eheart, B. (1982). Mother-child interactions with nonretarded and mentally retarded preschoolers. *American Journal of Mental Deficiency, 87,* 20–25.

Ellis, N. (1963). Stimulus trace and behavioral inadequacy. In N. Ellis (Ed.), *Handbook of mental deficiency.* New York: McGraw-Hill.

Ellis, N. (1970). Memory processes in retardates and normals. In N. Ellis (Ed.), *International review of research in mental retardation* (Vol. 4). New York: Academic.

Ellis, N., Deacon, J., Harris, L., Poor, A., Angers, D., Diorio, M., Watkins, R., Boyd, B., & Cavalier, A. (1982). Learning, memory, and transfer in profoundly, severely, and moderately mentally retarded persons. *American Journal of Mental Deficiency, 87,* 186–196.

Ellis, N., Deacon, J., & Wooldridge, P. (1985). On the nature of short-term memory deficit in mentally retarded persons. *American Journal of Mental Deficiency, 89,* 393–402.

Ellis, N., Woodley-Zanthos, P., & Dulaney, C. (1989). Memory for spatial location in children, adults, and mentally retarded persons. *American Journal on Mental Retardation, 93,* 521–527.

Emery, G., & Ramey, C. (1976). Maternal teaching styles as a function of mothers' level of education. Paper presented at fourth biennial Southeastern Conference on Human Development, Nashville.

Engle, R., & Nagle, R. (1979). Strategy training and semantic encoding in mildly retarded children. *Intelligence, 3,* 17–30.

Ervin-Tripp, S. (1973). Some strategies for the first two years. In T. Moore (Ed.), *Cognitive development and the acquisition of language*. New York: Academic.

Evans, D. (1977). The development of language abilities in Mongols: A correlational study. *Journal of Mental Deficiency Research, 21,* 103–117.

Evans, R., & Bilsky, L. (1979). Clustering and categorical list retention in the mentally retarded. In N. Ellis (Ed.), *Handbook of mental deficiency: Psychological theory and research*. Hillsdale, NJ: Lawrence Erlbaum Associates.

Ezell, H., & Goldstein, H. (1991). Comparison of idiom comprehension of normal children and children with mental retardation. *Journal of Speech and Hearing Research, 34,* 812–819.

Feldman, H. M., Evans, J. L., Brown, R. E., & Wareham, N. L. (1992). Early language and communicative abilities of children with periventricular leukomalacia. *American Journal on Mental Retardation, 97,* 222–234.

Fenson, L., Dale, P., Reznick, S., Thal, D., Bates, E., Hartung, J., Pethnick, S., & Reilly, J. (1993). *MacArthur Communicative Development Inventories*. San Diego, CA: Singular.

Fewell, R., & Langley, M. (1984). *Developmental Activities Screening Inventory*. Austin, TX: Pro-Ed.

Forehand, R., & Atkeson, B. (1977). Generality of treatment effects with parents as therapists: A review of assessment and implementation procedures. *Behavior Therapy, 8,* 575–593.

Frailberg, S. (1979). Blind infants and their mothers: An examination of the sign system. In M. Bullowa (Ed.), *Before speech*. New York: Cambridge University Press.

Frank, H., & Rabinovitch, M. (1974). Auditory short-term memory: Developmental changes in rehearsal. *Child Development, 45,* 397–407.

Fristoe, M., & Lloyd, L. (1980). Planning an initial expressive sign lexicon for persons with severe communication impairment. *Journal of Speech and Hearing Disorders, 45,* 170–180.

Giattinno, J., Pollack, E., & Silliman, E. (1978). Adult input in language impaired children. Paper presented at the American Speech and Hearing Association Annual Convention, San Francisco.

Glidden, L. (1977). Stimulus relations, blocking, and sorting in the free recall and organization of EMR adolescents. *American Journal of Mental Deficiency, 82,* 250–258.

Glidden, L., & Warner, D. (1985). Semantic processing and serial learning by EMR adolescents. *American Journal of Mental Deficiency, 89,* 635–641.

Goetz, L., Gee, K., & Sailor, W. (1985). Using a behavior chain interruption strategy to teach communication skills to students with severe disabilities. *Journal of the Association for Persons with Severe Handicaps, 10,* 21–30.

Goldberg, S. (1977). Social competence in infancy: A model of parent-infant interaction. *Merrill-Palmer Quarterly, 23,* 163–177.

Goossens, C. (1984). Assessment for nonspeech. Paper presented at the annual conference of American Association on Mental Deficiency, Minneapolis.

Graham, J., & Graham, L. (1971). Language behavior of the mentally retarded: Syntactic characteristics. *American Journal of Mental Deficiency, 73,* 623–629.

Greenfield, P., & Smith, J. (1976). *The structure of communication in early language development*. New York: Academic.

Greenspan, S. (1979). Social intelligence in the retarded. In N. Ellis (Ed.), *Handbook of mental deficiency: Psychological theory and research*. Hillsdale, NJ: Lawrence Erlbaum Associates.

Greenwald, C., & Leonard, L. (1979). Communicative and sensorimotor development of Down's syndrome children. *American Journal of Mental Deficiency, 84*, 296–303.

Grossman, H. (1983). *Classification in mental retardation*. Washington, DC: American Association on Mental Deficiency.

Guess, D., Koegh, W., & Sailor, W. (1978). Generalization of speech and language behavior: Measurement and training tactics. In R. Schiefelbusch (Ed.), *Bases of language intervention*. Baltimore: University Park Press.

Guess, D., Sailor, W., & Baer, D. (1976). *Functional speech and language training for the severely handicapped*. Lawrence, KS: H and H Enterprises.

Gullo, F., & Gullo, J. (1984). An ecological language intervention approach with mentally retarded adolescents. *Language, Speech and Hearing Services in Schools, 15*, 182–191.

Gutmann, A., & Rondal, J. (1979). Verbal operants in mothers' speech to nonretarded and Down's syndrome children matched for linguistic level. *American Journal of Mental Deficiency, 83*, 446–452.

Gutowski, W., & Chechile, R. (1987). Encoding, storage, and retrieval components of associative memory deficits of mildly mentally retarded adults. *American Journal of Mental Deficiency, 92*, 85–93.

Hagerman, R., Kemper, M., & Hudson, M. (1985). Learning disabilities and attentional problems in boys with the Fragile X syndrome. *American Journal of Diseases of Children, 139*, 674–678.

Halle, J., Alpert, C., & Anderson, S. (1984). Natural environment language assessment and intervention with severely impaired preschoolers. *Topics in Early Childhood Special Education, 4*, 36–56.

Hanley-Maxwell, C., Wilcox, B., & Heal, L. (1982). A comparison of vocabulary learning by moderately retarded students under direct instruction and incidental presentation. *Education and Training of Mentally Retarded, 3*, 214–221.

Hanna, R., Lippert, E., & Harris, A. (1982). *Developmental Communication Curriculum Inventory*. San Antonio, TX: Psychological Corporation.

Hanzlik, J., & Stevenson, M. (1986). Interaction of mothers with their infants who are mentally retarded, with cerebral palsy, or nonretarded. *American Journal of Mental Deficiency, 90*, 513–520.

Harding, C. (1984). Acting with intention: A framework for examining the development of the intention to communicate. In L. Feagans, C. Garvey, & R. Golinkoff (Eds.), *The origins and growth of communication*. Norwood, NJ: Ablex.

Hargis, K., & Blechman, E. (1979). Social class and training of parents as behavior change agents. *Child Behavior Therapy, 1*, 69–74.

Haring, N., & Bricker, D. (1976). Overview of comprehensive services for the severely/profoundly handicapped. In N. Haring & L. Brown (Eds.), *Teaching the severely handicapped*. New York: Grune & Stratton.

Harris, D. (1982). Communicative interaction processes involving nonvocal physically handicapped children. *Topics in Language Disorders, 2*, 21–38.

Harris, D., Lippert, J., Yoder, D., & Vanderheiden, G. (1977). Blissymbolics: An augmentative symbol communication system for non-vocal severely handicapped children. In R. York & E. Edgat, (Eds.), *Teaching the severely handicapped* (Vol. 4). Seattle: Special Press.

Harris-Vanderheiden, D., Brown, W., MacKenzie, P., Reinen, S., & Schiebel, C. (1975). Symbol communication for the mentally handicapped. *Mental Retardation, 13*, 34–37.

Hayes, C., & Koch, R. (1977). Interpersonal distance behavior of mentally retarded and nonretarded children. *American Journal of Mental Deficiency, 82*, 207–209.

Heifetz, L. (1980). From consumer to middleman: Emerging roles for parents in the network of services for retarded children. In R. Abidin (Ed.), *Parent education and intervention handbook*. Springfield, IL: Charles Thomas.

Hess, R., & Shipman, V. (1965). Early experience and the socialization of cognitive modes in children. *Child Development, 36*, 886–896.

Hockey, R. (1973). Rate of presentation in running memory and direct manipulation of input processing strategies. *Quarterly Journal of Experimental Psychology, 25*, 104–111.

Hogg, J. (1975). Normative development and educational program planning for severely educationally subnormal children. In C. Kiennan & F. Woodford (Eds.), *Behavior modification with the severely retarded*. Amsterdam, The Netherlands: Associated Scientific.

Horstmeier, D., & MacDonald, J. (1978). *Environmental Prelanguage Battery.* San Antonio, TX: Psychological Corporation.

Houghton, J., Bronicki, G., & Guess, D. (1987). Opportunities to express preferences and make choices among students with severe disabilities in classroom settings. *Journal of the Association for Persons with Severe Handicaps, 12*, 18–27.

Hoy, E., & McKnight, J. (1977). Communication style and effectiveness in homogeneous and heterogeneous dyads of retarded children. *American Journal of Mental Deficiency, 81*, 587–598.

Humphreys, L., & Parsons, C. (1979). Piagetian tasks measure intelligence and intelligence tests assess cognitive development: A reanalysis. *Intelligence, 3*, 369–382.

Hunt, N. (1967). *The world of Nigel Hunt: The diary of a mongoloid youth.* New York: Garret.

Hunt, P., Goetz, L., Alwell, M., & Sailor, W. (1986). Using an interrupted behavior chain strategy to teach generalized communication responses. *Journal of the Association for Persons with Severe Handicaps, 11*, 196–204.

Ingalls, R. (1978). *Mental retardation: The changing outlook.* New York: Wiley.

Ingram, D. (1972). Transivity in child language. *Language, 47*, 888–910.

Jarman, R. (1978). Patterns of cognitive ability in retarded children: A reexamination. *American Journal of Mental Deficiency, 82*, 344–348.

Jarman, R., & Das, J. (1977). Simultaneous and successive synthesis and intelligence. *Intelligence, 1*, 151–169.

Johnson-Martin, N., Jens, K., Attermeier, S., & Hacker, B. (1991). *Carolina Curriculum for Infants and Toddlers with Special Needs.* Baltimore, MD: Paul H. Brookes.

Johnston, J., & Schery, T. (1976). The use of grammatical morphemes by children with communication disorders. In D. Morehead & A. Morehead (Eds.), *Normal and deficient child language*. Baltimore: University Park Press.

Jones, O. (1977). Mother-child communication with prelinguistic Down's syndrome and normal infants. In H. Schaffer (Eds.), *Studies in mother–infant interaction*. New York: Academic.

Jones, P. (1972). Home environment and the development of verbal ability. *Child Development, 43*, 1081–1086.

Kahn, J. (1975). Relationship of Piaget's sensorimotor period to language acquisition of profoundly retarded children. *American Journal of Mental Deficiency, 79*, 640–643.

Kahn, J. (1977). A comparison of manual and oral language training. *Mental Retardation, 15*, 21–23.

Kamhi, A. (1981). Developmental vs. different theories of mental retardation: A new look. *American Journal of Mental Deficiency, 86*, 1–7.

Kamhi, A., & Masterson, J. (1989). Language and cognition in mentally handicapped people: Last rites for the difference-delay controversy. In M. Beveridge, G. Conti-Ramsden, & I. Leudar (Eds.), *Language and communication in mentally handicapped people*. London: Chapman & Hall.

Kangas, K., & Lloyd, L. L. (1988). Early cognitive skills as prerequisites to augumentative and alternative communication use: What are we waiting for? *Augumentative and Alternative Communication, 4*, 211–221.

Karen, R., Astin-Smith, S., & Creasy, D. (1985). Teaching telephone-answering skills to mentally retarded adults. *American Journal of Mental Deficiency, 89*, 595–609.

Karrer, R., Nelson, M., & Galbraith, G. (1979). Psychophysiological research with the mentally retarded. In N. Ellis (Ed.), *International review of research in mental retardation* (Vol. 7). New York: Academic.

Kearsley, R. (1979). Latrogenic retardation: A syndrome of learned incompetence. In R. Kearsley & I. Sigel (Eds.), *Infants at risk: Assessment of cognitive functioning*. Hillsdale, NJ: Lawrence Erlbaum Associates.

Kellas, G., Ashcroft, M., & Johnson, N. (1973). Rehearsal processes in the short-term memory performance of mildly retarded adolescents. *American Journal of Mental Deficiency, 77*, 670–679.

Kendall, C., Borkowski, J., & Cavanaugh, J. (1980). Maintenance and generalization of an interrogative strategy by EMR children. *Intelligence, 4*, 255–270.

Kernan, K. (1990). Comprehension of syntactically indicated sequence by Down's syndrome and other mentally retarded adults. *Journal of Mental Deficiency Research, 34*, 169–178.

Kintsch, W., & van Dijk, T. (1978). Toward a model of text comprehension and productions. *Psychological Review, 85*, 363–394.

Klaus, M., & Kennell, J. (1976). *Maternal–infant bonding*. St. Louis: Mosby.

Klein, M., & Briggs, M. (1987). *Observation of communicative interactions*. Los Angeles: Mother–Infant Communication Project, California State University.

Klink, M., Gerstman, L., Raphael, L., Schlanger, B., & Newsome, L. (1986). Phonological process usage by young EMR children and nonretarded preschool children. *American Journal of Mental Deficiency, 91,* 190–195.

Kogan, K., Wimberger, H., & Bobbitt, R. (1969). Analysis of mother-child interaction in young mental retardates. *Child Development, 40,* 799–812.

Kohl, F. (1981). Effects of motoric requirements on the acquisition of manual sign responses by severely handicapped students. *American Journal of Mental Deficiency, 85,* 396–403.

Kohl, F., Karlan, G., & Heal, L. (1979). Effects of pairing manual signs with verbal cues upon the acquisition of instruction-following behaviors and the generalization to expressive language with severely handicapped students. *AAESPH Review, 4,* 291–300.

Konstantases, M., Oxman, J., & Webster, C. (1917). Simultaneous communication with autistic and other severely dysfunctional nonverbal children. *Journal of Communication Disorders, 10,* 267–282.

Krupski, A. (1977). Role of attention in the reaction-time performance of mentally retarded adolescents. *American Journal of Mental Deficiency, 82,* 79–83.

Lackner, J. (1968) A developmental study of language behavior in retarded children. *Neuropsychologia, 6,* 301–320.

LaGreca, A., Stone, W., & Bell, C. (1983). Facilitating the vocational-interpersonal skills of mentally retarded individuals. *American Journal of Mental Deficiency, 88,* 270–278.

Lamberts, F. (1981). Sign and symbol in children's processing of familiar auditory stimuli. *American Journal of Mental Deficiency, 86,* 300–308.

Layton, T., & Sharifi, H. (1979). Meaning and structure of Down's syndrome and nonretarded children's spontaneous speech. *American Journal of Mental Deficiency, 83,* 439–445.

Leahy, R., Balla, D., & Zigler, E. (1982). Role-taking, self-image, and imitativeness of mentally retarded and nonretarded individuals. *American Journal of Mental Deficiency, 86,* 372–379.

Lee, L. (1974). *Developmental sentence analysis.* Evanston, IL: Northwestern University Press.

Leonard, L. B. (1987). Is specific language impairment a useful construct? In S. Rosenburg (Ed.), *Advances in applied psycholinguistics* (Vol. 1, pp. 1–39). Cambridge, UK: Cambridge University Press.

Leonard, L., Cole, B., & Steckol, K. (1979). Lexical usage of retarded children: An examination of informativeness. *American Journal of Mental Deficiency, 84,* 49–54.

Leonard, L., Steckol, K., & Panther, K. (1983). Returning meaning to semantic relations: Some clinical applications. *Journal of Speech and Hearing Disorders, 48,* 25–35.

Levine, H., & Langness, L. (1985). Everyday cognition among mildly mentally retarded adults: An ethnographic approach. *American Journal of Mental Deficiency, 90,* 18–26.

Liebert, A., & Baumeister, A. (1973). Behavioral variability among retardates, children, and college students. *The Journal of Psychology, 83,* 57–65.

Lincoln, A., Courchesne, E., Kilman, B., & Galambos, R. (1985). Neuropsychological correlates of information-processing by children with Down syndrome. *American Journal of Mental Deficiency, 89,* 403–414.

Lobato, D., Barrera, R., & Feldman, R. (1981). Sensorimotor functioning and prelinguistic communication of severely and profoundly mentally retarded individuals. *American Journal of Mental Deficiency, 85,* 489–496.

Lobb, H. (1974). Effects of verbal rehearsal on discrimination learning in moderately retarded nursery-school children. *American Journal of Mental Deficiency, 79,* 449–454.

Longhurst, T., & Berry, G. (1975). Communication in retarded adolescents: Response to listener feedback. *American Journal of Mental Deficiency, 80,* 158–164

Looney, P. (1980). Instructional intervention with language-disordered learners. *Directive Teacher, 2,* 30–31.

Love, R. J., & Webb, W. G. (1986). *Neurology for the speech-language pathologist.* Stoneham, MA: Butterworth.

Luftig, R., & Johnson, R. (1982). Identification and recall of structurally important units in prose of mentally retarded learners. *American Journal of Mental Deficiency, 86,* 495–502.

Luria, A. (1975). Basic problems of language in the light of psychology and neurolinguistics. In E. Lenneberg & E. Lenneberg (Eds.), *Foundations of language development: A multidisciplinary approach.* New York: Academic.

MacDonald, J. (1978a). *Environmental Language Inventory.* San Antonio, TX: Psychological Corporation.

MacDonald, J. (1978b). *Environmental Language Intervention Program.* Columbus, OH: Merrill/Macmillan.

MacDonald, J. (1985). Language through conversation: A model for intervention with language-delayed persons. In S. Warren and A. Rogers-Warren (Eds.), *Teaching functional language* (pp. 89–122). Baltimore: University Park Press.

MacDonald, J., Blott, J., Gordon, K., Spiegal, B., & Hartmann, M. (1974). An experimental parent-assisted treatment program for preschool language-delayed children. *Journal of Speech and Hearing Disorders, 39,* 295–415.

MacDonald, J., & Gillette, Y. (1978). *Environmental Communication System (ECO).* San Antonio, TX: Psychological Corporation.

MacDonald, J., & Gillette, Y. (1982). *ECO, ecological communication system: A clinical handbook for parents and teachers.* Columbus, OH: Nisonger Center.

MacMillan, D. (1972). Paired-associate learning as a function of explicitness of mediational set by EMR and nonretarded children. *American Journal of Mental Deficiency, 76,* 686–691.

Macnamara, J. (1972). Cognitive basis of language learning in infants. *Psychological Review, 79,* 1–13

Mahoney, G., Fors, S., & Wood, S. (1990). Maternal directive behavior revisited. *American Journal on Mental Retardation, 94,* 398–406.

Mahoney, G., Glover, A., & Finger, I. (1981). Relationship between language and sensori-motor development of Down syndrome and nonretarded children. *American Journal of Mental Deficiency, 86,* 21–27.

Mahoney, G., & Snow, K. (1983). The relationship of sensorimotor functioning to children's response to early language training. *Mental Retardation, 21,* 248–254.

Mahoney, G., & Weller, E. (1980). An ecological approach to language intervention. *New Directions for Exceptional Children, 2,* 17–33.

Malgady, R., Barcher, R., Towner, G., & Davis, J. (1979). Language factors in vocational evaluation of mentally retarded workers. *American Journal of Mental Deficiency, 83,* 432–438.

Manolson, A. (1983). *It takes two to talk.* Toronto: Hanen Early Language Resource Centre.

Marcell, M., & Armstrong, V. (1982). Auditory and visual sequential memory of Down syndrome and nonretarded children. *American Journal of Mental Deficiency, 87,* 86–95.

Marcell, M., & Jett, D. (1985). Identification of vocally expressed emotions by mentally retarded and nonretarded individuals. *American Journal of Mental Deficiency, 89,* 537–545.

Marcell, M., & Weeks, S. (1988). Short-term memory difficulties and Down's syndrome. *Journal of Mental Deficiency Research, 32,* 153–162.

Marshall, N., Hegrenes, J., & Goldstein, S. (1973). Verbal interactions: Mothers and their retarded children vs. mothers and their nonretarded children. *American Journal of Mental Deficiency, 77,* 415–419.

Maurer, H., & Sherrod, K. (1987). Context of directives given to young children with Down syndrome and nonretarded children: Development over two years. *American Journal of Mental Deficiency, 91,* 579–590.

McCarver, R., & Craig, E. (1974). Placement of the retarded in the community: Prognosis and outcome. In N. Ellis (Ed.), *International review of research in mental retardation* (Vol. 7). New York: Academic.

McCormick, L. (1986). Keeping up with language trends. *Teaching Exceptional Children, 18,* 123–129.

McLean, J., & Snyder-McLean, L. (1978). *A transactional approach to early language training.* Columbus, OH: Merrill/Macmillan.

McLean, L. K., Brady, N. C., McLean, J. E., & Behrens, G. A. (1999). Communication forms and functions of children and adults with severe mental retardation in community and institutional settings. *Journal of Speech, Language, and Hearing Research, 42,* 231–240.

McLeavey, B., Toomey, J., & Dempsey, P. (1982). Nonretarded and mentally retarded children's control over syntactic structures. *American Journal of Mental Deficiency, 86,* 485–494.

McNutt, J., & Leri, S. (1979). Language differences between institutionalized and non-institutionalized retarded children. *American Journal of Mental Deficiency, 83,* 339–345.

Meador, D. (1984). Effects of color on visual discrimination of geometric symbols by severely and profoundly mentally retarded individuals. *American Journal of Mental Deficiency, 89,* 275–286.

Mehrabian, A., & Williams, M. (1971). Piagetian measures of cognitive development for children up to age two. *Journal of Psycholinguistic Research, 1,* 113–126.

Menyuk, P. (1974). Early development of receptive language: From babbling to words. In R. Schiefelbusch & L. Lloyd (Eds.), *Language perspectives—Acquisition, retardation and intervention.* Baltimore: University Park Press.

Mercer, C., & Snell, M. (1977). *Learning theory research in mental retardation.* Columbus, OH: Merrill/Macmillan.

Merrill, E. (1985). Differences in semantic processing speed of mentally retarded and nonretarded persons. *American Journal of Mental Deficiency, 90,* 71–80.

Merrill, E., & Bilsky, L. (1990). Individual differences in the representation of sentences in memory. *American Journal on Mental Retardation, 95,* 68–76.

Merrill, E. C., & Jackson, T. S. (1992). Degree of associative relatedness and sentence processing by adolescents with and without mental retardation. *American Journal on Mental Retardation, 97,* 173–185.

Merrill, E., & Mar, H. (1987). Differences between mentally retarded and nonretarded persons' efficiency of auditory sentence processing. *American Journal of Mental Deficiency, 91,* 406–414.

Mervis, C. B. (1988). Early lexical development: Theory and application. In L. Nadel (Ed.), *The psychology of Down's syndrome* (pp. 104–144). Cambridge, MA: MIT Press.

Miller, A., & Miller, F. (1973). Cognitive developmental training with elevated boards and sign language. *Journal of Autism and Childhood Schizophrenia, 3,* 65–68.

Miller, A., & Newhoff, M. (1978). Language disordered children: Language disordered mothers? Paper presented at the American Speech and Hearing Association Annual Conference, San Francisco.

Miller, J. (1980). *Assessing language production in children.* Baltimore: University Park Press.

Miller, J., Chapman, R., & MacKenzie, H. (1981). Individual differences in the language acquisition of mentally retarded children. *Proceedings from the Second Wisconsin Symposium on Research in Child Language Disorders.* Madison: University of Wisconsin.

Miller, J. F., Sedey, A. L., & Miolo, G. (1995). Validity of parent report measures of vocabulary development for children with Down syndrome. *Journal of Speech and Hearing Research, 38,* 1037–1044.

Miller, J., & Yoder, D. (1974). An ontogenetic language teaching strategy for retarded children. In R. Schiefelbusch & L. Lloyd (Eds.), *Language perspectives—Acquisition, retardation, and intervention.* Baltimore: University Park Press.

Miller, S., & Sloan, H. (1976). The generalization effects of parent training across stimulus settings. *Journal of Applied Behavior Analysis, 9,* 355–370.

Mindell, C., & Budd, K. (1977). Issues in the generalization of parent training across settings. Paper presented at the annual meeting of the American Psychological Association.

Mittler, P. (1974). Language and communication. In A. Clarke & A. Clarke (Eds.), *Mental deficiency: The changing outlook.* London: Methuen.

Mittler, P. (1976) Assessment for language learning. In P. Berry (Ed.), *Language and communication in the mentally handicapped.* Baltimore: University Park Press.

Mirenda, P., & Locke, P. (1989). A comparison of symbol transparency in nonspeaking persons with intellectual disabilities. *Journal of Speech and Hearing Disorders, 54,* 131–140.

Montague, J., Hutchinson, E., & Matson, E. (1975). Comparative computer content analysis of the verbal behavior of institutionalized and noninstitutionalized retarded children. *Journal of Speech and Hearing Research, 18,* 43–57.

Moran, M., Money, S., & Leonard, D. (1984). Phonological process analysis of the speech of mentally retarded adults. *American Journal of Mental Deficiency, 89,* 304–306.

Muma, J. (1978). *Language handbook: Concepts, assessment, intervention.* Englewood Cliffs, NJ: Prentice Hall.

Mundy, P., Kasari, C., Sigman, M., & Ruskin, E. (1995). Nonverbal communication and early language acquisition in children with Down syndrome and in normally developing children. *Journal of Speech and Learning Research, 38,* 157–167.

Musselwhite, C., & St. Louis, K. (1982). *Communication programming for the severely handicapped: Vocal and non-vocal strategies.* Houston: College-Hill.

Naremore, R., & Dever, R. (1975). Language performance of educable mentally retarded and normal children at five age levels. *Journal of Speech and Hearing Research, 18,* 82–95.

Newfield, M. (1966). A study of the acquisition of English morphology by normal and EMR children. Master's thesis, Ohio State University, Columbus.

Newfield, M., & Schlinger, B. (1968) The acquisition of English morphology in normal and educable mentally retarded children. *Journal of Speech and Hearing Research, 11,* 693–706.

Nigro, G., & Roak, R. (1987). Mentally retarded and nonretarded adults' memory for spatial location. *American Journal of Mental Deficiency, 91,* 392–397.

Nugent, P., & Mosley, J. (1987). Mentally retarded and nonretarded individuals' attention allocation and capacity. *American Journal of Mental Deficiency, 91,* 598–605.

Nussvaum, R., & Ledbetter, D. (1986). Fragile X syndrome: A unique mutation in man. *Annual Review of Genetics, 20,* 109–145.

O'Connor, N., & Hermelin, B. (1978). *Seeing and hearing and space and time.* New York: Academic.

Ogletree, B. T., Wetherby, A. M., & Westling, D. L. (1992). Profile of the prelinguistic intentional communicative behavior of children with profound mental retardation. *American Journal on Mental Retardation, 97,* 188–196.

Oller, D., & Seibert, J. (1988). Babbling of prelinguistic mentally retarded children. *American Journal on Mental Retardation, 92,* 369–375.

Olswang, L., Stoel-Gammon, C., Coggins, T., & Carpenter, R. (1987a). *Assessing Linguistic Behavior (ALB).* Seattle: University of Washington Press.

Olswang, L., Stoel-Gammon, C., Coggins, T., & Carpenter, R. (1987b). *Assessing prelinguistic behaviors in developmentally young children.* Seattle: University of Washington Press.

O'Regan-Kleinert, J. (1980). Pre-speech/language therapeutic techniques for the handicapped infant. Paper presented at the American Speech-Language-Hearing Association Convention, Detroit.

O'Regan-Kleinert, J., Rosenwinkel, P., & Robbins, R. (1979). Remediation of severe language disorders: A pre-speech sensorimotor developmental model. Paper presented at the American Speech-Language-Hearing Association Convention, Atlanta.

Osofosky, J., & O'Connell, E. (1972). Daughter's effects upon mother's and father's behavior. *Developmental Psychology, 7,* 157–168.

Owens, R. E. (1978). Speech acts in the early language of non-delayed and retarded children: A taxonomy and distributional study. Unpublished doctoral dissertation, The Ohio State University.

Owens, R. (1982a). *Caregiver Interview and Environmental Observation.* San Antonio, TX: Psychological Corporation.

Owens, R. (1982b). *Developmental Assessment Tool.* San Antonio, TX: Psychological Corporation.

Owens, R. (1982c). *Diagnostic Interactional Survey.* San Antonio, TX: Psychological Corporation.

Owens, R. (1982d). *Program for the Acquisition of Language with the Severely Impaired* (PALS). San Antonio, TX: Psychological Corporation.

Owens, R. E. (1999). *Language disorders: A functional approach to assessment and intervention* (3d ed.). Boston: Allyn & Bacon.

Owens, R. (2001). *Language development: An introduction* (5th ed.). Boston: Allyn & Bacon.

Owens, R., & House, L. (1984). Decision-making processes in augmentative communication. *Journal of Speech and Hearing Disorders, 49,* 18–25.

Owens, R., & MacDonald, J. (1982). Communicative uses of the early speech of non-delayed and Down syndrome children. *American Journal of Mental Deficiency, 86,* 503–510.

Owens, R., McNerney, C., Bigler-Burke, L., & Lepre-Clark, C. (1987). The use of language facilitators with residential retarded populations. *Topics in Language Disorders, 7*(3), 47–63.

Owens, R. E., & Rogerson, B. S. (1988). Adults at the presymbolic level. In S. Calculator & J. Bedrosian (Eds.), *Communicative assessment and intervention for adults with mental retardation* (pp. 189–230). San Diego, CA: College-Hill.

Owings, N., & Guvette, T. (1982). Communication behavior assessment and treatment with the adult retarded: An approach. In N. Lass (Ed.), *Speech and language: Advances in basic research and practice* (Vol. 7). New York: Academic.

Page, J., & Horn, D. (1987). Comprehension in developmentally delayed children. *Language, Speech and Hearing Services in Schools, 18,* 63–71.

Papania, N. (1954). A qualitative analysis of vocabulary responses of institutionalized mentally retarded children. *Journal of Clinical Psychology, 10,* 361–365.

Paul, R. (2000). Facilitating transitions in language development for children using AAC. *Augmentative and Alternative Communication, 13,* 139–148.

Peter, D. (2000). Dynamics of discourse: A case study illuminating power relations in mental retardation. *Mental Retardation, 38,* 354–362.

Petersen, G., & Sherrod, K. (1982). Relationship of maternal language to language development and language delay of children. *American Journal of Mental Deficiency, 86,* 391–398.

Phillips, I., & Williams, N. (1975). Psychopathology and mental retardation: 1. Psychopathology. *American Journal of Psychiatry, 132,* 1265–1271.

Phillips, J., & Balthazar, E. (1979). Some correlates of language deterioration in severely and profoundly retarded long-term institutionalized residents. *American Journal of Mental Deficiency, 83,* 402–408.

Pickett, J., & Flynn, P. (1983). Language assessment tools for mentally retarded adults: Survey and recommendations. *American Journal of Mental Deficiency, 21,* 244–247.

Platt, J. & Coggins, T. (1990). Comprehension of social-action games in prelinguistic children. *Journal of Speech and Hearing Disorders, 55,* 315–326.

Polk, X., Schilmoeller, G., Embry, L., Holman, J., & Baer, D. (1976). Prompted generalization through experimenters' instructions: A parent training study. Paper presented at the annual meeting of the Midwestern Association of Behavior Analysis, Chicago.

Poulson, C. (1988). Operant conditioning of vocalization rate of infants with Down syndrome. *American Journal on Mental Retardation, 93,* 57–63.

Prater, R. (1982). Functions of consonant assimilation and reduplication in early word productions of mentally retarded children. *American Journal of Mental Deficiency, 86,* 399–404.

Prior, M., Minnes, P., Coyne, T., Golding, B., Hendy, J., & McGillivray, J. (1979). Verbal interactions between staff and residents in an institution for the young mentally retarded. *Mental Retardation, 17,* 65–70.

Pruess, J., Vadasy, P., & Fewell, R. (1987). Language development in children with Down syndrome: An overview of recent research. *Education and Training in Mental Retardation, 22,* 44–55.

Prutting, C. (1979). Process: The action of moving forward progressively from one point to another on the way to completion. *Journal of Speech and Hearing Disorders, 44,* 3–30.

Prutting, C., & Kirchner, D. (1983). Applied pragmatics. In T. Gallagher & C. Prutting (Eds.), *Pragmatic assessment and intervention issues in language.* San Diego, CA: College-Hill.

Realon, R., Lewallen, J., & Wheeler, A. (1983). Verbal vs. verbal feedback plus praise: The effects on direct care staff's training behaviors. *Mental Retardation, 21,* 209–213.

Rees, N. (1978). Pragmatics of language: Applications to normal and disordered language development. In R. Schiefelbusch (Ed.), *Bases of language intervention.* Baltimore: University Park Press.

Rees, N., & Wollner, S. (1981). Toward a taxonomy of pragmatic abilities in children. Paper presented at the ASHA Northeast Regional Conference, Philadelphia.

Reese, R., & Serna, L. (1986). Planning for generalization and maintenance in parent training: Parents need IEPs too. *Mental Retardation, 24,* 87–92.

Reich, R. (1978). Gestural facilitation of expressive language in moderately/severely retarded preschoolers. *Mental Retardation, 16,* 113–117.

Reichle, J. (1990). Intervention with presymbolic clients: Setting up an initial communication system. Paper presented at the New York State Speech-Language-Hearing Association Annual Convention, Kiamesha Lake, NY.

Reichle, J., & Sigafoos, J. (1991). Establishing an initial repertoire of requesting. In J. Reichle, J. York, & J. Sigafoos (Eds.), *Implementing augmentative and alternative communication*. Baltimore: Paul H. Brookes.

Reid, G. (1980). Overt and covert rehearsal in short-term motor memory of mentally retarded and non-retarded persons. *American Journal of Mental Deficiency, 85,* 69–77.

Rein, R., & Kernan, K. (1989). The functional use of verbal perseveratives by adults who are mentally retarded. *Education and Training in Mental Retardation, 24,* 381–389.

Reiss, S., Levitan, G., & Szyszko, J. (1982). Emotional disturbance and mental retardation: Diagnostic overshadowing. *American Journal of Mental Deficiency, 86,* 567–574.

Reiter, S., & Levi, A. (1980). Factors affecting social integration of noninstitutionalized mentally retarded adults. *American Journal of Mental Deficiency, 85,* 25–30.

Rescorla, L. (1989). The Language Development Survey: A screening tool for delayed toddlers. *Journal of Speech and Hearing Disorders, 54,* 587–599.

Rheingold, H., & Eckerman, C. (1975). Some properties for unifying the study of social development. In M. Lewis & M. Rosenblum (Eds.), *Friendship and peer relations*. New York: Wiley.

Richmond, G., & Lewallen, J. (1983). Facilitating transfer of stimulus control when teaching verbal labels. *Education and Training of Mentally Retarded, 18,* 111–115.

Riley, A. (1984). *Evaluating acquired skills in communication.* Tucson, AZ: Communication Skill Builders.

Robinson, L. A., & Owens, R. E. (1995). Functional augmentative communication and positive behavior change. *Augmentative and Alternative Communication, 11,* 207–211.

Robinson, N., & Robinson, H. (1976). *The mentally retarded child: A psychological approach* (2d ed.). New York: McGraw-Hill.

Romer, L., & Schoenberg, B. (1991). Increasing requests made by people with developmental disabilities and deaf-blindness through the use of behavior chain interruption strategies. *Education and Training in Mental Retardation, 26,* 70–78.

Romski, M., Sevcik, R., Pate, J., & Rumbaugh, D. (1985). Discrimination of lexigrams and traditional orthography by nonspeaking severely mentally retarded persons. *American Journal of Mental Deficiency, 90,* 185–190.

Romski, M., Sevcik, R., & Rumbaugh, D. (1985). Retention of symbolic communication skills by severely mentally retarded persons. *American Journal of Mental Deficiency, 89,* 441–443.

Rondal, J. (1976). *Maternal speech to normal and Down's syndrome children matched for mean length of utterance* (Research Report No. 98). Washington, DC: BEH (Contract No. 300–76–0036).

Rondal, J. (1978). Maternal speech to normal and Down's syndrome children matched for mean length of utterances. In C. Meyers (Ed.), *Quality of life in severely and profoundly mentally retarded people*. Washington, DC: American Association on Mental Deficiency.

Rondal, J., Ghiotto, M., Bredart, S., & Bachelet, J. (1988). Mean length of utterance of children with Down syndrome. *American Journal on Mental Retardation, 93,* 64–66.

Rosin, M., Swift, E., Bless, D., & Vetter, D. (1988). Communication profiles of adolescents with Down syndrome. *Journal of Childhood Communication Disorders, 12,* 49–64.

Ross, D., & Ross, S. (1979). Cognitive training for the EMR child: Language skills prerequisite to relevant-irrelevant discrimination tasks. *Mental Retardation, 17,* 3–7.

Rossetti, L. (1990). *Infant-Toddler Language Scale.* East Moline, IL: LinguiSystems.

Russell, A., & Tanquay, P. (1981). Mental illness and mental retardation: Cause or coincidence? *American Journal of Mental Deficiency, 85,* 570–574.

Ryan, J. (1975). Mental subnormality and language development. In R. Lenneberg & E. Lenneberg (Eds.), *Foundations of language development* (Vol. 2). New York: Academic.

Sacks, J., & Young, E. (1982). Infant Scale of Communication Intent. *Pediatrics Update, 7,* 1–5.

Salzberg, C., & Villani, T. (1983). Speech training by parents of Down syndrome toddlers: Generalization across settings and instructional contexts. *American Journal of Mental Deficiency, 87,* 403–413.

Schiefelbusch, R. (Ed.). (1963). Language studies in mentally retarded children. *Journal of Speech and Hearing Disorders, Monograph Supplement No. 10.*

Scruggs, T., Mastropieri, M., & Levin, J. (1985). Vocabulary acquisition of mentally retarded students under direct and mnemonic instruction. *American Journal of Mental Deficiency, 89,* 546–551.

Seitz, S., & Riedel, G. (1974). Parent-child interactions as the therapy target. *Journal of Communication Disorders, 7,* 295–304.

Semmel, M. (1967). Language behavior of mentally retarded and culturally disadvantaged children. In J. Magary & R. McIntyre (Eds.), *Distinguished lectures in special education.* Berkeley: University of California Press.

Semmel, M., Barritt, L., & Bennett, S. (1970). Performance of EMR and non-retarded children on a modified cloze task. *American Journal of Mental Deficiency, 74,* 681–688.

Semmel, M., & Herzog, B. (1966). The effects of grammatical form class on the recall of Negro and Caucasian educable retarded children. *Studies of Language and Language Behavior, 3,* 1–9.

Shane, H., & Bashir, A. (1980). Election criteria for the adoption of an augmentative communication system: Preliminary considerations. *Journal of Speech and Hearing Disorders, 45,* 408–414.

Shane, H., Lipshultz, R., & Shane, C. (1982). Facilitating the communicative interaction of nonspeaking persons in large residential settings. *Topics in Language Disorders, 2,* 73–84.

Shane, H., & Wilbur, R. (1980). Potential for expressive signing based on motor control. *Sign Language Studies, 29,* 331–347.

Sharav, T., & Shlomo, L. (1986). Stimulation of infants with Down syndrome: Long-term effects. *Mental Retardation, 24,* 81–86.

Share, J. (1975). Developmental progress in Down's syndrome. In R. Koch & F. de la Cruz (Eds.), *Down's syndrome.* New York: Bruner Mazel.

Shepard, G., & Marshall, J. (1976). Perceptions of interpersonal communication of EMR adolescents and their mothers. *Education and Training of Mentally Retarded, 11,* 106–111.

Shriberg, L., & Widder, C. (1990). Speech and prosody characteristics of adults with mental retardation. *Journal of Speech and Hearing Research, 33,* 627–653.

Siegel, G. (1975). The use of language tests. *Language, Speech and Hearing Services in Schools, 6,* 211–217.

Silverman, F. (1980). *Communication for the speechless.* Englewood Cliffs, NJ: Prentice Hall.

Simic, J., & Bucher, B. (1980). Development of spontaneous mending in language deficient children. *Journal of Applied Behavior Analysis, 13,* 523–528.

Skinner, B. F. (1957). *Verbal behavior.* New York: Appleton-Century-Crofts.

Smith, L., & Hagen, V. (1984). Relationship between the home environment and sensorimotor development of Down syndrome and nonretarded infants. *American Journal of Mental Deficiency, 89,* 124–132.

Snart, F., O'Grady, M., & Das, J. (1982). Cognitive processing of subgroups of moderately mentally retarded children. *American Journal of Mental Deficiency, 86,* 465–472.

Snell, M. (1979). Higher functioning residents as language trainers of the mentally retarded. *Education and Training of Mentally Retarded, 14,* 77–84.

Snow, C., & Ferguson, C. (1977). *Talking to children.* New York: Cambridge University Press.

Snyder, L. (1978). Communicative and cognitive abilities and disabilities in the sensorimotor period. *Merrill-Palmer Quarterly, 24,* 161–180.

Sokolov, J. L. (1992). Linguistic imitation in children with Down syndrome. *American Journal on Mental Retardation, 97,* 209–221.

Sommers, R., Patterson, J., & Wildgren, P. (1988). Phonology of Down syndrome speakers, ages 13–22. *Journal of Childhood Communication Disorders, 12,* 65–91.

Sommers, R., & Starkey, K. (1977). Dichotic verbal processing in Down's syndrome children having qualitatively different speech and language skills. *American Journal of Mental Deficiency, 82,* 44–53.

Spiegel, B. (1983). The effect of context on language learning by severely retarded young adults. *Language, Speech and Hearing Services in Schools, 14,* 252–259.

Spitz, H. (1966). The role of input organization in the learning and memory of mental retardates. In N. Ellis (Ed.), *International review of research in mental retardation* (Vol. 2). New York: Academic.

Spitz, H. (1979). Beyond field theory in the study of mental deficiency. In N. Ellis (Ed.), *Handbook of mental deficiency: Psychological theory and research.* Hillsdale, NJ: Lawrence Erlbaum Associates.

Spradlin, J. (1963). Language and communication of mental defectives. In N. Ellis (Ed.), *Handbook of mental deficiency.* New York: McGraw-Hill.

Spradlin, J., & Siegel, G. (1982). Language training in natural and clinical environments. *Journal of Speech and Hearing Disorders, 47,* 2–6.

Steffens, M. L., Oller, D., Lynch, M., & Urbano, R. C. (1992). Vocal development in infants with Down syndrome who are developing normally. *American Journal on Mental Retardation, 97,* 235–246.

Stephens, B., & McLaughlin, J. (1974). Two-year gains in reasoning by retarded and non-retarded persons. *American Journal of Mental Deficiency, 79,* 116–126.

Stephens, W. (1972). Equivalence formation by retarded and nonretarded children at different mental ages. *American Journal of Mental Deficiency, 77,* 311–313.

Sternberg, L., Pegnatore, L., & Hill, C. (1983). Establishing interactive communication behaviors with profoundly mentally handicapped students. *TASH Journal, 8,* 39–46.

Stevenson, M., & Lamb, M. (1979). Effects of infant sociability and the caretaking environment on infant cognitive performance. *Child Development, 50,* 340–349.

Stillman, R. (1978). *Callier-Azusa Scale.* Dallas: Callier Center, University of Texas.

Stoneman, Z., Brody, G., & Abbott, D. (1983). In-home observations of young Down syndrome children with their mothers and fathers. *American Journal of Mental Deficiency, 87,* 591–600.

Stowitschek, J., McConaughy, E., Peatross, D., Salzberg, C., & Lignngaris/Kraft, B. (1988). Effects of group incidental training on the use of social amenities by adults with mental retardation in work settings. *Education and Training in Mental Retardation, 23,* 202–212.

Sudhalter, V., Cohen, I., Silverman, W., & Wolf-Schein, E. (1990). Conversational analysis of males with Fragile X, Down syndrome, and autism: Comparison of the emergence of deviant language. *American Journal on Mental Retardation, 99,* 431–441.

Switsky, H., Rotatori, A., Miller, T., & Freagon, S. (1979). The developmental model and its implications for assessment and instruction for the severely/profoundly handicapped. *Mental Retardation, 17,* 167–170.

Szymanski, L., & Tanquay, P. (Eds.). (1980). *Emotional disorders of mentally retarded persons.* Baltimore: University Park Press.

Tannock, R. (1988). Mothers' directiveness in their interactions with their children with and without Down syndrome. *American Journal on Mental Retardation, 93,* 154–165.

Tannock, R., Girolametto, L., & Siegel, L. S. (1992). Language intervention with children who have developmental delays: Effects of an interactive approach. *American Journal on Mental Retardation, 97,* 145–160.

Taylor, A., & Turnure, J. (1979). Imagery and verbal elaboration with retarded children: Effects on learning and memory. In N. Ellis (Ed.), *Handbook of mental deficiency: Psychological theory and research.* Hillsdale, NJ: Lawrence Erlbaum Associates.

Tizard, B., Cooperman, O., Joseph, A., & Tizard, J. (1973). Environmental effects on language development: A study of young children in long stay residential nurseries. *Annual Progress in Child Psychiatry & Child Development, 13,* 705–728.

Trotter, R. (1983, August). Baby face. *Psychology Today,* pp. 14–20.

Turner, L., & Bray, N. (1985). Spontaneous rehearsal by mildly mentally retarded children and adolescents. *American Journal of Mental Deficiency, 90,* 57–63.

Ullman, D. (1974). Breadth of attention and retention in mentally retarded and intellectually average children. *American Journal of Mental Deficiency, 78,* 640–648.

Van Biervliet, A. (1977). Establishing words and objects as functionally equivalent through manual sign training. *American Journal of Mental Deficiency, 82,* 178–186.

Van Borsel, J. (1988). An analysis of the speech of five Down's syndrome adolescents. *Journal of Communication Disorders, 21,* 409–421.

Van Der Gagg, A. (1989). The view from Walter's window: Social environment and the communicative competence of adults with a mental handicap. *Journal of Mental Deficiency Research, 33,* 221–227.

Vanderheiden, G. (1982). *Computers can play a dual role for disabled individuals.* Madison: University of Wisconsin, Trace Center.

Variety Pre-Schooler's Workshop. (1987). *Parent/Professional Preschool Performance Profile (5Ps).* Syosset, NY: Variety Pre-Schooler's Workshop.

Varnhagen, C., Das, J., & Varnhagen, S. (1987). Auditory and visual memory span: Cognitive processing by TMR individuals with Down syndrome or other etiologies. *American Journal of Mental Deficiency, 91,* 398–405.

Vihman, M. (1978). Consonant harmony: Its scope and function in child language. In J. Greenberg (Ed.), *Universals of human language: Vol. 2. Phonology.* Stanford, CA: Stanford University Press.

Volpe, R. (1976). Orthopedic disability, restriction, and role-taking activity. *The Journal of Special Education, 10,* 371–381.

Watkins, O., & Watkins, M. (1980). The modality effect and echoic persistence. *Journal of Experimental Psychology: General, 109,* 251–278.

Weiss, B., Weisz, J., & Bromfield, R. (1986). Performance of retarded and non-retarded persons on information-processing tasks: Further tests of the similar structure hypothesis. *Psychological Bulletin, 100,* 157–175.

Welch, S., & Pear, J. (1979). Generalization by autistic-type children of verbal responses across settings. *Journal of Applied Behavior Analysis, 12,* 273–282.

Westby, C. (1980). Assessment of cognitive and language abilities through play. *Language, Speech and Hearing Services in Schools, 11,* 154–168.

Wetherby, A., & Prizant, B. (1993). *Communication and Symbolic Behavior Scales.* Chicago: Riverside.

Whatmough, J. (1956). *Language: A modern synthesis.* New York: American Library.

White, B., Watts, J., Barnett, I., Kahan, B., Marmor, J., & Shapiro, B. (1973). *Experience and environment: Major influences on the development of the young child* (Vol. 1). Englewood Cliffs, NJ: Prentice Hall.

Wilcox, M., & Campbell, P. (1983). Assessing communication in low-functioning multihandicapped children. Paper presented at the American Speech-Language-Hearing Association Annual Convention, Cincinnati, OH.

Wilkinson, K. M., & Romski, M. A. (1995). Responsiveness of male adolescents with mental retardation to input from nondisabled peers: The summoning power of comments, questions, and direct prompts. *Journal of Speech and Hearing, 38,* 1045–1053.

Windle, C. (1962). Prognosis of mental subnormals. *American Journal of Mental Deficiency* (Monograph Supplement).

Winitz, H. (1983). Use and abuse of the developmental approach. In H. Winitz (Ed.), *Treating language disorders.* Baltimore: University Park Press.

Wolf-Schein, E., Sudhalter, V., Cohen, I., Fisch, G., Hansen, D., Pfadt, A., Hagerman, R., Jenkins, E., & Brown, W. (1987). Speech-language and Fragile X syndrome. *ASHA, 29,* 35–38.

Wolfensberger, W. (1967). Counseling the parents of the retarded. In A. Baumeister (Ed.), *Mental retardation: Appraisal, education, and rehabilitation.* Chicago: Aldine.

Wolfensberger, W., Mein, R., & O'Connor, N. (1963). A study of the oral vocabularies of severely subnormal patients: III. Core vocabulary, verbosity and repetitiousness. *Journal of Mental Deficiency Research, 7,* 38–45.

Wolff, P., Gardner, J., Lappen, J., Paccia, J., & Meryash, D. (1988). Variable expression of the Fragile X syndrome in heterozygous females of normal intelligence. *American Journal of Medical Genetics, 30,* 213–225.

Woodward, M., & Stern, D. (1963). Developmental patterns of severely subnormal children. *British Journal of Educational Psychology, 33,* 10–21.

Wulbert, M., Inglis, S., Kreigsmann, E., & Mills, B. (1975). Language delay and associated mother-child interactions. *Developmental Psychology, 11,* 61–70.

Wulz, S., Hall, M., & Klein, M. (1983). A home-centered instructional communication strategy for severely handicapped children. *Journal of Speech and Hearing Disorders, 48,* 2–10.

Yoder, D., & Miller, J. (1972). What we may know and what we can do: Input toward a system. In J. McLean, D. Yoder, & R. Schiefelbusch (Eds.), *Language intervention with the retarded.* Baltimore: University Park Press.

Yoder, P. J., & Davies, B. (1992). Do children with developmental delays use more frequent and diverse language in verbal routines? *American Journal on Mental Retardation, 97,* 197–208.

Yoder, P. J. & Feagans, L. (1988). Mothers' attributions of communication to prelinguistic behavior of developmentally delayed and mentally retarded children. *American Journal on Mental Retardation, 93,* 36–43.

Zeaman, D., & House, B. (1963). The role of attention in retardate discrimination learning. In N. Ellis (Ed.), *Handbook of mental deficiency.* New York: McGraw-Hill.

Zeaman, D., & House, B. (1979). A review of attention theory. In N. Ellis (Ed.), *Handbook of mental deficiency: Psychological theory and research.* Hillsdale, NJ: Lawrence Erlbaum Associates.

Zetlin, A., & Gallimore, R. (1983). The development of comprehension strategies through the regulatory function of teacher questions. *Education and Training of Mentally Retarded, 18,* 176–183.

Zigler, E. (1967). Mental retardation technical comment. *Science, 157,* 578.

Zigler, E. (1971). The retarded person as a whole person. In H. Adams & W. Boardman (Eds.), *Advances in experimental clinical psychology.* New York: Pergamon.

Autism Spectrum Disorders

Ellenmorris
Tiegerman-Farber
Adelphi University

Learning to Communicate

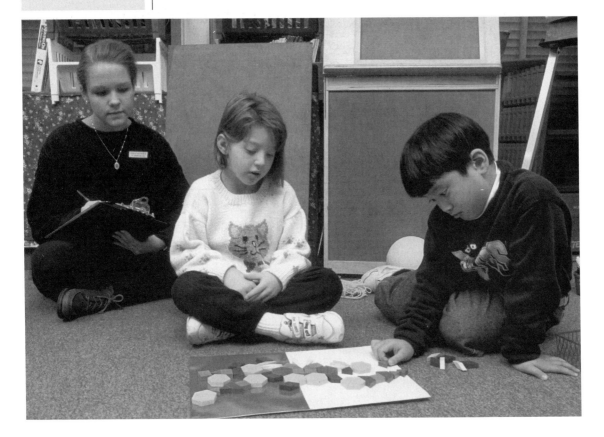

- Identify theoretical and etiological perceptions of the underlying cause(s) of autism spectrum disorders (ASD)
- Understand therapeutic programming provided for children with autism
- Discuss the setting(s) within which children with autism are educated and the reality of inclusion
- Discuss the changing role of the speech-language pathologist in serving children with autism across multiple settings
- Discuss the changing role of the parent as a primary teacher for the child with autism spectrum disorders
- List our expectations of how the individual with autism can function within society
- Understand the relationship between autism and language acquisition theory

Each child with autism has unique learning needs. Just as there are differences in normal language learners, so too are there individual differences in children with language disorders. It is unrealistic, therefore, to view children with autism spectrum disorders (ASD) as a homogenous population. Children with autism spectrum disorders present language, cognitive, communicative, behavioral, and social learning problems. Autism spectrum disorders include five disorders that share varying degrees of deficit across three domain areas: social, communication, and behavioral functioning. The disorders are autism, Rett's disorder, childhood disintegrative disorder (CDD), Asperger syndrome, and pervasive developmental disorder (PDD) (Shriver, Allen, & Mathews, 1999).

Kanner (1943) was the first to describe children with autism as being a distinct category. Since that time, autism has been the subject of much clinical investigation and research, yet the nature of its causes, manifestations, and treatment remains in dispute. Kanner defined the cause as an innate inability to form biologically affective contact with people. He attributed this inability to an emotional deprivation resulting from rigidity of the parents, who were characterized by obsessive meticulousness and intellectualization. Controlled studies have failed to demonstrate significant differences in parental psychopathology and early mother–child interaction between groups of children with and without psychotic brain damage. For a long time, the psychoanalytic view that the mother–child relationship was the cause of autism was widely accepted; however, support for that view has gradually declined as newer research has uncovered evidence of an organic basis for the disorder.

Greenspan and Wieder (1997) proposed that the symptoms that characterize autism spectrum disorders may be due to an underlying neuropsychological dysfunction in the connection between affect (or intent) and the sequencing of motor patterns and verbal symbols. Autism spectrum disorders, which include a range of affective and communicative disorders from more (autism) to less (pervasive developmental disorder) severe, have been increasing, from 1 in 2,500 to 1 in 500 in the last decade (Gillberg, 1990). Presently, the criteria described by Kanner (1943) have been more broadly defined to include degrees of dysfunction in reciprocal interaction, relating, and symbolic communication in the Diagnostic and Statistical Manual of Mental Disorders (DSM-IV) published by the American Psychiatric Association (APA).

One related issue involves how children are classified with developmental disabilities. Within the medical model, the underlying cause for a disorder is considered of primary importance. Historically, this point of view has carried over to the public school domain. As a result, many children with disabilities are assigned to educational placements based on etiological labels (mental retardation, autism, neurological impairment, etc.). Certainly there are advantages and disadvantages to both the etiological and the nonetiological models. One advantage of a nonetiological approach to disorders in the schools might be the classification of children by characteristics such as communication and language behaviors, the approach described in this chapter. The identification of language/communication deficits provides critical information about the unique educational needs of children with autism spectrum disorders. What information is provided by a label?

A discussion of autism research, more than research concerning any other population within the educational system, reveals the many theoretical and therapeutic changes that have occurred recently in the area of child language acquisition. In addition, it is my theoretical position that children with autism are severely language-disordered learners, rather than behaviorally impaired children. It should also be noted that the language learning characteristics of children with autism are also evident in the language patterns of other language-disordered children. To the extent that the language needs are the same, children with autism should be educated in the same manner as other children with language and communication disorders (LCD). As the chapters in this part are studied, it is important to compare the language/communication characteristics across children with different educational labels. Does the use of educational labels provide as much information?

ETIOLOGY: CENTRAL LANGUAGE DISORDER

Specific theories relating to the cause of ASD have been proposed but not proven (Wing, 1997). The range of etiological views of autism extends from a psychoanalytic perspective of the parent–child relationship to neurological, genetic, and biochemical causes. Bettelheim, in *The Empty Fortress* (1967), also proposed a psychological model. He suggested that the mother does not produce autism, but, rather, that autism is the child's reaction to her attitudes. The child with autism fears maternal destruction and rejects his mother. The child retreats within himself even further, and reality becomes so fearful that inactivity is the only available response; autism develops. The symptoms of autism have been attributed to problems with early interpersonal relationships, motivation, and emotionality resulting in a diagnosis of emotional disturbance.

About 75 percent of the children with autism have IQs in the severely retarded range; as a result, mental retardation is often associated with this disorder. Wetherby and Gaines (1982), however, did not observe the similarity in levels of cognitive and linguistic ability that is typical in children with mental retardation. In the children with autism, cognitive abilities exceeded linguistic abilities in several areas. The authors suggested that the relationship between cognition and language is dynamic rather than static; the interdependence varies over time with development. Whereas cognitive development may be necessary for intentional communication, "cognitive development may not be sufficient for more advanced language development" (p. 69).

Loveland, Landry, Hughes, Hall, and McEvoy (1988) described autism as a pervasive developmental disorder characterized by severe deficits in language, cognition, and social development. The language of children with autism is severely delayed and is often described as disordered. In many cases, functional language does not develop at all. Verbal language, when it does develop, is usually rigid, ritualistic, and stereotypical. Children with autism develop verbal routines that rarely change in form and are used over and over again in a variety of related and somewhat related contexts. Even though the language and gestures of children with autism are pragmatically deficient, they can be communicative despite the use of unconventional forms. Loveland and colleagues showed that, when compared to children of similar mental age and language level, children with autism present a different pattern of use of gesture and language. Children with autism produce fewer communicative acts than children with language delays. In addition, the children with autism showed some performance heterogeneity in their ability to produce communicative acts and to produce acts that served a range of interactive functions. The researchers suggested that although children with autism have difficulties initiating interaction, they seem to have less difficulty responding to the directions of another communicator. Their data support the idea that children with autism are relatively poor at engaging another person's attention or introducing a topic or taking turns in an interaction. The authors hypothesized, "The ability to initiate communication is closely tied to underlying social-pragmatic skills that are impaired in autism." In the child with autism who is learning language, the degree of communication initiation may reflect the degree of social-pragmatic impairment. Children with autism in the study had a lower level of pragmatic abilities than normally developing 2-year-olds. Language level, mental age, and IQ could not account for the children's pragmatic interactional deficits. The researchers concluded that there is an asynchrony in development between content areas (pragmatic and semantic) and structural areas (syntax and phonology). The language development of children with autism spectrum disorders follows a sequence that is quite different from that of other children with disabilities.

Along with the discussions of underlying central language disorder and heterogeneity of language characteristics in children with autism is their relationship to children with specific language impairment (SLI). Miller (1996) noted that SLI is not a static but a dynamic condition that evolves with developmental time. Although the patterns of strengths and weaknesses change as a function of intervention, there are only a limited number of profiles of language strengths and weaknesses in children with SLI. Conti-Ramsden and Botting (1999) noted in their investigation of children with specific language impairment that the profiles of difficulties in language impairment are stable even though individual children may be moving across subgroups. "When changes occurred and children moved to a different subgroup, the profiles of such children became similar to the profiles of the children belonging to a different group . . . children's profiles of difficulties continued to fall into a limited number of patterns already observed" (p. 8). Since children with SLI seem to fall into distinct subgroups, what are the implications for children with autism who also have language disorders? If the same classification system used to describe children with SLI can be applied to children with autism spectrum disorders, then would the system also be reliable over time for children with autism? Do children with autism spectrum disorders present a different pattern of language changes than children with SLI?

Related Factors

Four factors have contributed to the changing ways in which children with autism spectrum disorders have been viewed in the past several years. First, the Autism Society of America has heightened society's awareness of the needs of children with autism. This awareness has affected the direction of legislation in state and federal funding of educational programs. Second, Public Laws 94-142 and 99-457 have had profound implications for the development of curricula, due to the mandate that children with disabilities be educated in the least restrictive environment (LRE). As a result, there have been increasing funds available for the development of educational programs for children with autism spectrum disorders in early intervention programs and in public school settings. Third, recent developments in research have suggested neurological differences in processing (visual, auditory, linguistic, and cognitive) between children with autism spectrum disorders and other populations of children (Bailey, Phillips, & Rutter, 1996). Neurological differences suggest an etiological explanation other than emotional disturbance; specifically, that the underlying cause for the disorder relates to perceptual, cognitive, and information-processing differences. These characteristic differences result in language patterns that develop differently.

Gilger (1995) suggested that behavioral genetic research can be applied to language sciences. Since SLI shares some characteristics with autism, are the disorders genetically related? Although it is still unclear whether specific aspects of language are inherited and species-wide regardless of environmental variations, questions are being raised about genetic etiology for autism spectrum disorders. Folstein and Mankoski (2000) stated that the evidence from twin and family studies indicated that both autism and SLI are believed to be genetically mediated. "Not only are there more than the expected number of families who have children with both disorders, but there are some cases in which the features of both autism and SLI overlap." Other studies demonstrated the familiality of speech and language problems (Bishop, North, & Donlan, 1995; Lewis, Cox, & Byard, 1993). "In studies where families were selected through an individual with language impairment (i.e., the proband), an overage of approximately 20% to 50% of the first degree relatives of the proband also exhibited or reported a history for speech and language difficulties . . . clearly above expectations for the normal population (i.e., 2% to 7%). Brothers and sisters of language impaired probands were, respectively, 30 and 16 times more likely to have language problems than siblings of control probands" (Gilger, 1995, p. 14). The fourth and final factor involves the recent research in child language development. The changing perspectives in language theory and therapy have affected the view that the communication and language deficits in children with autism are of critical importance, suggesting that pragmatic/semantic deficits may serve to explain behavioral problems. The interplay among these factors has resulted in the progressive attempt to develop language and educational programs for children with autism spectrum disorders in more natural environments.

Since the goal of this chapter is to describe children with autism spectrum disorders in terms of characteristic behaviors, many aspects of developmental learning are presented: language, cognition, play, social interaction, and so forth. These characteristics provide a comprehensive picture of the child with autism spectrum disorders as one who has a language/communication disorder. The chapter also provides comparisons between children with autism and children with typical language development.

BEHAVIORAL CHARACTERISTICS

The population of individuals with autism spectrum disorders is heterogeneous. Children vary in the number and severity of characteristics exhibited, so, for the sake of description, all of the characteristics presented in this chapter are discussed in terms of Adam, who has been diagnosed as a preschool child with autism. As children exhibit fewer of the characteristics, they may be classified as having pervasive developmental disability (PDD). Children with very mild autism, recently called Asperger syndrome, have normal structural language but are highly rigid behaviorally and socially. Some of these characteristics will be discussed more fully in later sections dealing with communication and language.

Gaze Aversion

Bornstein and Brown (1996) described the development of attention in early infancy. Between 3 and 5 months after birth, infant attention patterns show stability. Whether the explanations are attributed to endogenous aspects within the child, such as perceptual acumen or persistent temperament style, or exogenous influences such as maternal responsiveness, attention behavior serves a critical communication function in child language development. Looking or gaze behavior serves as a signal to the adult that the child is ready to engage in interaction. In a similar fashion, when the child looks away or averts his gaze, the child communicates that the interaction has been terminated. Gaze interaction becomes one of the earliest dyadic means of communicative exchange between mother and child. In addition, the mother functions as a continuously gazing listener who is "turned on and off" by the infant. Later on, linguistic forms are mapped onto this early conversational exchange with the eyes. This earliest of communicative dialogues does not seem to occur or progress in children with autism. The clinical data needed at 3 to 6 months would require early identification of diagnostically significant atypical gaze patterns in infants.

Perhaps the most salient characteristic of autism is the lack of eye contact with other people during the communication exchange process. This characteristic more than any other has resulted in children with autism being described as aloof, distant, withdrawn, and nonrelating. Children with autism do not look at or facially orient their gaze toward another person; they avert their eyes when someone talks to them.

In fact, attempts by a communication partner to get the child to look are met with physical resistance, particularly when that person is physically near the child. As children with autism move farther away from another person, they exhibit a greater number of gazes oriented to that person. Another difference concerns the physical orientation of the child. Unless one is sneaking a look, the bodies of both speaker and listener are normally lined up shoulder to shoulder. Children with autism turn their entire body (and head) away from the speaker and emit infrequent, fleeting gazes from the corners of their eyes.

Consider Adam's gaze pattern during an interactional exchange. Even after having been trained to look at the speaker, Adam would change the orientation of his body. The more he focused on the speaker facially, the more of his body was turned away. When the speech-language pathologist (SLP) held his head so that face-to-face interaction could take place, his eyes shifted from corner to corner (side to side).

Ritualistic Behavior

Rituals are a normal part of the daily routines and patterns of life for most children and adults. There are, however, differences between the rituals exhibited by typical children (Jeremy) and children with autism. For the child with autism, the ritual is a sequence or pattern of behavior that must be exhibited in the same way and in the same order; there is little room for change. The chair must be placed just so in the living room. The child can only drink from the Snoopy cup. When there is a change in the environment, children spin records, twirl wires, bang objects, and turn lights on and off incessantly. They do not manipulate objects appropriately in a functional way; often an object manipulation (twirling the telephone wire) is repeated for hours. There are also rituals in which the child rocks back and forth in a corner. These repetitive behaviors are frequently referred to as self-stimulatory behaviors. They are presumably the child's attempt to maintain sameness or to get attention. Let us consider several rituals:

- *Jeremy's ritual:* Take bottles and Binkies (pacifiers) upstairs. Put bottles and Binkies in bed. Put Superdog in bed. Cover Superdog. Give Superdog his bottle. Give Superdog his Binky. Jeremy drinks bottle. Jeremy takes his own Binky (ritual pattern exhibited every night).
- *Ellenmorris's ritual:* "Hi, Adam. Come on, let's go play." Offers hand to Adam. Walk hand-in-hand to therapy room (ritual pattern exhibited before every therapy session).

What are the differences between normal ritual patterns and those that characterize autism? First, with a child who is developing normally, the ritual pattern represents only a small part of the child's performance or interaction repertoire. Because children with autism have very restricted performance repertoires, their ritual patterns constitute a much larger proportion. Children with autism develop many ritualized patterns of behavior. "Everything becomes a ritual," noted Adam's mother.

The second difference is that it is very difficult to change the ritualized patterns in the child with autism. Any minute change in a ritual can result in a catastrophic reaction from the child. Many parents note that the resulting violent temper tantrums are so aversive that they hesitate to, and often do not, change environmental sequences or events. Jeremy might balk a bit if something were performed differently or left out of his nightly sequence (e.g., not giving Superdog his Binky), but the result would not be a catastrophic reaction.

The third difference is that ritualized patterns, referred to as adultomorphisms by Piaget (1962), are indicative of a child's relational knowledge of experiences and events within his environment. The child's ritualized patterns show progressive and developmental changes; they incorporate the child's changing perceptions and conceptions of the world. Therefore, for the typically developing child, the ritual indicates an attempt to integrate and synthesize observed environmental sequences. For the child with autism, however, the ritualized pattern represents an attempt to maintain a systematic order within the environment.

Temper Tantrums

There are responses to the natural environment that develop and maintain ritualized patterns. Let us reconsider Ellenmorris's ritual, described previously, with regard to temper tantrums.

- *Ellenmorris's ritual:* One afternoon, therapy was running late. Because I was getting ready to see Adam, a graduate student volunteered to meet Adam in the waiting room of the Speech and Hearing Center. A few minutes later, Adam was wildly screaming in the hall. I walked into the hall to see Adam pounding the sides of his head with his fists. The therapy session was, to say the least, difficult. Before Adam's mother left, she was asked if anything had happened on the way to the center, and if Adam were feeling all right. She said that he was perfectly all right until the graduate student had met him in the waiting room.

For the two years that Adam had been enrolled at the Speech and Hearing Center, I had gone to the waiting room to bring him to the therapy room. In essence, a ritualized pattern had developed. As a result of this experience, my clinical staff attempted to identify the existence of other ritual patterns in their interactions with Adam. The purpose of the investigation was to modify the staff's and the child's patterns of ritualized interaction. Adam's response (a temper tantrum) was typical of how children with autism react to attempts to introduce change into their world. The temper tantrum is the autistic child's catastrophic reaction to change (Shriver, Allen, & Mathews, 1999a).

Temper tantrums can be either self-abusive or aggressive in form. Self-abusive and aggressive behaviors exhibited by children can include any of the following: pulling hair, biting, scratching, head banging, pinching, head butting, and so on. The difference between self-abusive and aggressive behaviors is the direction of the behavior—toward self or toward others. One of the difficulties related to temper tantrums is the intensity of the child's reaction to even a slight environmental change; a minute change in a ritual can result in a violent outburst. Children with autism can become physically uncontrollable; obviously, the older and the bigger the child gets, the harder it is for a parent or a teacher to manage such behaviors (Kobayashi & Murata, 1998).

Self-Stimulatory Behavior

Self-stimulation includes high-frequency behaviors that have been traditionally described as noncommunicative and noninteractional. They are often emitted when the child seeks to withdraw from the environment. This withdrawal pattern occurs when the child with autism cannot cope with direct input from teaching or instruction. Self-stimulatory behaviors are non-progressive. They interfere with the child's learning, especially in the classroom. What should the speech-language pathologist or teacher do about these behaviors? Behavioral approaches to training have proposed eliminating or decreasing the frequency of self-stimulatory behaviors by means of aversive consequences. However, the child's repertoire includes so many self-stimulatory behaviors that eliminating them would leave very few emitted behaviors.

Hypo- versus Hypersensitivity to Stimuli

Children with autism do not indicate the same response threshold to environmental stimuli as other children with and without disabilities. A reduced sensitivity to stimuli is called hyposensitivity. Adam's mother would say, "I could clap a pair of cymbals next to my child's ears and he would not blink." Children with autism do not react to, or seem in any way to recognize, sounds and environmental stimuli consistently. It is not surprising that many children at some point in their history have been identified as hearing impaired or deaf. Many parents describe the autistic child as being "here and there." Whenever Adam was responsive during a therapy session, his mother would say, "He's come in for a landing." The child's inconsistent responding is complicated by his inconsistent and often extreme reaction to even the slightest change in input. Heightened or excessive sensitivity to stimuli is called hypersensitivity. Adam would place his hands over his ears and eyes to block out input. The inconsistency in responding, with the ever-present possibility of a catastrophic temper tantrum, reduces the child's behavior (i.e., determining how he is going to react) to a guessing game for parents, speech-language pathologists, and teachers.

Mutism

Mutism includes a range of behavior, from periods of total silence to the production of meaningless sounds (i.e., used for self-stimulatory rather than communicative purposes). Most, if not all, children with autism progress through a period of mutism. Some autistic children remain mute all their lives. Hurford (1991) posited that there is a critical period for language acquisition. The clinical and developmental concern is that if a functional language system is not acquired by 5 years of age, there is little probability of it developing thereafter. Often, when the child becomes verbal, his initial words or phrases are quite intelligible. There seems to be a quantum leap or change in the child's performance that cannot as yet be explained. The child with autism does not evidence the progressive developmental changes in pragmatics, phonology, semantics, and syntax during the first 36 months that are seen in the typically developing child. Most of the information accumulated about this period of time comes from parent interviews. Parents provide critical information about the child's behavior and skills in natural settings with adults and peers that may not be directly observable by the speech-language pathologist, teacher, or psychologist. Parents can also provide information on developmental history because the age of onset is an important diagnostic factor. The child's medical history may assist in ruling out other developmental disabilities such as traumatic brain injury, deafness, cerebral palsy (Shriver, Allen, & Mathews, 1999b). Researchers are not sure why some children progress to the next stage—echolalic behavior—and some do not; nor is there agreement about the prerequisite changes within the child that result in transition to the next stage. For example, Adam's developmental history represents a dramatic and unexplainable change from one stage to another. Mute until the age of 4 years 3 months, Adam produced only meaningless grunts. When he started to speak, his productions were long, imitated utterances, such as "Open door please" and "Time go home now." His productions were, as his mother described, "as clear as a bell." It is important to note that during this phase, many SLPs and parents discuss the use of alternative systems of communication (see the section on alternative therapies). In Adam's case, a sign language system was introduced and used for many months quite successfully. Adam did acquire a core lexicon of signs, which he used appropriately to communicate his basic needs.

In Adam's case, the transition from the use of sign language to oral language forms was difficult to explain. The end result of this mute period was echolalic behavior. Adam's "eureka" experience—as his mother called it—occurred one day when he came to language therapy producing (very clearly) a verbal label in place of a learned sign. In the next 4 weeks, he replaced his sign productions with verbal productions. Sign training seems to have facilitated Adam's development of verbal production. Once a sign was replaced with a verbal production, the sign was never used again. His communication system, therefore, consisted of several forms: words, sign forms, and interchangeable sign/verbal forms. These interchangeable forms indicated a transition—a replacement of sign by word. Use of each new word form increased as use of the sign decreased. This replacement process emphasizes that, like a learner with a typical development, Adam indicated a systematic learning pattern. Perhaps the pattern represented an unique or idiosyncratic pattern of learning, but it was a pattern nonetheless, and when identified, provided some insight into how Adam learned.

Some children with autism never develop speech or language. The incidence of muteness ranges from 28 percent (Lotter, 1967) to 61 percent (Fish, Shapiro, & Campbell, 1966), the variability being a function of the difficulties with terminology and the issues discussed at the beginning of this chapter. Bartak and Rutter (1976) found that approximately 80 percent of all children with autism spectrum disorders were misdiagnosed as deaf at one time in their developmental history. DeMyer, Barton, DeMyer, Norton, Allen, and Steele (1973) noted that about 65 percent of the children who were mute at age 5 were still mute several years later. A large proportion of children with autism never develop conventional communicative and/or linguistic interactions within the environment. Why do so many children with autism remain nonverbal?

Echolalia

Echolalia has been defined traditionally as the meaningless repetition of someone else's words. As a result, some researchers have advocated that the behavior should be eliminated or decreased through therapy. Echolalia also has been described traditionally as a transition period between muteness and the evidence of linguistic knowledge, but research on children's progress through the various learning stages is limited. Is the child's imitation meaningless? If not, what function does it serve? Prizant and Duchan (1981) noted that, to determine what echolalic utterances mean, one must analyze them within a natural communicative environment. It is important to understand how the child functions within the communicative context—specifically, how children with autism use whatever behavior they have developed for the purpose of communication. In order to determine the communicative intent of the child's message, the SLP and parent must analyze the communicative context within which the utterance occurs. In such cases, eliminating echolalia would actually decrease the occurrence of communicative behavior. It thus becomes important to determine if the echolalic form represents the child's communicative intention. The following interactions illustrate that Adam's dramatic jump to an echolalic period revealed the need to assess the child's meaning within context. The examples indicate how this child manipulated various linguistic and nonlinguistic behaviors to convey communicative intentions. Adam's mother was, to say the least, thrilled when her son started to "talk"; however, her exuberance quickly wore away. She described Adam as her "talking shadow." A typical exchange between mother and child is presented to highlight the difficulty, confusion, and frustration in an exchange with a child who is echolalic.

> *Mother:*   Adam, are you ready?
>
> *Adam:*   Adam, are you ready?
>
> *Mother:*   Go open the door.
>
> *Adam:*   Go open the door.
>
> *Mother:*   Where is your coat?
>
> *Adam:*   Your coat.

To determine if Adam's imitations were meaningful, several aspects of his behavior could be analyzed within the context. For example, let us analyze the following exchange:

> *Mother:*   Go open the door.
>
> *Adam:*   Go open the door.
>
> *Nonverbal behavior:*   Adam looks at the door, then gets up and opens it.

Adam indicated by means of his behavior that, although he echoed his mother's production, he understood the meaning of her message and its related action. The nonverbal behavior (i.e., gaze behavior, gestures, and actions) of children with autism provides an indication of their understanding of the linguistic message and whether their echoic utterance was meaningful (Tiegerman-Farber & Radziewicz, 1998).

> *Mother:*   Where is your coat?
>
> *Adam:*   Your coat.
>
> *Nonverbal behavior:*   Adam looks at the coat, then goes to pull on the coat, which is lying across a chair.

In the second interchange, Adam's nonverbal behavior indicated his interpretation of the context. The interchange gives us additional information as well. First, the linguistic form of Adam's production was slightly different from that of his mother's utterance. Second, his intonation pattern, which was different from his mother's (upward inflection), indicated his ability to make changes in suprasegmental features. Third, he exhibited nonverbal behaviors that signaled he understood his mother's message. This interchange indicates several ways in which the child with autism can manipulate some of the components of the language process. These interchanges indicate how the form and function of the child's communicative behavior can be analyzed within the ongoing natural context (Tiegerman-Farber & Radziewicz, 1998). But many questions about the echolalic period still remain unanswered: Does the echolalic period incorporate several progressive stages? Does echolalic behavior change structurally and/or functionally over time? Does the echolalic period contribute to language and communication development in the child with autism?

Prizant and Wetherby (1987) proposed that, ordinarily, intentionality must combine with conventionality to develop communication. A close analysis of communicative intent might highlight the social and communicative functions in children with autism. Although they may not use conventional forms such as pointing or showing, children with autism may use idiosyncratic behaviors such as echolalia and self-stimulation to signal various communicative functions. One cannot assume that because the child with autism does not use conventional forms of communication, he cannot communicate. This position is as inappropriate as the one that assumes that the child's use of conventional forms reflects an intention to communicate. The meaning of the child's interaction can be determined only by analyzing the child's behavior within a social context. Such analysis of a child's unconventional communicative forms and functions requires multiple observations across different contexts; the ultimate challenge is to determine if the unconventional forms actually express communicative intentions.

Prizant and Rydell (1984) investigated the functions of delayed echolalia in children with autism. In delayed echolalia, children repeat utterances long after they originally heard them. The authors noted that "echolalic behaviors, both immediate and delayed, are best described as a continuum of behaviors in regard to exactness of repetition, degree of comprehension, and underlying communicative intent" (p. 183). Delayed echolalia has also been referred to as old forms applied to new situations. The use of echolalia as a form of communication is an unusual strategy in the typically developing child, but it serves several important functions in a child with autism. The fact that the child with autism uses old forms in new contexts indicates that on some associative level he establishes a relationship between a linguistic form (as rigid as it is) and an event. That is, the production of a delayed echolalic response indicates that the child perceived a relationship between a verbal utterance and a context. As the child's linguistic abilities increase, he is able to substitute, delete, and/or conjoin elements in the echoed response (delayed mitigated echolalia).

In addition, the child's unique ability to imitate sophisticated linguistic sentences and paragraphs verbally is often quite deceptive in terms of the child's actual spontaneous ability. In the Prizant and Rydell (1984) study, a production was considered a delayed echolalic utterance if it satisfied one or both of the following criteria: (1) the repetition was beyond the child's syntactic abilities and (2) the utterance consisted of a rigid and routinized string. The children in the study showed a marked discrepancy between the mean length of utterance (MLU) for echolalic and spontaneous productions. Whereas the children's spontaneous productions were primarily at a Phase 1 level of linguistic complexity, the echolalic utterances represented a much more sophisticated linguistic ability.

Whether the child uses immediate or delayed echolalia, his productions are generated for interactive purposes. Echolalia is not a simplistic or unitary form; it represents a continuum of interaction and comprehension. The adult's interpretation of the echolalic utterance is going to be based on knowledge of the child and characteristics of their shared context. For the child with autism, the use of unconventional forms interferes with the development of language's conventional forms and higher-order metalinguistic abilities. One of the most interesting findings of the Prizant and Rydell (1984) study was that some of the noninteractive echolalic utterances—those produced without communicative intent by the child—did serve meaningful purposes. Although some of the utterances served no specific functions, others served cognitive and/or conversational or turn-taking functions. Echolalia has been described as a transitional phase of development that signals movement from (1) echolalia without communicative intent, to (2) echolalia with the intent but limited linguistic competence, to (3) echolalia with intent and linguistic ability. This developmental pattern of linguistic and comprehension changes is similar to the communicative sequence exhibited by the typical child as he learns language.

Emotional/Behavioral Deficits

The child's experiences within the environment with agents, actions, and objects are important to the language learning process. Bryson, Landry, and Smith (1994) noted that children with autism exhibit deficits in social cognition, relationships with people and objects. These object deficits manifest themselves in a limited toy-play repertoire, self-stimulatory behavior, bizarre manipulation behaviors, and nonprogressive play skills. The interpersonal deficits manifest themselves as a lack of gaze interaction, decreased physical interaction, and severe limitations in cooperative play and social interaction. Children with autism have difficulty relating to and interacting with their communicators—peers and adults in the natural environment. Many children with autism withdraw from the approach and touch of others and become rigid or stiff when held or cuddled. Considering that communication and social learning involve interactional exchanges with peers and adults in the environment, one should not be surprised by the fact that the child's behavior negatively affects the emotions of parents and peers (Tiegerman-Farber & Radzewicz, 1998). Interaction implies reciprocity; there must be some reaction or response from the child to his parents and siblings. When the child does not respond to or withdraws from the adult's initiations, what is the adult's reaction? Is it a feeling of rejection? Is it a feeling of frustration? Consider how Adam's mother and Jeremy described their interaction with Adam.

Adam's mother: It is difficult to get close to a child who always pushes you away. Interaction is totally nonreinforcing.

Jeremy: Him no like me.

Notice that Adam's lack of responsiveness negatively affected the communicative initiations of these two individuals. Children with autism need to learn about the social context, yet their behavior leads to further isolation and they are often described as aloof.

Lainhart (1999) indicated that children with autism may have problems of mood and thought. Parents and siblings of children with autism may also experience affective difficulties because of stress and anxiety related to caring for the child and/or because of biological factors. The inability to communicate and emotionally relate to family members results in the child being further isolated emotionally and socially from natural events and experiences. The relationship between language and behavior has recently received a great deal of attention given the increasing demand for behavioral programs and treatments (Lovaas & Buch, 1997). Some behavioral intervention programs emphasize the primacy of behavior by (1) defining language as just another form of behavior, (2) minimizing the complexity of the language learning process into "discrete observable trials," (3) underestimating the significance of the language/communication deficits in children with autism by overemphasizing behavioral deficits, and (4) developing behavioral programs rather than language learning programs (Tiegerman-Farber, 1995). "Behavioral intervention programs for children who are perceived as habitually noncompliant that use reward systems to shape compliance have made the implicit assumption the children's noncompliance was due to oppositional behaviors, negativity or rebelliousness. The fact that at least some of the children's noncompliance could be due to their inability to understand instructions or directions or to use language to appropriately seek clarifications has been given insufficient attention. The relationship between language and noncompliance needs to be more fully understood given the prevalence of language disorders among children identified as having emotional/behavioral problems" (Gallagher, 1997, p. 7). This position reflects the philosophical approach to ASD presented in this chapter.

The child with autism has pervasive language deficits limiting his ability to express his feelings, talk about his thoughts, solve interpersonal problems, interpret the emotional behaviors of other communicators and encode/decode interpersonal language (Bloomquist, August, Cohen, Doyle, & Everhart, 1997). Intrapersonal and interpersonal functioning are interrelated and language dependent. The limited emotional vocabulary negatively affects his abilities to control his emotions and regulate his own behaviors. The child's emotional/behavioral problems should be viewed as a function of his pragmatic and semantic language deficits. This is not a minor issue given the implications for treatment recommendations and programs. Brinton and Fujiki (1993) noted that emotional/behavioral problems have been viewed as obstacles to language intervention that needed to be addressed prior to the initiation of language training. The assumption that language problems will decrease if emotional/behavioral problems decrease has not been supported. Current studies emphasize the critical role language serves in facilitating emotional/behavioral functioning (Gallagher, 1996; Prizant, Audet, Burke, Hummel, Maher, & Theadore, 1990). Given this perspective of the emotional/behavioral needs of children with autism, the speech-language pathologist will play a significant role on the inter/transdisciplinary teams of professionals developing language programs for children with autism spectrum disorders. It may be time to rethink temper tantrums and self-stimulatory behaviors as indicative of the child's pragmatic/semantic problems. These behaviors are socially penalizing and serve specific communicative needs for the child. By identifying those needs, the SLP can then substitute communicative alternatives that are functionally equivalent but more socially appropriate (Gallagher, 1999).

Early Onset/Assessment

The onset of autism relates to a parent's awareness of a problem. The diagnosis of autism becomes difficult if parents and professionals do not have access to standardized assessment tools. Assessing a child that may have autism requires the evaluation of several areas: language/communication, cognition, motor, and social skills. Public Law 99-457, which established the early intervention system, emphasizes a family-oriented approach to assessment and treatment. Part of the process is a family assessment that identifies the needs of the entire family as an ecological unit to support the child (Tiegerman-Farber & Radziewicz, 1998). The following tests can be used by the inter/transdisciplinary team as part of an assessment protocol:

1. Childhood Autism Rating Scale (CARS; Schopler, Reichler, & Rennet, 1998). The CARS is composed of 15 four-point scales on which a child's behavior is rated on a continuum from within normal limits (1) to severely abnormal (4). The CARS is best used as a screening measure.
2. Autism Diagnostic Interview—Revised (ADI—R; Lord, Rutter, & LeCouteur, 1994). The ADI—R is described as a semistructured, investigative-based interview for caregivers of children and adults for whom autism or pervasive development disorders is a possible diagnosis.
3. Autism Behavior Checklist (ABC; Krug, Arick, & Almond, 1993). The ABC is a behavior-rating checklist that is used when interviewing parents and teachers. It is considered most effective to use in contexts with direct observations across multiple domains.
4. Psychoeducational Profile—Revised (PEP—R; Schopler, Reichler, Bashford, Lansing, & Marcus, 1990). The PEP—R provides information on developmental functions as well as degrees of abnormality in relating and affect, play and interest in materials, sensory responses and language. The PEP—R is designed for children 6 months to 7 years of age or children under 12 years of age with developmental delays.
5. Pre-Linguistic Autism Diagnostic Observation Schedule (PL-ADOS; DiLavore, Lord, & Rutter, 1995). The PL-ADOS is designed for children under 6 years of age and as a standardized observational measure in which the examiner interacts with the child in structured situations.

Some parents describe their early awareness of a problem during the infant's first months of life. They note that the infant "could not be comforted." The younger the infant, the more tenuous the determination of disorder, unless there are neurological signs of impairment. Generally, parents proceed through the frustrations of a diagnostic evaluation as their child approaches the second birthday. One of the most important diagnostic variables—language—is often difficult to assess by standardized means before 24 months. It has only been within the past few years that early identification, focusing on the child between 2 and 3 years of age, resulted in intervention. Educational options are still rather limited for the preschool child with autism (Wagner & Lockwood, 1994).

According to Short and Schopler (1988), the onset of autism before age 30 months has been a central criterion in the differential diagnosis of autism. Their study indicated that in 76 percent of the autism cases, parents identified a problem before their child was 24 months of age. In 94 percent of the cases, parents identified a problem before their child was 36 months old. Parents who recognized a problem earlier tended to seek help sooner. In addition, early onset also related to developmental severity, particularly in behavioral functioning. Children with later developmental onset scored significantly higher on IQ tests than the early-onset children, suggesting that these "later" cases were less severe in terms of symptomatology characteristic of ASD. The authors recommended the need for further research into the differential diagnosis of two distinct groups within the late-onset category: (1) children with autism who experience a developmental regression after 30 months of age and (2) children with autism who are identified at a much later developmental period because their symptomatology is relatively mild.

Behavioral Characteristics: A Means of Discriminating among Children?

The nine characteristics of autism described previously can be used to differentiate between and among children. Table 11.1 highlights some of the performance differences between Adam's and Bryan's interactions within the environment.

There are some obvious developmental differences between the two children that might reflect language and processing differences. These differences are typical of children within the population and highlight the fact that children with ASD have very individual interactional patterns and styles. Developmental differences in gaze interaction, joint attention, and orientation to speech suggest that children with autism can be identified as early as one year of age. In addition to behavioral characteristics, communication, play, and linguistic behaviors provide insights into the most critical variable in autism—language functioning. The inability to interact and to communicate imposes a restriction on learning about language as a social process. Communication, play, and linguistic behaviors provide a more holistic picture of the child's unique interactional style within a complex social environment as well as a means of identifying the disorder earlier (Osterling & Dawson, 1994).

Communication Behaviors

In the communication exchange between the adult and the child, the two are participants in an ongoing interactive event. A 30-month-old child with autism does not evidence many of the communication behaviors exhibited by a typically developing 6-month-old. The child with autism does not exhibit the typical developmental progression in gaze, vocal, and gestural communication behaviors or the ability to coordinate these behaviors into complex patterns and sequences. Often parents are not aware that the child has autism until after infancy (between 18 and 36 months). By

TABLE 11.1	**A Comparison of Behavioral Performances**	

Behavior	Adam (40 months)	Bryan (40 months)
Gaze aversion	Gaze aversion	Gaze aversion, but does track a moving object
Imitation	Lack of motor and vocal imitation	Lack of vocal imitation, limited motor imitation
Ritualistic behavior	Feeding, dressing, and washing rituals	Constantly rearranging furniture in the room (and house)
Self-stimulatory behaviors	Walks on toes, flaps hands, rocks back and forth, makes grunting/guttural noises	Spins, opens and closes eyes rapidly, sticks finger down throat
Object performances	Nonfunctional and undifferentiated performances; spins, shakes, mouths, and bangs toys	Basically nonfunctional and undifferentiated; spins, shakes, mouths, and bangs toys. Some appropriate object-related performances: picks up telephone receiver and makes noises into receiver, puts baby in bed, stacks rings on stick, can replace pieces in Simplex puzzle
Temper tantrums	Self-abusive behavior: head-banging, handbiting. Aggressive behavior: pulls hair and scratches	No self-abusive behavior. Aggressive behavior: bites, scratches, pinches, kicks, butts his head, pulls hair, punches
Speech	Mute	Echolalia
Relational behavior	Turns and moves away when approached, stiffens when touched	Approaches people (adults and children), requests hugs, kisses, and tickles
Onset	Mother noted that something was wrong at 3 months of age. Psychiatric evaluation and diagnosis at 24 months.	Mother states that child progressed "normally" until 12 months of age and then withdrew. Child's behavior deteriorated. Psychiatric evaluation and diagnosis at 30 months.

this time, it has become clear that the child has not developed early communication and linguistic behaviors. The information concerning behavioral and communication development before the time of diagnosis is subjective and a function of the parents' interpretation and memory of early experiences with the child—although parents are reliable reporters.

The fact that communication behaviors are not present at 30 months of age does not mean that the behaviors were not present earlier. It is possible that early communication behaviors did develop during the first 9 to 12 months but deteriorated due to neurological deficits. Current diagnostic tools are not adequate to identify the communication behaviors—gaze, vocalization, and gesture—that are critical to the early identification of ASD. Research analyses and investigations of infants who are not acquiring early communication behaviors may provide important insights into the appearance and progression of ASD. The expanding knowledge of developmental processes between birth and 12 months will eventually result in the identification and diagnosis of ASD in younger and younger children. The ability to understand disorder is tied inextricably to our understanding of normal development. For the identification of autism to occur in infants between birth and 12 months of age, selected gaze, vocal, and gestural behaviors must be identified as diagnostic indicators (Wagner & Lockwood, 1994).

Play

It is generally acknowledged that play is important to the development of adaptability, learning, cognition, and social behavior (Lifter, Sulzer-Azaroff, Anderson, & Cowdery, 1993). The function of play is to exercise and develop manipulative and interactional strategies that children will later integrate into more sophisticated task-oriented sequences. A more general theory suggests that, in play, children learn to affect and control activities they are unable to execute or dominate in other contexts. In play, children develop control over animate and inanimate objects or contexts. Recent analyses of early social interactions suggest that play behavior influences the physical and interactional behaviors of all children involved in the experience (Stahmer, 1995). Thus, play has a cognitive, social, and integrative function in early development.

The underlying theory proposes that play begins with action manipulations directed by the child. As manipulative and physical abilities expand, children develop an increasing capacity to deal with objects and peers more actively (Koegel & Koegel, 1995). Children with autism, however, are limited in their social interaction with the environment and, because of their restricted experiences, they share many behavioral/learning problems with other children, whether the specific diagnosis is mental retardation, cerebral palsy, or brain damage. Children with autism withdraw from interactional experiences and learn to manipulate by means of temper tantrums and disruptive behaviors. Withdrawal from the environment makes it difficult to determine if they do not know how to play, if they lack the opportunity to do so, or both. Many researchers have suggested that there is a cyclical relationship between the children's bizarre manipulative performances and their inability to integrate experiences within the environment, causing even further withdrawal. The child's creation of an inner world is an attempt to establish and maintain an internal order that he or she cannot establish in the outside world; self-stimulatory and ritualistic behaviors may be a result of socio-affective deficits (Ozonoff, Pennington, & Rogers, 1991).

Play is a natural means of teaching children with autism social interactional skills. Play is a child-directed rather than a teacher-directed activity. Play facilitates children's choices for materials, activities, and peer partners. Within a play setting, the child with autism learns that specific behaviors lead to responses from peers.

Communicative behaviors and interactional exchanges are more likely to be learned and used in social settings if they lead to naturally reinforcing consequences for children with autism (Olley, 1999). Functional and symbolic play skills are associated with language abilities. In addition, specific nonverbal communication skills such as gestures are also correlated with language acquisition. Social interactional skills can be facilitated by typical peers-integrated preschool programs. The integrated classroom relies on play activities that involve child-based preferences for objects, creative interactions, and peer partners. The early-childhood curriculum emphasizes independent play and social interaction in naturally occurring routines. Social skills can be facilitated in play and in groups rather than the 1:1 instruction methodology described by behavioral specialists such as Lovaas. The early-childhood curriculum becomes part of an inclusion training model that uses circle time, story time, and activity centers to facilitate the development of communication (Strain & Cordisco, 1994). The controversy related to inclusive programming is discussed later in the chapter.

LANGUAGE COMPONENTS

In describing autism as a language/communication disorder (LCD), several components of language will be discussed: pragmatics, semantics, syntax, phonology, and cognition. Studying the interrelationship among these components can provide insight into the unique learning needs of children with ASD. An asynchronous pattern of development has been described with semantic and syntactic components progressing independently from one another; a child may evidence (1) more advanced or complex semantic skills while his syntactic abilities remain severely limited, or (2) more advanced syntactic skills while his semantic abilities remain severely limited. This uneven developmental pattern across language components is linked to the structures and functions of neuropsychology and to the development of different language processes (Tager-Flusberg, 1999). Uneven development indicates that different areas within the central nervous system are more or less impaired, which determines the level of functioning and the language abilities developed within the child. Language represents an integrated system; every component contributes to the development of the whole system. To understand the learning needs of children with language disorders, particularly children with ASD, it is important to compare and contrast development within and across components. The language and communication deficits evidenced in children with autism spectrum disorders might be caused by:

1. Uneven developments within and/or across the components of the learning system
2. An inability to interface and/or exchange developmental information across the components of the system

SOCIAL COGNITION

The relationships among perception, language, and cognition remain rather controversial. Current trends have been influenced by cognitive theories that stress the importance of early social and interactional experiences within the environment. In discussing cognitive development in children with autism, it is important to consider perceptual and cognitive processes as well as social interactional experiences. Harris, Handleman, Gordon, Kristoff, & Fuentes (1991) studied changes in intellectual and language functioning in children with autism and normally developing peers over the course of a year. The results indicated that, relative to their typical preschool peers, the preschool children with autism showed a greater increase in intellectual progress in the program. The typical preschool children maintained their cognitive functioning across the school year, but the preschool children with autism showed a significant increase in functioning. The 19-point increase in IQ provides support for the effectiveness of early intervention programming and the ability of children with autism to benefit from comprehensive programming.

Approximately 75 percent of children with autism are reported to function within the mentally retarded range (American Psychiatric Association, 1994). Differential diagnosis is further complicated by the fact that children with severe or profound mental retardation may exhibit behaviors similar to children with autism. Children with mental retardation exhibit quantitative delays in social interaction, communication, and behavior that are commensurate with their developmental level. In contrast, children with autism present qualitative differences in functioning that are not typically exhibited by other children with language delays. In addition, children with autism demonstrate a wide variability of skills. Sometimes the skill differences (i.e., splinter skills or savant abilities) result in exceptional abilities in one area while presenting significant deficits in other areas. Adam, for example, had excellent memory and rote recall. His ability, however, should be viewed in terms of his use of the skill within the social context. His remarkable recall was often used for noncommunicative and self-stimulatory purposes. Information was frequently extracted as a whole and not used for interactional purposes. Adam would sit in a corner of his room and recite verbatim the news report presented the previous night.

Identifying strengths, skills, or abilities is only an initial step; it is important to determine how children with ASD use and apply their skills within the learning context (see hyperlexia and phonology). Children with autism display significantly higher abilities on tasks that require the discrimination of concrete visual spatial relations and significantly lower abilities on tasks that require abstraction or the ability to organize concrete information on the basis of subtle conceptual relationships between stimuli. They also present integration deficits when stimuli increase in complexity and/or require cross-modal processing. Their difficulties identifying what is meaningful and relevant in a situation results in the rigid use of rules when interacting with the environment. Conceptual development is further compromised by their tendency to attend to, or fixate on, one aspect of a picture or story, often some irrelevant minutiae (Shriver, Allen, & Mathews, 1999a). All of these examples serve to describe an idiosyncratic pattern of interaction within the environment.

Sigman and Ungerer (1984) discussed the early cognitive deficits specific to the syndrome of autism. Although sensorimotor skills and language were positively correlated in children without disabilities, they were unrelated in the children with autism. The authors suggested that sensorimotor knowledge may be necessary but not sufficient for language development. The marked discrepancy between sensorimotor abilities and language disabilities in children with autism provides support for the argument that sensorimotor and symbolic knowledge may involve divergent development. Several hypotheses may explain the variation in deficits. The first theoretical possibility is that representational thought may require the interface of two subsystems. One such subsystem involves the development of sensorimotor skills with the ability to recall information for problem solving. The second subsystem involves the ability to translate experiences into symbols; it is with this area that children with autism have difficulty; cognitive deficits in children with autism are secondary to social deficits. The researchers also noted that "all the areas of specific cognitive deficit identified to date depend on social interaction for their development" (p. 301). This finding highlights the significance of the social learning process to other areas of development. The social experience becomes the "field with developmental areas such as play, cognition, imitation, and language facilitated on this field" (p. 301).

PERCEPTION

Little is known about how children with autism perceive their environments. Assumptions are made on the basis of their patterns of interaction in the environment—that is, the way in which they relate to agents, actions, and object. The behavioral characteristics described previously provide some indication of the child's internal operations and the resulting reactions to the impinging world. What is it that the child with autism sees and hears? One can only infer, based on observed responses and reactions, the child's difficulties and confusions. The child's behavior suggests that very little of what he sees and hears makes sense. Words, voices, faces, and gestures are no more than rapidly changing stimuli, like changes in color that are transient and difficult to grasp. People handle the child and do things to him; what does it mean? All those faces and changing expressions; what do they mean? Few things are recognizable to the child since everything is always changing. That the world appears confusing to the child with autism is not surprising. Nor is it surprising that the child maintains a ritualized, ordered environment and, indeed, struggles to continue that order and sameness. Finally, when the environment impinges beyond the management point, the child fights back and throws tantrums, which are the result of frustration and confusion. The child tries to create an inner world that is more understandable and consistent (Tiegerman-Farber & Radziewicz, 1998). Self-stimulation can be seen as an attempt to reestablish sameness. Many parents indicate that their child exhibits self-stimulatory behaviors when exposed to a new situation or experience. The child's perceptual deficits create further problems because they severely limit his interactional experiences with peers and adults. The child who sees the world in a distorted manner interacts with the world in a distorted manner. This cycle does not permit the child to experience the multiplicity of interactions that are the building blocks of conceptual development (Tager-Flusberg, 1999).

GENERALIZATION

Children with autism also have difficulty in generalizing learned behaviors from one context to another. Because these children cannot identify the relevant information within the complexities of a situation, they cannot identify what is important and what is not, creating a further problem in establishing conceptual or perceptual relationships. The ability to establish categories of any kind depends on the ability to discriminate differences as well as to determine how stimuli are associated and related to one another. Perceptual deficits contribute to the failure to generalize learning and to develop strategies for adapting to continually changing social contingencies. Social rigidity limits their ability to adjust to changing social contingencies, and perseverative responses interfere with the development of problem-solving skills (Russell, Mauthner, Sharpe, & Tidswell, 1991; Prior & Hoffmann, 1990).

Deficits in generalization indicate a cognitive impairment in children, a problem that seriously limits the ability to learn spontaneously and to benefit from more structured and formalized learning. The inability to develop conceptual relationships, to extract and use similarities across situations and to learn from past experiences condemns children with autism to repeated learning experiences. Typical children search for rules; in order to establish rules, they identify relevant and related stimuli within conceptual categories. Generalization involves the ability to identify the relationship between situation A and situation B, and then to apply the rule to situations A′ and B′. Without rule-governed behavior, children have difficulty processing, categorizing, and interpreting social events (Tager-Flusberg, 1999).

LANGUAGE PROCESSING

The roots of representational behavior are based on the child's interactional experiences within the environment; it is therefore important to examine the interrelationship between cognitive and communicative functioning. Research now supports the view that the unique acquisition and use of language by children with autism results from a cognitive processing style that differs from that of typical children. Children with autism have often been described as "language chunkers." Prizant (1983) suggested that the characteristics of ritualistic behavior and echolalia indicate a gestalt processing style. As a result of this gestalt preference, children with autism produce whole phrases and sentences without understanding the individual linguistic elements. This also means that children can not manipulate the building blocks of language to combine and recombine linguistic structures creatively. Although the gestalt processing style occurs as a part of normal language development, it is integrated with an analytic processing strategy. Echolalia and routinized rituals are better described as characteristics that relate to cognitive-linguistic processing styles in the child with ASD rather than deviant characteristics. The interface between these two processing approaches provides typical language learners with a creativity and flexibility that children with autism do not indicate in their language productions. Because they use a gestalt style of language processing, children with autism do not learn to break down long memorized strings into elemental units of language. Language development, production, and creativity depend on an analytic style of processing that offsets the gestalt processing style. Without a working knowledge of the meaningful units of language, the child with autism can form only surface associations between long language chunks and contexts. Often the meaning relationship between the memorized chunk and the context is tangential. The discrepancy between form and function presents a serious strain on the communication process. The listener must attempt to derive the child's communicative intent based on what the listener thinks the child means.

Theory of Mind and Meta Abilities

The development of "theory of mind" involves the ability to represent mental states. Research indicates that typical children realize that the actions of other people are related to what they think and believe and not necessarily to factual occurrences. A child's ability to take the perspective of another person, to understand another's point of view, begins in early childhood. Theory of mind research in autism refers to the ability to attribute mental states such as desire, knowledge and belief to oneself and other people as a means of explaining behavior. Pennington, Rogers, Bennetto, Griffith, Reed, and Shyu (1998) described a shift in theoretical perspective concerning the underlying origin of autism as a deficit in metarepresentation. "Meta" skills—metacognitive and metalinguistic—require intact language production and comprehension abilities in children. The metas involve the abilities to revise, reflect, and repair language rules. Metalinguistic skills represent a higher conceptual understanding of production and comprehension skills. When the child can "talk about talking," he is aware of language structures and can make judgments about their appropriateness. Metacognitive skills involve the ability to deal abstractly with one's thought processes in comprehension, memory, information processing, reasoning, and problem solving. For the child with autism, pervasive deficits in social interaction, language production, and comprehension limit the development of the more abstract meta skills (Mundy, Sigman, & Kasari, 1994). The majority of children with autism (60 to 70 percent) present limited development in the metarepresentational area; a minority (20 to 30 percent) appear to develop to a level equivalent to 3- to 4-year-old typical children by the time they reach their teenage years.

Investigations related to research in the area of "theory of mind" may provide another explanation; they propose that the communication, socialization, and mental imagery deficits characteristic of autism may be attributable to the inability to symbolize and conceptualize mental states—what Baron-Cohen (1995, 1998) refers to as "mindblindness." For example, children with autism present conceptual difficulties in connected situations requiring judgments about joking, lying, persuasion, and pretense (Happe, 1994). Children with autism may also have difficulty developing the behavioral strategies involving disengagement of attention from focal objects. The results of the Hughes and Russell (1993) research indicated that subjects with autism failed a test of strategic deception because they had difficulty mentally disengaging from a focal object and not because they were unable to perform a "theory of mind" task. The ability to disengage attention from a focal object is one of many mental operations referred to as executive functions. These functions "are separately necessary and jointly sufficient for volitional goal directed behavior; inhibition of perceptually triggered or inappropriate responses; and monitoring the success and failure of current strategies." The researchers further suggested that the results achieved from the tests traditionally used to assess "theory of mind" may have been confounded by the executive difficulties exhibited in children with autism. The theory of mind deficit in autism is part of the broader deficit in higher-order cognitive processes (Russell, 1997).

Pragmatics

For children with autism, the use of language for communicative purposes remains severely impaired in spite of developments in other language areas. Part of the problem relates to the interrelationship between social interaction and communication. Most children with autism do not develop a range of communicative functions, and as a result their communicative and social interactions are limited. Whereas the social context facilitates learning in the typically developing child, this is the environment that presents the most difficulty for the child with autism, who removes himself from the very context which teaches him about communication. Given the child's severe communication deficits, the social situation becomes of primary importance for further learning (Ogletree & Fischer, 1995).

In addition, the few interactive behaviors exhibited by children with autism are often part of specific and unusual routines. As noted previously, the established routine allows children with autism to maintain some control within their rapidly changing environment. The routine establishes predictability by maintaining a contextual sameness. Although children with autism indicate a preference for building such routines, these ritualized patterns further restrict social interaction. This added social limitation serves to maintain the communication deficit. By responding to a limited range of behaviors, children with autism selectively reinforce certain aspects of the adult's input. The adult's problem is the child's limited interactional responsiveness and tolerance for change. Frequently, for the sake of interaction, the adult continues to provide a highly restricted form of communication. As a result, social interaction tends to be inflexible, ritualistic, and rigidly routinized. In turn, these limited social and interactional patterns further affect the following aspects of communication: (1) initiating and terminating interaction, (2) maintaining conversational topics, (3) functioning within speaker and listener roles, and (4) using behavior for the purpose of communication (Piven, Harper, Palmer, & Arndt, 1996).

In general, children with autism present the following pragmatic problems: (1) they do not develop a range of communicative functions, (2) they do not develop gaze interaction skills, (3) they do not develop prototypical behaviors such as protodeclaratives or protoimperatives, (4) they do not develop attention and joint action schemes, (5) they do not develop an awareness of agent, action, or object contingencies, (6) they do not develop turn-taking or reciprocal action skills, and (7) they do not develop gestures or imitation behaviors. Prelinguistic behaviors such as pointing, showing, or turn taking typically are not present and, as a result, the communicative behavior in children with ASD is different from the communicative behavior in typical children. In addition, the differential aspects of each child tend to promote different patterns of responding and contingencies for interaction in peers and adults within the child's environment (Folstein, 1999).

Bernard-Opitz (1982) demonstrated that communicative performance is related to specific variables within the communicative context. The author analyzed how a child with autism used language with his mother, his clinician, and a stranger. The child's communicative style was different with each communication partner. With his mother, the child initiated communication by using requests as the primary speech act, whereas with the clinician the child used statements to interact. The communicative interaction with the stranger resulted in unintelligible and noncommunicative utterances. In addition, the adults had a tendency to use requests as the predominant speech act during interaction with the child. The author suggested that the differences in the child's communicative behavior might have been related to his familiarity with the listener. Also, the child did not typically respond to the requests of the adults, but rather generated another request by imitating the adult's syntactic structure. Another interesting aspect was the difference between the mother's and the clinician's response to the child's echolalic behavior. The mother reinforced the echolalic pattern by answering or clarifying the child's behavior. The clinician's response to unrelated utterances was to introduce another topic, redirecting the discourse rather than responding directly to the child's utterance. The description of children with autism as noncommunicative and noninteractive is not supported. Even with a limited range of communicative behaviors within his repertoire, the child responded differently to different interactional partners. So it is not that a child with autism cannot interact, but rather that his range of communicative options is limited (Calloway, Myles, & Earles, 1999).

Another factor that interferes with the child's communicative effectiveness involves idiosyncratic behaviors. The typical language learner develops conventional behaviors to communicate his needs; the child with autism uses unconventional behaviors and/or linguistic forms. The result is that the social communicators in the child's environment may misinterpret and misunderstand the child's intentions and meaning. Communicative functions and exchanges, rather than specific linguistic forms or structures, should be facilitated in children with autism. Given the learning style of children with autism, linguistic forms are often acquired as routinized chunks. Historically, clinical and educational programs have focused on teaching specific linguistic structures or forms, the result being that children with autism learned to reproduce rigid or "frozen" strings without a semantic-syntactic understanding of these utterances. Schwartz and Carta (1996) suggested that programmatic and instructional goals should focus on teaching children with autism the process of interactional communication rather than teaching them responses to specific questions or forms.

Children with ASD are quite diverse in their range of communication and language deficits. As already noted, children with autism appear to use various strategies in an attempt to interact, even with a limited repertoire of conventional forms. In addition, they develop a more limited range of communicative functions than typical children. In the typically developing child, communication does not occur consecutively from one function to another; some functions emerge concurrently. Linguistic structures develop from communicative functions; typical children talk about the interactional context and their manipulative experiences. It is the social process that provides the basis for the development of conventional forms. The synchronous development of communicative functions evident in typical children appears as a nonsequential pattern in children with autism. This suggests that the communicative pattern developed by children with autism is qualitatively, as well as quantitatively, different from the normal prelinguistic sequence. Children with ASD acquire communicative functions in a different developmental sequence, and as a result their linguistic abilities develop differently (Calloway et al., 1999). The following communicative characteristics describe the child with autism:

1. Communicative intent in gestural and vocal areas develops asynchronously.
2. The communicative profile is different from profiles in other children with language disorders.
3. The sequence of communicative development is different from that in typical children.
4. Communicative functions are limited.
5. Certain aberrant behaviors can be intentional, interactive, and communicative.
6. Children with ASD develop many behaviors that result in an environmental consequence but few behaviors that result in a social consequence.

Finally, educational techniques must take into consideration the communication learning style of the individual child (Cafiero, 1998). Children with autism do not readily develop the range of communicative intentions produced by typical children because of an inability to develop and coordinate the interactional behaviors described previously. If and when linguistic skills do develop, communicative deficits remain.

Communicative Acts

Do children with autism communicate? If yes, what is the nature of the interaction? Calloway et al. (1999) indicated that children with autism used communication as a means of requesting objects or controlling the behaviors of peers and adults rather than as a means of social initiation to show, share, comment, provide information and/or request information. Their findings indicated that as children with autism continue to develop communicative functions and means, more primitive communicative forms were replaced with more advanced forms. Although the progression of specific communicative functions varied, children showed consistent progress and development often following a pattern from behavior regulation to social interaction to joint attention. The only way to determine intentional behaviors is to observe and analyze how children with ASD behave within the social situation. What should the SLP look for in a child's behavior? Even the child with the most severe deficits has behaviors that can be identified as communicative if they are analyzed within the context (Prizant et al., 1990). Several incidents with Adam highlight this point.

Situation 1:

Clinician:	Clinician places a tightly sealed container of vanilla ice cream on the table.
Adam:	Adam walks over to the table, turns over the container, tries to pull open the top, bites on the container, and drops it on the

| | table. He walks away for several moments. He walks back to the table and picks up the container. He brings the container to the clinician and puts it in her lap. He walks away from the clinician and looks at her from across the room. (The clinician, of course, does nothing.) Adam approaches the clinician from the side, takes her hand, and places it on the ice cream. |
| *Interpretation:* | Adam is requesting that the clinician perform an action (open the ice cream) that he could not do himself. |

Situation 2:

Clinician:	Clinician approaches Adam and sits down next to him.
Adam:	Adam gets up and moves away from the clinician.
Interpretation:	Adam is rejecting interaction.

Situation 3:

Clinician:	Clinician talks to Adam.
Adam:	Adam puts his hands over his ears, turns away from the clinician, but does not move away. Periodically, he takes his hands off his ears. When the clinician stops talking, Adam turns back to the clinician.
Interpretation:	Adam does not want to engage in verbal interaction. The clinician learned that during these periods, Adam would participate in activities that could be maintained without discourse (e.g., puzzles, blocks, coloring).

Adam could communicate several different intentions and presented different combinations of behavior to indicate his responses to input from the environment. It becomes critical for adults and typical peers to "read" the child's behaviors within a contextual framework before attempting to interpret the child's reactions to the environment. In fact, the maternal variable of rich interpretation—in which the mother assumes that her infant reacts to the environment and treats the infant as an active listener and communicator—could facilitate the communication exchange process with the child with ASD. The assumption that children with autism do not have the ability to communicate results in a self-fulfilling prophesy. If it is believed that they cannot communicate, they are not treated as communicators and their behaviors are not analyzed to identify communicative interactions (Tiegerman-Farber, 1995).

Semantics

The linguistic term **semantics** refers to meaning as it is encoded in language. Semantic knowledge, therefore, refers to the meaning within a language that is linguistically coded. Conceptual knowledge affects the acquisition of the semantic component of language. Tager-Flusberg (1999) suggested that conceptual knowledge in typical children is transformed into semantic knowledge. The difficult task for children is to determine which aspects of these concepts are encoded within their particular linguistic system. Children's interactional experiences with agents, actions, and objects develop semantic relationships that code the content of language. Children with ASD have difficulty developing complex relationships and, as a consequence, establishing the underpinnings for symbolic forms of behavior, which provide the foundations for language. The ability to develop meaningful and relevant perceptual-conceptual relationships allows typical children to establish general categories—that is, to relate agents, actions, and objects to one another. General categories enable children to make cohesive and consistent sense of an environment, stimuli in the environment, and experiences within the environment that would otherwise be continually novel and changing. Categorical and organizational abilities provide children with the means of developing a schematic framework for their experiences. Language as a representation of reality begins within the microcosm of the child's social world. At a very basic semantic level, children with autism cannot understand how objects are functionally related or associated and as a result they cannot translate their real-world experiences into linguistic structures by using a semantically based processing strategy.

Ogletree and Fischer (1995) noted that the focus of research has shifted from the structural aspects of language (i.e., phonology, morphology, and syntax) to the development of meaning within social contexts. Brook and Bowler (1992) listed some of the semantic/pragmatic deficits presented by children with autism:

1. Confusion specific to the intent of communicative acts
2. Problems encoding meaning relevant to conversation
3. Difficulty with verbal/nonverbal cues of partners
4. Problems initiating or responding to questions
5. Impaired language comprehension
6. Too literal interpretations of verbal messages
7. Poor turn taking and topic maintenance
8. Inappropriate speech volume and intonational patterns
9. Semantic confusion specific to temporal sequencing
10. Poor sense of semantic relationships
11. Low rates of conversational repairs
12. Providing too little or too much information to conversational partners

Table 11.2 describes Adam's development of lexical items to express his semantic knowledge and ideas about the world. Adam's semantic development at this time (4 years 9 months) indicates his limited or restricted developmental use of functions. Adam developed lexical items within four semantic categories. Most of the lexical items were food related—specifically, desserts. Fewer action performances than objects were coded, and two of the action performances related to food (e.g., eat and drink). Analyzing the child's corpus in this way provides the SLP with insight into what is important to the child within his environment. The child's preferences can then be incorporated into therapeutic activities.

Old knowledge provides a framework for processing new information. With the analytic style, new information can be compared to old information to develop concepts—specifically, semantic concepts. Prizant (1983) noted that semantic memory involves the ability to conceptualize beyond any single or specific context. Here the child abstracts relevant information across situations to organize concepts for long-term memory. This semantic ability allows the child to represent and reconstruct an event symbolically. So, in order to learn language, a child must be able to reconstruct

TABLE 11.2	Adam's Early Lexicon

Semantic Functions	Lexical Entries
Object	Car, cookie, pretzel, juice, ice cream, milk, chip, M&M, hot dog, lolly, soda, popcorn, puzzle, Slinky, block, shoe, raisin, grape
Action	Open, push, eat, drink, throw, give
Negation: rejection	No
cessation	No
Recurrence	(Repeat of item label)
Agent	—
Action + object	—

sentence elements, not merely imitate them. The analytic style allows for linguistic generation with an understanding of semantic meaning as well as the related structural forms to express it. Children with ASD have a language pattern characterized by repetition of unanalyzed forms. This language pattern indicates an inability to use generative rules for production purposes and an inability to analyze the internal structure of another's production (Windsor & Doyle, 1994).

Prizant (1983) suggested that gestalt and analytic styles represent processing abilities on opposite ends of a continuum. Because children with ASD have an extreme style of gestalt processing, generative language development becomes a very difficult process. In particular, "those who remain primarily echolalic demonstrate a failure to move along the continuum toward analytic processing due to cognitive imitations" (p. 303). As spontaneous utterances increase, echolalia decreases; spontaneous productions indicate more flexibility in the use of combinatorial rules. This movement toward the analytic end of the processing continuum is necessary for the development of semantic-syntactic relations. To understand further the impact of the child's processing pattern on language learning, splinter abilities can be contrasted with idiosyncratic deficits. Children with autism have excellent memories, visual processing skills, visual-spatial abilities, numerical skills, and musical abilities. The gestalt learning style interferes with the analytic requirements for the development of semantic functions and semantic-syntactic relationships (Brook & Bowler, 1992).

Hyperlexia

The term **hyperlexia** has been used to describe children with ASD who present highly developed word-recognition skills, but little or no comprehension of the words that they recognize. There appears to be a disparity between this site-recognition ability and the underlying semantic comprehension that relates to the processing of meaning in language (O'Connor & Hermelin, 1994; Tirosh & Canby, 1993). Hyperlexia has been described as a savant skill in children with autism. Why certain children acquire this splinter skill and its overall relationship to other developmental areas of learning continues to be perplexing and interesting from an educational perspective. Many of the characteristics of autism involve highly idiosyncratic and fragmented abilities, including hyperlexia. These splinter skills present learning problems over time because they are not well integrated or cross-referenced with other areas of the child's learning; these skills do not represent functional behaviors that serve a social or communicative process (Patti & Lupinetti, 1993). Hyperlectic readers appear to be highly attuned to orthographic and phonological features; this visual–verbal decoding ability is not integrated with semantic and reading comprehension. As a result, the hyperlectic process in children with autism can be understood given the pervasive semantic deficits. Savant abilities and splinter skills highlight uneven and nonintegrated aspects of developmental learning, which appear to develop independently from areas of social communicative learning. Since the savant skill does not serve to facilitate communicative interaction, it poses an interesting problem for parents and teachers. In trying to understand an advanced reading ability or any savant skill in children with ASD the question becomes, how can this splinter skill be utilized educationally to facilitate the child's interactional abilities within the social context?

Syntax

The development of a normal linguistic system, in which structure is related to meaning, requires an interfacing of linguistic and nonlinguistic cognitive development. In typical children, lexical and relational semantic abilities are linked to broader conceptual developments but morphological and syntactic abilities are not. The aspects of language that are conceptually based and reflect pragmatic/semantic functioning are significantly impaired in children with ASD. The language/communication deficits presented by children with ASD are a result of a disintegrated developmental system in which advances in one component area do not seem to affect developments in other component areas of language (Conti-Ramsden & Botting, 1999). The language pattern in children with ASD indicates that pragmatic/semantic development occurs independently from the structural development of language. The separate development of components highlights the devastating impact of two language subsystems that do not "communicate" with each other. Linguistic aspects such as verb endings, past tense, and present progressive, which require syntactic structures, present significant difficulties to children with ASD because of their inability to understand the underlying meaning of "past tense." The more basic problem for children with autism is that they do not understand the conceptual ideas that underlie the formulation of language. They have difficulties using or manipulating certain linguistic forms of language because they do not understand their semantic counterparts. Bartak, Rutter, and Cox (1975) compared autistic with dysphasic children. The researchers found both groups comparable in mean length of utterance (one of the major measures of productive language development) and grammatical complexity. On a test of comprehension, however, the children with autism performed more poorly than the children with dysphasia. It seems that the syntactic delays in children with autism are related to their general developmental delays. These children present syntactic processing skills similar to those evidenced by children with other types of disorders.

Linguistic analyses indicated the use of rule-governed behavior, however, despite their limited production and comprehension of language.

Adam's productions are presented within the framework of various contextual and interactional situations to highlight his limited linguistic processing abilities. Consider Adam's use of the following morphemes: present progressive, past tense, personal pronouns, relative pronouns, copula, articles, and plurals.

> *Clinician:*   What is Mommy doing?
>
> *Adam:*   Mommy is opening juice.

Within the framework of an interaction with the adult, Adam was able to use the copula and present progressive morphemes within his own speech. He also responded to the adult's question by altering the inflectional form of the adult's utterance (i.e., he did not imitate the question's inflectional pattern).

> *Clinician:*   What did you do?
>
> *Adam:*   Adam ate three cookie.

Within the framework of this interaction with the adult, Adam responded to the question by referring to himself as Adam; he did not use any of the personal pronouns. He was not able to code (or use) the past-tense form. When Adam was not able to code the morphemic structures presented within the adult's production, he reduced his own utterance or reverted to a string of content words. Plural forms were coded by the use of number without the plural -*s*. In the preceding examples, there was a structural relationship between the linguistic input provided by the adult and the child's linguistic response: Adam based his response on the structure of the adult's input. The following interaction shows what happened to Adam's linguistic structure when the adult input was not provided:

> *Clinician:*   (has just poured Adam some juice)
>
> *Adam:*   Drink juice. (describing his own action)
>
> *Adam:*   More. (requesting more juice)
>
> *Adam:*   Pour juice. (directing clinician to perform an action)
>
> *Adam:*   Give. (requesting cup from clinician)

In this interaction, the clinician responded nonverbally to all of Adam's requests and directions. He did not, therefore, have the adult's linguistic input to rely on to structure his own utterances. The result was a reduction to the minimum use of forms that would "get the message across" effectively. This reduction process was quite typical of Adam's spontaneous, or self-initiated, speech. To understand the structural/syntactic abilities of children with autism, it is important to analyze if and how their linguistic structures change within various interactional situations. For Adam, the adult's input provided a syntactic framework for responses. Finally, Adam's productions required a close analysis of the context in order to disambiguate the meaning of his utterances. He rarely provided gestural support for his verbal productions.

During the third year of life, the typical language learner begins to encode meaning syntactically in the form of phrases, sentences, and finally, narratives. In the process of combining words, the child learns that words must be organized into sentences given specific linguistic rules. The child learns that ideas can be expressed by using specific sentence structures such as questions, negation, coordination, sequence, causality, and temporality. Conventional forms are important to the expression of ideas; by 3 years of age, the typical language learner has already integrated aspects of formal structure, semantic meaning, and communicative interaction. This can be contrasted with some striking statistics on children with autism. Newsom, Carr, and Lovaas (1979) estimated that 50 percent of all children with autism are mute, and that 75 percent of those who become verbal are echolalic by five years of age.

Phonology

Few studies have been conducted investigating phonological abilities in children with ASD, possibly because speech-language production is so limited (Wolk & Edwards, 1993). Adams and Gathercole (1995) indicated that 3-year-old children with good phonological memory skills produced speech that was grammatically more sophisticated than children with poorer phonological memory skills. This appears to be consistent with the speech production of children with autism, although utterances are imitated rather than spontaneous. Many children with autism have savant memory skills, resulting in the reproduction of large chunks of syntactically sophisticated utterances. The researchers also demonstrated that typical children with better phonological memory abilities were able to produce a wider array of grammatical forms in spontaneous speech. In addition, the ability to imitate utterances and retain them in short-term memory before they are incorporated into the child's syntactic knowledge appears to influence the development of syntactic forms. This certainly is not the case in children with autism: their spontaneous productions are severely limited and reflect significant semantic/syntactic deficits. Although children with autism have excellent memory skills:

1. Their sophisticated imitated utterances are not reflective of their understanding of the structural aspects of language.
2. Their memory abilities appear to be separated from the required phonological/morphological processing that occurs in normal development. Phonological and morphological development require analytic processing to identify phonemic and morphemic building blocks. Phonological memory may be necessary but it is not sufficient for the structural acquisition of language.
3. The imitation of new structural forms, no matter how many repetitions, is not conceptually understood by the child with autism. As a result, new forms will not be readily incorporated "into the store of knowledge about the syntactic forms of the native language" (Adams and Gathercole, 1995, p. 11).

The inability of the child to progressively develop more complex morphosyntactic structures relates to developments in subsystems—structure and meaning—that do not interface/overlap. So the schism between structure and meaning or form and function creates developmental differences at the phonological level as well as the syntactic level. In this case, the child with autism acquires a sound system apart from its meaning and its application. Large sound chunks are often tangentially related to contextual occurrences and social interactions. Long sound strings are produced like a foreign language student repeating an English phrase without understanding its meaning. The inability to utilize an analytic processing style prevents the child with ASD from acquiring the basic elemental sound/symbol units, which are finite but can be combined to generate an infinite number of speech productions. Fragmented language development results in growth without integration. The highest percentage of errors involves phonemes that are generally acquired later in typical children. The order of phonemic acquisition in children with autism seems to follow the typical developmental pattern in spite of the delay in the onset of speech. The phonological ability of children with autism contrasts markedly with their developmental delays in pragmatic/semantic areas.

THERAPEUTIC ISSUES AND STRATEGIES

The clinical view of the child with autism has changed in the past several years. Theoretical changes in the area of child language development have dramatically affected the content and context of therapeutic programs. Children with autism now undergo communication training rather than speech training. With the focus on communication learning, several related issues have been investigated by speech-language pathologists: parent language training, home training, alternative language systems, and language socialization in inclusive classrooms. These components present a more holistic approach to the language learning experience for children with autism (Schwartz & Carta, 1996).

Therapeutic programming varies from child to child, family to family, and clinician to clinician. It is this variety in training approaches and styles that provides our profession with its clinical strength. Given their developmental differences and needs, children with ASD present a number of challenges for educators, parents, and public officials. Children with ASD require an integrated educational model that facilitates the development of a life-cycle philosophical approach for home and school. ASD is after all, a life-long developmental disability. For a child with ASD, each social context represents an ecology with its place on life's learning continuum (Kohler & Strain, 1997). Research in the area of therapeutic methodologies stresses the need for adaptive communication in multiple contexts, integration of services, and development of inclusive social learning models. This "systems" view establishes programming and decision making across a long-term service continuum from birth through adulthood. In addition, the professional collaborative network must enhance the child's transition from one learning context to another and from one developmental stage to another. Finally, programming itself should focus on the process of learning rather than specific content (Pierce & Schreibman, 1997).

Alternative Therapies

A recent controversy within the clinical journals involves a therapeutic technique called facilitated communication (Hostler, 1996). In facilitated communication, an adult facilitator provides physical support to help the child with autism overcome his or her neuromotor difficulties. This physical support may be provided by helping the child to isolate his or her index finger and/or stabilizing his or her hand, wrist, or arm during a typing process. What is interesting about the technique is its underlying therapeutic premise. Basic to the use of facilitated communication is the supposition that the child with autism is not cognitively impaired but rather has a form of praxis. This motor-processing disorder interferes with the expression of language and communication, and the underlying etiology is clearly different from anything discussed earlier within this chapter (Eberlin, McConnachie, Ibel, & Volpe, 1993; Cabey, 1994; Duchan, 1993).

Biklen (1993) described the use of facilitated communication with a number of children with autism. He detailed a series of steps, similar to a successive approximation procedure, that gradually allows the child to become more independent in his or her use of this procedure. When facilitated communication was used with the subjects within his study, all demonstrated literacy skills. This suggests that children with autism have acquired a linguistic set of skills but cannot express the skills verbally. Facilitated communication provides a mechanism just as other alternative therapies do, to allow the child with autism to communicate by means of another system.

Facilitated communication represents a controversial form of therapeutic intervention for a number of reasons, as described by Calculator (1992). "This communication technique remains one that is characterized by its ambiguity (e.g., lack of specific teaching process), mystique, recording anecdotes and spiritual underpinning" (p. 18). Calculator noted that facilitated communication exploded on the therapeutic scene before its efficacy had been investigated experimentally. Thus, professionals and parents know little about how or why and/or with whom facilitated communication works or does not work. Calculator noted that experimental investigation is critical because this procedure suggests that we must reevaluate our perception of autism as a social, cognitive disability. This clearly has important implications for children with autism and other nonverbal, developmentally disordered children. In the process of analyzing results, advocates for facilitated communication must be responsible for their claims of success. This cannot be another panacea that over time leads parents, teachers, and professionals "down a chaotic road." One important question involves how the child with autism has learned to be literate despite severe communicative, behavioral, and social difficulties. Researchers describe ongoing theoretical and clinical issues related to methodological problems in facilitated communication with implications for the introduction of other alternative treatments that have not undergone empirical scrutiny. Researchers must be held accountable for unsubstantiated claims. The chaos created by the successes claimed by "facilitators" resulted in legal suits and damages.

The information-processing style of children with autism becomes an important issue when adaptive systems are being considered. There are no clear-cut conclusions on the efficacy of any of the intervention systems: sign language, Blissymbols, pictorial and written words, communication boards, microcomputers, and facilitated communication. The highly individualized learning styles of children with ASD must be taken into consideration. The introduction of an adaptive learning system does not mean that the communication learning problems will be resolved automatically. The gestalt processing style in children with autism suggests that the way information is processed must be incorporated into therapeutic decision making. Mirenda and Schuler (1988) suggested that "because of its dual spatial and temporal organization, sign language may have the potential to facilitate the transition from a simultaneous to a more sequential mode of processing" (p. 26). The communication difficulties of children with autism are often offset by extraordinary abilities in memory, visual processing, hyperlectic reading abilities, and mathematical and musical talents. Given the marked discrepancy between "the form and the function," the issue for SLPs becomes one of attempting to use and to integrate the child's skills in teaching communication. The variability in the population is compounded by the highly individualized splinter of skills in each child; intervention procedures must be matched to the child's learning style and needs.

Learning Contexts

Adam's training reflected the pragmatic/semantic issues raised in the literature during the 1990s. In the following program, there was an attempt to incorporate each environment (school, after-school therapy, home, and daycare) within the educational process. A set of operating principles was developed to coordinate intervention goals and therapeutic programming with inclusive education in mind. The identified learning contexts and communication behaviors represented a means of recreating communication experiences for Adam. The communication behaviors learned in therapy could be generalized to his home, preschool special education classroom, and daycare center.

Since Adam had been enrolled in the Speech and Hearing Center for early intervention services, I attended the Committee on Preschool Special Education meeting (CPSE) when he transitioned into the preschool system. The CPSE consisted of a special education teacher, a school psychologist, a speech/language pathologist from the local school district, Adam's mother, and me. The CPSE functioned as a collaborative team, reviewing all of Adam's evaluations and progress reports. The language training program that I presented to other members of the team was discussed to determine implementation issues within the recommended special education classroom. The CPSE recommended that Adam's mother and I meet with Adam's preschool teacher to discuss instructional and organizational changes within the classroom that would be required to implement the language program. The team recommended that I function as a teacher consultant within the classroom to provide teacher training and support. The CPSE also asked that I work with Adam's SLP, because language therapy was recommended three times per week as a related service. Adam's mother informed the CPSE that in the afternoon Adam would be attending an integrated/early childhood program. The coordination of programming and services was not only complicated but time consuming. To ensure the implementation of the program, the generalization of skills from context to context and the development of an inclusion program, I met with all of the professionals and the mother on a regular basis. It is important to know that because Adam was receiving progammatic services across diverse settings—preschool special education classroom, early childhood classroom, individual speech language therapy, and private speech language therapy—the collaborative team consisted of the special education teacher, the early childhood teacher, a parent, the SLP, and myself.

TABLE 11.3   **An Example of a Learning Context**

Place	Activity/Context	Materials	Routine	Communicative Behavior
Therapy room	Making bubbles	Bubbles	Get bubbles	Point to object
	Large Bubble	Wand	Open bubbles	Gaze at object/adult
		Fan	Get wand	Sign for object
			Pour bubbles (or action)	Consistent vocalization for object (or action)
			Turn fan on	Word
			Make bubbles	Some combination of these behaviors

The following operating principles were used to develop Adam's learning contexts:

1. A learning context was defined as any activity that provided an interactional framework, that is, an opportunity for interchange between the adult and the child. The activity was then described in terms of the type of (a) interactions to be developed, (b) communicative behaviors to be learned, and (c) semantic functions to be closed (see Table 11.3).

2. Each learning context established a task structure to develop an anticipation and sequence of events in the routine.

3. The learning context facilitated action and interaction; it allowed for the development of reversible role relationships between adult and child.

4. A core lexicon was developed within each learning context to consistently and systematically focus communication and language training across all the adults working with the child.

5. The core lexicon was based on the development of those communicative behaviors that appear earliest in child language. These communicative behaviors were used across a variety of learning contexts to generalize language and communication relations.

6. Communicative interaction was stressed above production of stereotypic/routinized utterances.

7. Learning contexts developed were relevant and functional to the child. To facilitate interaction and communication, the adult focused on activities that the child preferred.

8. Input to the child was limited in complexity and mean length of utterance. Adult input was functional and relevant to the immediate context and semantically related to the child's vocal, verbal, and nonlinguistic behavior.

9. The child was presented with a choice of learning contexts; at any time, the child could maintain or terminate an activity. Verbal, vocal, and nonverbal

behaviors were analyzed within the learning contexts to determine communicative intentions.

10. The child was trained first to participate and interact within the context and second to "talk" about his social experiences.

11. Every adult working with Adam was given a copy of the communication/language description of each learning context. Thus, each teacher provided consistent input within and across activities (see Table 11.4).

12. Echolalic behavior was used to develop language behaviors. With the knowledge that the child would imitate, the adult would code, for instance, a nonlinguistic event:

    Event: Adam opening the bubbles
    Adult: Adam open bubbles.
    Adam: Adam open bubbles.

The clinical goals identified for Adam's training included:

1. Development of imitative interaction skills
2. Expansion of object manipulation skills (semantic knowledge)
3. Development of sign/gesture forms
4. Use of interactional behaviors that signal communicative intentions
5. Generalization of communication behaviors

TABLE 11.4	An Example of a Communication/Language Description of a Learning Context (Context: Bubbles; Materials: Bottle of Bubbles, Bubble Maker, Fan)

Semantic Functions	Forms Trained/Adult Input
1. Object	Bubbles, fan
2. Action	Open, blow, give, turn on
3. Agent	Ellen, Adam, Mommy, Daddy
4. Agent + agent	Adam open, Ellen open Adam blow, Ellen blow
5. Action + object	Make bubbles, pour bubbles, open bubbles
6. Recurrence	Bubbles . . . bubbles . . . bubbles, more, more bubbles
7. Negation Rejection Cessation (action)	No, no bubbles Stop, no more, no more bubbles No pour, no blow
8. Agent + action + object	Adam open bubbles Ellen open bubbles Mommy open bubbles Adam pour bubbles Ellen pour bubbles Adam blow bubbles Ellen blow bubbles Mommy blow bubbles

The goals and procedures described in this section were developed, given the need to individualize language and communication programming for Adam. The pragmatic/semantic content was applicable to other children with ASD as well as other children with language disorders. The skills developed in individual therapy needed to become part of the special education classroom curriculum. The primary goal within the classroom, which was highly structured, was to provide opportunities for Adam to engage in social interactions with peers. As a result, the preschool classroom was organized around group activities that facilitated communicative interactions, peer-related behaviors, and functional play. Children with LCD who present disruptive behaviors tend to be less responsive to peers and do not initiate interactions; this was certainly the case with Adam. The development of social competence was critical if Adam was going to engage in positive interactions with typical peers in daycare. Adam needed to develop a level of social performance comparable to children without disabilities if social interaction was going to occur (Odom, 2000; Brown & Odom, 1999). The pragmatic/semantic program was the starting point for Adam.

Communication interaction would be the result of "predictable interaction routines" between two or more people. Once Adam learned to operate within these familiar contexts, event sequences could be altered. Adam's awareness of the environment was noted by observing his reactions to unanticipated change and his attempts to repair the situation. This provided opportunities to facilitate the development of communicative behaviors and interactions between adult and child or child and child. It was important to provide Adam with opportunities to initiate and to regulate actions, people, and events in his environment. Adam needed to develop a contingency relationship between his behavior and that of his peers; reciprocal interaction was based on such a consequence-based conceptualization (Odom et al., 1999b).

In attempting to teach Adam to express his needs, the teacher manipulated contextual events to create the need and facilitate its expression.

Context:	Ice cream container cannot be opened by the child.
Adult:	"Ellen open ice cream."
Adam:	"Ellen open ice cream."
Consequence:	Ellen performs action.

It was important to identify a number of situational contexts that created communicative need. These situations provided Adam with the opportunity to intentionally direct the course of events within the environment. The ultimate goal was teaching Adam that language is a tool, a vehicle, a means to affect the behavior of other interactants. To achieve this goal, Adam had to experience himself as an effective communicator with his peers.

Generalization of Communication Behaviors through Home Training

A home training program can be used to help children generalize the learning experience to various environments (Tiegerman-Farber & Radziewicz, 1998). In Adam's case, the home provided a training experience within a more natural environment. Part of the home training program developed for Adam included training parents and siblings as communication facilitators. In addition, a dedicated group of volunteers was trained to work within the framework of the program and to provide extensive training 7 days a week—after school and on weekends. The home training program can be contrasted to the more traditional therapy experience provided for Adam in school. Family members could not participate in sessions during the school day, whereas at home the parent training model incorporated everyone's participation (Schopler, 1995). His mother was present and integrated into the framework of each session. She was carefully trained by the speech-language pathologist to work with Adam at home (Simpson, 1995).

The home and school training experiences were different in terms of the amount of stimulation provided (Harn, Bradshaw, & Ogletree, 1999). The home-based program was developed to be a language training program for as long as Adam was awake. In school, the SLP provided language training outside the classroom for 30 minutes three times a week. Coordinating training goals with the classroom teacher was possible but difficult. Another difference concerned the nature of the training experience itself. The home training program focused on the development of language and communication behaviors within all of the training contexts (see Table 11.3). Activities were identified to facilitate interaction and communication. The activity provided a means to an end: adult–child interaction; nothing had to be simulated. Activities were meaningful and relevant to the child's daily living needs and the immediate context.

As a language learning experience, the home training program presented certain advantages for Adam. First, family members were trained to function as communication facilitators. Second, various activities within the home provided the means to integrate language behavior with relevant nonlinguistic experiences. Third, the use of communicative behaviors was generalized across learning contexts. Fourth, the orientation of the program emphasized the child's language and communication needs. These components were not available to Adam within the traditional special education classroom. The home training program proved to be an important addition to traditional learning.

The educational setting has a responsibility to develop parent language training programs to formally provide parents with academic and procedural knowledge (Tiegerman-Farber, 1995). Training parents to function as communication facilitators for children with ASD extends the educational process beyond 3 p.m. to the home context. Parents need to understand language development, language disorders, and language intervention issues if they are going to assist in the educational development of their children; teaching parents about language and the language needs of their children gives them the tools to do so. To teach parents to understand their children is the greatest responsibility and the greatest gift of education (Wehman, 1998).

Social Problems and Behavioral Technology

Because of the extensive behavioral difficulties characteristic of children with autism, many clinicians and parents use behavioral procedures to train targeted behaviors such as self-care and daily-living skills. The behavioral approach is also used as part of an educational program to deal with inappropriate and injurious behaviors exhibited within the classroom (Risley, 1996). The classroom teacher may utilize a behavior-modification model because of the need to operationalize classroom procedures and training goals. Underlying the behavioral approach is the identification of an observable and measurable targeted performance (e.g., sitting, looking, or vocalizing). For example, rather than targeting attention as a training performance, the clinician or teacher would identify all of the descriptive behaviors of attention: sitting, physical orientation, eye contact, and so on. These identified behaviors are then trained by means of a successive approximation procedure.

The management difficulties presented by children with ASD impact significantly upon the abilities of educators and parents to integrate these children (Yell & Drasgow, 2000). The behavior problems often exhibited by children with autism—aggression, self-injurious behavior, unanticipated explosive behaviors, self-stimulation, and extraneous verbal-vocal behaviors—often interfere with their acceptance by others within natural settings and complex community contexts (Lord, 1995). The management of severe behavior problems may initially require a combined treatment approach utilizing highly individualized training schedules by means of behavior analysis. Children's behavior can be assessed and functionally analyzed to determine the most appropriate management schedule within the educational setting, at home and within the community. The management of intrusive behaviors requires the identification of contingent stages that will be utilized by a multidisciplinary team of professionals across various learning settings. The combined behavioral approach emphasizes the identification of target behaviors and also emphasizes the need for developing appropriate social learning skills that will be maintained and reinforced by adults and peers (Kohler & Strain, 1997). The disruptive behaviors of children with ASD often result in social rejection by peers, which further interferes with the educational learning process in integrated settings. The identification of training procedures may vary from child to child, but the behavioral needs of children with ASD suggest targeted programming and instruction within the special education classroom. This is necessary if the child with ASD is going to be ultimately mainstreamed to less restrictive educational and environmental placements. Research has documented that preschool special education programs are including many more children with autism, behavioral-emotional, and pervasive developmental disabilities (Odom, 2000).

Peer-Mediated Communicative Intervention

The integration of children with ASD in less restrictive classrooms and early childhood programs requires a high degree of specialized programming and teacher training (Odom et al., 1999a). Researchers advocating for full inclusive programming propose peer-mediated social strategies as a mechanism for facilitating social skills and integration in children with autism. The process of teaching children to teach children provides the opportunity to integrate children with ASD in a socially meaningful way. The proviso, however, is the child's level of social performance comparable to other children without disabilities in the classroom. The greater the discrepancy, the greater is the need for highly individualized instruction and the greater the possibility for peer rejection (Tiegerman-Farber & Radziewicz, 1998). If specialists seek to achieve social rather than physical integration of children with ASD, typical peers must be trained. Guralnick (1999) noted that the point of "child benefit" is not clearly defined for either the child with a disability or his typical peer. Teachers are much more comfortable with the inclusion process when children with mild disabilities are involved—Adam was a challenge. Cooperative learning and peer tutoring, in which learners with and without disabilities are brought together to interact and socialize, provide an opportunity for students to develop a social awareness of peer roles, responsibilities, and skills as socialization becomes a primary focus for instruction (Tiegerman-Farber & Radziewicz, 1998).

The typical language learner can provide peer instruction and modeling for the child with autism. It becomes important, however, for teachers and adults to educate typical peers and ready them for this peer instructional opportunity (Odom et al., 1999b). The early-childhood classroom plays an important role in the social learning process for many children with developmental disabilities. The child with ASD presents a unique set of learning needs in social and communicative areas. In the effort to improve peer acceptance, it becomes important for early intervention programs to develop a peer training program; normal learners must be "readied" and trained to accept learners with different language and social skills (Odom & Diamond, 1998). Activities, interactional experiences, learning contingencies, and educational procedures must all be defined with peer partners in mind. The typical peer and a more socially challenging environment provides an opportunity for language learning and natural environmental contingencies. The preschool classroom provides the opportunity for naturalistic learning. Milieu teaching approaches include naturalistic language intervention techniques (Rule, Losardo, Dinnebeil, Kaiser, & Rowland, 1998). Communicative interactions are facilitated within the context of social activities and conversational interchanges. Clinical research has clearly evidenced a change in intervention technologies to focus on child specific, contextual, and interactional variables as underpinnings for teaching communication between the child with autism and typical peers (Frea, Craig, Odom, & Johnson, 1999).

For the child who presents with severe language and communication deficits, early peer experiences by means of dyadic and triadic interchanges provide an opportunity for social learning. Peer-mediated communicative interventions provide a means of facilitating social interactions in children with ASD (Odom, 2000). Children with autism usually remain on the outside of social play situations that would naturally provide the very learning stimulation needed. In addition, children with autism are provided with few opportunities to interact with typical peers, given their pervasive behavioral deficits. Peers can be trained to use specific interactional strategies to engage children with autism in various activities and thereby facilitate the social learning process (Taylor & Levin, 1998).

Social scripts can provide the means for controlled interactions between children with and without autism. Each child learns about the script story and then his or her own role. The script provides the format and the structure for the social interactions among the "players" (Tiegerman-Farber & Cartusciello-King, 1995). The rehearsal of the script is very similar to the early social games that mothers engage in with their infants. The game provides a limited semantic domain and clearly defined roles for the interactants. With the sociodramatic play scripts, typical children can model for the child with ASD and provide ongoing gestural and verbal cues. The research indicates that in integrated preschool classrooms:

1. Training peers to act as social agents resulted in higher rates of communicative interaction in preschoolers with disabilities.
2. Children with disabilities were equally responsive to teacher and peer input, suggesting that young children without disabilities can take on more directive responsibility for facilitating intervention with peers with ASD.

However, early childhood programs and schools attempting to provide inclusive opportunities for children with autism will require organizational changes and funding supports for the following (Tiegerman-Farber & Radziewicz, 1998):

- The collaborative development of an inclusion mission for parents and teachers
- Physical reconstruction of classrooms and buildings to remove structural barriers to inclusion
- Teacher training and staff development for regular education and special education teachers on instructional management of diverse learners (Bennett, DeLuca, & Bruns, 1997)
- Development of an inclusion curriculum that provides modified instruction for children with autism in the general education classroom
- Parent education programs that incorporate families within the educational decision-making process (Guralnick, 1999)

Educational Considerations

The treatment of ASD has presented parents with significant emotional and financial problems, because many of the treatments are based on anecdotal reports and not on experimental investigations. Treatments such as sensory integration therapy, auditory integration training, medications, diets, and megavitamins may offer some benefits to selected behaviors, but they do not improve general areas of functioning for children with ASD on a consistent basis (Heflin & Simpson, 1998). How do parents make a decision about these alternative treatments?

The trend in educational programming involves the use of applied behavioral analysis (ABA), because there has been a great deal of scientific support for its limited effectiveness. Clearly there are individual differences in children with autism that will affect how they respond to behavioral treatment. Many schools and parents feel that applied behavioral analysis is the treatment of choice because (1) behavioral changes are observable and measurable; (2) parents must be part of the training program to generalize results to natural settings; (3) aside from the management of disruptive behavior, another primary goal is independent functioning (Lovaas, 1999). One issue however, is the changing role of the speech-language pathologist given the significance of language to all other developmental areas. Since language/communication deficits remain to be the central problem for children with ASD, there needs to be a collaboration among the behavioral specialist, the speech-language pathologist, and the parent. Applied behavioral analysis may provide a procedural methodology for how some children are taught, but a language learning curriculum determines what children should be taught. ABA is one methodological or instructional approach; there are many others that should be considered, given the diversity of needs within the ASD population (Prizant & Rubin, 1999). Just as there is a continuum of severity within ASD, there is a continuum of instructional approaches that should be investigated. ABA is not effective for every child with ASD. Another way to view ABA given other treatment interventions is to consider a diversity of methodologies, ABA being one of many. The SLP must work as a collaborator and consultant to ensure that language and communication behaviors are facilitated by other professionals. The underlying controversy with ABA can best be described by saying that language has structural form, but behavior is not language.

The California Departments of Education and Developmental Services formed a Collaborative Work Group that recommended that curriculum should be organized around normal developmental expectations by using predictable routines in areas such as social engagement, language, coping, and behavior management. The curriculum focused on skills that are typically deficient in children with ASD, such as socialization and communication. Often a discussion of curriculum includes teaching methodology; in reality, educators need to develop curricula for early childhood through adolescence (Wolery & Winterling, 1997). Finally, given the increasing demands from parents for inclusion and services within local public schools, some state departments of education have developed clinical guides for children with autism spectrum disorders to establish consensus recommendation on best-practice procedures.

Given the fact that autism is now understood to be a severe language and communication disorder, the level of "speech therapy" services has been described as dramatically inadequate. Language learning must become the primary goal for classroom instruction and not just another related service. The educational curriculum and IEP should include language-communication goals and procedures. In addition, special education teachers have very limited academic training in language development and language disorders. Many educational programs are now placing speech-language pathologists in classrooms rather than employing them as individual service providers. At the School for Language and Communication Development in New York, the speech-language pathologist is the primary classroom teacher. Clearly, the language learning needs of children with autism require more than what the traditional education model has provided in the past.

Finally, the use of an etiological placement approach provides serious educational problems for children with autism. Adam's mother noted that "a class of six autistic children is really six one-child classes." Six children who cannot interact and communicate also cannot serve as facilitators for one another. If the need is communication, children with autism must be provided with child models who can facilitate such interactional development. A nonetiological educational approach to placement would certainly address this issue. It would also provide children with a less restrictive educational placement and the opportunity to interact with higher-functioning social peers. Peer facilitation would allow for language modeling in the special education classroom. The placement of children with ASD should be based on language level of functioning rather than etiological label. To make this a reality, however, state education departments across the United States would have to change their disability categories and their (etiologically based) educational placement processes. The enactment of PL 99-457 in 1986 mandated educational services for preschool children with disabilities. Infants and preschoolers now can receive educational services. The need for early intervention has moved from a dream to a reality. Society will finally actualize the findings of research proving that children with disabilities have a better prognosis the earlier intervention occurs.

The Inclusion Mandate

There is a great deal of legal and social support for the inclusion of all students, including those with severe developmental disabilities, within regular classroom settings (Wisniewski & Alpert, 1994; Polansky, 1994; Rock, Rosenberg, & Carran, 1995). Several research studies support the notion that students with severe developmental disabilities can be provided with appropriate educational services in general education classrooms. These studies also document the fact that students with severe disabilities can benefit from an inclusive setting, given the expanded opportunities for communication and social interactions between children with and without disabilities. The IDEA (1997) emphasizes that inclusive programming during the preschool years in which children with and without disabilities are integrated by means of socialization experiences may represent the best point in time to integrate and to manage behavioral-social problems in children with ASD. The early childhood curriculum focuses on daily-living skills, language learning skills, play skills, peer interactions, self-awareness, and independence (Wolfberg & Schuler, 1993). The preschool process also provides an important link between educational programming between the classroom and the home environment. Preschool programs often coordinate their goals across educational and therapeutic services by collaborating with parents. Educational and instructional needs identified at home and at school provide the basis for parent-teacher coordination of social and behavioral planning (Clark & Smith, 1999).

Children with autism have great difficulty generalizing learned behaviors to new contexts and situations, so educational programming must begin early. The focus on socialization, peer interactions, and communication behaviors will provide the child with a repertoire of social skills. The child's ability to remain within the social context of the classroom, the restaurant, the playground, the mall, and other natural environments is based on the generalized use of social-communicative behaviors. Early intervention programs emphasize learning during a critical period for children with ASD. Children with severe developmental disabilities can be provided with appropriate social and language models from age-appropriate peers. Children without disabilities will have the humanistic opportunity to acquire an understanding of social values that relate to learning differences between people. Children need to be provided with a curriculum that addresses positive attitudes about a variety of multi-cultural learners, including children with disabilities.

The failure to include students with severe disabilities underscores the difficulties within the public school system to implement and to achieve full inclusion. What is the least restrictive environment for the child with ASD (Tiegerman-Farber & Radziewicz, 1998)? Children with autism present severe language and communication deficits, social relational problems, and behavioral management problems. The principle of normalization that is often raised about inclusive education suggests that the child with ASD will benefit from the regular education experience. Although there may be an attempt to maintain the child with ASD within ongoing social and academic activities such as reading, math, social studies, and science, the differences in learning require major modifications in teacher instruction, classroom procedures, and peer sensitivity-awareness. Part of the decision concerning the appropriateness of a regular classroom for the child with autism should be the ability of educators to substantiate the educational benefit of inclusion for children with and without disabilities. What does benefit mean to the child with ASD? How do you measure benefit? Is it social benefit or academic benefit that parents are being offered? What if inclusion can provide social benefit and not academic benefit? One criticism of the regular classroom involves the fact that the child's education may not be individualized to the same degree as it would be in a special education classroom. Parents and teachers must carefully consider the individual needs of the child by reviewing various learning options. Inclusion is one of many educational options; it is not the only option. It certainly is not the option for every child. Finally, parents should never be forced to place their child in a setting that they believe will not be educationally beneficial to the child. The challenges for educators are whether the regular classroom can be redesigned and restructured as a learning environment that can handle the diverse needs of severely behaviorally impaired children. Odom (2000) suggests that education must focus on identifying what is in the best interest of the child. The integration and inclusion of the child with autism into a regular classroom requires a great deal of reorganization and commitment from parents, teachers, and administrators. One significant change within the regular classroom may be to change the responsibilities of paraprofessionals from collecting data to facilitating the integration of children with autism into less restrictive environments by teaching functional skills. In light of changing service delivery systems, the roles and responsibilities of paraprofessionals will also change. The paraprofessional's role will involve implementing instructional programs in school and community environments where these skills will be used (Boomer, 1994). It will be interesting to see in the next several years whether speech assistants are utilized in the same way by SLPs. Given our professional concerns about educational standards and requirements for licensure, SLPs may not agree with the statement, "The speech assistant is a support to the speech/language program but is not a replacement for the speech/language pathologist." In some communities a licensed speech-language pathologist supervises several speech assistants, because that is more cost effective. The instructional and financial demands of inclusive programming in schools may result in this kind of service delivery model. As professionals, the more we understand language development and learning, the greater will be the role of the SLP in educational decision making.

CASE STUDY

The significance of language has broad implications not only in education but in other related areas such as the law. I recently received a legal brief describing a young man (A.J.) diagnosed with Asperger syndrome who was being tried for murder and for whom the death penalty was being considered. A group of legal specialists contacted me concerning A.J.'s competency and sanity to stand trial, given his Asperger disorder. Competency is a threshold requirement that involves an individual's ability to participate in his own defense and *understand* the implications of his actions. If the court deems that an individual is competent to stand trial, the next phase is the potential determination of mental illness—insanity by means of psychiatric evaluations. Competency is obviously a lower standard; an individual may be competent to stand trial but later found to be insane. The definition of insanity is as follows:

> A person is not criminally responsible for conduct if at the time of such conduct as a result of mental disease or defect, he lacks substantial capacity:
>
> a. to know or appreciate the wrongfulness of the conduct, or
> b. to conform his conduct to the requirements of the law. (New York Penal Law Section 40.15)

How does this relate to the young man with Asperger syndrome? Asperger syndrome is one of several disorders on the autism spectrum continuum. Individuals with ASD, as was discussed in this chapter, present with three primary areas of impairment: social behavior, language, and stereotypical patterns of behavior. The critical relationship between language and cognition is underscored by the research findings related to "theory of mind." The key question for consideration is, "What do individuals with disabilities understand and think as a function of their language deficits?" Theory of mind refers to the ability to attribute mental states to one's self and other people as a means of understanding behavior. Research has indicated that children with ASD perform worse on theory-of-mind tests than language- or mental age-matched comparison children. The research results present strong evidence that children with ASD have a specific impairment in interpreting human action within a mentalistic framework—what Baron-Cohen (1995) refers to as "mindblindness." In addition, the deficits in theory of mind are closely related to language deficits: "A deficit in theory of mind is central to how we interpret autism because human and social behavior depends on our understanding that people with whom we interact are intentional mental beings" (Tager-Flusberg, 1999, p. 4).

The young man with Asperger syndrome had been diagnosed with a disability as a preschool child. Over the years, as his behavior became progressively more disruptive, he was reevaluated using various psychological measures. It is my contention that the competency/insanity definitions cannot be applied to individuals with Asperger syndrome for the following reasons. Competency to stand trial is based on an IQ test, and insanity is based on a psychiatric interview. An IQ test does not adequately measure language deficits and certainly cannot determine specific impairments such as mindblindness. The determination of competency, based on an IQ test, does not identify a spectrum of language and social problems. The assumption of competency is based on a performance level on an IQ test as well as the individual's understanding of his behavioral conformance. An individual with a disability could present with an average IQ but could also have a severe language/communication disorder (mindblindness) or other disability, which the IQ test would not measure or identify. The present definition of competency should apply only to individuals who do not have a documented history of developmental disabilities, because it makes accommodations for (1) the individual with insanity (mental disease) who would be disqualified by means of a psychiatric evaluation or (2) the individual with mental retardation (lacks capacity to understand) who would be disqualified by means of the IQ test. The problem for the individual with Asperger syndrome is that if a disorder such as mindblindness is not tested for, it does not exist and as a result he or she would be considered competent to stand trial. This clearly discriminates against the individual with ASD and other disabilities. The issue is thus A.J.'s capacity to *understand*.

Questions:

1. Does the IQ test measure a language disorder?
2. Does a psychiatric evaluation measure a language disorder?

The legal history related to competency/insanity evolved prior to the passage of IDEA (PL 94-142) in 1975. Can the competency/insanity standard be appropriately applied to individuals with disabilities without additional standardized assessments? The competency/insanity standard was developed to rule out individuals who did not understand the implications of their actions. The IDEA requires a multidisciplinary evaluation to determine disability. The tests utilized by the courts to determine competency—IQ tests and psychiatric evaluations, either individually or in combination—would not be considered sufficient to determine a developmental disability by IDEA standards. As a result, given the fact that A.J. was classified as developmentally disabled under IDEA, how can the court utilize: (1) a less comprehensive standard of review to determine competency—a lower standard; and (2) an assessment protocol that could not have been utilized to identify A.J.'s disabilities to begin with. The IQ test and psychiatric evaluations cannot be used to identify the fact that A.J. has a disability or his specific impairment of mindblindness. If A.J.'s disability cannot be identified by the present protocol, is he competent to stand trial? The implication here is that the process of determination to stand trial *and* to be considered for the death penalty is less comprehensive than the process of determination for a developmental disability. It is "easier" to classify someone as competent to stand trial and to be considered for the death penalty than classify that individual as developmentally disabled—something is seriously wrong with the logic.

Analyzing this scenario from another direction, consider the fact that A.J. had been classified as having a disability since he was a preschooler. Even with this information, the court used only an IQ test and a psychiatric evaluation to determine his competency and sanity to stand trial. Should consideration have been given to the fact that A.J. had (1) a developmental disability and, more specifically, (2) a condition referred to as "mindblindness," which could have affected his "capacity" to *know* the wrongfulness of his conduct and to conform his conduct to the requirements of the law? It is also important to the remember that the "theory of mind" research, as well as the impairment "mindblindness," represent relatively new areas of inquiry and investigation. There are few specialists who now understand this impairment and even fewer assessment measures to identify the impairment.

Based on the little that is known about "mindblindness" and the inadequacy of the competency/insanity protocol to identify such disabilities, should not the court reconsider its decision? The ability of the court to assess A.J.'s *understanding* was limited by tests that cannot evaluate his "mindblindness" impairment. I would have to argue that A.J.'s understanding and, as a result, his competency to stand trial should be reevaluated.

I believe that the terms competency/insanity as they are presently defined discriminate against individuals with disabilities, particularly those with language and social impairments not appropriately assessed by IQ tests and psychiatric evaluations, which result in deficits such as mindblindness. It is my recommendation that competency, which is a lower standard of review, must be replaced by a more stringent IDEA standard of review for individuals with disabilities. Our expanding knowledge of language disorders presents a case for a legal reconsideration of what is meant by "competent" to stand trial.

SUMMARY

This chapter has emphasized the unique language learning problems presented by children with ASD. Children with autism have traditionally been described as a single population, but the research cited in this chapter has stressed the heterogeneity exhibited within this group, suggesting that the etiological label is misleading. In addition, the use of this label detracts from the central problem related to the disorder, the inability to integrate communicative functions with other aspects of language. The research describes a schism between "form and function" in children with basic language disturbances in pragmatic and semantic skills; phonological and syntactic skills develop relatively intact. In fact, literature describing the language of higher-functioning children with ASD indicates severe communicative deficits in contrast to the almost-normal acquisition of structural linguistic skills. Such communicative incompetence includes ongoing problems with initiating and terminating interaction, deficits in topic maintenance, and speaker/listener roles.

ASD requires language-based educational programming during the infant and preschool years—the earlier, the better! The changes in child language theory have contributed greatly to the new therapeutic approaches used with children such as Adam. In a way, Adam is a product of the pragmatic era and the communication revolution. At this point, the impact of these theoretical and therapeutic changes on children with ASD can only be imagined. Finally, the SLP has a central role to play in the educational programming developed for children with ASD. There is no other professional who can better understand the language and communication deficits underlying this disorder.

REFERENCES

Adams, A., & Gathercole, S. (1995). Phonological working memory and speech. Production in preschool children. *Journal of Speech & Hearing Research, 38*(2), 403. Retrieved from the World Wide Web: http://www.ehostvgw6.epnet.com/

American Psychiatric Association. (1994). Diagnostic and statistical manual of mental disorders (4th ed., rev.). Washington, DC: American Psychiatric Association.

Bailey, A., Phillips, W., & Rutter, M. (1996). Autism: Towards an integration of clinical, genetic, neuropsychological, and neurobiological perspectives. *Journal of Child Psychology and Psychiatry, 37,* 89–126.

Baron-Cohen, S. (1995). *Mindblindness: An essay on autism and theory of mind.* Cambridge, MA: MIT Press.

Baron-Cohen, S. (1998). Does the study of autism justify minimal innate modularity? *Learning and Individual Differences, 10*(3), 179.

Bartak, L., & Rutter, M. (1976). Differences between mentally retarded and normally intelligent autistic children. *Journal of Autism and Childhood Schizophrenia, 6,* 109–120.

Bartak, L., Rutter, M., & Cox, A. (1975). A comparative study of infantile autism and specific developmental receptive language disorder. 1. The children. *British Journal of Psychiatry, 126,* 127–145.

Bennett, T., DeLuca, D., & Bruns, D. (1997). Putting inclusion into practice: Perspectives of teacher and parents. *Exceptional Children, 64,* 115–131.

Bernard-Opitz, V. (1982). Pragmatic analysis of the communicative behavior of an autistic child. *Journal of Speech and Hearing Disorders, 47,* 99–109.

Bettelheim, B. (1967). *The empty fortress: Infantile autism and the birth of the self.* New York: Free Press.

Biklen, D. (1993). *Communication unbound: How facilitated communication is challenging traditional views of autism and ability/disability* (Special Education Series #13). New York: Teachers College Press.

Bishop, D., North, T., & Dolan, C. (1995). Genetic basis of specific language impairment: Evidence from a twin study. *Developmental Medicine and Child Neurology, 37,* 56–71.

Bloomquist, M., August, G., Cohen, C., Doyle, A., & Everhart, K. (1997). Social problem solving in hyperactive-aggressive children: How and what they think in conditions of automatic and controlled processing. *Journal of Clinical Child Psychology, 26*(2), 127–180.

Boomer, L. (1994). The utilization of paraprofessionals in programs for students with autism. *Focus on Autistic Behavior, 9*(2), 1.

Bornstein, M., & Brown, E. (1996). Patterns of stability and continuity in attention across early infancy. *Journal of Reproductive and Infant Psychology, 14*(3), 195.

Brinton, B., & Fujiki, M. (1993). Language, social skills and socioemotional behavior. *Language, Speech and Hearing Services in Schools, 24,* 194–198.

Brook, S., & Bowler, D. (1992). Autism by another name? Semantic and pragmatic impairments in children. *Journal of Autism and Development Disorders, 22,* 61–81.

Brown, W., & Odom, S. (1999). Ecobehavioral assessment in early childhood programs: A portrait of preschool inclusion. *Journal of Special Education, 33*(3), 138.

Bryson, S., Landry, R., & Smith, I. (1994). Brief report: A case study of literacy and socioemotional development in a mute autistic female. *Journal of Autism and Developmental Disorders, 24*(2), 225–230.

Cabey, M. (1994). Brief report: A controlled evaluation of facilitated communication using open-ended and fill-in questions. *Journal of Autism and Developmental Disorders, 24*(4), 517–526.

Cafiero, J. (1998). Communication power for individuals with autism. *Focus on Autism & Other Developmental Disabilities, 13*(2), 113.

Calculator, S. (1992). Perhaps the emperor has clothes after all: A response to Biklen (1992). *American Journal of Speech Language Pathology,* 18–20.

Calloway, C., Myles, B., & Earles, T. (1999). The development of communicative functions and means in students with autism. *Focus on Autism and Other Developmental Disabilities, 14*(3), 140.

Clark, D., & Smith, S. (1999). Facilitating friendships: Including students with autism in the early elementary classroom. *Intervention in School and Clinic, 34*(4), 248.

Conti-Ramsden, G., & Botting, N. (1999). Classification of children with specific language impairment: Longitudinal considerations. *Journal of Speech, Language and Hearing Research, 42*(5), 1195. Retrieved from the World Wide Web: http://www.ehostvgw6.epnet.com/

DeMyer, M., Barton, S., DeMyer, E., Norton, J., Allen, J., & Steele, R. (1973). Prognosis in autism: A follow-up study. *Journal of Autism and Childhood Schizophrenia, 3,* 199–216.

DiLavore, P., Lord, C., & Rutter, M. (1995). The Pre-linguistic Autism Diagnostic Observation Schedule. *Journal of Autism and Developmental Disorders, 25,* 355–379.

Duchan, J. (1993). Issues raised by facilitated communication for theorizing and research on autism. *Journal of Speech and Hearing Research, 36,* 1108–1119.

Eberlin, M., McConnachie, G., Ibel, S., & Volpe, L. (1993). Facilitated communication: A failure to replicate the phenomenon. *Journal of Autism and Developmental Disorders, 23*(3), 507–530.

Fish, B., Shapiro, T., & Campbell, M. (1966). Long-term prognosis and the response of schizophrenic children to drug therapy: A controlled study of trifluoperazine. *American Journal of Psychiatry, 123,* 32–39.

Folstein, S. (1999). Autism: Autistic children. *International Review of Psychiatry, 11*(4), 269.

Folstein, S., & Mankoski, R. (2000). Chromosome 7q: Where autism meets language disorder? *American Journal of Human Genetics, 67,* 278–281.

Frea, W., Craig, L., Odom, S., & Johnson, D. (1999). Differential effects of structured social integration and group friendship activities for promoting social interaction with peers. *Journal of Early Intervention, 22,* 230–242.

Gallagher, P. (1997). Promoting dignity: Taking the destructive D's out of behavior disorders. *Focus on Exceptional Children, 29*(9), 1–19.

Gallagher, T. (1996). Social-interactional approaches to child language intervention. In J. Beitchman and M. Konstatareas (Eds.), *Language, learning and behavior problems: Emerging perspectives* (pp. 418–435). Cambridge, UK: Cambridge University Press.

Gallagher, T. (1999). Interrelationships among children's language, behavior, and emotional problems. *Topics in Language Disorders, 19*(2), 1–15.

Gilger, J. (1995). Behavioral genetics: Concepts for research and practice in language development and disorders. *Journal of Speech and Hearing Research, 38*(5), 1126–1142. Retrieved from the World Wide Web: http://www.ehostvgw6.epnet.com/

Gillberg, C. (1990). Infantile autism: Diagnosis and treatment. *Acta Psychiatrica Scandanavica, 81,* 209–215.

Greenspan, S., & Wieder, S. (1997). Learning to interact. *Scholastic Early Childhood Today, 12*(3), 23–24.

Guralnick, M. (1999). The nature and meaning of social integration for young children with mild developmental delays in inclusive settings. *Journal of Early Intervention, 22,* 70–86.

Happe, F. (1994). *Autism: An introduction to psychological theory.* London: University College London Press.

Harn, W., Bradshaw, L., & Ogletree, B. (1999). The speech-language pathologist in the schools: Changing roles. *Intervention in School & Clinic, 34*(3), 163.

Harris, S., Handleman, J., Gordon, R., Kristoff, B., & Fuentes, F. (1991). Changes in cognitive and language functioning of preschool children with autism. *Journal of Autism and Developmental Disorders, 21,* 281–290.

Heflin, L., & Simpson, R. (1998). Interventions for children and youth with autism: Prudent choices in a world of exaggerated claims and empty promises. Part I: Intervention and treatment option review. *Focus on Autism and Other Developmental Disabilities, 13,* 194–211.

Hostler, S. (1996). Facilitated communication. *Pediatrics, 97*(4), 584.

Hughes, C., & Russell, J. (1993). Autistic children's difficulty with mental disengagement from an object: Its implications for theories of autism. *Developmental Psychology, 29*(3), 498–510.

Hurford, J. (1991). The evolution of the critical period for language acquisition. *Cognition, 40,* 159–201.

Individuals with Disabilities Education Act of 1997 (IDEA), 20 U.S.C. Sec. 1400 et seq.

Kanner, L. (1943). Autistic disturbances in affective contact. *Nervous Child, 2,* 217–250.

Kobayashi, R., & Murata, T. (1998). Behavioral characteristics of 187 young adults with autism. *Psychiatry and Clinical Neuroscience, 52,* 383–390.

Koegel, R., & Koegel, L. (1995). Teaching children with autism: Strategies for initiating positive interactions and improving learning opportunities. Baltimore: Paul H. Brookes.

Kohler, F., & Strain, P. (1997). Merging naturalistic teaching and peer-based strategies to address the IEP objectives of preschoolers with autism: An examination of structural and child behavior outcomes. *Focus on Autism and Other Development Disabilities, 12*(4), 196.

Krug, D., Arick, J., & Almond, P. (1993). Austim Screening Instrument for Educational Planning (2d ed.), Examiner's manual. Austin, TX: Pro-Ed.

Lainhart, J. (1999). Psychiatric problems in individuals with autism, their parents and siblings. *International Review of Psychiatry, 11*(4), 278.

Lewis, B., Cox, N., & Byard, P. (1993). Segregation analysis of speech and language disorders. *Behavior Genetics, 23,* 291–299.

Lifter, K., Sulzer-Azaroff, B., Anderson, S., & Cowdery, G. (1993). Teaching play activities to preschool children with disabilities: The importance of developmental considerations. *Journal of Early Intervention, 17*(2), 139–159.

Lord, C. (1995). Facilitating social inclusion. In E. Schopler and G. B. Mesibov (Eds.), *Learning and cognition in autism* (pp. 221–240). New York: Plenum.

Lord, C., Rutter, M., & LeCouteur, A. (1994). Autism Diagnostic Interview—Revised (ADI—R): A revised version of a diagnostic interview for caregivers of individuals with possible pervasive developmental disorders. *Journal of Autism and Developmental Disorders, 24,* 659–685.

Lotter, V. (1967). Epidemiology of autistic conditions in young children: Some characteristics of parents and children. *Social Psychiatry, 1,* 163–181.

Lovaas, O. (1999). Experimental design and cumulative research in early behavioral intervention. In *Johns Hopkins 20th Annual Spectrum in Developmental Disabilities.* Timonium, MD: York.

Lovaas, O., & Buch, G. (1997). Intensive behavioral intervention with young children with autism. In N. N. Singh (Ed.), *Prevention and treatment of severe behavior problems: Models and methods in developmental disabilities* (pp. 61–86). Pacific Grove, CA: Brooks/Cole.

Loveland, K., Landry, S., Hughes, S., Hall, S., & McEvoy, R. (1988). Speech acts and the pragmatic deficits of autism. *Journal of Speech and Hearing Research, 31,* 593–604.

Miller, J. (1996). The search for the phenotype of disordered language perfomance. In M. Rice (Ed.), *Toward a genetics of language* (pp. 297–314). Mahwah, NJ: Lawrence Erlbaum Associates.

Mirenda, P., & Schuler, A. (1988). Augmenting commenting for persons with autism: Issues and strategies. *Topics in Language Disorders, 9,* 24–43.

Mundy, P., Sigman, M., & Kasari, C. (1994). Nonverbal communication, developmental level and sympton presentation in autism. *Development and Psychopathology, 6,* 389–401.

Newsom, C., Carr, E., & Lovaas, O. (1979). The experimental analysis and modification of autistic behavior. In R. S. Davidson (Ed.), *Modification of pathological behavior.* New York: Gardener.

O'Connor, N., & Hermelin, B. (1994). Two autistic savant readers. *Journal of Autism and Developmental Disorders, 24*(4), 501–514.

Odom, S. (2000). Preschool inclusion: What we know and where we go from here. *Topics in Early Childhood Special Education, 20*(1), 20.

Odom, S., & Diamond, K. (1998). Inclusion of young children with special needs in early childhood education: The research base. *Early Childhood Research Quarterly, 13,* 3–25.

Odom, S., Horn, E., Marquart, J., Hanson, M., Wolfberg, P., Beckman, P., Lieber, J., Li, S., Schwartz, I., Janko, S., & Sandall, S. (1999). On the forms of inclusion: Organizational context and service delivery models. *Journal of Early Intervention, 22,* 185–199.

Odom, S., McConnell, S., McEvoy, M., Peterson, C., Ostrosky, M., Chandler, L., Spicuzza, R., Skellenger, A., Creighton, M., & Favazza, P. (1999). Relative effects of interventions supporting the social competence of young children with disabilities. *Topics in Early Childhood Special Education, 19,* 75–91.

Ogletree, B., & Fischer, M. (1995). An innovative language treatment for a child with high-functioning autism. *Focus on Autistic Behavior, 10*(3), 10.

Olley, J. (1999). Curriculum for students with autism. *School Psychology Review, 28*(1), 595.

Osterling, J., & Dawson, G. (1994). Early recognition of children with autism: A study of first birthday home videotapes. *Journal of Autism and Developmental Disorders, 24*(3), 247–256.

Ozonoff, S., Pennington, B., & Rogers, S. (1991). Executive function deficits in high-functioning autistic individuals: Relationship to theory of mind. *Journal of Child Psychology and Psychiatry, 32,* 1081–1105.

Patti, P., & Lupinetti, L. (1993). Brief report: Implications of hyperlexia in an autistic savant. *Journal of Autism and Developmental Disorders, 23*(2), 397–404.

Pennington, B., Rogers, S., Bennetto, L., Griffith, E., Reed, D., & Shyu, V. (1998). Validity test of the executive dysfunction hypothesis of autism. In J. Russell (Ed.), *Executive functioning in autism.* Oxford, UK: Oxford University Press.

Piaget, J. (1962). *Play, dreams, and imitation in childhood.* New York: Norton.

Pierce, K., & Schreibman, L. (1997). Using peer training to promote social behavior in autism: Are they effective at enhancing multiple social modalities? *Focus on Autism and Other Developmental Disabilities, 12*(4), 207.

Piven, J., Harper, J., Palmer, P., & Arndt, S. (1996). Course of behavioral changes in autism: A retrospective study of high-IQ adolescents and adults. *Journal of the American Academy of Child and Adolescent Psychiatry, 35*(4), 523–529.

Polansky, H. (1994). The meaning of inclusion. Is it an option or a mandate? *School Business Affairs, 66,* 27–29.

Prior, M., & Hoffmann, W. (1990). Brief report: Neuropsychological testing of autistic children through an exploration with frontal lobe tests. *Journal of Autism and Developmental Disorders, 20,* 581–590.

Prizant, B. (1983). Language acquisition and communicative behavior in autism: Toward an understanding of the "whole" of it. *Journal of Speech and Hearing Disorders, 46,* 241–249.

Prizant, B., Audet, L., Burke, G., Hummel, L., Maher, S., & Theadore, G. (1990). Communication disorders and emotional/behavioral disorders in children and adolescents. *Journal of Speech and Hearing Disorders, 55,* 179–192.

Prizant, B., & Duchan, J. (1981). The functions of immediate echolalia in autistic children. *Journal of Speech and Hearing Disorders, 46,* 241–249.

Prizant, B., & Rubin, E. (1999). Contemporary issues in interventions for autism spectrum disorders: A commentary. *Journal of the Association for Persons with Severe Handicaps, 24*(3), 199–208.

Prizant, B., & Rydell, P. (1984). Analysis of functions of delayed echolalia in autistic children. *Journal of Speech and Hearing Research, 27,* 183–192.

Prizant, B., & Wetherby, A. (1987). Communicative intent: A framework for understanding social-communicative behavior in autism. *Journal of the American Academy of Child and Adolescent Psychiatry, 26,* 472–479.

Risley, T. (1996). Get a life. In R. Koegel, L. Koegel, & G. Dunlap (Eds.), *Positive behavior support* (pp. 425–437). Baltimore: Paul H. Brookes.

Rock, E., Rosenberg, M., & Carran, D. (1995). Variables affecting the reintegration rate of students with serious emotional disturbance. *Exceptional Children, 61*(3), 254–268.

Rule, S., Losardo, A., Dinnebeil, L., Kaiser, A., & Rowland, C. (1998). Translating research on naturalistic instruction into practice. *Journal of Early Intervention, 21,* 283–293.

Russell, J. (1997). How executive disorders can bring about an inadequate theory of mind. In J. Russell (Ed.), *Autism as an executive disorder.* Oxford, UK: Oxford University Press.

Russell, J., Mauthner, N., Sharpe, S., & Tidswell, T. (1991). The "window task" as a measure of strategic deception in preschoolers and autistic subjects. *British Journal of Developmental Psychology, 9,* 331–349.

Schopler, E. (1995). *Parent survival manual: A guide to crisis resolution in autism and related developmental disorders.* New York: Plenum.

Schopler, E., Reichler, R., Bashford, A., Lansing, M., & Marcus, L. (1990). *Psychoeducational Profile Revised (PEP—R).* Austin, TX: Pro-Ed.

Schopler, E., Reichler, R., & Rennet, B. (1998). *The Childhood Autism Rating Scale (CARS).* Los Angeles, CA: Western Psychological Services.

Schwartz, I., & Carta, J. (1996). Examining the use of recommended language intervention practices in early childhood special education classrooms. *Topics in Early Childhood Special Education, 16*(2), 251.

Short, A., & Schopler, E. (1988). Factors relating to age of onset in autism. *Journal of Autism and Developmental Disorders, 18,* 207–216.

Shriver, M., Allen, K., & Mathews, J. (1999a). Effective assessment of the shared and unique characteristics of children with autism. *School Psychology Review, 28*(1), 538.

Shriver, M., Allen, K., & Mathews, J. (1999b). Introduction to the mini-series: Assessment and treatment of children with autism in the schools. *School Psychology Review, 28*(1), 535.

Sigman, M., & Ungerer, J. (1984). Cognitive and language skills in autistic, mentally retarded, and normal children. *Developmental Psychology, 20,* 293–302.

Simpson, R. (1995). Individualized Education Programs for students with autism: Including parents in the process. *Focus on Autistic Behavior, 10*(4), 11.

Stahmer, A. (1995). Teaching symbolic play skills to children with autism using pivotal response training. *Journal of Autism and Developmental Disorders, 25,* 123–141.

Strain, P., & Cordisco, L. (1994). LEAP preschool. In S. L. Harris and J. S. Handleman (Eds.), *Preschool education programs for children with autism* (pp. 225–244). Austin, TX: Pro-Ed.

Tager-Flusberg, H. (1999). A psychological approach to understanding the social and language impairments in autism. *International Review of Psychiatry, 11*(4), 235. Retrieved from the World Wide Web: http://www.ehostvgw6.epnet.com/

Taylor, B., & Levin, L. (1998). Teaching a student with autism to make verbal initiations: Effects of a tactile prompt. *Journal of Applied Behavior Analysis, 31*(4), 651–654.

Tiegerman-Farber, E. (1995). *Language and communication intervention in preschool children.* Boston: Allyn & Bacon.

Tiegerman-Farber, E., & Cartusciello-King, R. (1995). The classroom as language laboratory. In E. Tiegerman-Farber (Ed.), *Language and communication intervention in preschool children* (pp. 186–215). Boston: Allyn & Bacon.

Tiegerman-Farber, E., & Radziewicz, C. (1998). *Collaborative decision making: The pathway to inclusion.* Upper Saddle River, NJ: Prentice Hall.

Tirosh, E., & Canby, J. (1993). Autism with hyperlexia: A distinct syndrome? *American Journal on Mental Retardation, 98*(1), 84–92.

Wagner, A., & Lockwood, S. (1994). Pervasive developmental disorders: Dilemmas in diagnosing very young children. *Infants and Young Children, 6*(4), 21–32.

Wehman, T. (1998). Family-centered early intervention services: Factors contributing to increased parent involvement. *Focus on Autism & Other Developmental Disabilities, 13*(2), 80.

Wetherby, A., & Gaines, B. (1982). Cognition and language development in autism. *Journal of Speech and Hearing Research, 47,* 63–71.

Windsor, J., & Doyle, S. (1994). Language acquisition after mutism: A longitudinal case study of autism. *Journal of Speech and Hearing Research, 37*(1), 96.

Wing, L. (1997). The autistic spectrum. *Lancet, 350,* 1761.

Wisniewski, L., & Alpert, S. (1994). Including students with severe disabilities in general education settings. *Remedial and Special Education, 15*(1), 4–13.

Wolery, M., & Winterling, V. (1997). Curricular approaches to controlling severe behavior problems. In N. N. Singh (Ed.), *Prevention and treatment of severe behavior problems: Models and methods in developmental disabilities* (pp. 87–120). Pacific Grove, CA: Brooks/Cole.

Wolfberg, P., & Schuler, A. (1993). Integrated play groups: A model for promoting the social and cognitive dimensions of play in children with autism. *Journal of Autism and Developmental Disorders, 23*(3), 467–488.

Wolk, L., & Edwards, M. (1993). The emerging phonological system of an autistic child. *Journal of Communication Disorders, 26,* 161–177.

Yell, M., & Drasgow, E. (2000). Litigating a free appropriate public education: The Lovaas hearings and cases. *Journal of Special Education, 33*(4), 205.

12

Christine Radziewicz
School for Language and Communication Development

Susan Antonellis
St. John's University

Considerations and Implications for Habilitation of Hearing-Impaired Children

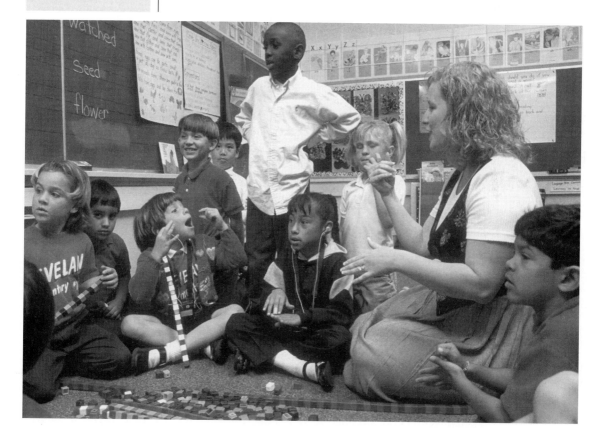

....

When you finish this chapter you should be able to

....

- Define and explore the type, classification and degree of hearing loss
- Discuss the efforts of the government and professionals toward early identification of hearing loss and the parent's role in this cause
- Explore the intricate details of an audiological evaluation and discuss each parameter that encompasses it, including otoacoustic emission testing
- Consider the adjustments and special tests needed in preparing for the pediatric evaluation
- Identify the proper management needed after diagnosis of hearing loss, whether it be a permanent sensorineural hearing loss or a temporary conductive hearing loss
- Understand the educational needs of the hearing impaired, including reading, written language, whole language, sign language, and bilingualism
- Discuss the mainstreaming option and its impact on the hearing-impaired child
- Identify several techniques that facilitate successful inclusion of preschool hearing-impaired children with normal hearing peers
- Identify challenges to family-professional collaboration related to cultural diversity and socioeconomic status
- Identify those factors successful in inclusion of school-aged hearing-impaired children in regular educational settings
- Identify those factors that put hearing-impaired children at educational risk
- Identify the differences between mainstreaming and inclusion

The identification and rehabilitation of a child with a hearing impairment is an enormous and important task. Research and recent government legislation has certainly confirmed the importance of early identification along with the profound effects of chronic otitis media on speech and language.

Rehabilitating children with hearing impairments encompasses the instrumentation, the methods, and the follow-up. Technology has miniaturized the amplification systems available and opened up fitting choices with the latest computer software. We have gone from the bulky body aid to the completely-in-the canal aid, from the hardwire induction loop to the personal FM unit, and from preschool screening to otoacoustic emissions on neonates.

The educational setting has also changed for hearing-impaired children. In the past, education routinely took place in residential schools for the deaf. Today, children with hearing impairments are more often educated in regular classrooms, exercising the inclusion option.

Educating children with hearing impairments has been accomplished through either an aural/oral approach or an approach incorporating manually coded English. Over the last thirty years a tremendous body of research has been accumulated highlighting the advantages of each. An aural/oral approach incorporates speech and speechreading as the primary communication channels. The total communication approach incorporates manual communication or sign language with speech and speechreading. In 1979 Jordan, Gustason, and Rosen reported that approximately 65 percent of deaf children in the United States were taught using some combination of manual and oral communication. Today, however, with hearing-impaired children being identified earlier and cochlear implantation more accessible, this may no longer be the case. There is a trend for implanted children to be mainstreamed into regular education settings earlier. Support services may or may not include manual communication interpreting.

TYPE, CLASSIFICATION, AND DEGREE OF HEARING LOSS

Hearing loss should be considered in terms of type, classification, and degree. Hearing loss falls into three types: conductive hearing loss, sensorineural hearing loss, and mixed hearing loss. This section describes each of these types, then presents a classification system used to define degree of loss.

Conductive Hearing Loss

Conductive hearing loss results from any barrier to sound present in the outer ear or middle ear (Martin & Clark, 2000); the inner ear functions normally. Conductive hearing loss never exceeds a hearing threshold of 60 decibels (dB) (hearing thresholds are discussed shortly) and is generally medically treatable. A common disorder found in children associated with conductive impairment is otitis media. Otitis media is defined as inflammation of the middle ear resulting predominantly from eustachian tube dysfunction (Stach, 1997). Medically, otitis media needs to be looked at more specifically. *Acute* otitis media is an active inflammation and/or infection of the middle ear space. The presence of a bulging tympanic membrane is evidence of acute otitis media. *Serous* otitis media is the presence of a thin, watery, clear fluid in the middle ear space and is usually an early sign of eustachian tube dysfunction. *Chronic* otitis media is an infection of the middle ear space with purulent fluid (pus) persisting beyond the time limit of acute otitis media. Also, whereas acute otitis media can be quite painful and develop over a short period of time, chronic otitis media is not generally accompanied by pain and therefore can go untreated. *Secretory* otitis media refers to a condition associated with a thick, gluelike fluid found in the middle ear space.

Chronic otitis media has its effects in the early childhood years, most often during the critical years of speech and language development. Chronic otitis media is linked with fluctuating hearing loss ranging anywhere from 10 to 40 dB. Presumably, hearing will return to normal after the episode is over. Because otitis media occurs most frequently during the first 3 years of life, it can have a dramatic effect on speech and language during these years. It is during these years that "the infant moves from being a communicator to being a competent (although not fully competent) user of the speech and language categories of the language" (Menyuk, 1986).

Conductive hearing loss can also occur as a result of a totally blocked air conductive pathway, as in atresia, stenosis, complete stapes fixation, or ossicular discontinuity.

Sensorineural Hearing Loss

Sensorineural hearing loss results from damage to the sensory end organ, the cochlear hair cells, or the auditory nerve (damage may have occurred during development of the ear, from injury of infection, from individual environment, or from the degenerative effects of aging). Sensorineural hearing losses may easily be overlooked upon physical examination, because the external auditory canal and tympanic membrane will appear normal. This type of hearing loss is not medically treatable and is almost always irreversible.

Mixed Hearing Loss

Mixed hearing loss can occur in children as well as adults. It is a problem that occurs simultaneously in both the conductive and sensorineural mechanisms. This results in a loss via bone conduction due to the sensorineural component and an even greater loss of sensitivity by air conduction.

Classification System

The following is a audiometric scale, suggested by Martin and Clark (2000), for defining hearing loss. This scale also can be used to describe the degree of hearing loss and refers to the ANSI-1996 scale.

Pure Tone Average	Degree
−10 to 15 dB	None
16 to 25 dB	Slight
26 to 40 dB	Mild
41 to 55 dB	Moderate
56 to 70 dB	Moderately severe
71 to 90 dB	Severe
91 dB +	Profound

Intensity of sound is measured in decibels (dB). Hearing is also affected by the frequency of the sound wave; higher-pitched sounds have higher frequencies (measured in hertz, Hz). This classification system is based on a pure tone average, that is, the average of the thresholds of 500, 1,000, and 2,000 Hz, respectively. These frequencies, commonly known as the **speech frequencies,** are known to be important for hearing speech. Pure tone thresholds are discussed more fully later in this chapter.

HEARING LOSS AND LANGUAGE DEVELOPMENT

Describing the speech and language behaviors of children with hearing impairments is a difficult task. Various factors influence the development of language in the presence of hearing loss (Quigley & Kretschmer, 1982). These variables include

- Degree of hearing loss
- Age of onset of loss
- Slope of hearing loss
- Age of identification of hearing loss
- Age of habilitation

- Amount of habilitation
- Type of habilitation

As noted, degree of hearing loss refers to the severity of the hearing loss and is easily measured. According to Knauf (1972), the hearing threshold is frequently the first measurement available for estimating the impact of the child's hearing impairment. In the past, it was generally assumed that the greater would be the hearing loss, the greater the impact on speech and language development. Although a severe hearing loss of 71 to 90 or 95 dB does have a devastating effect on speech and language development, we cannot assume that a mild hearing loss of 26 to 40 dB will always have a minimal effect or that a profound loss of 96 dB or above will have the most detrimental effect on speech and language development.

To emphasize this point, Northern (1984) referred to the case report of a 13-year-old patient who had suffered from frequent bouts of otitis media. Over a period of 7 years, from age 6 to age 13, the air conduction thresholds fluctuated from normal to mild to moderate levels. Over the 7 years, five myringotomies were performed. However, the child's repeated attacks of serous otitis media resulted in a progressive sensorineural hearing loss with bone conduction thresholds of 25 dB at 4,000 Hz in one ear and 30 and 45 dB at 2,000 Hz and 4,000 Hz in the other ear. In this case, not only the degree of hearing loss but also the age of onset, the age of identification, and the type of habilitation were critical factors affecting the severity of the language deficit. Although this child's loss was not discovered until the age of 6, he probably had suffered from chronic otitis media earlier in his life. Age of onset could have occurred more than 5 years before age of identification and therefore could have included the critical language learning years. Furthermore, habilitation involved surgical myringotomies without habilitative speech and language therapy. Northern concluded his description of this case by stating that when the 13-year-old patient was given a hearing aid for habilitation, it was already 13 years too late. This child was evidencing a delay in speech and language that was irreversible.

The degree of hearing loss, although the most salient variable, is not necessarily the most critical. The combination and interplay of all the aforementioned variables determine the effect of hearing loss on speech and language development. Because of the interdependency of variables, one can never predict with certainty the detrimental effects of hearing loss on speech and language from degree of impairment alone. The only certainty is that hearing loss in any form (conductive, sensorineural, or mixed) and of any degree (mild to profound) can have a devastating effect on speech and language development.

IDENTIFICATION AND HABILITATION

Early identification of hearing loss and the delivery of appropriate services are critical factors in the habilitation of children with hearing impairments. Because language development begins at the time a child is born, there is an urgent need for an organized infant screening procedure to identify those infants who may have hearing losses. Identification of hearing-impaired infants can be facilitated through neonatal screenings of infants with a high risk of hearing loss. In 1997 the National Institute on Deafness and Other Communication Disorders (NIDCD) Workshop on Universal Newborn Hearing Screening was held in Maryland. This group recommended that universal newborn hearing screenings be conducted in the United States. To date, thirty-two states have enacted legislation that provides universal hearing screening to newborns. This leaves eighteen states plus the District of Columbia without any newborn hearing screening provisions. Approximately two to three children per 1,000 children born in the United States are born with significant hearing impairment. Given the annual birth rate of approximately 4 million infants per year, this translates into thirty-three children per day born with hearing impairment. At present, many such children are not identified until their second year of life or even later. This delay in identification results in a significant negative impact on spoken language, academic performance, and vocational choices. If newborn children are screened for hearing loss in hospital nurseries before discharge, there will be a greater likelihood that a child with a hearing impairment will enjoy academic, social and vocational success (NIDCD, 1997). Yoshinaga-Itano and Apuzzo (1998b) conducted a study in Colorado and found that language development is significantly delayed when a hearing loss is not identified until after a child is 6 months of age. If infants do not receive hearing screenings shortly after birth and while still in the hospital, there is a good likelihood that if these children have a hearing impairment it will not be identified until long after 6 months of age. In another study by Yoshinaga-Itano and Apuzzo (1998a) it was found that children who were identified with a hearing loss before 6 months of age and who received early home intervention performed significantly better in measurements of expressive language, comprehension of language, and development of concepts than children who were identified after 6 months of age.

Early Parent–Infant Interaction

Early language development of the infant with normal hearing has been of great interest to researchers. These investigations have shown that normal-hearing children have a basic capacity for perceiving speech behaviors in the environment and also are sensitive to the social and affective aspects of the context of language (Eimas, 1974; Miller & Morse, 1976; Miller, Morse, & Dorman, 1977; Morse, 1972). Bloom and Lahey (1978) have stated that one of the precursors of language use occurs when infants begin to exchange gaze and vocalizations with their mothers. Bateson (1975) also described this mutual gaze or eye contact between mother and infant and called it protoconversation. Jaffe, Stern, and Peery (1973) studied the infant–mother dyad and found mother–infant gazing to be analogous to the rhythms of adult dialogue. Behaviors such as these are all continuous with eventual development of speech and language, which begins in the second year of life. Although infants with hearing impairments do not have the perceptual capabilities to receive and discriminate speech sounds as well as children with normal hearing, they do have a residual amount of hearing that allows for some discrimination when amplification is used. In addition, they are able to extract the social and affective aspects of the context of language (Bloom & Lahey, 1978).

Brown (1975) stated that the most important form of concept learning for the infant is probably socially mediated. The first social contact of the infant is the parents. They are the most responsible for the development of the behaviors that lead to language growth in the normally developing child, and they are the major forces in the habilitation of the hearing impaired child. Because studies have demonstrated that mothers of normal hearing children play a vital role in the development in speech and language, it becomes obvious that mothers of hearing-impaired infants play an even more crucial role.

Greenstein, Bush, McConville, and Stellini (1977) examined the mother–infant communication dyad and its effect on language acquisition in infants with hearing impairments. They found that affective aspects of mother–infant interaction were central to the language acquisition of the hearing-impaired child. All other aspects of the mother's language input to the child were far less significant than the existence of a good mother–infant bond. This bond frequently was broken by the mother's discovery of the child's hearing impairment. Vorce (1974) believed that the social relationships that exist between the mother and child stimulate the infant's early vocalizations, and therefore this relationship should be emphasized.

Because speech and language development begins with the earliest social exchanges between mother and infant, and because the affective aspects of mother–infant interaction are crucial to future language acquisition, programs that enhance mother–infant communication are invaluable in effective intervention for children with hearing impairments. Parent–infant programs, first developed during the 1970s, educate parents about their critical role in the development of their hearing-impaired child. Parents are taught to make everyday experiences language-enhancing experiences. They learn to understand the implications of hearing impairment on speech and language development and how to deal with their feelings about the hearing loss in their child. Furthermore, they are taught how to incorporate auditory training into the child's daily life and how to employ language learning strategies when they are interacting with their child. Parent and infant come to the parent–infant center at least once a week for training, and the teacher/speech-language pathologist makes weekly visits to the home. Parents frequently meet with other professionals such as psychologists and audiologists for additional training and support.

The teacher/speech-language pathologist employs a variety of training techniques. For example, videotapes have been used in many ways to enhance communication between parents and hearing-impaired infants. Cole and St. Clair-Stokes (1984) analyzed videotaped caregiver–child interactions to identify interactive behaviors promoting development of early language. Radziewicz (1985) used videotapes as a technique to train parents to incorporate more effective communicative behaviors in their interactions with their infants. The use of videotapes has resulted in clearer understanding of hearing loss and more appropriate communicative interactions.

When hearing-impaired children and their parents are enrolled in a parent–infant program, that child's education begins during the critical speech and language learning years. Intervention during the first year increases the child's chances of developing more typical speech and language. Parents can gain insights into management and effective communication behaviors that will facilitate language development in their child. They can be trained to model and develop interactive language learning opportunities during all their parent–child interactions. Recent research has emphasized the degree to which parents and infants respond to and influence each others' behaviors (Koester & Meadow-Orlans, 1999). Parents and children have individual temperament patterns, and these patterns can have either positive or negative impacts on the child's development (Chess & Thomas, 1996). Early infant behavioral characteristics such as repetitive motor activity and eye gaze behaviors are ways an infant communicates. Parents need to be trained early to interpret behaviors as well as shape them into communicative interactions. As the child grows and develops, the parents learn how to make each and every activity a language learning experience for their deaf child. As the parents become more skilled in enhancing language development, their children develop more language.

In today's multicultural society, children from diverse cultural communities are frequently identified as having language disorders. It is important that bilingual evaluators and interpreters be used when evaluating these children. However, once these children are identified, it is imperative that the parents and professionals participate when developing Individualized Education Plans (IEPs) and Individualized Family Service Plans (IFSPs). When large differences—such as socioeconomic status and differences in values and beliefs—exist between families and professionals, this collaborative partnership becomes more fragile and poses challenges to all team members. For early intervention to be successful, the early interventionist must work on everyday activities that are part of the family's cultural customs and must be viewed by the family as appropriate. The extent to which the family has been exposed to the customs of the dominant society will determine the level of conflicts that may occur between the family and the professionals working with them (Hanson et al., 1990). A recent study by DeGangi, Wietlisbach, Poisson, Stein, and Royeen (1994) identified the challenges to family–professional collaboration related to cultural diversity and socioeconomic status (SES). It was found that families from lower SES and educational backgrounds often were concerned with basic survival needs and deferred to professional judgments when setting goals; had difficulty identifying their child's needs; and showed reluctance in sharing information. With all this in mind, it is imperative that professionals working collaboratively with families recognize the impact of culture and socioeconomic status on the collaborative process.

AUDIOLOGICAL ASSESSMENT

The routine audiological evaluation consists of pure tone findings, speech audiometry yielding speech reception thresholds and speech discrimination scores, and aural acoustic immittance testing. Because not all testing procedures can be used with very young children, pediatric evaluation is considered separately.

Pure Tone Findings

The search for accurate pure tone thresholds is no small feat, particularly with small children. Before the options and procedures for finding threshold are discussed, it is necessary to define threshold. A **pure tone threshold** is the level at which the tone is so soft that it can be perceived only 50 percent of the time it is presented (Stach, 1997).

Two techniques are used to measure threshold. In the ascending method, the person being tested is exposed to stimuli that range from inaudible to audible. In the descending method, the stimuli go from audible to inaudible. In determining pure tone threshold by air conduction, proper earphone placement is essential. The diaphragm of the earphone must be placed directly over the opening of the external canal. If placement is not secure, test results could be invalid.

Having discussed threshold and the method for obtaining the result, consider the step-by-step procedure in obtaining the pure tone findings:

1. Instruct patient to respond when a tone is heard, even if the tone is very soft.
2. Place the earphones on the head of the patient with proper positioning as discussed previously. A specific earphone is used for the right and left ears.
3. Test the better ear first, in case masking is needed.
4. Start with a 1,000-Hz tone and allow the patient to hear what it sounds like; that is, present the tone at an audible level for the patient.
5. Find threshold at 1,000-Hz by presenting the signal using an "up 5, down 10" method.
6. Use the same procedure for the other audiometric frequencies, following this order: 2,000, 4,000, 8,000, 500, and 250 Hz.
7. Follow the same procedure for the second ear, but do not start at 1,000 Hz.
8. Plot each threshold obtained on the audiogram (see Figure 12.1).
9. Find the pure tone average of each ear (average 500, 1,000, and 2,000 Hz).
10. Conduct bone conduction testing in the same manner, using the bone oscillator. Proper placement of the oscillator on the mastoid process is important for accuracy.

Speech Audiometry

The speech audiometry portion of the audiological evaluation consists primarily of determining the speech recognition threshold, speech detect threshold, and the word recognition score.

The **speech recognition threshold** (SRT) typically refers to the threshold level of speech, which is the lowest level (in decibels) at which the listener is able to identify approximately 50 percent of spondaic words (Stach, 1997).

The SRT is administered by having the patient hear examples of test words through the earphones. This test can be performed with live voice or a recorded speech signal. The pure tone average of each ear allows the technician to choose an audible level to begin the test procedure.

Speech audiometry has been used in pediatric audiologic assessment for many purposes. As a stimulus, speech has been found to be useful with infants and young children because it has high interest value and a complex spectrum (Gravel & Hood, 1999).

The second portion of speech testing is the evaluation of the speech recognition score. This test is a significant one, because a common complaint is "I hear, but I

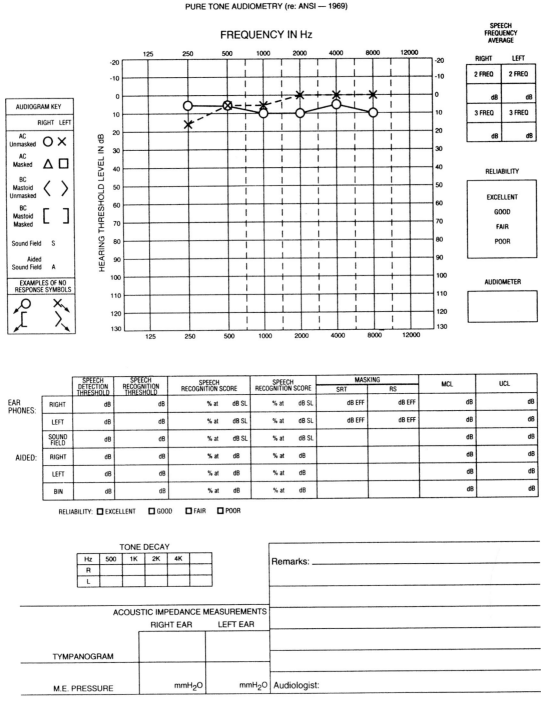

FIGURE 12.1

Pure Tone Thresholds Plotted on Audiogram

don't understand." **Word recognition** is a measure of the ability to perceive and identify a word, word discrimination, and word intelligibility (Stach, 1997).

Aural Acoustic Immittance Testing

In view of the major role the middle ear plays in audiological diagnosis, the importance of aural acoustic immittance testing must be considered.

Aural acoustic immittance testing is an essential piece of the audiological assessment. It consists of tympanometry, acoustic reflexes, and eustachian tube evaluation. For our purposes, we will not discuss eustachian tube evaluation at this time.

Tympanometry is the procedure used in the assessment of middle ear function in which the immittance of the tympanic membrane and middle ear is measured as air pressure delivered to the ear canal is varied (Stach, 1997). Tympanometry testing produces a chart of results called a tympanogram. Figure 12.2 illustrates several possible tympanogram results:

1. Type A tympanogram—normal tympanic membrane.
2. Type B tympanogram—middle ear effusion, patent ventilating tubes, or perforation.
3. Type C tympanogram—eustachian tube dysfunction, retracted tympanic membrane; effusion may be present.
4. Type A_s tympanogram—stiff tympanic membrane.
5. Type A_d tympanogram—flaccid tympanic membrane or ossicular discontinuity.

It is important in looking at a tympanogram that we observe three parameters: pressure (*x* axis), amplitude (*y* axis), and shape. Pressure is measured in milliliters of H_2O, which creates either positive or negative pressure within the canal (see Figure 12.2).

The **acoustic reflex** is the reflexive contraction of the intra-aural muscles (tensor tympani and stapedius) in response to loud sound, dominated by the stapedius muscle in humans (Stach, 1999). The diagnostic significance of the acoustic reflex lies in helping detect the presence or absence of pathology. One pathology to consider is middle ear pathology, which is the most common. Others are central pathology and nonorganic hearing loss.

It is apparent in this discussion of pure tone findings, speech audiometry, and aural acoustic immittance testing that the audiological evaluation consists of a network of intricate pieces that produce a holistic picture of the auditory system of an individual.

Pediatric Evaluation

Early detection of hearing loss in an infant is imperative, yet this is not an easy task. Although the audiological evaluation can yield a wealth of information about an individual's auditory system, many of the tests described cannot be successfully administered to the infant or preschooler. In view of this, it is necessary to discuss options in the evaluation process for the young pediatric population.

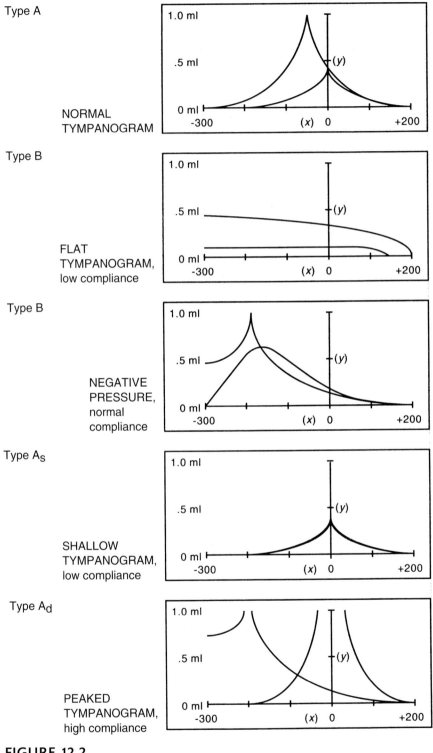

FIGURE 12.2

Possible Tympanogram Results

Note: x axis = air pressure; y axis = compliance.

First and foremost, a discussion with the parents and people closely associated with the child before actual testing plays an important role in the audiological assessment. Second, the clinician needs to establish a pleasant relationship with the child.

As the degree of diagnostic difficulty increases, the input from these individuals is important. Parents, care providers, teachers, and therapists can provide valuable insights (Gravel & Hood, 1999).

The "cross-check principle" has worked in our profession over the years, evolving from the work of Jerger and Hayes in 1976. This principle states that the results of any single audiometric test cannot be considered valid without independent verification from another test (Gravel & Hood, 1997). Technology has certainly added a new dimension to the pediatric evaluation, but one measure alone should not be used to assess a child's hearing.

Many factors can affect pediatric assessment, including otitis media. As stated previously, the tympanometry portion of the evaluation must be considered when interpreting audiological findings.

Behavioral Assessment

According to Gravel and Hood (1999), behavioral assessment is useful for two purposes. When used for audiometric purposes, behavioral methods should provide a means for quantifying hearing sensitivity—determining thresholds across the speech range (minimum 500–4,000 Hz). When used for functional purposes, the auditory assessment is used to examine the child's auditory behaviors qualitatively, determining whether they are typical for age.

Infants (Birth to Age Two)

Testing of infants requires an adequate sound room, a quiet state, and measured stimuli (Northern & Downs, 1984). It is appropriate to seat the mother with the baby in her lap in the middle of the sound room. The audiologist should get the baby's attention straight ahead by moving a toy back and forth. Next, a noisemaker is introduced without the baby seeing it. Responses to watch for are eye widening, eyes turning, a rapid eye blink, and, if the child is at least 4 months old, a rudimentary head turn. At about 5 to 7 months, the infant will turn her head toward the side of a signal. The audiologist continues this procedure using speech stimuli and warble tones. As the child reaches 9 months, the audiologist can obtain a speech awareness threshold by repeating a phrase such as "Bye-bye Amy," slowly reducing the level of presentation until the child ceases to respond. As the child's age increases, additions are made to the evaluation process. For example, the child may be asked to recognize or point to familiar pictures.

Children (Ages Two to Five)

The procedure known as play conditioning can be used for children 2 to 5 years old. The 2-year-old will probably need to sit in his mother's lap for the procedure, but the 4- or 5-year-old most likely can sit alone. The audiologist introduces the procedure as a game, using motivational toys such as pegs or building blocks. The peg or block is placed in the child's hand, and the child is instructed to listen for a little sound (presented in the sound field). When a sound is heard, the child is guided in putting the peg into a bucket or box. Once the child can do the task alone, the sounds can be presented to the child through earphones. This procedure is followed for pure tones, as discussed in the "Audiological Assessment" portion of this chapter. It is necessary to move rapidly with small children, because their attention span is generally short.

Speech audiometry can be accomplished through various picture pointing tasks. Objective testing, such as auditory brainstem response audiometry (ABR), is most assistive in diagnosing the difficult-to-test child. This testing includes responses observed by way of electrical impulses of the cerebral cortex. Responses are recorded on a graph.

Otoacoustic Emissions

The twentieth century has brought with it the birth of otoacoustic emissions. In 1978, Kemp made an extraordinary discovery, using the simple technique of coupling a small microphone to the external ear canal and recording the sound present in the canal during and after the presentation of click stimuli. Kemp's microphone system was similar to that used in clinical immittance instruments. Kemp's observations revealed that low-intensity sounds could be detected in the ear canal for several milliseconds after the presentation of each click. The procedure is similar to the way auditory brainstem responses are obtained. These sounds provided a quick view of the cochlea's active response to sound, a response that involves the addition of energy to that provided by the stimulus arriving at the ear. Outer hair cells are thought to play a major role. Kemp's recordings represent one form of emission of acoustic energy from the cochlea. Collectively, these sounds are known as **otoacoustic emissions** (OAE) (Glattke & Kujawa, 1991).

Otoacoustic emissions are particularly important in evaluating infants who are free of external and/or middle ear pathology (Lafraniere, Smurzynski, Jung, Leonard, & Kim, 1993). Measurement of the OAE in the external ear canal, regardless of the type of OAE, is dependent on the integrity of the middle ear system as well as the cochlea. Emissions amplitude increases from newborn to ages of 1 to 9 months, while decreases in amplitude have been observed in children ages 4 to 13 years (Widen, 1997). Although OAE testing is a very sensitive measure of cochlea function and plays an important role in the early identification and diagnosis of dysfunction in the pediatric population, this test is not a test of hearing and cannot replace the audiogram (Hall, 2000).

AUDIOLOGICAL MANAGEMENT

Diagnosis of a child with a hearing loss is only the beginning. A child with a hearing impairment must have adequate audiological management to be successful educationally, psychologically, and socially.

Amplification Devices

When a family first learns that their child is hearing impaired, the primary concern is: "What can be done? What physician do we see?" The child first must be seen by an otolaryngologist to provide medical clearance for amplification. The audiologist then conducts an ongoing evaluation to find the appropriate type of amplification for the individual child. In the young child, it can take anywhere from 6 months to 1 year before a final fitting is decided. In the interim, the child may be fitted with a loaner hearing aid.

A hearing aid is an electronic amplifier that has three main components: a microphone, an amplifier, and a loudspeaker (Stach, 1998). All hearing aids are powered by a battery.

There are various types of amplification, ranging from the body aid to the canal aid and from the linear circuit to the digital signal processing circuit.

- *Body aid.* About the size of a pocket radio, the body aid is connected to an earmold in the ear by a receiver wire. In the past, only a body aid could provide adequate power to benefit those with more than a moderate hearing loss. Today, amplifiers with high power can be fit into a small space and the body aid is used rarely; however, due to its large size, it still provides more power than other hearing aid types, and more flexibility as far as circuitry and controls. Most people who use a body aid are fitted monaurally (one ear).
- *Behind-the-ear Aid.* The behind-the-ear (BTE) hearing aid is also known as the postauricular hearing aid. This type of aid rests over and behind the pinna and has a plastic earhook at one end near the receiver. A small piece of plastic tubing connects the hook to the earmold. The BTE hearing aid also provides flexibility as far as circuitry and control options.
- *Eyeglass aid.* The eyeglass aid is not as popular as it was years ago; in fact, it accounts for few hearing aid sales today. The components of the hearing aid are built into the temples of the eyeglasses, and a small metal pin holds the plastic tubing connected to the earmold.
- *CROS (contralateral routing of signal) aid.* This type of hearing aid is designed for unilateral loss, in which a microphone is placed on the poor ear, and the signal is routed to a hearing aid on the better ear (Stach, 1997). The CROS aid can be obtained as an in-the-ear aid, a behind-the-ear aid, or an eyeglass aid. These instruments are recommended for people who have an ear that is unaidable. A variation of this aid is the BiCROS (bilateral contralateral routing of signal).
- *In-the-ear/canal aid.* The in-the-ear aid was the most popular form in the 1990s. Modern technology and miniaturization have allowed for more power in a small space. This type of hearing aid holds all components in one shell. Many people choose this type of hearing aid for cosmetic reasons. In-the-ear instruments are not always the best choice for small children, however, because the ear grows rapidly and modifications are needed more often.
- *Completely-in-the canal (CIC) aid.* As the in-the-ear hearing aid and the canal hearing aid have been the most popular amplification used, we now have the emergence of the CIC hearing aid. This type of hearing aid requires a deep air impression and produces a hearing aid that is completely in the canal and virtually invisible.

As we have seen growth in miniaturization, we are also seeing sophisticated new circuitry options. These come under the basic categories known as programmable and digital hearing aid technology.

Programmable technology gives the user flexible control of hearing aid characteristics and multiple memories for programming various parameters for different situations—for example, the child at home doing homework in a quiet room versus the child listening for directions in a noisy lunchroom.

Digital technology provides more exact and flexible frequency shaping, better feedback reduction, more complex compression parameters, and enhanced noise reduction.

Hearing aids open a new world to the hearing-impaired child, but some problems can occur with the use of a hearing aid. Common problems are acoustic feedback, distorted signal, intermittent signal, noisy sound, or hearing aid dysfunction. Because these problems do exist, audiological follow-up is important.

Cochlear Implants

Children who cannot benefit from conventional amplification are good candidates for cochlear implants. The first reports on this technology were not promising; the most encouraging results were that speech signals were perceived as speech, but were not intelligible. As research progressed, however, and as the sophistication of signal processing increased, reports of patients with good—sometimes markedly improved—speech recognition abilities surfaced.

Cochlear implants provide auditory sensations by electrically stimulating residual nerve fibers in the ears of the profoundly deaf, and the most important function is to provide some level of speech recognition for the user. Various designs are available that perform the task of representing speech signals as electrical stimuli (Tartter, Hellman, & Chute, 1992). Stach (1997) states that the strategies for cochlear implants are numerous and complex, but all are based on extracting frequency intensity and temporal cues from the speech signals and translating them to the electrode array in a manner that can be effectively processed by the residual neurons of the auditory nerve.

Auditory Trainers

In addition to hearing aids and cochlear implants, various other assistive devices can give extra help to a child with a hearing loss, particularly in the educational setting. Auditory trainers operate like a hearing aid and are used in the classroom or at a particular site as a training device. Because they are used collectively on site, size and appearance are not important considerations. Their large size enables them to be equipped with larger components and special circuitry that produce better fidelity.

There are four basic types of auditory trainer systems: desk trainers, hardwire units, induction loop units, and FM units.

- *Desk trainers.* The desk trainer is built into a case and is usually found on the student's desk. The components are distributed in the case. The child can carry the desk trainer from one location to another. A disadvantage of the device is that its signal-to-noise ratio (the ratio between the intensity of the signal and the intensity of the noise present) is poor if there is a distance between the teacher and the student. These trainers are beneficial in training sessions with one child but are not particularly recommended in a classroom of hearing-impaired children.

- *Hardwire units.* Hardwire units are also placed on children's desks, and each child has an individual volume control. The signal-to-noise ratio is good because the teacher speaks directly into a microphone. A disadvantage of hardwire units is that they are not portable.

- *Induction loop unit.* The loop system involves a wire loop around the room, installed under carpeting or under the floor. It conducts electrical energy from an amplifier, then creates a magnetic field; current flow from the loop is induced in the induction coil at the hearing aid telecoil (Stach, 1997). Each child in the room wears a hearing aid in the telephone position. The telephone coil in the hearing aid will pick up the signal and present it to the ear. The signal-to-noise ratio is excellent, but children can hear only the teacher and not the other children or themselves. Today, there are hearing aids available with a switch in which the microphone and telephone setting can be used simultaneously. The loop system is flexible within the room itself.

- *FM units.* A wireless unit, the FM auditory trainer is the most widely used trainer. The teacher wears a microphone-transmitter, and the child wears an FM receiver with the hearing aid. The teacher transmits directly to the child's unit on a frequency-modulated radio carrier wave. The signal-to-noise ratio is generally good. Ross (1987) stated: "In my judgement, the advent of the FM Auditory Training System has been the most significant educational tool for the average hearing-impaired child since the initial appearance of modern hearing aids. Indeed, historically, they may be the most powerful such tool we've ever had."

Other Considerations in Audiological Management

Audiological management does not end with the fitting of a hearing aid or the use of an auditory trainer. A child who is hearing impaired needs to be monitored and followed throughout the educational years.

A child suffering from conductive hearing loss due to acute otitis media needs to be monitored as well as a child exhibiting a sensorineural hearing loss. Because of the high incidence of otitis media in young children, Feagans (1986) recommended that daycare centers be places for early intervention and follow-up. The model she recommended contains four components:

1. Workshops for staff to educate them on the high incidence and long-term effects of otitis media
2. Routine hearing screenings to determine thresholds, in addition to ear checks by professionals
3. Routine developmental assessments, including a battery of cognitive, attention, and language measures, for children who have persistent recurrences of otitis media
4. Intervention, including training in sustained attention to language, and reorganization of day care setting and structure, including modification of classrooms to permit smaller groups and thus reduce noise characteristics

A child with sensorineural hearing loss who is fitted with amplification needs to be followed routinely. Once the child has been fitted with hearing aids, monitoring techniques must be implemented. First, the parents of the young child should be trained in use, care, and maintenance of the instruments. Second, the child needs to be seen by the audiologist at least every six months to be sure the earmolds are still secure and do not need to be remade. The tubing in the earmolds may need to be replaced or cleaned. Moisture, dirt, and wax buildup can cause the hearing aid to be dysfunctional. Third, the child should receive an audiological assessment at least once a year. Lastly, the teachers of the hearing impaired child must be made aware of the child's needs and issues involving the hearing aid.

EDUCATION OF THE HEARING IMPAIRED

The educational performance of hearing-impaired children in the United States has been a cause of concern to educators for some time. In 1921, Reamer reported on the educational achievement of 2,500 deaf students. He found that they were academically delayed on an average of four to five years when compared with hearing peers. A 1968–1970 annual survey (Gentile & DiFrancesca, 1969) gathered statistical information on the educational performance of hearing-impaired persons in preschool through college. This survey revealed that, on the whole, children and youth with hearing impairments demonstrated an average educational lag of four years. Their highest levels of performance were in the areas of spelling and arithmetic computation (Martin & Clark, 2000). However, it must be noted that arithmetic concepts and performance on word problems still presented much difficulty, as they inherently included the ability to decode written language. The area of greatest lag in achievement was reading, with the average reading comprehension for 15- to 16-year-olds at the 3.5 grade level. Later studies by the Office of Demographic Studies at Gallaudet University confirmed this delay in reading achievement (King & Quigley, 1985). Specifically, Trybus and Karchmer (1977) reported that the median reading level for deaf students at age 20 was grade 4.5. In 1994, Allen calculated the average reading achievement of deaf students completing school to be at the fourth-grade level. Thus, the majority of students who are deaf or hard of hearing exhibit English language and reading difficulties (Paul, 1998; Paul & Jackson, 1993). This becomes even more troubling now that 80 percent of all hearing-impaired or deaf students attend public school (Luetke-Stahlman, Griffiths, & Montgomery, 1999).

Poor performance in most academic subjects is not surprising, considering that reading comprehension plays a major role in academic learning and that the understanding of written language relates directly to the understanding of spoken language. From about the third or fourth grade, students are expected to read to learn; this task becomes extremely difficult for the hearing-impaired child who does not have an adequate language base. In fact, the majority of children with severe hearing impairments do not develop the adequate language skills that would make them efficient decoders of written language. Because of this, their comprehension of written language is significantly delayed when compared with that of normal hearing children (Robbins, 1986). This is probably related to the fact that hearing-impaired children take longer to reach the final stage of comprehension development of spoken language, in which they attend to syntactic and morphological aspects of sentences rather than to paralinguistic cues (Robbins, 1986). Furthermore, it has been suggested that children with hearing impairments use different strategies for comprehension of verbal language (Davis & Blasdell, 1975).

Reading

Learning to read is a complex task that requires the integration of syntactic, semantic, and pragmatic skills, as well as the ability to decode words. Once words are decoded, the reader must translate them into a more usable form. For the person with normal hearing, this form consists of phonetic elements. For the person who is hearing impaired, this form depends on the language input model and may be either phonetic forms, signs, fingerspelling, or visual orthography. In addition, the reader must have the ability to abstract both explicit and implicit meaning from the text through inferencing and hypothesizing (Kretschmer, 1989). This is further complicated by text variables such as vocabulary, syntax, figurative language, and discourse.

There are four basic approaches to teaching reading in programs for children with hearing impairments: the basal reader approach, the language experience approach (LEA), programmed instruction, and an individualized approach. In the LEA, the most frequently used approach in primary grades, children use their own language to write stories; that is, a child dictates a story and the teacher writes it. The story is then used in reading instruction. The LEA has been expanded to include modifying the child's dictated story in order to model and incorporate English syntactical forms. Once the child has achieved some writing skills, these written samples are incorporated into the reading program. The stories that children either dictate or write are based on personal interaction and represent the children's experiences with their social environment. This approach is most interesting in that it bridges the processes of reading and writing (King & Quigley, 1985).

Computer-based instruction has also been used to facilitate development of reading skills. Unfortunately, there have been relatively few studies that clearly support the use of computers with hearing-impaired children. However, a study by Prinz, Nelson, and Stedt (1982) highlighted improvement in word recognition and identification for 3- to 6-year-old deaf children who were trained to use the ALPHA Program, a sight-word computer program. This program utilized words, pictures, and manual sign representations and therefore could be used by children whose primary form of communication was sign language. Further studies (Nelson, Prinz, & Dalke, 1989; Prinz & Nelson, 1985) on deaf children 3 and 11 years old supported the use of computer-based instruction for reading and writing. More recently Prinz, Nelson, Loncke, Geysels, and Willems (1993) have continued to support computer-based instruction with elementary-age hearing-impaired children. Basically, all of these above-mentioned studies espoused the use of multimodality and multimedia reading programs for young deaf children.

Before formal training in reading begins, hearing-impaired children must have developed language skills. An excellent way to develop language is through storytelling, which exposes children to story structure, print, and common cultural themes (Snow, 1983; Wells, 1985). A recent study by Schick and Gale (1995) examined storytelling with preschool deaf and hard-of-hearing children who used some form of manually coded English during three different language conditions: using pure ASL, using pure SEE2, and using SEE2 with ASL features and ASL structures. SEE2 is a form of manually coded English, while ASL is a sign language that is typically used by deaf adults. Interestingly, it was found that children participated more and initiated more interactions when stories contained ASL signing. This study is important when considering educational approaches for children using manually coded English. It suggests that including ASL in the deaf child's programming may promote more interest in communication and increase incidents of child-initiated interactions. A more recent study by Strong and Prinz (1997) highlights the strong positive impact that learning ASL has on reading achievement. It was found that deaf students who use ASL as a primary mode of communication achieve higher levels of English literacy skills than their peers who do not utilize ASL.

Because of the strength of the research that supports ASL as a facilitator of literacy development, subtle changes are occurring in deaf education. Because ASL is an independent language from English, it makes sense to approach the teaching of reading to ASL communicators using bilingual education approaches. The theory is that the deaf child who uses ASL is a fluent "speaker." Therefore, this child has a language base that can be used in parallel with learning a second language, English.

Other research by Kelly (1996) and Paul (1996) indicates that vocabulary skills and syntactical skills are important factors in the reading process. The stronger these skills are, the better a child's reading comprehension will be.

Whole Language

During the late 1980s, a whole-language methodology gained acceptance among teachers of the nondisabled population. Whole language is an educational philosophy that incorporates all areas of language in the acquisition process. It is based on a developmental view of language acquisition (Schory, 1990). Advocates of whole language propose that children fail to become facile readers and writers because reading and writing have traditionally been taught as discrete skills separate from language. They espouse the integration of speaking, reading, and writing in the learning process and consider learning to be an active, constructive process during which new information is continuously incorporated into existing knowledge (Norris & Damico, 1990).

This philosophy can be incorporated into habilitative strategies when working with children who are hearing impaired. Intervention should incorporate the following whole-language assumptions (Norris & Samico, 1990):

1. Language exists in order to comprehend our environmental interactions and to convey meaning about ourselves and our world.
2. All components of language interact simultaneously (phonology, syntax, morphology, pragmatics, semantics) and cannot be parceled out and taught as separate units.
3. Language occurs in context—without context, there is no meaning.

4. Language learning is an active process that incorporates new knowledge with existing knowledge in order to develop complex schemata of knowing.

With these premises in mind, the speech-language pathologist/teacher must carefully organize and plan language learning activities that promote the discovery of various communication functions. Activities must be interesting and meaningful to the child as she relates to her environment, and they must encourage and optimize opportunities for social interaction (for specific teaching strategies, see Krashen, 1982; Norris & Damico, 1990; Sulzby, 1985).

Nevertheless, while keeping this content focus in mind, we must recognize that deaf and hearing-impaired children still need specific work to develop vocabulary and syntax skills in order to become literate.

Sign Language and Bilingualism

As already noted, children with hearing impairments have generally been educated via either an aural/oral program, emphasizing speechreading and speech and using no sign systems, or a total communication program, using signs, speechreading, and speech. A variety of sign systems have been used to educate children who are deaf. For example, Signing Essential English (Anthony, 1971) and Signing Exact English (Gustason, Pfetzing, & Zawolkow, 1972) consist of manual productions of spoken English and adhere to the syntactical and grammatical forms of spoken English. Educators who use this type of sign system are actually attempting to teach English as a first language through the use of a visual system.

During the 1970s a body of research evolved around American Sign Language (ASL), the sign language used by deaf adults (Bellugi & Fischer, 1972; Bellugi & Klima, 1975; Bellugi, Klima, & Siple, 1974; Wilbur, 1979). ASL is a language in its own right, with its own syntax and idioms. ASL is just as different from English as is Spanish or Russian or any other language. Thus, researchers have suggested that hearing-impaired/deaf children born to hearing-impaired/deaf parents who use ASL at home should be taught spoken and written English in a different manner than hearing-impaired/deaf children born to parents with normal hearing. The premise is that the children exposed to ASL have already achieved a primary language base—ASL. When they are exposed to English in the educational setting, English is their second language, and therefore the educational approach must be a bilingual one. In addition, these hearing-impaired/deaf children have also been exposed to a deaf culture, with its traditions and customs. This makes them bicultural and strengthens the position for teaching them with an ASL/ESL (English as a second language) approach. The idea of taking a bilingual approach in the education of hearing-impaired and deaf children is based on the work of Cummins (1981), who hypothesized that if a child is proficient in one language, he or she will have more success in developing a second language. Thus, if a deaf child is proficient with ASL, then that child will more easily acquire English literacy skills.

Today, a bilingual approach to educating children who are deaf or hearing impaired has not been implemented to any great extent. Reasons for this include the following:

1. ASL is not the native language of the majority of deaf children.
2. ASL has no written form.
3. There are few trained teachers who know ASL.
4. Bilingual education in general is controversial.
5. Few ASL curricula have been published.
6. Some educators question the true language status of ASL (Strong, 1988).

In spite of these obstacles, there have been attempts to document and justify the use of a bilingual approach in education. An experimental curriculum described by Michael Strong (1988) uses a storytelling format to introduce ASL into the classroom setting. English is then taught via ASL. This program is particularly interesting because it emphasizes metalinguistic awareness.

More recently, Prinz and Strong (1998) developed an ASL proficiency and English literacy within a bilingual deaf education model of instruction. They found that there was a positive connection between ASL and reading and writing in English and emphasize the need for more research and curriculum model development in this area. The national Council on Education of the Deaf (CED) and the National Association of the Deaf (NAD) support the idea of a bilingual educational approach when educating deaf students.

Considering the difficulty with which hearing-impaired/deaf children acquire language and the poor academic performance common among many of these children, it seems possible and practical to adopt a second-language acquisition approach in the educational setting. However, much more careful and systematic research is needed before extensive use of such an approach can be recommended.

Inclusionary Education

Today, many educational options are available for the young child who is hearing impaired. Whereas the choice was once limited to segregated settings such as residential schools for the deaf and day schools for the hearing impaired, changes in federal legislation have brought forth new options, including day classes, resource rooms, itinerant programs, and team teaching.

Early inclusion of deaf and hard-of-hearing children with normal-hearing peers provides considerable educational benefits for the hearing-impaired child. Three types of preschool integration placement options are available today (Luetke-Stahlman, 1994):

1. Enrolling normal-hearing preschoolers in early childhood programs specifically set up for children who are deaf or hard of hearing (reverse mainstreaming)
2. Placing children who are deaf or hard of hearing in self-contained early intervention programs for part of the day and then in child care centers for additional socialization experiences
3. Placing children who are deaf or hard of hearing in preschool classes comprised of normal hearing peers, with sufficient support services to enable the hearing-impaired child to participate fully in all activities with the other preschoolers throughout the day

Clearly, integrating hearing-impaired preschoolers into mainstreamed environments poses considerable challenges. Peer interactions between hearing-impaired and normal-hearing children is generally limited, because the communication attempts of the hearing-impaired child are often inadequate and ineffective (Vendell & George, 1981). Children who are hearing impaired learn language by participating in conversational exchanges (Kretschmer & Kretschmer, 1989). If their conversational attempts are unreinforced due to unresponsive peers, placement in integrated settings will have little benefit unless specific facilitative strategies are employed to ensure rich reciprocal conversation. Such conversations will result not only in language learning, but also in socially interactive complex play as well. In order to facilitate good interaction between hearing-impaired children and their normal-hearing peers, several strategies can be employed, such as encouraging hearing-impaired children to articulate more clearly, encouraging hearing peers to increase their communicative interactions with the hearing-impaired children, and, if the hearing-impaired children sign, to insist that they utilize simultaneous speech and sign (Luetke-Stahlman, 1991).

In the 1980s the main thrust of special education was to facilitate mainstreaming, which is an educational attempt to serve children with disabilities in a regular school environment with the aid of supportive personnel (Nicolosi, Harryman, & Kresheck, 1978). Supportive personnel may include a speech-language pathologist, an audiologist, a teacher of the hearing impaired, and others. Birch (1976) recommended that children who are deaf should be mainstreamed only after thorough preparation, with sensitivity to the needs of all parties, and with careful monitoring and support. Inherent in the concept of mainstreaming is the expectation that the student can perform at the regular classroom educational level.

For mainstreaming to be successful, the child placed in a regular classroom must also receive personalized instruction and supportive services necessary to benefit from an Individualized Educational Plan or IEP. The IEP is confirmation for children with hearing impairments that a more objective and scientific educational decision-making process will be followed (Northern & Downs, 1984).

Bricker (1978) suggested that "integration is a means of eliminating the deleterious effects of segregation and the stigma often attached to the handicapped student." Flexer, Wray, and Ireland (1989) reported that for a hearing-impaired child to be able to survive in a regular classroom, three issues must be addressed: understanding the nature of hearing and consequences of hearing loss, the essential use of technology to enhance the signal-to-noise ratio, and educational management strategies.

Mainstreaming of a child who is hearing impaired can take several forms. Complete mainstreaming occurs when the child remains in the regular classroom for all academic instruction, which is given by the regular classroom teacher. In this instance, the child relies on speechreading and amplification for instructional input. A modification of this complete mainstreaming option includes the use of a sign language interpreter in the classroom. In 1982, this type of educational support option was challenged by the Hendrick Hudson Board of Education in New York. The case was heard by the Supreme Court in *Hendrick Hudson Board of Education v. Rowley* (1982). The court ruled that Amy did not need an interpreter; however, it upheld the argument that PL 94-142 entitled students with disabilities to personalized instruction such as interpreter services.

Other mainstreaming options include part-time placement in regular classes with some special classes, and part-time placement in a resource room with some regular classes (McCortney, 1984).

Once a mainstreaming option is selected for a child, it is necessary to consider what factors will lead to success. Reynolds and Birch (1977) highlight the following as necessary components for mainstreaming success:

1. The regular classroom teacher is given a choice as to whether he or she wants to have the hearing-impaired child in the class.
2. Mainstreaming begins early, at the preschool level.
3. The educational setting has a teacher of the hearing impaired on staff.
4. In-service training is provided for all staff who work with the hearing-impaired child.
5. The classroom environment is well equipped with necessary amplification units.
6. Separation of the hearing-impaired child from the regular educational setting is minimal.
7. All the professionals who work with the mainstreamed child meet regularly to review the child's progress and make modifications as needed.

More recently, educators have been considering the concept of inclusion. In its purest form, inclusion is the meaningful involvement of all students in their neighborhood, school, and community (Progorzelski & Kelly, 1995). For the most severely handicapped students the emphasis of inclusion is on socialization, not academics, and academics are modified for the special-needs student. For hearing-impaired children who are capable of acquiring age-appropriate academics, the concept of inclusion must not erode the integrity of academic programming and expectations. If hearing-impaired students require presentation of academic material via sign language such as ASL, then full inclusion means that both a regular education teacher and an ASL-proficient teacher of the deaf collaborative within the regular education classroom.

With this in mind, consider the advantages of inclusionary programming for hearing-impaired/deaf children. The advantages of the mainstreamed setting are:

1. It is stimulating, and the highly verbal setting provides models for hearing-impaired children.
2. The mainstreamed setting includes interaction with typical peers, thereby exposing the hearing-impaired child to social, academic, and communicative behaviors of those typical peers.
3. There are many opportunities for technological support, peer-to-peer instruction, high expectations, and exposure to varied ideas and experiences (Brackett, 1997).

CASE HISTORY

Hearing loss has a negative impact on the development of speech and language. G.D. is a child who has a history of ear infections since 6 months of age. Between the ages of 6 months and 40 months he has had nine ear infections, which were treated with antibiotics and resolved. The insertion of pressure-equalization tubes is being considered by the family. Most recent audiological testing reveals a bilateral conductive hearing loss with slightly depressed speech-recognition scores. Middle ear pathology is present bilaterally (see Figure 12.3). Recommendations include the use of an auditory

Child: G.D.

Age: 3.4

HX—Child was born @4.7 lbs. Premature—35 week gestation. Delivered by Caesarean Section. Speech and language is delayed. Motor development is age appropriate. Child has a history of ear infections since 6 months old, treated with antibiotics and resolved. Parents are contemplating insertion of pressure equalization tubes.

No family history of hearing loss.

Name	G.D.	Referred by:	ENT	Date:	11/9/00
Age	3.4	Examined by:	S.A.	Audiometer:	GSI 61

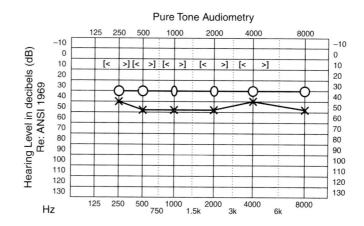

Speech Audiometry

	SRT	Discrim Scores	PBK
Right	25	84%	65 dB
Left	40	90%	80 dB

Reflexes

	500	1000	2000	4000
Right	Absent			
Left	Absent			

Speech Audiometry

Ear	Two Frequencies	Three Frequencies
Right		30 dB
Left		50 dB

Tympanogram

	Type	M.E.P.
Right	B	—
Left	B	—

Results:

Child presents with a bilateral conductive hearing loss with slightly depressed speech recognition scores. Middle ear pathology present bilaterally.

Recommendations

1. Otologic consult
2. Auditory trainer use during speech/language therapy, to compensate for fluctuations in hearing.
3. Periodic recheck post medical intervention.

FIGURE 12.3

G.D.'s Audiogram

FIGURE 12.4

G.D.'s Language Assessment Instrument

Name: G. D.

Age: 3.4

Preschool Language Scale—3 (PLS—3)

Auditory comprehension
Standard Score 58
Percentile 1st
Age Equivalent 1 year 3 months

Expressive Communication
Standard Score 58
Percentile 1st
Age Equivalent 1 year 2 months

Total Language Score 53
Percentile 1st
Age Equivalent 1 year 3 months

trainer during speech/language therapy. G.D.'s speech/language testing (Preschool Language Scale—3 (PLS—3) (see Figure 12.4) reveals severe delays in both the understanding of language and the production of spoken language. On the auditory comprehension portion of the PLS—3 he received a standard score of 58, a percentile of 1, and an age equivalent of 1 year 3 months. On the expressive communication portion he received a standard score of 58, a percentile of 1 and an age equivalent of 1 year 2 months. Total language score on the PLS—3 of 53, with a percentile of 1 and an age equivalent of 1 year 3 months. G.D. has a lexicon of approximately fifty words, and he does use a few two-word phrases such as "drink juice" and "go bye bye." He does not consistently respond to people or yes/no questions, and he inconsistently follows one-step commands. His eye contact is somewhat fleeting, and he can label a few familiar objects and pictures of a few animals. G.D. does not consistently use language to communicate with his peers or adults in his environment. The structure and function of the oral peripheral speech mechanisms appear adequate for production of speech and vegetative purposes. Habitual open mouth posture is noted. Because of a paucity of verbalizations, voice rate and fluency cannot be accurately assessed at this time.

The Committee for Preschool Special Education (CPSE) received the assessment information for G.D. The CPSE found G.D. to be a preschool child with a disability and recommended placement in a full-day special education preschool with individual speech language therapy for 30 minutes per session three times a week.

SUMMARY

The acquisition of literacy skills, reading and writing, involves the complex integration of many areas of learning, including speaking, listening, and critical thinking. An oral or manual language system must be intact if a hearing-impaired child is to learn to read and write. Learning to read and write involves the ability to store up word meanings, remember vocabulary, and make abstract judgments about causal relationships (Streng, 1964). A solid language foundation is a prerequisite for literacy skills.

Individuals with hearing impairments have the same innate abilities to develop speech and language as persons in the normal-hearing population. Often, however, because of the severity of their hearing loss, they cannot acquire language through audition alone. Consequently, overall delays in language development can result, and hearing-impaired children are at a great educational disadvantage. Only through application of normal language development theory can educators devise more effective methodology for educating students with hearing impairments. Their challenge is to be creative as well as effective. In addition, passage of recent legislation and the mandate for the least restrictive environment (LRE) further challenge the professional working with hearing-impaired children in the mainstreamed setting. Children who are hearing impaired should not necessarily be segregated. Instead, they should be educated in the LRE with normal-hearing peers. It is up to the educator to ensure that children who are hearing impaired benefit from instruction in the mainstreamed setting. Only through careful planning, monitoring, and a team approach can that occur.

In diagnosing hearing impairments in the pediatric population, the clinician needs to remember the importance of early detection and intervention. The complete audiological assessment needs to include pure tone findings, speech findings, and aural acoustic immittance testing. Otoacoustic emission testing should also be used in conjunction with behavior testing. Appropriate test parameters must be based on the age of the child. Accuracy and reliability are significant variables. The objective tests available and their use as a screening tool is inevitable in assisting to ensure early detection.

Each child with a hearing impairment has unique management needs. In general, children suffering from chronic otitis media need routine medical and audiological follow-up. Children exhibiting sensorineural hearing loss have different management needs. These children must be fitted properly with amplification, appropriate assistive devices must be selected for the school setting, and an appropriate educational setting must be considered.

Major changes have taken place in the education of children who are hearing impaired. Continual research and application of effective rehabilitative and educational theory will ensure that professionals can continue to meet the challenges of educating the children with hearing impairment.

STUDY QUESTIONS

1. What are the three types of hearing loss?
2. What are the effects of chronic otitis media on speech and language?
3. What is the speech recognition threshold?
4. What is tympanometry?
5. What are the benefits of the FM auditory trainer unit?
6. What are three types of preschool integration placement options available today?
7. What activity is most beneficial in developing language skills in young hearing impaired children? Why?
8. How does a hearing loss affect educational achievement?
9. What are the reasons that a bilingual educational approach is not routinely used when educating children with severe hearing impairments?

10. Who are candidates for cochlear implants?
11. How has hearing aid technology changed in the new millennium?
12. What impact has the cochlear implant had on children in the educational setting?
13. How have otoacoustic emissions affected the early detection of hearing loss in neonates?

GLOSSARY

Acoustic reflex   The bilateral contraction of the intra-aural muscles (tensor tympani and stapedius) in response to sound.

Acute otitis media   An active inflammation and/or infection of the middle ear space.

ASL (American Sign Language)   Typically used by deaf adults, ASL has its own syntax and grammar and is recognized as a language separate from English.

Aural/oral approach   A philosophy of educating deaf/hearing impaired children that emphasizes the use of speechreading and audition only for the development of speech and language.

Chronic otitis media   An infection of the middle ear space with purulent fluid (pus) persisting beyond the time limit of acute otitis media.

Conductive hearing loss   Interference of any sort in the transmission of sound from the external auditory canal to the inner ear.

IEP (Individual Education Plan)   A plan generated by a Committee for Special Education for eligible children ages 3 years through age 21.

IFSP   (Individualized Family Service Plan) A plan for providing services to an eligible child, birth up to age 3, and the child's family.

Inclusion   The legal right of handicapped children to be accommodated in the natural school environment regardless of their physical or educational limitations.

Mainstreaming   An educational attempt to serve children with disabilities in a regular school environment; students who are mainstreamed should be able to handle academics in a manner comparable to their regular education classmates.

Mixed hearing loss   A problem that occurs simultaneously in both the conductive and sensorineural mechanisms.

Otoacoustic emissions   The low-intensity sounds detected in the ear canal, which represent the cochlea's active response to sound, a response involving the addition of energy to that provided by the stimulus arriving at the ear.

Pure tone average   The average of the thresholds of 500, 1,000, and 2,000 Hz.

Pure tone threshold   The faintest tone a person can hear 50 percent of the time.

Secretory otitis media   A condition associated with a thick, gluelike fluid found in the middle ear space.

SEE2 (Signing Exact English 2)   A manually coded English sign system.

Sensorineural hearing loss   Damage to the sensory end organ, the cochlear hair cells, or the auditory nerve.

Serous otitis media   The presence of a thin, watery, clear fluid in the middle ear space, usually an early sign of eustachian tube dysfunction.

Speech recognition A measure of the ability to differentiate between various speech sounds, such as nonsense syllables, monosyllabic words, and multisyllabic words.

Speech recognition threshold The threshold of intelligibility, which is the lowest level (in decibels) at which the listener is able to identify approximately 50 percent of spondiac bisyllabic words.

Total communication A philosophy of educating deaf/hearing-impaired children that requires the use of signs, speech, gestures, and facial expressions for the development of speech and language.

Tympanometry The measurement of the resistance to the flow of acoustical energy at the tympanic membrane during various pressure changes.

SUGGESTED READING

Clattke, T. J., Kujawa, S. (1991, November). Otoacoustic emissions. *American Journal of Audiology, 2,* 29–37.

Greenberg, J. (1985). *What is the sign for friend?* New York: F. Watts.

Kavanagh, J. F. (Ed.). (1986). *Otitis media and child development.* Parkton, MD: York.

Kretschmer, R. (1989). Pragmatics, reading, and writing: Implications for hearing impaired individuals. *Topics in Language Disorders, 9*(4), 17–32.

Northern, J. (Ed.). (1984). *Hearing disorders* (2nd ed.). Boston: Little, Brown.

Prieve, B. A. (1992). Otoacoustic emission in infants and children: Basic characteristics and clinical application. *Seminars in Hearing, 13*(1), 37–52.

Schow, R., & Nerbonne, M. (Eds.). (1989). *Introduction to aural rehabilitation* (2d ed.). Baltimore: University Park Press.

REFERENCES

Allen, T. E. (1994). Who are the deaf and hard of hearing students leaving high school and entering postsecondary education? Unpublished manuscript, Gallaudet University Center for Assessment and Demographic Studies, Washington, DC.

American National Standards Institute. (1996). American National Standard specifications for audiometers, ANSI S3.6-1996. New York: Author.

Anthony, D. (1971). *Signing Essential English* (vols. 1 and 2). Anaheim, CA: Educational Division, Anaheim Union School District.

Bateson, M. C. (1975). Mother–infant exchanges: The epigenesis of conversational interaction. In M. Aaronson & R. Reiber (Eds.), *Annals of the New York Academy of Sciences:* Developmental psycholinguistics and communication disorders.

Bellugi, U., & Fischer, S. (1972). A comparison of sign language and spoken language. *Cognition, 1,* 173–200.

Bellugi, U., & Klima, E. (1975). Aspects of sign language and its structure. In J. Kavanagh and J. Cutting (Eds.), *The role of speech in language* (pp. 171–203). Cambridge, MA: MIT Press.

Bellugi, U, Klima, E., & Siple, P. (1974). Remembering in signs. *Cognition, 3,* 93–125.

Birch, J. W. (1976). Mainstream education for hearing impaired pupils: Issues and interviews. *American Annals of the Deaf, 121,* 69–71.

Blennerhasset, L. (1984). Communicative styles of a 13-month-old hearing impaired child and her parents. *Volta Review, 86,* 217–228.

Bloom, L, & Lahey, M. (1978). *Language development and language disorders.* New York: Wiley.

Brackett, D. (1997). Intervention for children with hearing impairment in general education settings. *Language, Speech, and Hearing Services in Schools, 28*(4), 355–371.

Bricker, D. D. (1978). A rationale for the integration of handicapped and non-handicapped preschool children. In N.J. Guralnich (Ed.), *Early intervention and the integration of handicapped and non-handicapped children.* Baltimore: University Park Press.

Brown, R. (1975). *Social psychology.* New York: Free Press.

Bruner, J. (1975). The ontogenesis of speech acts. *Journal of Child Language, 2,* 1–19.

Chess, S., & Thomas, A. (1996). *Temperament: theory and practice.* New York: Brunner/Mazel.

Cole, E. B., & St. Clair-Stokes, J. (1984). Caregiver–child interactive behaviors: A videotape analysis procedure. *Volta Review, 86,* 200–216.

Cummins, J. (1981). The role of primary language development in promoting educational success for language minority students. In California State Department of Education, *Schooling and language minority students: A theoretical framework.* Los Angeles: Evaluation, Assessment and Dissemination Center.

Davis, J. M., & Blasdell, R. (1975). Perceptual strategies by normal hearing and hearing-impaired children in the comprehension of sentences containing relative clauses. *Journal of Speech and Hearing Research, 18,* 281–295.

DeGangi, G., Wietlisbach, S., Poisson, S., Stein, E., & Royeen, C. (1994). The impact of culture and socioeconomic status on family–professional collaboration: Challenges and solutions. *Topics in Early Childhood Special Education, 14*(4), 503–520.

Eimas, P. (1974). Auditory and linguistic processing cues for place of articulation by infants. *Perceptual Psychology, 16,* 513–521.

Feagans, L. (1986). Otitis media: A model for longterm effects with implications for intervention. In J. F. Kavanagh (Ed.), *Otitis media and child development* (pp. 192–210). Parkton, MD: York.

Flexer, C., Wray, D., & Ireland, J. (1989). Preferential seating is not enough: Issues in classroom management of hearing impaired students. *Language, Speech and Hearing Services in Schools, 20*(1), 11–21.

Geers, A., Moog, J., & Schick, B. (1984). Acquisition of spoken and signed English by profoundly deaf children. *Journal of Speech and Hearing Disorders, 49,* 378–388.

Gentile, A., & DiFrancesca, S. (1969, Spring). *Academic achievement test performance of hearing impaired students: United States* (Series D, No. 1). Washington, DC: Gallaudet College, Office of Demographic Studies.

Glattke, T. J., & Kujawa, S. (1991, November). Otoacoustic emissions. *American Journal of Audiology, 2,* 29–37.

Gravel, J., & Hood, L. (1999). Pediatric audiologic assessment. In F. Musiek, and W. Rintelmann (Eds.), (pp. 305–323). Boston: Allyn & Bacon

Greenstein, J. M., Bush, B., McConville, K., & Stellini, L. (1977). *Mother–infant communication and language acquisition in deaf infants.* New York: Lexington School for the Deaf.

Gustason, G., Pfetzing, D., & Zawolkow, E. (1972). *Signing Exact English.* Rossmoor, CA: Modern Sign Press.

Hall, J., III (2000). *Handbook of otoacoustic emissions.* San Diego/London: Singular.

Hanson, M., Lynch, E. W., & Wayman, K. L. (1990). Honoring the culture diversity of families when gathering data. *Topics in Early Childhood Education, 10*(1), 112–131.

Hanson, V. L., & Padden, C. A. (In press). Computers and videodisc technology for bilingual ASL/English instruction of deaf children. In D. Nix and R. Spiro (Eds.), *Cognition, education, and multimedia: Exploring ideas in high technology.* Hillsdale, NJ: Lawrence Erlbaum Associates.

Hendrick Hudson School District v. Rowley, 458 U.S. 176, 102 S. Ct. 3034, 73 L. Ed. 2d 690 (1982).

Hopkinson, N. (1978). Speech reception threshold. In J. Katz (Ed.), *Handbook of clinical audiology* (2d ed.) (pp. 141–148). Baltimore: Williams & Wilkins.

Jaffe, J., Stern, D., & Peery, J. (1973). "Conversational" coupling of gaze behaviors in prelinguistic human development. *Journal of Psycholinguistic Research, 2*, 321–328.

Jerger, J., and Hayes, D. (1976). The cross-check principle in pediatric audiometry. *Archives of Otolaryngology, 702*, 614–620.

Jordan, I., Gustason, G., & Rosen R. (1979). Current communication trends at programs for the deaf. *American Annals of the Deaf, 124*, 350–357.

Kelly, L. (1996). The interaction of syntactic competence and vocabulary during reading by deaf students. *Journal of Deaf Studies and Deaf Education, 1*, 75–90.

Kemp, D. T. (1978). Stimulated acoustic emissions from within the human auditory system. *Journal of the Acoustic Society of America, 64*, 1386–1391.

King, C. M., & Quigley, S. P. (1985). *Reading and deafness.* San Diego, CA: College-Hill.

Knauf, V. H. (1972). Meeting speech and language needs for the hearing impaired. In J. Katz (Ed.), *Handbook of clinical audiology* (2nd ed.) (pp. 733–777). Baltimore: Williams & Wilkins.

Koester, L. S., & Meadow-Orlans, K. P. (1999). Responses to interactive stress: Infants who are deaf or hearing. *American Annals of the Deaf, 144*, 295–403.

Krashen, S. (1982). *Principles and practices in second language acquisition.* New York: Pergamon.

Kretschmer, R. (1989). Pragmatics, reading, and writing. *Topics in Language Disorders, 9*(4), 17–32.

Kretschmer, R., & Kretschmer, L. (1989). Communication competence: Impact of the pragmatics revolution on education of hearing impaired individuals. *Topics in Language Disorders, 9*(4), 1–16.

Lafreniere, O., Smurzynski, J., June, M. D., Leonard, G., & Kim, D. O. (1993). Otoacoustic emissions in full-term newborns at risk for hearing loss. *Laryngoscope, 103*, 1334–1341.

Luetke-Stahlman, B. (1991). Hearing impaired students in integrated child care. *Perspectives,* 9(1), 8–11.

Luetke-Stahlman, B. (1994). Procedures for socially integrating preschoolers who are hearing, deaf, and hard of hearing. *Topics in Early Childhood Special Education, 14*(4), 472–487.

Luetke-Stahlman, B., Griffiths, C., & Montgomery, N. (1999). A deaf child's language acquisition verified through text retelling. *American Annals of the Deaf, 144,* (3), 270–280.

Mahon, W. (1987). U.S. hearing aid sales summary. *The Hearing Journal, 40,* 9–14.

Martin, F., & Clark, J. (2000). *Introduction to audiology.* Boston: Allyn & Bacon.

Mavilya, M. (1969). *Spontaneous vocalization and babbling in hearing-impaired infants.* Doctoral dissertation, Teacher's College, Columbia University, New York.

McCortney, B. (1984). Education in the mainstream. In R. Stoker & J. Spear (Eds.), *Hearing-impaired perspectives on living in the mainstream* (pp. 41–52). Washington, DC: Alexander Graham Bell Association for the Deaf.

Menyuk, P. (1986). Predicting speech and language problems with persistent otitis media. In J. F. Kavanagh (Ed.), *Otitis media and child development* (pp. 83–98). Parkton, MD: York.

Miller, C., & Morse, P. (1976). The "heart" of categorical speech discrimination in young infants. *Journal of Speech and Hearing Research, 19,* 578–589.

Miller, C., Morse, P., & Dorman, N. (1977). Cardiac indices of infants' speech perception: Orienting and burst discrimination. *Quarterly Journal of Experimental Psychology, 29,* 533–545.

Morse, P. (1972). The discrimination of speech and speech stimuli in early infancy. *Journal of Experimental Psychology, 14,* 477–492.

Myklebust, H. R. (1960). *The psychology of deafness.* New York: Grune & Stratton.

National Institutes of Health, National Institute on Deafness and other Communication Disorders (NIDCD). (1997). www.nih.gov/nidcd.

Nelson, K., Prinz, P., & Dalke, D. (1989). Transitions from sign language to text via an interactive micro-computer system. In B. Woll (Ed.), *Papers from the Seminar on Language Development and Sign Language* (Monograph 1, International Sign Linguistics Association). Bristol, UK: Centre for Deaf Studies, University of Bristol.

Nicolosi, L., Harryman, E., & Kresheck, J. (1978). *Terminology of communication disorders-speech-language-hearing.* Baltimore: Williams & Wilkins.

Norris, J., & Damico, J. (1990). Whole language in theory and practice: Implications for language intervention. *Language, Speech and Hearing Services in Schools, 21,* 212–220.

Northern, J. (Ed.). (1984). *Hearing disorders* (2d ed.). Boston: Little, Brown.

Northern, J., & Downs, M. (1984). *Hearing in children.* Baltimore: Williams & Wilkins.

Padden, C. (1980). The deaf community and the culture of deaf people. In C. Baker & R. Battison (Eds.), *Sign language and the deaf community.* Washington, DC: National Association for the Deaf.

Paul, P. (1996). Reading, vocabulary knowledge, and deafness. *Journal of Deaf Studies and Deaf Education, 1,* 3–15.

Paul, P. (1998). *Literacy and deafness.* Boston: Allyn & Bacon.

Paul, P., & Jackson, D. (1993). *Towards a psychology of deafness: Theoretical and empirical perspectives.* Boston: Allyn & Bacon.

Prinz, P., & Nelson, K. (1985). Alligator eats cookie: Acquisition of writing and reading skills by deaf children using the microcomputer. *Applied Psycholinguistics, 6,* 283–306.

Prinz, P., Nelson, K., Loncki, F., Geysels, G., & Willems, C. (1993). A multimodality and multimedia approach to language, discourse and literacy development. In F. Coninx & B. Elsendoorn (Eds.), *Interactive learning technology for the deaf.* New York: Springer-Verlag.

Prinz, P., Nelson, K. A., & Stedt, J. (1982). Early reading in young deaf children using microcomputer technology. *American Annals of the Deaf, 127,* 529–535.

Prinz, P., & Strong, M. (1998). ASL proficiency and English literacy within a bilingual deaf education model of instruction. *Topics in Language Disorders, 18*(4), 47–60.

Progorzelski, G., & Kelly, B. (1995). *Inclusion: The collaborative process.* Buffalo, NY: United Educational Services, Inc.

Quigley, S. P., & Kretschmer, R. E. (1982). *The education of deaf children.* Baltimore: University Park Press.

Radziewicz, C. (1985). *The use of videotapes as a means of parent training for parents of hearing-impaired infants.* Unpublished doctoral dissertation, Adelphi University, Garden City, NY.

Reamer, J. C. (1921). Mental and educational measurement of the deaf. *Psychological Monographs,* No. 132.

Reynolds, M. C., & Birch, J. W. (1977). *Teaching exceptional children in all America's schools.* Reston, VA: Council for Exceptional Children.

Robbins, A. M. (1986). Language comprehension in young children. *Topics in Language Disorders, 6,* 12–23.

Ross, M. (1987). FM auditory training systems as an educational tool. *Hearing Rehabilitation Quarterly, 12*(4), 4–6.

Schick, B., & Gale, E. (1995). Preschool deaf and hard of hearing students' interactions during ASL and English storytelling. *American Annals of the Deaf, 140,* 363–370.

Schory, M. E. (1990). Whole language and the speech-language pathologist. *Language, Speech and Hearing Services in Schools, 21,* 206–211.

Simmons, B. (1966). Electrical stimulation of the auditory nerve in man. *Archives of Otolaryngology, 84,* 2–54.

Snow, C. (1983). Literacy and language relationships during the preschool years. *Harvard Educational Review, 53,* 165–189.

Stach, B. A. (1997). Comprehensive dictionary of audiology. *The Hearing Journal.* Baltimore: Williams & Wilkins.

Stach, B. A. (1998). *Clinical audiology.* San Diego/London: Singular.

Streng, A. (1964). *Reading for deaf children.* Washington, DC: Alexander Graham Bell Association for the Deaf.

Strong, M. (Ed.). (1988). *Language learning and deafness.* New York: Cambridge University Press.

Strong, M., & Prinz, P. (1997). A study of the relationship between ASL and English literacy. *Journal of Deaf Studies and Deaf Education, 2*(1), 37–46.

Sulzby, E. (1985). Children's emergent reading of favorite storybooks: A developmental study. *Reading Research Quarterly, 20,* 45–81.

Tartter, V. C., Hellman, S. A., & Chute, P. M. (1992). Vowel perception strategies of normal-hearing subjects and patients using Nucleus Multichannel and 3M/house cochlear implants. *Journal of Acoustical Society of America, 92,* 1269–1283.

Trybus, R., & Karchmer, M. (1977). School achievement scores of hearing impaired children: National data on achievement status and growth patterns. *American Annals of the Deaf Directory of Programs and Services, 122,* 62–69.

Vendell, D. L., & George, L. B. (1981). Social interaction in hearing and deaf students: Success and failures in initiations. *Child Development, 52,* 627–635.

Vorce, E. (1974). *Teaching speech to deaf children.* Washington, DC: Alexander Graham Bell Association for the Deaf.

Wedell-Monning, J., & Westerman, T. B. (1977, September). *Mothers' language to deaf and hearing infants: Examination of the feedback model.* Paper presented at the Second Annual Boston University Conference on Language Development, Boston.

Wells, G. (1985). Preschool literacy related activities and success in school. In D. Olson, N. Torrance, & A. Hildyard (Eds.), *Literacy, language and learning: The nature and consequences of reading and writing* (pp. 229–255) New York: Cambridge University Press.

Widen, J. E. (1997). Evoked otoacoustic emission in evaluating children. In M. S. Robinette and T. J. Glattke (Eds.), *Otoacoustic emissions: Clinical applications* (pp. 271–306). New York: Thieme.

Wilbur, R. B. (1979). *American Sign Language and sign systems.* Baltimore: University Park Press.

Woodford, C. M., Feldman, A. S., & Wright, H. N. (1975) Stimulus parameters, the acoustic reflex and clinical implications. *NYS Speech and Hearing Review, 7,* 29–37.

Yoshinaga, C. (1983). *Syntactic and semantic characteristics in the written language of hearing impaired and normally hearing school-aged children.* Unpublished doctoral dissertation, Northwestern University, Evanston, IL.

Yoshinaga-Itano, C. (1986). Beyong the sentence level: What's in a hearing impaired child's story? *Topics in Language Disorders, 6*(3), 71–83.

Yoshinaga-Itano, C., & Apuzzo, M. R. (1998a). The development of deaf and hard of hearing children identified early through the high-risk registry. *American Annals of the Deaf, 143,* 416–424.

Yoshinaga-Itano, C., & Apuzzo, M. R. (1998b). Identification of hearing loss after 18 months is not early enough. *American Annals of the Deaf, 143,* (380–387).

Yoshinaga-Itano, C., & Snyder, L. (1985). Form and meaning in the written language of hearing impaired children. In R. R. Kretschmer (Ed.), *Learning to write and writing to learn* [Monograph]. *Volta Review, 87*(5), 75–90.

Index